Handbook of Zoonotic Diseases

Handbook of Zoonotic Diseases

Editor: Gustavo Shaw

Callisto Reference
www.callistoreference.com

Callisto Reference,
118-35 Queens Blvd., Suite 400,
Forest Hills, NY 11375, USA

Visit us on the World Wide Web at:
www.callistoreference.com

ISBN: 978-1-64116-843-4 (Hardback)

Cataloging-in-Publication Data

Handbook of zoonotic diseases / edited by Gustavo Shaw.
p. cm.
Includes bibliographical references and index.
ISBN 978-1-64116-843-4
1. Zoonoses. 2. Animals as carriers of disease. 3. Communicable diseases. I. Shaw, Gustavo.
SF740 .H36 2023
636.083 2--dc23

Table of Contents

Preface

Zoonotic diseases are the infectious diseases in humans, which are transmitted from animals to humans. They can be caused due to infectious agents such as prion, bacteria, parasites, or viruses. Zoonotic diseases can be transmitted directly from animal hosts to humans by media such as air or through saliva or bite of the host. The indirect transmission of zoonotic diseases occurs through transmission by intermediate species or vectors, which may carry the pathogen. The genetics of the host plays a significant role in determining which animal viruses have the capability to replicate themselves in humans. Those animal viruses which require less number of mutations for replicating themselves in the human cells are considered to be more dangerous. This book provides significant information to help develop a good understanding of zoonotic diseases. Also included herein is a detailed explanation of the hosts and vectors associated with zoonotic diseases. This book will prove to be immensely beneficial to students and researchers studying these diseases.

Significant researches are present in this book. Intensive efforts have been employed by authors to make this book an outstanding discourse. This book contains the enlightening chapters which have been written on the basis of significant researches done by the experts.

Finally, I would also like to thank all the members involved in this book for being a team and meeting all the deadlines for the submission of their respective works. I would also like to thank my friends and family for being supportive in my efforts.

Editor

TABLE 1 | Municipalities where *Atelerix algirus* were captured in Tenerife (Canary Islands, Spain), number of animals per area, and pathogens found.

Municipality	Number of samples analyzed	FilmArray Results (number of positive samples)
La Laguna	11	*Cryptosporidium* sp. (2), enteropathogenic *E. coli* (5), *Campylobacter* sp. (3), *Salmonella* (7), *Clostridioides difficile* (5), *Shigella*/enteroinvasive *E. coli* (1)
Santa Cruz	8	Enteropathogenic *E. coli* (8), enterotoxigenic *E. coli lt/st* (1), *Salmonella* (4), *Clostridioides difficile* (2), *Campylobacter* sp. (1)
Arona	7	*Clostridioides difficile* (2), enteropathogenic *E. coli* (4), enterotoxigenic *E. coli lt/st* (1), *Salmonella* sp. (5), *Campylobacter* sp. (2)
El Rosario	7	*Clostridioides difficile* (1), *Salmonella* sp. (6), enteropathogenic *E. coli* (5), *Campylobacter* sp. (2), enterotoxigenic *E. coli lt/st* (1), *Vibrio* sp. (1)
La Orotava	2	*Cryptosporidium* (1), *Clostridioides difficile* (2), *Salmonella* sp. (1), enteropathogenic *E. coli* (1), *Plesiomonas shigelloides* (1)
San Miguel	3	*Clostridioides difficile* (1), *Salmonella* sp. (3), enteropathogenic *E. coli* (3)
Granadilla	2	Enteropathogenic *E. coli* (1), *Campylobacter* sp. (2)
Adeje	2	*Clostridioides difficile* (1), *Salmonella* sp. (2), enteropathogenic *E. coli* (2)
Tacoronte	1	*Clostridioides difficile* (1), *Salmonella* sp. (1), enteropathogenic *E. coli.* (1)
Güímar	1	*Salmonella* sp. (1)., enteropathogenic *E. coli* (1), norovirus GI/GII (1)
Fasnia	1	Enteropathogenic *E. coli* (1)
Total	45	*Campylobacter* sp. (10), *Clostridioides difficile* (15), *Plesiomonas shigelloides* (1), *Salmonella* sp. (30), *Vibrio* sp. (1), enteropathogenic *E. coli* (32), enterotoxigenic *E. coli lt/st* (3), *Shigella*/enteroinvasive *E. coli* (1), *Cryptosporidium* (3), Norovirus GI/GII (1)

DISCUSSION

The introduction of invasive species in a delicate ecosystem like the Canary Islands not only implies a potential danger to the environment, as more than 500 endemic species inhabit the archipelago (8), but also can contribute to the dispersion of different diseases. The results of this study show a wide distribution of causative agents of diarrhea in Tenerife, as the majority of the hedgehogs included in this study were found in the most populated areas of Tenerife, since La Laguna and Santa Cruz are the biggest cities of the island and Arona, San Miguel, and Adeje are highly touristic municipalities. The finding of causative agents of human diarrhea in the hedgehogs from the wildlife of these areas could imply a risk of transmission to humans, specially taking into consideration that in the Canarian archipelago, *A. algirus* is commonly adopted from the environment without any veterinary control.

Regarding the pathogens found in this study, the finding of *Salmonella* sp. in exotic animals of Spain is not unusual, as in 2013 it was found in free-living turtles of Eastern Spain, with a prevalence of 11% (9), although this is the first time this bacterial genus is found in *A. algirus*. The high prevalence of *Salmonella* and *Campylobacter* species in *A. algirus* may be due to the fact that this hedgehog species is mainly an insectivore, although its diet may vary according to availability and weather conditions (10), and some studies have shown that insects can act as carriers of *Salmonella* and *Campylobacter* species (11). The high prevalence of both bacteria found in this study compared to other wildlife species may imply that insects of the Canary Islands are probably carriers of these pathogens and *A. algirus* feeding habits facilitates their infection. Apart from the acute gastroenteritis that both bacteria cause, campylobacteriosis can sometimes lead to long-term sequelae such as Guillain–Barré syndrome, irritable bowel syndrome, or reactive arthritis (9).

The prevalence found in this study regarding *Cryptosporidium* sp. is similar to those found in pigeons of the Canary Islands in 2009, in which 28 wild pigeons were captured in Santa Cruz and its feces were posteriorly analyzed by PCR for the presence of *Cryptosporidium*, with 5.9% of them being positive (12). Further investigations in the presence of *Cryptosporidium* in wildlife species of the Canary Islands should be done in order to prevent risk focuses of cryptosporidiosis, a disease that can cause severe enteritis and malabsorption (13).

The presence of *P. shigelloides* in a hedgehog from La Orotava is also remarkable, a bacterium capable of causing sepsis and meningitis to immunosuppressed hosts, specially babies, in which 12 cases has been described, 6 of whom died due to the infection (14). Besides, the presence of *C. difficile* may be one of the most problematic among the bacteria found in this study, as its infection is transmitted by spores resistant to acid, antibiotics, or even heat and are commonly found in the environment. Also, elderly people, cancer patients and other diseases seem to be risk factors for the susceptibility to this bacterium, which may cause colitis. It is important to note that 40% of the community acquired infections of *C. difficile* requires hospitalization (15). The finding of this bacterium in the feces of animals that can potentially be adopted constitutes a risk of transmission to its owners, which is specially concerning in the case of immunosuppressed individuals.

The finding of *Vibrio* sp. (*parahaemolyticus* or *vulnificus*) in a hedgehog of Tenerife is also interesting, as these bacteria species are usually transmitted by seafood, with *V. vulnificus* being of special concern as it is responsible for more than 95% of seafood-related death in the United States, usually in individuals with liver disease or those who are immunocompromised (16). Besides, both *V. parahaemolyticus* and *V. vulnificus* are the most common causative agents isolated when *Vibrio* spp. are isolated from skin and soft tissue infections, which range from bullous skin lessons to severe necrotizing of the tissue with secondary septicemia (17). In the Canary Islands, one case of skin and soft tissue infection due to *Vibrio* sp. was reported in a patient with cancer and diabetes mellitus type II (17); the presence of this genera of bacteria in the wildlife, especially in a species that usually lives in close contact with humans, could constitute a high risk for immunocompromised individuals, as well as people presenting chronic diseases such as cancer and diabetes.

Regarding the *E. coli* strains found in this study, the prevalence of EPEC found in hedgehogs was considerably higher than other wildlife species studied along mainland Spain (18). That is why hedgehogs should be considered as an important wildlife reservoir of this bacterium, as nearly three quarters of the animals studied hosted EPEC.

In the particular case of Norovirus, one third of the people infected are asymptomatic; however, elderly, children, and immunocompromised people are at greater risk for severe symptoms and complications, such as acute renal failure leading to hemodialysis, cardiac complications including arrhythmias, acute graft organ rejection in transplant recipients, and death (19). The finding of Norovirus GI/GII in animals that can potentially be adopted by families may constitute a risk focus for this viral infection.

Another factor to take into consideration is that hedgehogs present a behavior named anting or anointing, which consist in moistening their spines with saliva (20). The fact that hedgehogs showed high prevalence of gastrointestinal pathogens implies a risk for humans to get in contact with them only by touching the animals, even more taking into consideration that coinfection was commonly found in these animals, so multiple pathogens can be transmitted. Also, further investigations should be done in the islands of the Canary archipelago where *A. algirus* presence has been spotted, as this is the first study on the zoonotic pathogens that this species hosts in the archipelago.

In mainland Spain, two species of hedgehogs inhabiting the country, *Atelerix albiventris* (Wagner, 1841) and *Hemiechinus auratus* (Gmelin, 1770), are included in the catalog of exotic invasive species (RD 63/2013, de 2 de Agosto) (21), which allows the competent authorities to control the population. Management strategies as well as educative measurements should be applied in order to reduce the impact that this species may be having in the Canary archipelago.

In conclusion, the lack of management measurements, the non-controlled selling, and the fact that some of the hedgehogs included in this study belonged to highly populated areas of Tenerife imply a high risk of transmission of pathogens to humans.

PERMISSION TO REUSE AND COPYRIGHT

The original image from the figure in this article was acquired from https://commons.wikimedia.org/wiki/File:Santa_Cruz_de_Tenerife_-_Mapa_municipal.svg in which the permission to copy, distribute, or modify it is established. It was later edited in photoshop CS6 by Izquierdo-Rodríguez.

AUTHOR CONTRIBUTIONS

EI-R and NM-C were responsible for the collection of the samples as well as the analysis. PF coordinated the relationships between the wildlife recovery center and the laboratory, as well as supervised the analysis and the writing of the article. BV and PF obtained the funding for the study and supervised the work. EI-R did the main writing of the article. All authors have read and approved the final manuscript.

ACKNOWLEDGMENTS

We would like to thank the workers from the Wildlife Recovery Centre of La Tahonilla for their essential contribution to this study.

REFERENCES

1. Arechavaleta M, Rodríguez S, Zurita N, García A. *Lista de Especies Silvestres de Canarias. Hongos, Plantas y Animales Terrestres.* Santa Cruz de Tenerife: Gobierno de Canarias (2010). p. 579.
2. Medina FM. First record of Algerian hedgehog *Atelerix algirus* (Lereboullet, 1842) in La Palma Island biosphere reserve. *Galemys.* (2016) 28:61–2. doi: 10.7325/Galemys.2016.N3
3. Tomás-Pérez M, Khaldi M, Riera C, Mozo-León D, Ribas A, Hide M, et al. First report of natural infection in hedgehogs with *Leishmania* major, a possible reservoir of zoonotic cutaneous leishmaniasis in Algeria. *Acta Trop.* (2014) 135:44–9. doi: 10.1016/j.actatropica.2014.03.018
4. Khaldi M, Socolovschi C, Benyettou M, Barech G, Biche M, Kernif T, et al. Rickettsiae in arthropods collected from the North African Hedgehog (*Atelerix algirus*) and the desert hedgehog (*Paraechinus aethiopicus*) in Algeria. *Comp Immunol Microb.* (2012) 35:117–12. doi: 10.1016/j.cimid.2011.11.007
5. Paredes-Esquivel C, Sola J, Delgado-Serra S, Puig Riera M, Negre N, Miranda MA, et al. *Angiostrongylus cantonensis* in North African hedgehogs as vertebrate hosts, Mallorca, Spain, October 2018. *Euro Surveill.* (2019) 24:1900489. doi: 10.2807/1560-7917.ES.2019.24.33.1900489
6. Foronda P, López-González M, Miquel J, Torres J, Segovia M, Abreu-Acosta N, et al. Finding of *Parastrongylus cantonensis* (Chen, 1935) in Rattus Rattus in Tenerife, Canary Islands (Spain). *Acta Trop.* (2010) 114:123–7. doi: 10.1016/j.actatropica.2010.02.004
7. Martin-Alonso A, Abreu-Yanes E, Feliu C, Mas-Coma S, Bargues MD, Valladares B, et al. Intermediate hosts of *Angiostrongylus cantonensis* in Tenerife, Spain. *PLoS ONE.* (2015) 10:e0120686. doi: 10.1371/journal.pone.0120686
8. Morales Matos G, Pérez González R. *Gran Atlas Temático de Canarias.* Santa Cruz de Tenerife: Interinsular Canaria (2000). p. 97.
9. Marin C, Ingresa-Capaccioni S, González-Bodi S, Marco-Jiménez F, Vega S. Free-living turtles are a reservoir for Salmonella but not for *Campylobacter. PLoS ONE.* (2013) 8:e72350. doi: 10.1371/journal.pone.0072350
10. Mouhoub-Sayah C, Djoudad-Kadji H, Kletty F, Malan A, Robin J-P, Saboureau M, et al. Seasonal variations in the diet and food selection of the Algerian hedgehog *Atelerix algirus. Afr Zool.* (2018) 53:1–10. doi: 10.1080/15627020.2017.1419072
11. Skov MN, Spencer AG, Hald B, Petersen L, Nauerby B, Carstensen B, et al. The role of litter beetles as potential reservoir of *Salmonella enterica* and *Thermophilic Campylobacter* spp. between brolier flocks. *Avian Dis.* (2004) 48:9–18. doi: 10.1637/5698
12. Abreu-Acosta N, Foronda-Rodríguez P, López M, Valladares B. Occurrence of *Cryptosporidium hominis* in pigeons. *Acta Parasitol.* (2009) 54:1–5. doi: 10.2478/s11686-009-0008-4
13. Flanigan T, Whalen C, Turner J, Soave R, Toerner J, Havlir D, et al. Cryptosporidium infection and CD4 counts. *Ann Intern Med.* (1992) 116:840–2. doi: 10.7326/0003-4819-116-10-840
14. Xia F-Q, Liu P-N, Zhou Y-H. Meningoencephalitis caused by *Plesiomonas shigelloides* in a Chinese neonate: case report and literature review. *Ital J Pediatr.* (2015) 41:3. doi: 10.1186/s13052-014-0107-1
15. Leffer DA, Lamont JT. *Clostridium difficile* infection. *N Eng J Med.* (2015) 372:1539–48. doi: 10.1056/NEJMra1403772
16. Elmahdi S, DaSilva LV, Parveen S. Antibiotic resistance of *Vibrio*

parahaemolyticus and *Vibrio vulnificus* in various countries: a review. *Food Microbiol.* (2016) 57:128–34. doi: 10.1016/j.fm.2016.02.008
17. Aguinaga A, Portillo ME, Yuste JR, del Pozo JL, García-Tutor E, Pérez-Gracia JL, et al. Non-O1 *Vibrio cholerae* inguinal skin and soft tissue infection with bullous skin lesions in a patient with a penis squamous cell carcinoma. *Ann Clin Microbiol Antimicrob.* (2009) 8:1–4. doi: 10.1186/1476-0711-8-17
18. Andrea Alonso C, Mora A, Díaz D, Blanco M, González-Barrio D, Ruiz-Fons F, et al. Occurrence and characterization of STX and/or EAE-positive *Escherichia coli* isolated from wildlife, including a typical EPEC strain from a wild boar. *Vet Microbiol.* (2017) 207:69–73. doi: 10.1016/j.vetmic.2017.05.028
19. Cardemil CV, Parashar UD, Hall AJ. Norovirus infection in older adults, epidemiology, risks factors, and opportunities for prevention and control. *Infect Dis Clin N Am.* (2017) 31:839–70. doi: 10.1016/j.idc.2017.07.012
20. Fairley JA, Suchniak J, Paller AS. Hedgehog hives. *Arch Dermatol.* (1999) 135:561–3. doi: 10.1001/archderm.135.5.561
21. España. Real Decreto 630/2013, de 2 de agosto, por el que se regula el Catálogo español de especies exóticas invasoras. *Boletín Oficial del Estado* (2013, August 3). p. 56764–86.

2

Pet Reptiles: A Potential Source of Transmission of Multidrug-Resistant *Salmonella*

Clara Marin[1]*, *Laura Lorenzo-Rebenaque*[1], *Omar Laso*[1], *José Villora-Gonzalez*[2] *and Santiago Vega*[1]

[1] *Facultad de Veterinaria, Instituto de Ciencias Biomédicas, Universidad Cardenal Herrera-CEU, CEU Universities, Alfara del Patriarca, Spain,* [2] *Selvätica Veterinary Clinic, Valencia, Spain*

***Correspondence:**
Clara Marin
clara.marin@uchceu.es

Salmonella spp. is widely considered one of the most important zoonotic pathogens worldwide. The close contact between reptiles and their owners provides favourable conditions for the transmission of zoonotic pathogen infections, and ~6% of human salmonellosis cases are acquired after direct or indirect contact with reptiles. Moreover, antimicrobial resistance is one of the most important health threats of the twenty-first century and has been reported in *Salmonella* strains isolated from pet reptiles, which could entail therapeutic consequences for their owners and breeders. The aim of this study was to assess *Salmonella* carriage by pet reptiles in pet shops and households, and their role in the transmission of antimicrobial resistance, to inform the owners about the possible risks factors. During the period between January 2019 and December 2019, 54 reptiles from pet shops and 69 reptiles from households were sampled in the Valencian Region (Eastern Spain). Three different sample types were collected from each reptile: oral cavity, skin, and cloacal swabs. *Salmonella* identification was based on ISO 6579-1:2017 (Annex D), serotyped in accordance with Kauffman-White-Le-Minor technique, and antibiotic susceptibility was assessed according to Decision 2013/652. The results of this study showed that 48% of the pet reptiles examined from households and pet shops carry *Salmonella* spp. All the strains isolated presented resistance to at least one antibiotic, and 72% were multidrug-resistant strains, the most frequently observed resistance patterns being gentamicin-colistin and gentamicin-colistin-ampicillin. The present study demonstrates that pet reptiles could be a source of human multidrug-resistant *Salmonella* infection. In this context, the most optimal prevention of multidrug-resistant *Salmonella* infections necessarily involves strict control of the sanitary status of reptile pet shops and hygienic handling by the individual owners at home.

Keywords: reptile-associated salmonellosis, multidrug-resistant *Salmonella*, pet reptiles, One Health, zoonosis, *Salmonella*

INTRODUCTION

Salmonella is widely considered one of the most important zoonotic pathogens worldwide. This pathogen has become an important public health concern with a significant economic impact, which has been estimated at 3.6 billion dollars annually (1, 2). In Europe, salmonellosis was responsible for 94,203 human cases, of which 9.3% corresponded to Spain (3). The infection usually causes self-limited diarrhoeal illness, although severe illness and death may occur, especially in children, elderly or immunocompromised adults (4). However, the overall epidemiological pattern of human salmonellosis cases is related to *Salmonella*-contaminated food from animal origin, especially eggs and poultry meat, and ~6% of human salmonellosis cases are acquired after direct or indirect contact with reptiles (3, 4).

In the last few years, exotic reptiles have risen in popularity as pets, with a population of over 7 million in European households (5). This increase in "living presents for children" is resulting in a trade of non-conventional species around the world, with Europe as the leading reptile importer (6, 7). The close contact between reptiles and their owners provides favourable conditions for the transmission of zoonotic pathogens infections, constituting a public health concern, as these pets have been considered as potential *Salmonella* carriers (7–11). Reptiles are natural reservoirs of *Salmonella*, which can hold a wide variety of serovars simultaneously without symptoms (12–14). However, reptile-associated salmonellosis seems to be responsible for more serious complications, with invasive disease and hospitalisation, especially in children (14, 15). From a public health standpoint, pet reptiles represent a persistent source of salmonellosis in households (16–19).

In addition, *Salmonella* multi-resistant strains emerge as a potential concern for public health safety, with implications of increased disease severity, longer hospitalisations and higher cost rates (20, 21). In this context, the World Health Organisation deemed antimicrobial resistance (**AMR**) one of the most important health threats, which could cause 10 million deaths a year by 2050, ahead of other diseases such as cancer (22, 23). In this sense, *Salmonella* has been included in the World Health Organisation priority list of twelve antibiotic-resistant bacteria (24). Interest in the role of reptiles as an antibiotic-resistant *Salmonella* reservoir has increased in recent years (7, 25, 26). Moreover, AMR had been reported in *Salmonella* isolated from captive reptiles, and their release could entail therapeutic consequences for their owners and breeders (16, 27). Moreover, the widespread use of antibiotics against *Salmonella* has been described in the international trade of pet reptiles, in order to prevent economical loses, as well as in animal welfare in crowded farms and long-distance transport (28–30). Therefore, more information on AMR in pet reptiles is needed in view of One Health (31).

In this context, the objective of the present study is to assess *Salmonella* carriage by pet reptiles in pet stores and households in Eastern Spain (Valencia Region) and gain more in-depth knowledge of their role in AMR transmission, in order to inform the owners about the possible risk factors.

MATERIALS AND METHODS

All animals were handled according to the principles of animal care published by Spanish Royal Decree 53/2013 (32).

Sample Collection

During the period between January 2019 and December 2019, a total of 349 samples from 123 different reptile species from households and pet shops reptiles were taken. Previously, the owners were contacted by advertising the project through the University community (Universidad Cardenal Herrera-CEU, and Universidad Politécnica de Valencia) and veterinary clinics of the Valencian Region (Eastern Spain).

A total of 37 species were identified from the 123 of the reptiles sampled (**Table 1**). From these species, 12 were classified as chelonians (order *Chelonia*), 16 as lizards (suborder *Sauria*) and 9 as snakes (suborder *Ofidia*) (**Table 1**). According to the individuals sampled from each group, 43.9% (54/123), 39.0% (48/123), and 17.1% (21/123) were chelonians, lizards and snakes, respectively (**Table 1**).

For each individual, whenever possible, samples from oral cavity (n = 114), skin (n = 123), and cloaca (n = 112) were taken using sterile cotton swabs (Cary Blair sterile transport swabs, DELTALAB®) (33). All individuals sampled were healthy and none of them presented clinical symptoms such as diarrhoea at the moment of sampling. In addition, an epidemiological questionnaire was filled in. The questionnaire contained information related to species, diet and the number of reptiles that cohabit in the same terrarium. The diet was classified as food from animal origin (including live prey, fresh meat and frozen meat), food of vegetable origin (including fruit and vegetables) and processed (including commercially manufactured reptile food). Moreover, the number of reptiles coexisting in the same terrarium was recorded as reptiles that inhabit alone, or reptiles that cohabit with two or more reptiles.

Detection of *Salmonella* spp.

The collected samples were analysed within 24 h of collection according to ISO 6579-1:2017 (Annex D) recommendations (34). Samples were pre-enriched in 1:10 vol/vol Buffered Peptone Water 2.5% (BPW; Scharlau, Barcelona, Spain), and then incubated at 37 ± 1°C for 18 ± 2 h. The pre-enriched samples were transferred onto Semi-Solid Modification Rappaport Vassiliadis (MSRV; Difco, Valencia, Spain), and incubated at 41.5 ± 1°C for 24–48 h. For the positive plates, the cultures obtained in MSRV were inoculated onto two specific agar plates for *Salmonella* spp. detection: Xylose Lysine Deoxycholate Agar (XLD; Liofilchem, Valencia, Spain) and a selective chromogenic agar medium specific for detection of C8-esterase activity (ASAP, bioMérieux, Marcy l'Étoile, France), then incubated at 37 ± 1°C for 24 h. After incubation, one typical colony was collected and inoculated into a pre-dried nutrient agar plate (Scharlau, Barcelona, Spain), then incubated at 37 ± 1°C for 24 h. Finally, an API (API-20-E; bioMérieux, Madrid, Spain) biochemical test was performed to confirm *Salmonella* spp. The *Salmonella* isolates were stored at −80°C for further serotyping and antimicrobial susceptibility testing.

TABLE 1 | *Salmonella* isolated from reptiles in relation to reptile species.

Category	Reptile species	Number of reptiles examined	Number of positive reptiles (%)
Suborder *Sauria*	*Zonosaurus ornatus*	1	1 (100)
	Hemitheconyx caudicinctus	2	1 (50.0)
	Correlophus ciliatus	1	1 (100)
	Eublepharis macularius	21	11 (52.4)
	Paroedura picta	2	2 (100)
	Iguana	2	2 (100)
	Tupinambis teguixin	1	1 (100)
	Physignathus cocincinus	5	5 (100)
	Petrosaurus thalassinus	2	2 (100)
	Pogona vitticeps	4	4 (100)
	Chamaleo calyptratus	2	1 (50.0)
	Varanus glauerti	1	1 (100)
	Varanus albigularis	1	1 (100)
	Phelsuma grandis	1	0
	Pseudopus apodus	1	0
	Gecko gecko	1	0
Suborder *Ofidia*	*Python regius*	5	5 (100)
	Boa constrictor imperator	1	1 (100)
	Gongylophis colubrinus	1	1 (100)
	Acrantophis madagascariensis	1	1 (100)
	Elaphe guttata	7	5 (71.4)
	Spalerosophis diadema	2	2 (100)
	Lampropeltis getula	2	1 (50.0)
	Basiliscus plumifrons	1	0
	Heterodon nasicus	1	0
Order *Chelonia*	*Graptemys pseudographica*	5	3 (60.0)
	Testudo marginata	1	1 (100)
	Testudo hermanni	11	5 (45.5)
	Testudo horsfieldii	8	1 (12.5)
	Trachemys scripta elegans	5	0
	Pelusios	1	0
	Mauremys reevesii	3	0
	Cuora flavomarginata	1	0
	Pelomedusa subrufa	1	0
	Stigmochelis pardalis	1	0
	Testudo graeca	16	0
	Pseudemys nelsoni	1	0

Serotyping and Antimicrobial Susceptibility Testing

From each individual, the serotyping was performed from a cloacal strain, and when not present, a strain from the skin or oral cavity was analysed. Thus, all the strains were unfrozen and revived (ASAP) and the selected isolates were serotyped at the National Reference Laboratory for Animal Health (Algete, Madrid, Spain). The method used for serotyping was antigenic agglutination with specific antisera according to the White-Kauffmann-Le Minor scheme (35).

From all strains, *Salmonella* antimicrobial susceptibility was tested according to the European Committee on Antimicrobial Susceptibility Testing guidelines (36). *Salmonella* strains were inoculated into Mueller-Hinton agar (Scharlab, S.L.) to form a bacterial lawn and were allowed to dry for 30 min at ambient (25°C) temperature; then, the antibiotic discs were applied and plates were incubated at 37°C for 24 h. The antimicrobial agents selected were those set out in Decision 2013/652 (37), including three b-lactams: ampicillin (AMP, 10 μg), cefotaxime (CTX, 30 μg) and ceftazidime (CAZ, 30 μg); two quinolones: ciprofloxacin (CIP, 5 μg) and nalidixic acid (NA, 30 μg); one phenicol: chloramphenicol (CHL, 5 μg); one potentiated sulfonamide: trimethoprim-sulfamethoxazole (SXT, 1.25/23.75 μg); one polymyxin: colistin (COL, 10 μg); one macrolide: azithromycin (AZM, 15 μg); one glycylcycline: tigecycline (TGC, 15 μg); one aminoglycoside: gentamicin (GM, 10 μg); and one pyrimidine: trimethoprim (TM, 5 μg). The source for zone diameters used for interpretation of the test and plates after incubation at 37°C for 24 h was the European Committee on Antimicrobial Susceptibility Testing (EUCAST) (http://www.eucast.org/clinical_breakpoints/), and where this was not possible, according to Clinical and Laboratory Standards Institute (CLSI) indications (https://clsi.org/media/2663/m100ed29_sample.pdf) (38). The isolate strains were categorised as susceptible (S) or resistant (R), based on EUCAST imperative criteria (39). Multidrug resistance (MDR) was defined as acquired resistance to at least one agent in two or more antimicrobial classes (40).

Statistical Analysis

A Generalised Linear Model, which assumed a binomial distribution for *Salmonella* shedding, AMR and MDR, was fitted to the data to determine whether there was an association with the categorical variables (species and order or suborder of reptile, the habitat of the reptile, sample type, diet and number of reptiles that cohabit in the same terrarium). A reptile was considered *Salmonella* positive if one or more samples collected (oral cavity, skin and/or cloacal) tested positive. A $P \leq 0.05$ was considered to indicate a statistically significant difference. Data are presented as least squares means ± standard error of the least squares means. In addition, a descriptive analysis has been done to assess the subespecies isolated in this study. Analyses were carried out using a commercially available software application (SPSS 24.0 software package; SPSS Inc., Chicago, IL, 2002).

RESULTS

From all samples collected during this study, 25.2 ± 2.3% (88/349) tested positive for *Salmonella*. The type of sample taken was significantly associated with *Salmonella* carriage ($P = 0.000$), with higher positive samples from cloaca (38.0 ± 4.6%, 43/112) than from skin (22.0 ± 3.7%, 27/123) and oral cavity (16.0 ± 3.4%, 18/114).

Salmonella spp. was detected in 48.0 ± 4.5% (59/123) of individuals sampled, with significant differences between snakes (76.0 ± 9.3%, 16/21) and lizards (69.0 ± 6.7%, 33/48), compared to chelonians (19.0 ± 5.3%, 10/54) ($P = 0.000$).

The reptiles sampled in this study inhabited households with private owners (56.1%, 69/123), as well as pet shops (43.9%, 54/123) in the Valencian Region (Eastern Spain). Significant differences for *Salmonella* isolation were found among the different reptile habitats (owners vs. pet shops) ($P = 0.000$), being higher in pet shop reptiles (67.0 ± 6.4%, 36/54) than in household pets (33.0 ± 5.7%, 23/69).

Moreover, the number of reptiles cohabiting the same terrarium were known for 111 of the 123 reptiles analysed, 49 for pet shops and 66 for households. In pet shops, significant differences were found between the number of reptiles present in the same terrarium and *Salmonella* shedding ($P = 0.008$). Thus, 89 ± 7.4% of reptiles that cohabit in terrariums with two or more reptiles were positive for *Salmonella* (16/18), while 58 ± 8.9% of reptiles that inhabit terrariums alone were positive for the bacterium (18/31). In contrast, for private owners' reptiles, no significant differences were observed between reptiles that cohabit in terrariums with two or more reptiles or alone and *Salmonella* shedding ($P = 0.064$), 21.0 ± 7.8% (16/38) and 42.0 ± 8.0% (6/28), respectively.

The diet was significantly associated with *Salmonella* carriage ($P = 0.000$), with higher frequency in reptiles that were fed with food from animal origin (65.0 ± 5.6%, 47/72), in contrast to reptiles that were fed with food from vegetable origin, and processed (24.0 ± 6.6%, 10/42, and 22.0 ± 13.9%, 2/9, respectively).

From the 59 strains selected for serotyping, 51 were viable after culture and were serotyped. All *Salmonella* isolates were classified as *Salmonella enterica*. The most represented subspecies were *S. enterica* (56.9%, 29/51), *S. houtenae* (19.6%, 10/51), *S. diarizonae* (11.8%,6/51), *S. salamae* (9.8%, 5/51) and *S. arizonae* (2.0%, 1/51). Fifteen different serovars of *S. enterica* subspecies were identified (**Table 2**). From all the strains serotyped, one *Salmonella enterica* serovar was indeterminate.

Seventy-five out of 88 *Salmonella* strains isolated were viable after culture and included in the antimicrobial susceptibility study. All strains analysed were resistant to at least one out of the twelve antibiotics tested ($n = 75/75$). The highest percentages of AMR were found to COL (97.3%, $n = 73$), followed by GM (84.0%, $n = 63$), AMP (46.7%, $n = 35$) and TGC (42.7%, $n = 32$), AZM (26.7%, $n = 20$), NAL (12.0%, $n = 9$), CHL (9.3%, $n = 7$), SXT and TM (8.0%, $n = 6$, both), and finally CAZ (6.7%, $n = 5$), CTX (4.0%, $n = 3$), and CIP (1.3%, $n = 1$) ($P = 0.000$). Antimicrobial resistance of the different *Salmonella enterica* serovars was summarised in **Table 3**.

Furthermore, a total of 72.0% (54/75) *Salmonella* isolates were resistant to two or more antimicrobials. No significant differences in MDR rates were shown between lizards (78.0%, 32/41), chelonians (73.3%, 11/15) and snakes (57.9%, 11/19) ($P = 0.206$). Although the type of sample collected was not significantly associated with MDR carriage, oral cavity (75.0%, 12/16), skin (77.3%, 17/22) and cloacal samples (67,6%, 25/37) ($P = 0.692$), significant differences were found between the type of sample and the different types of reptiles, except for lizards (**Table 4**, $P < 0.05$). Moreover, no significant differences were found between the habitat (pet shop and household), diet (food from animal origin, vegetable origin, and processed) and MDR *Salmonella* carriage ($P = 0.065$ and $P = 0.432$, respectively)

TABLE 2 | *Salmonella* serovars isolated from private owners and pet shops.

Sample origin	Subspecies	Serovar	*n*
Private Owner	*enterica*	Albany 8,20:z4,z24	2
		Cerro 18: z4,z23	1
		Lattenkamp 45:z35:1,5	3
		Newport 6,8:e,h:1,2	1
		Paratyphi 4,12:b:1,2	1
	diarizonae	60:r:e,n,x,z15	1
		48:z53	1
		50:z52:z35	1
		47:z10:z35	1
		47:i:z53	1
	arizonae	44:z4,z23	1
	houtenae	11:z4,z23	1
	salamae	13, 22:z29:1,5	1
Pet Store	*enterica*	Cotham 28:i:1,5	2
		Fresno 9,46:z38	1
		Hadar 6,8:z10:e,n,x	3
		Hvittingfoss 16:b:e,n,x	1
		Muenster 3,15:e,h:1,5	2
		Newport 6,8:e,h:1,2	2
		Panama 9,12:l,v:1,5	1
		Pomona 28:y:1,7	3
		Sandiego 4,12:e,h:e,n,z15	1
		Vitkin 28:1,v:e,n,x	4
	houtenae	11:z4,z23	6
		16:z4,z32	2
		16:z36	1
	salamae	30:l,z28:z6	2
		21:g,s,t	1
		52:g,t	1
	diarizonae	42:k: z35	1

n: Number of strains isolated.

Overall, 25 different resistance patterns were observed. The combination of GM-COL (18.7%, 14/75) was the most frequently observed pattern, followed by GM-COL-AMP and GM-COL-TGC (10.7%, 8/75, both), COL alone (9.3%, 7/75) and GM-COL-AMP-TGC (8.0%, 6/75).

DISCUSSION

The present study demonstrates that 48% of the pet reptiles examined from households and pet shops carry *Salmonella* spp. All the strains isolated showed resistance to at least one antibiotic and 72% were multidrug-resistant strains. To our knowledge, this is the first study in the literature evaluating the prevalence and the antimicrobial resistance of this zoonotic pathogen from a considerable sample size in pet reptiles of Eastern Spain (Valencia Region).

TABLE 3 | Percentage of antimicrobial resistance of *Salmonella enterica* isolated from pet reptiles.

Salmonella enterica serovars	*n*	AMP	CTX	CAZ	CIP	NA	CHL	SXT	COL	AZM	TGC	GM	TM
Albany	2	100	0	0	0	100	100	100	100	0	100	100	100
Cerro	1	0	0	0	0	0	0	0	100	0	0	100	0
Cotham	2	100	0	0	0	0	0	0	100	0	100	100	0
Fresno	1	0	0	0	0	0	0	0	100	0	0	100	0
Hadar	3	66.7	0	0	0	0	0	0	100	100	66.7	100	0
Hvittingfoss	1	100	0	0	0	0	0	0	100	0	100	100	0
Lattenkamp	3	0	0	0	0	0	0	0	66.7	0	0	33.3	0
Muenster	2	100	0	0	0	0	0	0	100	50	50	100	0
Newport	3	0	0	0	0	0	0	0	100	0	33.3	66.7	0
Panama	1	0	0	0	100	0	0	0	100	0	0	100	0
Paratyphi	1	0	0	0	0	0	0	0	100	0	0	100	0
Pomona	3	100	0	33.3	0	0	0	0	100	66.7	0	100	0
Sandiego	1	100	0	0	0	0	0	0	100	100	100	100	0
Vitkin	4	50	0	25	0	0	0	0	100	0	75	75	0

n: Number of samples. The resistance was determined by disc diffusion. AMP, Ampicillin (10 μg); CTX, Cefotaxime (30 μg); CAZ, Ceftazidime (30 μg); CIP, Ciprofloxacin (5 μg); NA, Nalidixic acid (30 μg); CHL, Chloramphenicol (5 μg); SXT, Trimethoprim-sulfamethoxazole (1.25/23.75 μg); COL, Colistin (10 μg); AZM, Azithromycin (15 μg); TGC, Tigecycline (15 μg); GM, Gentamicin (10 μg); TM, Trimethoprim (5 μg).

TABLE 4 | Multidrug-resistant *Salmonella* isolated according to the type of sample collected in the different type of reptiles.

Reptile classification	Type of sample	*n*	MDR rate
Suborder *Sauria*	Oral cavity	9	89.0 ± 10.5
	Skin	13	79.0 ± 9.4
	Cloacal	19	69.0 ± 12.8
Suborder *Ofidia*	Oral cavity	3	0.0 ± 0.0^{a}
	Skin	23	100.0 ± 0.0^{b}
	Cloacal	13	62.0 ± 13.5^{c}
Order *Chelonia*	Oral cavity	4	100.0 ± 0.0^{a}
	Skin	6	83.0 ± 15.2^{ab}
	Cloacal	5	40.0 ± 21.9^{b}

Data are presented as least squares means ± standard error of the least squares means. [a,b,c]Different superscripts in each file means significant differences in the same reptiles' classification with a $P < 0.05$. MDR, Multidrug resistance. n, Number of samples.

Reptiles have been known to be important carriers of *Salmonella* spp. worldwide, which may pose a health hazard as a source of human infection, particularly in children (4, 16, 41–43). However, there is a lack of consensus regarding the role of reptile shops on MDR *Salmonella* strains spreading. The results of this study showed that *Salmonella* strains isolated in reptiles from shops were twice as high as those from private owners (67 vs. 33%) (44, 45). This may be due to poor hygienic management of terrariums, especially in pet shops where they are usually occupied and ensuring a proper cleaning and disinfection procedure is not easy (45). This fact could facilitate that MDR strains remain in the shop environment among different reptile batches. In addition, the reptiles' stress related to cohabiting with individuals of different ages and origins could result in an increase in the bacterial infection, shedding in the terrarium and reptile-to-reptile transmission (45, 46). Conversely, reptiles from private owners are exposed to better hygiene practises and less stressful environments, leading to lower *Salmonella* shedding (45).

In reptiles, *Salmonella* is spread by faecal-oral route with an asymptomatic natural colonisation of the enteric tract, so in this study cloacal swabs collected were more sensitive for *Salmonella* isolation than other samples collected, such as skin or oral cavity. However, it is important to highlight that because *Salmonella* is excreted through faeces, it could contaminate the reptile's skin, oral cavity and the environment, being a source of infection for humans who handle the reptile or who are exposed to the reptile's environment (11, 46–50). Moreover, the *Salmonella* serovars most frequently detected in this study have been cited previously in reptile studies (51, 52), as well as in human outbreaks (3, 51–55). In addition, it has been reported that cold-blooded animals could be the major reservoir for the subspecies *houtenae*, *diarizonae*, *salamae*, and *arizonae* (56, 57).

The results of this study showed higher *Salmonella* prevalence among snakes and lizards compared to chelonians, in accordance with previous research (11, 31, 52, 58, 59). Particular attention has recently been given to snakes and lizards, as human interaction with these reptiles has become increasingly common in domestic environments (11, 60). In this sense, it is important to highlight that these reptiles are mainly fed with food from animal origin, which represents an important source of *Salmonella* (49, 61, 62). Previous studies carried out in the United Kingdom reported the important role of commercial feeder rodents in bacterial transmission among reptiles, and even their owners (63, 64). Thus, handling *Salmonella*-contaminated feeder rodents, as well as cross-contamination in the kitchen due to the rodents being kept in the freezer and thawed in microwaves, also in contact with food for human consumption, have been linked to human *Salmonella* outbreaks (63, 65). In this context, to avoid *Salmonella* infection of reptiles, control of food products of animal origin has to be mandatory for the food suppliers (64).

On the other hand, special attention must be given to chelonians, due to their popularity as a pet for children. In this context, several countries, such as the US, have implemented strict bans in an attempt to curtail chelonian-associated salmonellosis; however, in Europe there are not many regulations to control its prevalence (53, 66). In the present study, *Salmonella* has been isolated from 18.5% of the chelonians tested. Seasonal effects, such as hibernation or season of sampling, have been speculated by previous studies to explain the low isolation rate of *Salmonella* in chelonians compared to other reptiles (31). Moreover, the diet may also have an important role (43, 49) because, as reported above, a large proportion of the chelonians are fed with food from vegetable origin or processed, and not from animal origin, frequently related with *Salmonella* outbreaks (11, 31, 67).

The increase in MDR *Salmonella* strains is of worldwide interest because it enhances the risk of therapeutic failure in cases of life-threatening salmonellosis in human and veterinary medicine (68, 69). In fact, it has been estimated that AMR could be the main cause of human mortality in 2050 (22). One of the most relevant outcomes in this study was the level of MDR isolated from pet reptiles, the most frequently observed resistance patterns being GM-COL and GM-COL-AMP. The high resistance against GM could be explained due to the indiscriminate use of aminoglycosides in pet reptile breeders, especially in the chelonian industry (28, 70). The use of GM as prophylactic *Salmonella* treatment in eggs to ensure sanitary conditions is a common practise in the US, the main supplier country of live reptiles for the EU (28, 71). Indeed, this practise has contributed to the finding of high-level plasmid-mediated gentamicin resistance in *Salmonella* isolated in its breeder farms (28).

Polymyxins have been widely used against Gramme-negative infections in animals, especially in animal production, the origin of several products involved in reptile feeding (72, 73). Currently, polymyxins such as COL represent the last line of defence against severe resistant infections in humans (72). Thus, it is highly restricted for animal infection treatments, and it is expected that resistance to this antibiotic will decrease in the coming years (74–76).

AMP was the third most frequent resistance shown in this study of *Salmonella* reptile strains, in line with a previous study conducted on species of gecko in Italy (10). This antibiotic is the most widely used in human medicine in Spain (76) and could thus be implicated in possible transmission of resistance from humans to reptiles, as a consequence of the direct and indirect contact between reptiles and their owners (75, 77, 78).

On the other hand, the level of resistance to NAL, CHL, SXT, TM, CAZ, CTX, and CIP in reptile *Salmonella* strains was relatively low. Resistance to CAZ contrasts with a survey conducted on geckos by Russo et al. (10), who showed a high resistance of *Salmonella* species to this antimicrobial, that is used in reptiles to treat infections or prophylactically after a traumatic injury (79). Moreover, it is important to note that fluoroquinolones (e.g., CIP) are the drugs of choice for invasive salmonellosis infections in humans (adults) and cephalosporins (e.g., CTX and CAZ) in children (21), although both are implicated in a reduced effectiveness of *Salmonella* treatment (77).

Should be essential to inform pet reptile owners about the risks of wrongly handling these animals (60). Proper hygienic management measures should be taken, such as the use of gloves when cleaning the reptile, and even during cleaning and disinfection of the surfaces that come in contact with the pet reptile (13). Moreover, it is important to thorough hand washing after handling the reptiles, especially the wounds due to bites or scratch (13). Reptiles and its feed should keep away from the kitchen and areas where the owners prepare their own food (64). Besides, before introducing a new reptile in the household, microbiological exams should be carried out to avoid cross-infection (13). Finally, it highlights the importance of extreme caution with young children and immunocompromised patients, because they are especially susceptible to *Salmonella* spp. infections (60).

CONCLUSIONS

The present study clearly demonstrates that pet reptiles could be a source of human MDR *Salmonella* infection. The problem of MDR in reptiles could start with the shops, where *Salmonella* presence is extremely high, and seems to be linked with the origin of reptile food. In this context, the most optimal prevention of MDR *Salmonella* infections involves strict control of the sanitary status of reptile pet shops and hygienic handling of the individuals in the household. Nevertheless, it is important to highlight that the number of included samples is relatively small, which may restrict the interpretation of our results to Eastern Spain. Further studies are needed to validate our results in a larger study sample.

AUTHOR CONTRIBUTIONS

CM, OL, and SV: conceptualisation. OL, JV-G, CM, and SV: data curation. LL-R, CM, OL, and JV-G: methodology. CM and SV: investigation, writing–review and editing, and funding acquisition. CM and LL-R: writing–original draft preparation. SV: project administration. All authors: have read and agreed to the published version of the manuscript.

ACKNOWLEDGMENTS

The authors wish to thank the reptile owners, veterinary clinics and pet shops for allowing access to their reptiles to enable this work to be carried out. Also, the authors wish to thank the "Improvement of Production System-related Food Safety and End Products" research group (Veterinary Faculty, University Cardenal Herrera-CEU) for the technical support. The English text version was revised by N. Macowan English Language Service.

REFERENCES

1. USDA (United States Department of Agriculture). *USDA ERS—Cost Estimates of Foodborne Illnesses.* (2014). Available online at: https://www.ers.usda.gov/data-products/cost-estimates-of-foodborne-illnesses.aspx (accessed April 24, 2020).
2. WHO (World Health Organization). *Interventions for the Control of Non-typhoidal Salmonella spp.* 30th ed. L. Thorgeir Rome: Microbiological Risk Assessment Series (2016).
3. EFSA and ECDC. The European Union One Health 2018 zoonoses report. *EFSA J.* (2019) 17:1–276. doi: 10.2903/j.efsa.2019.5926
4. Mermin J, Hutwagner L, Vugia D, Shallow S, Daily P, Bender J, et al. Reptiles, amphibians, and human *Salmonella* infection: a population-based, case-control study. *Clin Infect Dis.* (2004) 38:S253–61. doi: 10.1086/381594
5. FEDIAF (The European Pet Food Industry). *FEDIAF Annual Report 2019. RunSignup.* (2019). p. 60.
6. Bush ER, Baker SE, Macdonald DW. Global trade in exotic pets 2006-2012. *Conserv Biol.* (2014) 28:663–76. doi: 10.1111/cobi.12240
7. Bertelloni F, Chemaly M, Cerri D, Le Gall F, Ebani VV. *Salmonella* infection in healthy pet reptiles: bacteriological isolation and study of some pathogenic characters. *Acta Microbiol Immunol Hung.* (2016) 63:203–16. doi: 10.1556/030.63.2016.2.5
8. Stockman JA. Multistate outbreak of *Salmonella* infections associated with small turtle exposure, 2007–2008. *Yearb Pediatr.* (2011) 2011:288–9. doi: 10.1016/S0084-3954(10)79733-5
9. Jiménez RR, Barquero-Calvo E, Abarca JG, Porras LP. *Salmonella* isolates in the introduced asian house gecko (*Hemidactylus frenatus*) with emphasis on *Salmonella* Weltevreden, in two regions in Costa Rica. *Vector-Borne Zoonotic Dis.* (2015) 15:550–5. doi: 10.1089/vbz.2015.1785
10. Russo TP, Varriale L, Borrelli L, Pace A, Latronico M, Menna LF, et al. Salmonella serotypes isolated in geckos kept in seven collections in southern Italy. *J Small Anim Pract.* (2018) 59:294–7. doi: 10.1111/jsap.12808
11. Ramos CP, Santana JA, Morcatti Coura F, Xavier RGC, Leal CAG, Oliveira Junior CA, et al. Identification and characterization of *Escherichia coli*, *Salmonella* spp., *Clostridium perfringens*, and *C. difficile* isolates from reptiles in brazil. *Biomed Res Int.* (2019) 2019:1–9. doi: 10.1155/2019/9530732
12. Wikström VO, Fernström LL, Melin L, Boqvist S. *Salmonella* isolated from individual reptiles and environmental samples from terraria in private households in Sweden. *Acta Vet Scand.* (2014) 56:7. doi: 10.1186/1751-0147-56-7
13. Ebani VV. Domestic reptiles as source of zoonotic bacteria: a mini review. *Asian Pac J Trop Med.* (2017) 10:723–8. doi: 10.1016/j.apjtm,.2017.07.020
14. Dudek B, Ksiazczyk M, Krzyzewska E, Rogala K, Kuczkowski M, Wozniak-Biel A, et al. Comparison of the phylogenetic analysis of PFGE profiles and the characteristic of virulence genes in clinical and reptile associated *Salmonella* strains. *BMC Vet Res.* (2019) 15:1–12. doi: 10.1186/s12917-019-2019-1
15. Walters MS, Simmons L, Anderson TC, De Ment J, Van Zile K, Matthias LP, et al. Outbreaks of salmonellosis from small turtles. *Pediatrics.* (2016) 137:1–9. doi: 10.1542/peds.2015-1735
16. Seepersadsingh N, Adesiyun AA. Prevalence and antimicrobial resistance of *Salmonella* spp. in pet mammals, reptiles, fish aquarium water, and birds in Trinidad. *J Vet Med Ser B Infect Dis Vet Public Heal.* (2003) 50:488–93. doi: 10.1046/j.0931-1793.2003.00710.x
17. Lowther SA, Medus C, Scheftel J, Leano F, Jawahir S, Smith K. Foodborne outbreak of *Salmonella* subspecies IV infections associated with contamination from bearded dragons. *Zoonoses Public Health.* (2011) 58:560–6. doi: 10.1111/j.1863-2378.2011.01403.x
18. Gay N, Le Hello S, Weill FX, de Thoisy B, Berger F. *Salmonella* serotypes in reptiles and humans, French Guiana. *Vet Microbiol.* (2014) 170:167–71. doi: 10.1016/j.vetmic.2014.01.024
19. Kuroki T, Ishihara T, Nakajima N, Furukawa I, Une Y. Prevalence of *Salmonella enterica* subspecies enterica in red-eared sliders trachemys scripta elegans retailed in pet shops in Japan. *Jpn J Infect Dis.* (2019) 72:38–43. doi: 10.7883/yoken.JJID.2018.140
20. O'Neill J. Antimicrobial resistance: tackling a crisis for the health and wealth of nations. In: O'Neil, editor. *The Review on Antimicrobial Resistance Chaired.* London (2014).
21. EFSA (European Food Safety Authority). The European union summary report on antimicrobial resistance in zoonotic and indicator bacteria from humans, animals and food in 2017. *EFSA J.* (2019) 17:1–278. doi: 10.2903/j.efsa.2019.5598
22. O'Neill J. Tackling drug-resistant infections globally. *Rev Antimicrob Resist.* (2016) 7:110. doi: 10.4103/2045-080X.186181
23. WHO. *Ten Threats to Global Health in 2019.* (2019). Available online at: https://www.who.int/vietnam/news/feature-stories/detail/ten-threats-to-global-health-in-2019 (accessed May 12, 2020).
24. Tacconelli E, Carrara E, Savoldi A, Kattula D, Burkert F. *Global Priority List of Antibiotic-Resistant Bacteria to Guide Research, Discovery, and Development of New Antibiotics.* (2017). Available online at: http://www.cdc.gov/drugresistance/threat-report-2013/ (accessed April 24, 2020).
25. Gorski L, Jay-Russell MT, Liang AS, Walker S, Bengson Y, Govoni J, et al. Diversity of pulsed-field gel electrophoresis pulsotypes, serovars, and antibiotic resistance among *Salmonella.* isolates from wild amphibians and reptiles in the California Central Coast. *Foodborne Pathog Dis.* (2013) 10:540–8. doi: 10.1089/fpd.2012.1372
26. Zhang J, Kuang D, Wang F, Meng J, Jin H, Yang X, et al. Turtles as a possible reservoir of nontyphoidal *Salmonella* in Shanghai, China. *Foodborne Pathog Dis.* (2016) 13:428–33. doi: 10.1089/fpd.2015.2107
27. Wei Z, Xu X, Yan M, Chang H, Li Y, Kan B, et al. *Salmonella* Typhimurium and *Salmonella* Enteritidis infections in sporadic diarrhea in children: source tracing and resistance to third-generation cephalosporins and ciprofloxacin. *Foodborne Pathog Dis.* (2019) 16:244–55. doi: 10.1089/fpd.2018.2557
28. Díaz MA, Cooper RK, Cloeckaert A, Siebeling RJ. Plasmid-mediated high-level gentamicin resistance among enteric bacteria isolated from pet turtles in Louisiana. *Appl Environ Microbiol.* (2006) 72:306–12. doi: 10.1128/AEM.72.1.306-312.2006
29. Giacopello C, Foti M, Fisichella V, Latella G, Aleo A, Mammina C. Antibiotic resistance in *Salmonella* isolated from tegus (*Tupinambis* spp.). *J Exot Pet Med.* (2012) 21:328–31. doi: 10.1053/j.jepm.2012.09.008
30. Goławska O, Zajac M, Maluta A, Pristas P, Hamarová L, Wasyl D. Complex bacterial flora of imported pet tortoises deceased during quarantine: another zoonotic threat? *Comp Immunol Microbiol Infect Dis.* (2019) 65:154–9. doi: 10.1016/j.cimid.2019.05.007
31. Chen CY, Chen WC, Chin SC, Lai YH, Tung KC, Chiou CS, et al. Prevalence and antimicrobial susceptibility of salmonellae isolates from reptiles in Taiwan. *J Vet Diagnostic Investig.* (2010) 22:44–50. doi: 10.1177/104063871002200107
32. Spain. Royal Degree 53/2013, 1st of Febrary, por el que se establecen las normas básicas aplicables para la protección de los animales utilizados en experimentación y otros fines científicos, incluyendo la docencia. *Boletín Oficial del Estado.* (2013) 34:11370–421.
33. Pees M, Rabsch W, Plenz B, Fruth A, Prager R, Simon S, et al. Evidence for the transmission of *Salmonella* from reptiles to children in Germany, July 2010 to October 2011. *Eurosurveillance.* (2013) 18:1–10. doi: 10.2807/1560-7917.ES2013.18.46.20634
34. ISO. *Microbiology of Food and Animal Feeding Stuffs. Horizontal Method for the Detection of Salmonella spp. 6579-1:2017.* Genève: International Organization for Standardization (2017).
35. Grimont PAD, Weill FX. *Antigenic Formulae of the Salmonella Serovars.* 9th ed. Paris: WHO Collaborating Centre for Reference and Research on Salmonella (2007).
36. Matuschek E, Brown DFJ, Kahlmeter G. Development of the EUCAST disk diffusion antimicrobial susceptibility testing method and its implementation in routine microbiology laboratories. *Clin Microbiol Infect.* (2014) 20:O255–66. doi: 10.1111/1469-0691.12373
37. European Commission. *Commission Implementing Decision of 12 November 2013 on the Monitoring and Reporting of Antimicrobial Resistance in Zoonotic and Commensal Bacteria (Notified Under Document C(2013) 7145).* (2013). Available online at: https://eur-lex.europa.eu/legal-content/EN/TXT/?uri=CELEX%3A32013D0652 (accessed May 5, 2020).
38. CLSI. *Performance Standards for Antimicrobial Susceptibility Testing: Twenty—fourth Informational Supplement.* CLSI document M100—S24. Wayne, PA: s.n (2014).

39. EUCAST. *New Definitions of S, I and R from 2019.* (2019). Available online at: https://www.eucast.org/newsiandr/ (accessed May 1, 2020).
40. EFSA and ECDC. (European Food Safety Authority and European Centre for Disease Prevention and Control). *EU Protocol for Harmonised Monitoring of Antimicrobial Resistance in Human Salmonella and Campylobacter Isolates.* Stockholm: EFSA; ECDC (2016).
41. Gambino-Shirley K, Stevenson L, Wargo K, Burnworth L, Roberts J, Garrett N, et al. Notes from the field: four multistate outbreaks of human *Salmonella* infections linked to small turtle exposure—United States, 2015. *Morb Mortal Wkly Rep.* (2016) 65:655–6. doi: 10.15585/mmwr.mm6525a3
42. Kiebler CA, Bottichio L, Simmons L, Basler C, Klos R, Gurfield N, et al. Outbreak of human infections with uncommon *Salmonella* serotypes linked to pet bearded dragons, 2012–2014. *Zoonoses Public Health.* (2020) 67:425–34. doi: 10.1111/zph.12701
43. Sodagari HR, Habib I, Shahabi MP, Dybing NA, Wang P, Bruce M. Veterinary sciences a review of the public health challenges of salmonella and turtles. *Vet Sci.* (2020) 7:1–12. doi: 10.3390/vetsci7020056
44. Nakadai A, Kuroki T, Kato Y, Suzuki R, Yamai S, Yaginuma C, et al. Prevalence of *Salmonella* spp. in pet reptiles in Japan. *J Vet Med Sci.* (2005) 67:97–101. doi: 10.1292/jvms.67.97
45. Marin C, Vega S, Marco-Jiménez F. Tiny turtles purchased at pet stores are a potential high risk for *Salmonella* human infection in the Valencian Region, Eastern Spain. *Vector-Borne Zoonotic Dis.* (2016) 16:455–60. doi: 10.1089/vbz.2016.1950
46 Lukac M, Pedersen K, Prukner-Radovcic E. Prevalence of *Salmonella* in captive reptiles from Croatia. *J Zoo Wildl Med.* (2015) 46:234–40. doi: 10.1638/2014-0098R1.1
47. Ebani VV, Cerri D, Fratini F, Meille N, Valentini P, Andreani E. *Salmonella* enterica isolates from faeces of domestic reptiles and a study of their antimicrobial *in vitro* sensitivity. *Res Vet Sci.* (2005) 78:117–21. doi: 10.1016/j.rvsc.2004.08.002
48. Marin C, Ingresa-Capaccioni S, González-Bodi S, Marco-Jiménez F, Vega S. Free-living turtles are a reservoir for *Salmonella* but not for campylobacter. *PLoS ONE.* (2013) 8:e72350. doi: 10.1371/journal.pone.0072350
49. Clancy MM, Davis M, Valitutto MT, Nelson K, Sykes JM. *Salmonella* infection and carriage in reptiles in a zoological collection. *J Am Vet Med Assoc.* (2016) 248:1050–9. doi: 10.2460/javma.248.9.1050
50. Guyomard-Rabenirina S, Weill FX, Le Hello S, Bastian S, Berger F, Ferdinand S, et al. Reptiles in Guadeloupe (French West Indies) are a reservoir of major human *Salmonella* enterica serovars. *PLoS ONE.* (2019) 14:e0220145. doi: 10.1371/journal.pone.0220145
51. Ricard C, Mellentin J, Ben Abdallah Chabchoub R, Kingbede P, Heuclin T, Ramdame A, et al. Méningite à Salmonelle chez un nourrisson due à une tortue domestique. *Arch Pediatr.* (2015) 22:605–7. doi: 10.1016/j.arcped.2013.09.019
52. Bjelland AM, Sandvik LM, Skarstein MM, Svendal L, Debenham JJ. Prevalence of *Salmonella* serovars isolated from reptiles in Norwegian zoos. *Acta Vet Scand.* (2020) 62:3. doi: 10.1186/s13028-020-0502-0
53. De Jong B, Andersson Y, Ekdahl K. Effect of regulation and education on reptile-associated salmonellosis. *Emerg Infect Dis.* (2005) 11:398–403. doi: 10.3201/eid1103.040694
54. Jones SB, Spalloni W, Ferreccio F, Postigo J, Fernández A, Porte L, et al. *Salmonella* spp. Gastroenteritis associated to pet turtles in three infants. *Rev Chil Infectol.* (2015) 32:334–8. doi: 10.4067/S0716-10182015000400013
55. Bosch S, Tauxe RV, Behravesh CB. Turtle-associated salmonellosis, United States, 2006-2014. *Emerg Infect Dis.* (2016) 22:1149–55. doi: 10.3201/eid2207.150685
56. Briones V, Téllez S, Goyache J, Ballesteros C, Del Pilar Lanzarot M, Domínguez L, et al. *Salmonella* diversity associated with wild reptiles and amphibians in Spain. *Environ Microbiol.* (2004) 6:868–71. doi: 10.1111/j.1462-2920.2004.00631.x
57. Bauwens L, Vercammen F, Bertrand S, Collard JM, De Ceuster S. Isolation of *Salmonella* from environmental samples collected in the reptile department of Antwerp Zoo using different selective methods. *J Appl Microbiol.* (2006) 101:284–9. doi: 10.1111/j.1365-2672.2006.02977.x
58. Abalem De Sá IV, and Solari CA. *Salmonella* in Brazilian and imported pet reptiles. *Brazilian J Microbiol.* (2001) 32:293–7. doi: 10.1590/S1517-83822001000400007
59. Geue L, Löschner U. *Salmonella* enterica in reptiles of German and Austrian origin. *Vet Microbiol.* (2002) 84:79–91. doi: 10.1016/S0378-1135(01)00437-0
60. Whiley H, Gardner MG, Ross K. A review of *Salmonella* and squamates (Lizards, snakes and amphisbians): implications for public health. *Pathogens.* (2017) 6:1–15. doi: 10.3390/pathogens6010001
61. Fuller CC, Jawahir SL, Leano FT, Bidol SA, Signs K, Davis C, et al. A multistate *Salmonella* Typhimurium outbreak associated with frozen vacuum-packed rodents used to feed snakes. *Zoonoses Public Health.* (2008) 55:481–7. doi: 10.1111/j.1863-2378.2008.01118.x
62. Vrbova L, Sivanantharajah S, Walton R, Whitfield Y, Lee C, Picard I, et al. Outbreak of *Salmonella* Typhimurium associated with feeder rodents. *Zoonoses Public Health.* (2018) 65:386–94. doi: 10.1111/zph.12442
63. Kanagarajah S, Waldram A, Dolan G, Jenkins C, Ashton PM, Carrion Martin AI, et al. Whole genome sequencing reveals an outbreak of *Salmonella* Enteritidis associated with reptile feeder mice in the United Kingdom, 2012-2015. *Food Microbiol.* (2018) 71:32–8. doi: 10.1016/j.fm.2017.04.005
64. Marin C, Martelli F, Rabie A, Davies R. Commercial frozen mice used by owners to feed reptiles are highly externally contaminated with *Salmonella* Enteritidis PT8. *Vector-Borne Zoonotic Dis.* (2018) 18:453–7. doi: 10.1089/vbz.2018.2295
65. Cartwright EJ, Nguyen T, Melluso C, Ayers T, Lane C, Hodges A, et al. A multistate investigation of antibiotic-resistant *Salmonella* enterica serotype I 4,[5],12:i:-Infections as part of an International Outbreak Associated with Frozen Feeder Rodents. *Zoonoses Public Health.* (2016) 63:62–71. doi: 10.1111/zph.12205
66. Cohen ML, Potter M, Pollard R, Feldman RA. Turtle-associated salmonellosis in the United States. Effect of Public Health Action, 1970 to 1976. *JAMA.* (1980) 243:1247–9. doi: 10.1001/jama.1980.03300380027016
67. Wojdat E, Kwiatek K, Zasadny R. Microbiological quality of petfood in Poland. *Pol J Vet Sci.* (2004) 7:207–9.
68. Threlfall EJ, Fisher IS, Berghold C, Gerner-Smidt P, Tschäpe H, Cormican M, et al. Antimicrobial drug resistance in isolates of *Salmonella* enterica from cases of salmonellosis in humans in Europe in 2000: results of international multi-centre surveillance. *Euro Surveill.* (2003) 8:41–5. doi: 10.2807/esm.08.02.00400-en
69. Münch S, Braun P, Wernery U, Kinne J, Pees M, Flieger A, et al. Prevalence, serovars, phage types, and antibiotic susceptibilities of *Salmonella* strains isolated from animals in the United Arab Emirates from 1996 to 2009. *Trop Anim Health Prod.* (2012) 44:1725–38. doi: 10.1007/s11250-012-0130-4
70. Arnafia W, Ningrum SG, Adji RS, Lukman DW, Pasaribu FH, Wayan I, et al. Aislamiento de *Salmonella* en tiendas de mascotas de reptiles y su suceptibilidad a los antibioticos en Indonesia. *Hum Vet Med Int J Bioflux Soc Res Artic.* (2016) 8:177–88.
71. Auliya M, Altherr S, Ariano-Sanchez D, Baard EH, Brown C, Brown RM, et al. Trade in live reptiles, its impact on wild populations, and the role of the European market. *Biol Conserv.* (2016) 204:103–19. doi: 10.1016/j.biocon.2016.05.017
72. Sartelli M, Weber DG, Ruppé E, Bassetti M, Wright BJ, Ansaloni L, et al. Antimicrobials: a global alliance for optimizing their rational use in intra-abdominal infections (AGORA). *World J Emerg Surg.* (2016) 11:1–32. doi: 10.1186/s13017-016-0089-y
73. Elbediwi M, Li Y, Paudyal N, Pan H, Li X, Xie S, et al. Global burden of colistin-resistant bacteria: mobilized colistin resistance genes study (1980–2018). *Microorganisms.* (2019) 7:461. doi: 10.3390/microorganisms7100461
74. Aarestrup FM. The livestock reservoir for antimicrobial resistance: a personal view on changing patterns of risks, effects of interventions and the way forward. *Philos Trans R Soc B Biol Sci.* (2015) 370:20140085. doi: 10.1098/rstb.2014.0085
75. ECDC/EFSA/EMA (European Centre for Disease Prevention and Control/European Food Safety Authority/ European Medicines Agency). ECDC/EFSA/EMA second joint report on the integrated analysis of the consumption of antimicrobial agents and occurrence of antimicrobial resistance in bacteria from humans and food-producing animals: Joint Interagency Antimicrobial Consumption and Resistan. *EFSA J.* (2017) 15:1–135. doi: 10.2903/j.efsa.2017.4872
76. MAPA (Ministry of Agriculture, Fishing and Food). Informe JIACRA España. Primer análisis integrado del consumo de antibióticos y su relación

con la aparición de resistencia. AEMPS. Plan Nac. Resist. Antibióticos. (2018). p. 1–165. Available online at: http://www.resistenciaantibioticos.es/es/system/files/field/files/informe_jiacra-espana.pdf?file=1andtype=nodeandid=410andforce=0 (accessed April 24, 2020).

77. Crump JA, Sjölund-Karlsson M, Gordon MA, Parry CM. Epidemiology, clinical presentation, laboratory diagnosis, antimicrobial resistance, and antimicrobial management of invasive *Salmonella* infections. *Clin Microbiol Rev.* (2015) 28:901–37. doi: 10.1128/CMR.00002-15

78. EMA (European Medicines Agency). *Categorisation of Antibiotics in the European Union.* (2019). Ema/Cvmp/Chmp/682198/2017 31. Available online at: https://www.ema.europa.eu/en/documents/report/categorisation-antibiotics-european-union-answer-request-european-commission-updating-scientific_en.pdf (accessed May 1, 2020).

79. Cerreta AJ, Lewbart GA, Dise DR, Papich MG. Population pharmacokinetics of ceftazidime after a single intramuscular injection in wild turtles. *J Vet Pharmacol Ther.* (2018) 41:495–501. doi: 10.1111/jvp.12500

3

A Novel Sampling Model to Study the Epidemiology of Canine Leishmaniasis in an Urban Environment

Lucy A. Parker[1,2†], Lucrecia Acosta[3†], Mariana Noel Gutierrez[4], Israel Cruz[5], Javier Nieto[6], Enrique Jorge Deschutter[7] and Fernando Jorge Bornay-Llinares[3]*

[1] Departamento de Salud Pública y Ginecología, Universidad Miguel Hernández de Elche, Alicante, Spain, [2] CIBER Epidemiología y Salud Pública, Madrid, Spain, [3] Área de Parasitología, Departamento de Agroquímica y Medio Ambiente, Universidad Miguel Hernández de Elche, Alicante, Spain, [4] Veterinary Centre "Dame la Pata", Posadas, Argentina, [5] National School of Public Health, Instituto de Salud Carlos III, Madrid, Spain, [6] WHO Collaborating Centre for Leishmaniasis, Servicio de Parasitología, Centro Nacional de Microbiología, Instituto de Salud Carlos III, Madrid, Spain, [7] Facultad de Ciencias Exactas, Químicas y Naturales, Universidad Nacional de Misiones, Posadas, Argentina

***Correspondence:**
Lucrecia Acosta
lacosta@umh.es

†These authors have contributed equally to this work and share first authorship

Background: Visceral leishmaniasis (VL) is one of the most important parasitic diseases in the world. The domestic dog is the main reservoir of zoonotic VL and a high prevalence of canine leishmaniasis (CanL) is associated with transmission of infection to humans. Here we describe the methodology used to obtain a rapid and representative sample of domestic dogs in the city of Posadas, Misiones, and compare the prevalence of *Leishmania* infection with a sample of shelter dogs.

Methodology: We used the city land registry to make a random selection of homes and systematically recruited 349 domestic dogs from the selected properties. We also included all dogs from the main canine shelter within the city. Dogs were examined by two experienced veterinarians who recorded the presence of clinical signs common in CanL using a standardized protocol. We extracted a blood sample from each dog and performed four different serological tests to reveal the presence of anti-*Leishmania* antibodies.

Results: After clinical examination, 145 domestic dogs (41.5%) and 63 (90%) shelter dogs had clinical signs compatible with CanL ($p < 0.001$). The seroprevalence among domestic dogs was 20.1% (95% CI 16.1–24.6) which was significantly lower than among the abandoned dogs (38.6%, 95% CI 27.7–50.6, $p < 0.001$). The spatial distribution of infected dogs was fairly homogenous throughout the city. Among domestic dogs, we observed a positive association between where the dog slept and presence of anti-*Leishmania* antibodies ($p = 0.034$). Of the seropositive domestic dogs 38 (54.4%) were asymptomatic.

Conclusions: Our findings demonstrate how seroprevalence results can be highly influenced by sampling methodology. We demonstrate how the land registry can be used to estimate the prevalence of CanL in representative sample of domestic dogs in an urban setting, allowing decision makers to deepen their understanding the epidemiology of CanL in a timely and efficient manner for the development of plans to address both human and canine disease.

Keywords: visceral leishmaniasis, canine leishmaniasis, sampling, epidemiology, canine population

INTRODUCTION

Visceral leishmaniasis (VL) is one of the most important parasitic diseases in the world. The domestic dog is the main reservoir of zoonotic VL (ZVL) and a high prevalence of canine leishmaniasis (CanL) is associated with transmission of infection to humans (1, 2). ZVL is widespread in Latin America (3), where it is caused by *Leishmania infantum* (syn. *L. chagasi*) transmitted by phlebotomine sand flies of the genus *Lutzomyia* (Psychodidae) (4), and is an increasing public health problem (5).

It has a strong complex link with poverty mainly in rural and suburban areas but has been growing among urban populations in recent years (6). Emerging focuses of disease can be difficult to manage and have been associated with widespread culling of infected dogs although evidence supporting this approach is lacking (7). Many factors are thought to contribute to the expansion and urbanization of ZVL, such as environmental changes, changes in the ecology and biology of *Lutzomyia longipalpis* and population migration from rural to urban areas (8).

In Argentina, leishmaniasis is an emerging disease, with a growing number of human and canine clinical cases (9). In Posadas, in the province of Misiones, Argentina, the first human transmission of ZVL associated with dogs and *Lu. longipalpis* was reported in 2006 (10). The presence of *L. infantum* was further described in *Lu. longipalpis* sandflies and dogs using molecular methods (11, 12). In 2009, after human cases of Leishmania had been identified within the city, local health authorities were keen to understand the spread of canine infection within the city in a non-biased manner. Together with local health authorities, we set out to estimate the prevalence of *Leishmania* infection among the canine population in Posadas, by designing a rapid but robust sampling method to understand the epidemiology of the infection within the city using the available but limited resources. This current report shares the methods we used and demonstrate the importance of the adequate selection of the sample and its impact on the epidemiological interpretation of the disease.

In order to provide a valid estimation of disease prevalence it is necessary to include a representative sample of the total population. Ideally, estimates should be drawn through a simple random sample where all members of the population have an equal opportunity to be selected in the sample, but when it comes to dog populations it can be logistically difficult to determine the total population size let alone the probability of the inclusion of each animal in the sample (13). When recent canine censuses are available, prevalence studies are able to obtain a representative sample fairly easily by extracting a random sample from the census or performing the serosurvey alongside the census. Surveys of this type may be carried out due to the known presence of human or canine cases of VL (14). Even when canine censuses are present, limitations remain because they are rarely up to date and do not include free roaming dogs. Other options include the recruitment of animals through the local veterinary practices (15), or taking advantage of local rabies vaccination campaigns (16).

In Posadas, like many of the places in Latin America where CanL is widespread, there was no official census of canines that could be used to extract a random sample. Furthermore, there was a significant population of free-roaming dogs with no owner, and registration of the domestic dogs with local veterinary practices is far from comprehensive. For this reason, we needed to develop a novel strategy to extract a random sample of domestic dogs within the city, working with the information available. Furthermore, Misiones is one of the poorest provinces in Argentina and given the competing health problems in this area, we wanted to make the estimation as efficiently as possible, i.e., using the minimum number of dogs to make an accurate estimation with adequate precision.

In this paper, we describe the methodology used to obtain a representative sample of domestic dogs in the city of Posadas. We describe the presence of anti-*Leishmania* antibodies in domestic dogs and a systematic sample of dogs housed in a private dog shelter in the same region in the same time period. We identify variables related to infection in both populations. The main objective of this report is to share the methodology used to obtain a rapid and representative sample of domestic dogs in this urban setting. Furthermore, we aim to reveal how the sampling strategy can have major implications on the validity of epidemiological indicators for the development and monitoring of activities to address canine disease.

METHODS

Study Area

The surveys were conducted between 1st of October and 15th of November 2009 in the city of Posadas (27° 23′ S, 55° 53′ W), located in the southwest of Misiones province, northeast Argentina. In 2008, Posadas had an estimated population of 297,499 inhabitants. The surface area of the city is 324 Km^2, and it is characterized by a subtropical humid climate with an annual rainfall of 1,700 mm and an average temperature of 21.5°C.

Sample Size

To estimate the prevalence of *Leishmania* infection in domestic dogs in Posadas, we attempted to obtain a random sample of all domestic dogs in the city. We calculated a priori that we would need between 322 and 368 dogs to provide a reliable estimate with an error margin of ± 5%, at a 95% confidence level, using Epidat

3.1 software [Jan 2006; Servizo de Epidemioloxía da Dirección Xeral de Innovación e Xestión da Saúde Pública a Consellería de Sanidade (Xunta de Galicia) and the Pan American Health Organization (PAHO), http://dxsp.sergas.es]. This calculation required the following assumptions: (i) an estimated total dog population of 100,000 and (ii) an estimated prevalence of 30–40%. These assumptions were made after consultation with local government as to the expected size of the domestic dog population and observation for the prevalence obtained in similar settings in the region (3, 12).

Sampling Strategy

Given that it is unfeasible to carry out simple random sampling of the Posadas city domestic dogs, we used the City Land Registry Census to define our primary sampling unit. In this census, the city of Posadas is divided into almost 90,000 separate registries which mostly refer to individual properties. To allow for registry errors, non-urbanized entries on the land registry (e.g., parks, wasteland, recently flooded areas, etc.), dog owner's refusal to participate in the survey and ineligibility of the property (e.g., commercial properties or properties without a dog) we selected a total of 600 properties from the City Land Registry by simple random sampling. To minimize losses, it was decided a priori that if the initially selected property was ineligible (due to being commercial or not having a dog) the field workers would go to the residence located directly to the right. Furthermore, when more than one dog lived in the property all dogs were offered diagnosis but only one was selected at random to be included in the prevalence survey. Finally, 349 dogs were included in the survey. A detailed description of the selection process can be found in **Figure 1**. The location of the sampled dogs was plotted on the map of the city using a GPS point taken in the residence.

Finally, we also recruited 70 abandoned dogs from the "El Refugio" dog shelter, located in the outskirts of Posadas city. The sample constituted of all dogs present at the shelter when the study team visited. Repellent was not used at the dog shelter.

Clinical Observation and Data Collection

Each dog was examined by two experienced veterinarians who recorded clinical signs using a standardized protocol. Dogs were considered symptomatic if they had one or more of the following signs, common in canine leishmaniasis: alopecia, desquamations, skin ulcers, alterations in oral and nasal mucosa, apathy, weight loss, cachexia, bleeding, onychogryphosis, ocular signs (conjunctivitis, uveitis or any other), lymphadenopathy, hepatomegaly and splenomegaly. Other parameters recorded were age, sex, breed, the number of dogs in the residence, and whether the dog slept inside or outside the house. Dogs were grouped according to their age in four different groups: younger than 1 year, from 1 to 4 years, from 5 to 9 years and 10 years or over.

Biological Samples

After clinical examination 0.6 mL of peripheral blood was collected in a Multivette® 600 EDTA tube (Sarstedt AG & Co., Nümbrecht, Germany). Plasma was separated by centrifugation (5 min to 3,000 r.p.m. in a bench top micro centrifuge). Blood samples were analyzed at extraction time and the rest of the samples were stored at 4°C (Universidad Nacional de Misiones, UNaM) until shipment to the WHO Collaborating Centre for Leishmaniasis (WHO-CCL) in Madrid (Spain), where they were stored at −20°C until later analysis. All analysis were performed within 4 months of sample collection.

Detection of Anti-*Leishmania* Antibodies

Four different serological tests were performed to reveal the presence of anti-*Leishmania* antibodies, two of them based on the recombinant antigen rK39 (Kalazar Detect® immunochromatographic test, rK39-ICT, and an *in-house* enzyme linked immunosorbent assay, rK39-ELISA), and the other two based on whole antigen (a commercial direct agglutination test, DAT, and *in-house* immunofluorescence antibody test, IFAT) (17). A more detailed description of these methods can be found in the **Supplementary Data 1**. A dog was considered seropositive when it yielded a positive result for at least one serological method using total antigen (IFAT and/or DAT) as well as one using recombinant antigen (ICT whole blood and/or plasma and/or ELISA).

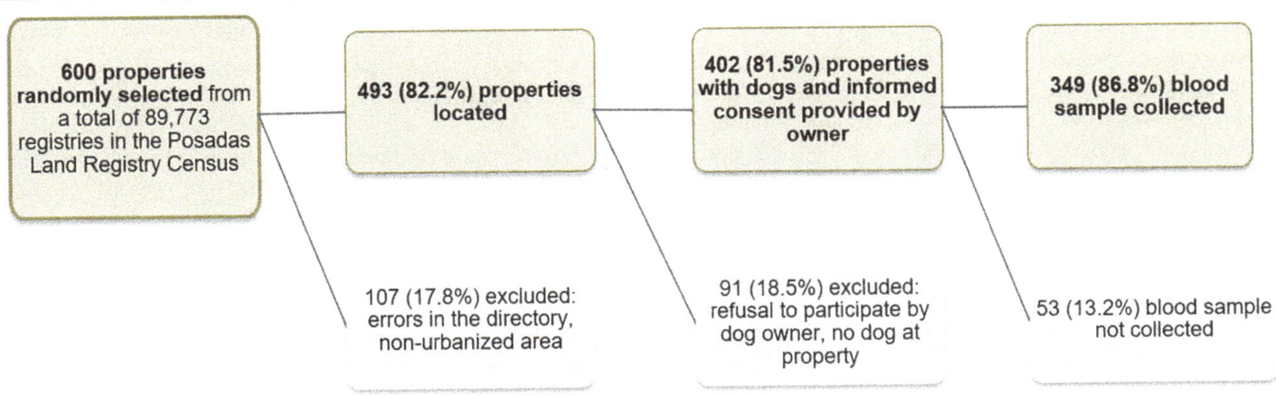

FIGURE 1 | Sampling strategy used to obtain a representative sample of domestic dogs in Posadas, Argentina, 2009.

Statistical Analysis

Data recorded from the surveys were entered into an Excel (Microsoft, Redmond, WA, USA) spread sheet and imported into Stata SE version 15.0 (StataCorp LLC, USA). The proportion of seropositive dogs was calculated with a 95% confidence interval. The relationship between the characteristics of the dog and seroprevalence was evaluated using Pearson's chi-square test and differences were considered statistically significant when the p-value was <0.05.

RESULTS

Of 600 randomly selected land registries, 107 (17.8%) were excluded because of errors in the registry or because they were non-urbanized plots of land. Of 493 registries with built properties, we further excluded 91 (18.5%) because there was no dog residing at the property, or because the dog owner refused to participate in the study. Finally, of 402 dog owners who agreed to participate and signed the informed consent, 52 (13.2%) were not included in the sero-survey because they did not attend the appointment with the veterinarians where biological samples were extracted and clinical signs recorded.

Finally, 349 domestic dogs were included aged between 4 months and 16 years, with a mean age of 5 years. The 70 dogs from the shelter were older, aged between 3 months and 10 years, with a mean age of 7.3 years ($p < 0.001$). **Table 1** shows the characteristics of the dogs from both survey populations. There were no significant differences in sex between the two populations, but the domestic dogs were more likely to be pure breed. After clinical examination, 145 domestic dogs (41.5%) and 63 (90%) shelter dogs had clinical signs suggestive of CanL ($p < 0.001$). The most common clinical sign observed in the dogs was lymphadenopathy, present in 124 (35.5%) of domestic dogs, and 52 (74.3%) of the shelter dogs. Other common signs observed in the dogs were onychogryphosis (51, 14.6% of domestic dogs and 43, 61.4% shelter dogs), desquamations (13.7 and 30%, respectively) and alopecia (12.6 and 52.9%, respectively).

The spatial distribution of the population in the study area are shown in **Figure 2**, along with the seroprevalence. We can observe a greater concentration of dogs, both with and without anti-*Leishmania* antibodies, in the north-east part of the city corresponding to the more densely populated city center. In less populated areas the selected dogs are more scattered.

The seroprevalence among domestic dogs was 20.1% (95% CI 16.1–24.6) which was significantly lower than among the abandoned dogs (38.6, 95% CI 27.7–50.6, $p = 0.001$). A detailed description of seroprevalence with regards to the sex, age group, breed, where dog slept, number of dogs in the house and clinical status of the dogs can be found in **Table 2**. We did not observe an association between seroprevalence and sex, age group and clinical status in either of the dog populations. Among domestic dogs, we observed a positive association between where the dog slept and presence of anti-*Leishmania* antibodies ($p = 0.034$). Among the dogs from the canine shelter, although there were few pure breed dogs, we observed that they were more likely to have anti-*Leishmania* antibodies ($p = 0.048$). Of the seropositive domestic dogs 38 (54.4%) were asymptomatic. Of the 204 asymptomatic domestic dogs, 38 (18.6%) were seropositive.

TABLE 1 | Characteristics of the dogs included in the sero-surveys according to sampling strategy.

Symptoms	Representative sample of domestic dogs *N* (%)	Systematic sample of shelter dogs *N* (%)	*P*-value[a]
Sex			0.756
Male	191 (54.9)	37 (52.8)	
Female	157 (45.1)	33 (47.1)	
Age group			<0.001
<1 year	21 (6.1)	2 (2.9)	
1–4 years	161 (46.5)	11 (15.7)	
5–9 years	118 (34.1)	29 (41.4)	
10+ years	46 (13.3)	28 (40.0)	
Breed			<0.001
Pure bred	94 (26.9)	5 (7.1)	
Mongrel	255 (73.1)	65 (92.9)	
Clinical status			<0.001
Asymptomatic	204 (58.4)	7 (10.0)	
Symptomatic	145 (41.5)	63 (90.0)	
Lymphadenopathy	124 (35.5)	52 (74.3)	<0.001
Onychogryphosis	51 (14.6)	43 (61.4)	<0.001
Desquamations	48 (13.7)	21 (30.0)	0.001
Alopecia	44 (12.6)	37 (52.9)	<0.001
Weight loss	39 (11.2)	22 (31.4)	<0.001
Hepatomegaly	32 (9.2)	22 (31.4)	<0.001
Splenomegaly	31 (8.9)	21 (30.0)	<0.001
Ocular signs	31 (8.9)	20 (28.6)	<0.001
Pale oral mucosa	28 (8.1)	14 (20.0)	0.002
Ulcers	25 (7.2)	13 (18.6)	0.002
Bleeding	11 (3.2)	4 (5.7)	0.292
Apathy	9 (2.6)	4 (5.7)	0.167
Alterations in nose mucosa	9 (2.6)	5 (7.1)	0.052
Cachexia	4 (1.2)	4 (5.7)	0.011
Total	349 (100)	70 (100)	

[a] *P-values are comparing the shelter dogs with the random sample of domestic dogs.*

DISCUSSION

The prevalence of antibodies for *Leishmania* in domestic dogs from the city of Posadas was 20.1% (95% CI 16.1–24.6), suggesting that at least one in every five domestic dogs in the city is infected or has been exposed to CanL. In the sample of shelter dogs, the observed seroprevalence of CanL was nearly double at 38.6% (95% CI 27.7–50.6). Although our sampling strategy was designed to obtain a random sample of domestic dogs, and not to make geographical comparisons between areas, it was noticeable that seropositive dogs show a fairly homogeneous distribution pattern throughout the city. Because the sampling unit we used was household, we can observe a greater concentration of dogs,

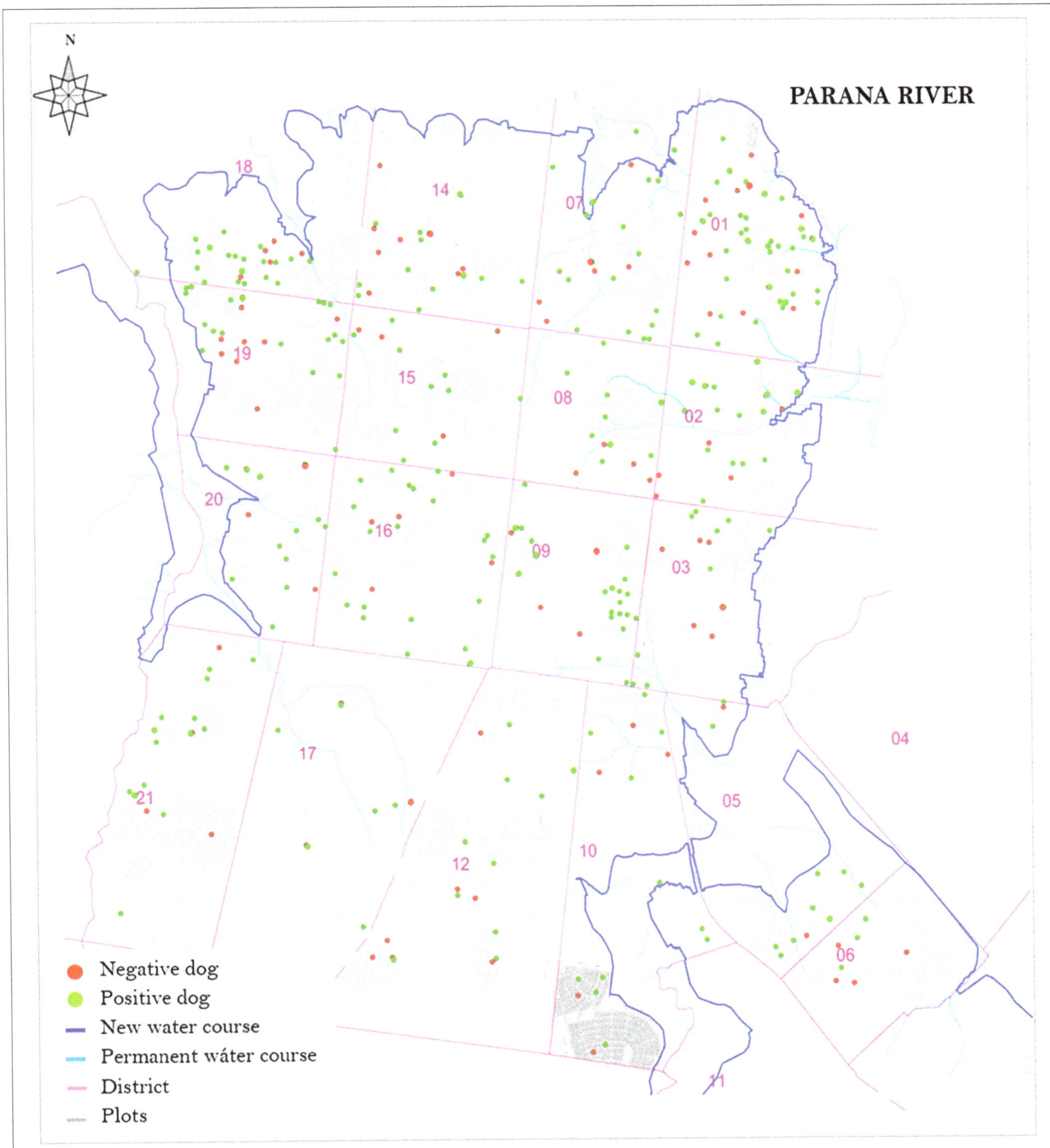

FIGURE 2 | Spatial distribution of the sample of domestic dogs included in the study, according to presence of anti-*Leishmania* antibodies. New water course: New permanent water course due to construction of the Yacyretá- Apipé hydroelectric power station downstream.

both with and without anti-*Leishmania* antibodies, in densely populated areas, while in less populated areas the selected dogs are more scattered. There is a stark contrast with suggestions of a relationship between the focal distribution of potential vectors in the presence of human clusters of infection in the city of Posadas (18). Even if the vector is clustered, the homogeneous distribution of the disease reservoir, perhaps associated with the high mobility of domestic dogs could have important

TABLE 2 | Seroprevalence of *Leishmania* infection according to sampling strategy and characteristics of the dogs, in Posadas, Argentina 2009.

	Representative sample of domestic dogs			Systematic sample of shelter dogs		
	Seropositivity *n* (%)	Total *n*	*P*-value	Seropositivity *n* (%)	Total *n* (%)	*P*-value
Sex			0.910			0.532
Male	38 (19.9)	191		13 (35.1)	37	
Female	32 (20.4)	157		14 (42.4)	33	
Age group			0.988			0.603
<1 year	4 (19.0)	21		0 (0)	2	
1–4 years	33 (20.5)	161		4 (36.4)	11	
5–9 years	23 (19.5)	118		13 (44.8)	29	
10+ years	10 (21.7)	46		10 (38.6)	28	
Breed			0.518			0.048
Pure bred	21 (22.3)	94		4 (80.0)	5	
Mongrel	49 (19.2)	255		23 (35.4)	65	
Where the dog slept			0.034			NA
Inside the house	7 (9.6)	73		–	–	
Outside the house	61 (23.2)	263		–	–	
Both	2 (15.4)	13		–	–	
Number of dogs in residence			0.075			NA
1	27 (15.7)	172		–	–	
2	32 (27.8)	115		–	–	
3	7 (15.9)	44		–	–	
>3	4 (22.2)	18		–	–	
Clinical status			0.429			0.567
Asymptomatic	38 (18.6)	204		2 (28.6)	7	
Symptomatic	32 (22.1)	145		25 (39.7)	63	
Total	70 (20.1)	349 (100)		27 (38.6)	70 (100)	

implications for control and may play an important role in the persistence of the disease in urban settings. Other studies have shown similar high prevalence of CanL is the surrounding area which has shown a decrease in recent years (19).

While seroepidemiological surveys are commonly used to measure the prevalence of leishmaniasis, there is a lot of variation in the methods used to recruit the canine study participants, and the details of how the sampling procedures are carried out is often lacking. For example, a recent study in Colombia (20) described how the sample being carried out in municipalities with increasing numbers of clinical cases reported by health authorities, but the procedures used to access the dog population is not provided. Some studies report using veterinary practices or samples extracted during a vaccination campaign (15, 16), but it can be difficult to determine if the sample if truly representative, Confounding factors could be that dogs participating in a vaccination campaign are less likely to be infected because of the behavioral factors associated with their care. Estimating the prevalence using a canine census can derive valid estimated of domestic dog infection but canine censuses are not always available, and it can be resource heavy ensuring they are up to date. In this study we used the land registry and simple random sample to obtain a representative sample of domestic dogs.

Our study is not without limitations. On the one hand the fact that we did not attempt to include free roaming dogs should be considered a limitation as it could lead to an underestimation of the true prevalence of CanL in the city. A higher prevalence of CanL among stray dogs compared to domestic dogs has been observed in other studies (21). We can expect free roaming dogs to be more similar to shelter dogs than domestic dogs, especially if we consider the higher prevalence in dogs sleeping outside the house, which has been observed in other studies (8). We observed a markedly higher prevalence among animals recruited from the shelter. A pilot study 3 years earlier with a convenience sample had observed a prevalence of 43.6% (12). Another limitation is the incomplete sampling of shelter dogs. We recruited all dogs from "El Refugio" animal shelter, which is one of two shelters in the city, and by far the largest shelter in the city. Although it is possible that the prevalence of CanL varies between the shelters, inclusion of this shelter was made due to interest and collaboration of the shelter owner, and the disease status of the dogs was not considered when deciding which shelter to include. The dogs from the canine shelter were significantly older, and more likely to be in poor health than the domestic dogs.

Many studies have pointed out the importance of identifying asymptomatic carriers in endemic areas (22–26). Some studies show that asymptomatic dogs may comprise several between 50 and 60% of all infected dogs in the area (27–29). What is striking in this study is that despite having randomly selected the domestic dogs from a normal population a total of 54.2% of seropositive dogs were asymptomatic and only the 7.4% on canine shelter. Otherwise, 22.1% of symptomatic domestic dogs were seropositive. Therefore, a diagnosis based only on the appearance of clinical signs related to the disease could overestimate the number of cases infected by *Leishmania* in this area.

We must also acknowledge that the study was carried out in 2009, which is a major limitation if one objective is to know the prevalence of infection in the city, but the purpose of this report here is to describe our methods and demonstrate the importance of the adequate sample and its impact on the epidemiological interpretation of the disease. We did not collect information about the use of insecticide. Some studies have shown how this can influence disease presence and it should be considered in future studied (30, 31).

We did not use a multi-stage or stratified sampling strategy because we were interested in observing the geographical spread of the disease in the entire city. We could have improved the efficiency of our strategy by undertaking a multistage sampling strategy where we take a first stage random sample of larger geographical units (sectors or parishes), and then sample a specific number of land registries within this sample. This would be logistically simpler and reduce the number of movements of the team within the city, which can be important especially when the geographical area is large. In this study we used the land registry census as our primary sampling unit, and there was a significant proportion of errors in the registry. Another attractive option would be to carry out geospatial sampling and obtain a the random selection of properties or animals using randomly generated GPS points or grid-squares (19, 32, 33). Such methods are highly valid but require users to be competent in using Geographical Information Systems (GIS) which may be a challenge in many low-resource settings. Here we propose a simpler strategy using available registries which can allow local stakeholders to obtain a valid estimation of disease prevalence with limited technology.

In response to the results from the study and the model used for epidemiological investigation of the disease, preventative and curative services for canine disease were strengthened throughout the municipality of Posadas. The local government implemented a control program where dog owners from low-income families were offered a free screening service for canine leishmaniasis. It is estimated that 40% of the dog owner population took part in the scheme. More recently, the city established a Centre for Vectorial and Zoonotic Diseases, with the support of the Municipality and the Ministry of Health. Tackling CanL in the city is a key line of work within the center.

CONCLUSIONS

Overall, the two prevalence estimations observed and the spatial distribution of the domestic dogs with anti-*Leishmania* antibodies suggest that this focus of disease was well-established in 2009. Our novel sampling strategy allowed us to obtain a representative sample of domestic dogs in an urban setting. The prevalence of CanL obtained was much lower than the prevalence among dogs from the animal shelter. Although this difference is not surprising, it is important to acknowledge how seroprevalence results are influenced by sampling methodology, and the fact that samples using convenience sampling may under or overestimate disease prevalence and can lead to misinformed decisions about control and management. We demonstrate how a representative sample can be obtained in a timely and efficient manner, allowing decision makers to deepen their understanding the epidemiology of CanL for the development of plans to address both human and canine disease, while protecting animal welfare.

AUTHOR CONTRIBUTIONS

IC, LA, and FB-L conceived the study. LA, LP, FB-L, and IC designed the study. LA and LP drafted the original draft, analyzed data and realized formal analysis and interpretation of data. IC and FB-L critically reviewed it and contributed to its design. FB-L and ED supervised and coordinated the study. LA, MG, and ED contacted dog owners to enroll the study. LA, MG, JN, FB-L, and IC carried out clinical examination and obtained biological samples from the dogs. JN and MG designed the protocol for clinical scoring of the dogs. IC, LA, and JN performed serological diagnosis. All authors revised and edited the different draft versions, and read and approved the submitted manuscript.

FUNDING

This work was supported by: Dirección General de Cooperación al Desarrollo, Generalitat Valenciana, Spain (Ref. 3014/2008) and European Commission 6th Framework Programme INCO-CT-2005-015407 [Control strategies for visceral leishmaniasis (VL) and mucocutaneous leishmaniasis (MCL) in South America: Applications of molecular epidemiology/LeishEpiNetSA].

ACKNOWLEDGMENTS

We especially acknowledge the essential collaboration of the health promoters, primary health care staff and drivers from the Ministry of Public Health in Posadas, Argentina, and the City Land Registry for their help. To Etelvina Sorghe, the canine shelter' responsible from the non-profit civil association El Refugio for her disinterested collaboration. Furthermore, we would like to thank Miguel Ángel Gutiérrez for developing the map, and Bernardo Acosta for their help with map editing.

REFERENCES

1. Fraga DBM, Solcà MS, Silva VMG, Borja LS, Nascimento EG, Oliveira GGS, et al. Temporal distribution of positive results of tests for detecting Leishmania infection in stray dogs of an endemic area of visceral leishmaniasis in the Brazilian tropics: a 13 years survey and association with human disease. *Vet Parasitol.* (2012) 190:591–4. doi: 10.1016/j.vetpar.2012.06.025
2. Moreno J, Alvar J. Canine leishmaniasis: epidemiological risk and the experimental model. *Trends Parasitol.* (2002) 18:399–405. doi: 10.1016/S1471-4922(02)02347-4
3. Dantas-Torres F. Canine leishmaniosis in South America. *Parasit Vectors.* (2009) 2 (Suppl. 1):S1. doi: 10.1186/1756-3305-2-S1-S1
4. Lanzaro GC, Ostrovska K, Herrero MV, Lawyer PG, Warburg A. Lutzomyia longipalpis is a species complex: genetic divergence and interspecific hybrid sterility among three populations. *Am J Trop Med Hyg.* (1993) 48:839–47. doi: 10.4269/ajtmh.1993.48.839
5. Pan American Health Organization. *Manual of Procedures for Leishmaniases Surveillance and Control in the Americas.* Washington, DC: Pan American Health Organization (2019). Available online at: https://iris.paho.org/handle/10665.2/51838 (accessed December 2, 2020).
6. Shaw J. The leishmaniases–survival and expansion in a changing world. A mini-review. *Mem Inst Oswaldo Cruz.* (2007) 102:541–7. doi: 10.1590/S0074-02762007000500001
7. Dantas-Torres F, Miró G, Baneth G, Bourdeau P, Breitschwerdt E, Capelli G, et al. Canine leishmaniasis control in the context of One Health. *Emerg Infect Dis.* (2019) 25:1–4. doi: 10.3201/eid2512.190164
8. Leal GG de A, Carneiro M, Pinheiro A da C, Marques LA, Ker HG, Reis AB, et al. Risk profile for Leishmania infection in dogs coming from an area of visceral leishmaniasis reemergence. *Prev Vet Med.* (2018) 150:1–7. doi: 10.1016/j.prevetmed.2017.11.022
9. Salomón OD, Sosa Estani S, Rossi GC, Spinelli GR. Lutzomyia longipalpis and leishmaniasis visceral in Argentina. *Medicina.* (2001) 61:174–8.
10. Salomon O, Sinagra A, Nevot M, Barberian G, Paulin P, Estevez J, et al. First visceral leishmaniasis focus in Argentina. *Mem Inst Oswaldo Cruz.* (2008) 103:109–11. doi: 10.1590/S0074-02762008000100018
11. Acardi SA, Liotta DJ, Santini MS, Romagosa CM, Salomón OD. Detection of *Leishmania infantum* in naturally infected *Lutzomyia longipalpis* (Diptera: Psychodidae: Phlebotominae) and Canis familiaris in Misiones, Argentina: the first report of a PCR-RFLP and sequencing-based confirmation assay. *Mem Inst Oswaldo Cruz.* (2010) 105:796–9. doi: 10.1590/S0074-02762010000600011
12. Cruz I, Acosta L, Gutiérrez MN, Nieto J, Cañavate C, Deschutter J, et al. A canine leishmaniasis pilot survey in an emerging focus of visceral leishmaniasis: Posadas (Misiones, Argentina). *BMC Infect Dis.* (2010) 10:342. doi: 10.1186/1471-2334-10-342
13. Belo VS, Werneck GL, da Silva ES, Barbosa DS, Struchiner CJ. Population estimation methods for free-ranging dogs: a systematic review. *PLoS ONE.* (2015) 10:e0144830. doi: 10.1371/journal.pone.0144830
14. Lopes JV, Michalsky ÉM, Pereira NCL, Paula AJV de, Souza AGM, Pinheiro LC, et al. Canine visceral leishmaniasis in area with recent Leishmania transmission: prevalence, diagnosis, and molecular identification of the infecting species. *Rev Soc Bras Med Trop.* (2020) 53:e20200141. doi: 10.1590/0037-8682-0141-2020
15. Velez R, Ballart C, Domenech E, Abras A, Fernández-Arévalo A, Gómez SA, et al. Seroprevalence of canine Leishmania infantum infection in the Mediterranean region and identification of risk factors: the example of North-Eastern and Pyrenean areas of Spain. *Prev Vet Med.* (2019) 162:67–75. doi: 10.1016/j.prevetmed.2018.10.015
16. Pires H, Martins M, Matos AC, Cardoso L, Monteiro F, Roque N, et al. Geospatial analysis applied to seroepidemiological survey of canine leishmaniosis in east-central Portugal. *Vet Parasitol.* (2019) 274:108930. doi: 10.1016/j.vetpar.2019.108930
17. Bray RS. Immunodiagnosis of leishmaniasis. In: Chang KP, Bray RS, editorS. *Leishmaniasis.* Amsterdam, The Netherlands: Elsevier Ltd. (1985). p. 177–182.
18. Fernández MS, Salomón OD, Cavia R, Perez AA, Acardi SA, Guccione JD. Lutzomyia longipalpis spatial distribution and association with environmental variables in an urban focus of visceral leishmaniasis, Misiones, Argentina. *Acta Trop.* (2010) 114:81–7. doi: 10.1016/j.actatropica.2010.01.008
19. Lamattina D, Berrozpe PE, Casas N, Moya SL, Giuliani MG, Costa SA, et al. Twice upon a time: the progression of canine visceral leishmaniasis in an Argentinean city. Munderloh UG, editor. *PLoS ONE.* (2019) 14:e0219395. doi: 10.1371/journal.pone.0219395
20. Picón Y, Almario G, Rodríguez V, Garcia NV. Seroprevalence, clinical, and pathological characteristics of canine leishmaniasis in a central region of Colombia. *J Vet Res.* (2020) 64:85–94. doi: 10.2478/jvetres-2020-0011
21. Shokri A, Fakhar M, Teshnizi SH. Canine visceral leishmaniasis in Iran: a systematic review and meta-analysis. *Acta Trop.* (2017) 165:76–89. doi: 10.1016/j.actatropica.2016.08.020
22. Alvar J, Cañavate C, Molina R, Moreno J, Nieto J. Canine leishmaniasis. *Adv Parasitol.* (2004) 57:1–88. doi: 10.1016/S0065-308X(04)57001-X
23. Dantas-Torres F, Brandão-Filho SP. Visceral leishmaniasis in Brazil: revisiting paradigms of epidemiology and control. *Rev Inst Med Trop Sao Paulo.* (2006) 48:151–6. doi: 10.1590/S0036-46652006000300007
24. Chargui N, Amro A, Haouas N, Schönian G, Babba H, Schmidt S, et al. Population structure of Tunisian *Leishmania infantum* and evidence for the existence of hybrids and gene flow between genetically different populations. *Int J Parasitol.* (2009) 39:801–11. doi: 10.1016/j.ijpara.2008.11.016
25. Rondon FCM, Bevilaqua CML, Franke CR, Barros RS, Oliveira FR, Alcântara AC, et al. Cross-sectional serological study of canine Leishmania infection in Fortaleza, Ceará state, Brazil. *Vet Parasitol.* (2008) 155:24–31. doi: 10.1016/j.vetpar.2008.04.014
26. Solano-Gallego L, Koutinas A, Miró G, Cardoso L, Pennisi MG, Ferrer L, et al. Directions for the diagnosis, clinical staging, treatment and prevention of canine leishmaniosis. *Vet Parasitol.* (2009) 165:1–18. doi: 10.1016/j.vetpar.2009.05.022
27. Abranches P, Silva-Pereira MC, Conceição-Silva FM, Santos-Gomes GM, Janz JG. Canine leishmaniasis: pathological and ecological factors influencing transmission of infection. *J Parasitol.* (1991) 77:557–61. doi: 10.2307/3283159
28. Solano-Gallego L, Riera C, Roura X, Iniesta L, Gallego M, Valladares JE, et al. Leishmania infantum-specific IgG, IgG1 and IgG2 antibody responses in healthy and ill dogs from endemic areas. Evolution in the course of infection and after treatment. *Vet Parasitol.* (2001) 96:265–76. doi: 10.1016/S0304-4017(00)00446-5
29. Brandonisio O, Carelli G, Ceci L, Consenti B, Fasanella A, Puccini V. Canine leishmaniasis in the Gargano promontory (Apulia, South Italy). *Eur J Epidemiol.* (1992) 8:273–6. doi: 10.1007/BF00144813
30. Gálvez R, Miró G, Descalzo MA, Nieto J, Dado D, Martín O, et al. Emerging trends in the seroprevalence of canine leishmaniosis in the Madrid region (central Spain). *Vet Parasitol.* (2010) 169:327–34. doi: 10.1016/j.vetpar.2009.11.025
31. Martín-Martín I, Molina R, Rohoušová I, Drahota J, Volf P, Jiménez M. High levels of anti-Phlebotomus perniciosus saliva antibodies in different vertebrate hosts from the re-emerging leishmaniosis focus in Madrid, Spain. *Vet Parasitol.* (2014) 202:207–16. doi: 10.1016/j.vetpar.2014.02.045
32. Rinaldi L, Biggeri A, Carbone S, Musella V, Catelan D, Veneziano V, et al. Canine faecal contamination and parasitic risk in the city of Naples (southern Italy). *BMC Vet Res.* (2006) 2:29. doi: 10.1186/1746-6148-2-29
33. Barnard S, Ippoliti C, Di Flaviano D, De Ruvo A, Messori S, Giovannini A, et al. Smartphone and GPS technology for free-roaming dog population surveillance - a methodological study. *Vet Ital.* (2015) 51:165–72. doi: 10.12834/VetIt.233.2163.3

4

Trends in the Epidemiology of Leishmaniasis in the City of Barcelona (1996–2019)

David Palma[1,2†], *Lilas Mercuriali*[1†], *Jordi Figuerola*[2,3*], *Tomás Montalvo*[1,2], *Rubén Bueno-Marí*[4,5], *Joan-Pau Millet*[1,2], *Pere Simón*[1], *Eva Masdeu*[1] *and Cristina Rius*[1,2]

[1] Agència de Salut Pública de Barcelona (ASPB), Barcelona, Spain, [2] Centro de Investigación Biomédica en Red en Epidemiología y Salud Pública (CIBER-ESP), Madrid, Spain, [3] Estación Biológica de Doñana (EBD-CSIC), Sevilla, Spain, [4] Department of Research and Development (R&D), Laboratorios Lokímica, Valencia, Spain, [5] Parasitology Area, Department of Pharmacy and Pharmaceutical Technology and Parasitology, University of Valencia, Valencia, Spain

***Correspondence:**
Jordi Figuerola
jordi@ebd.csic.es

†These authors have contributed equally to this work and share first authorship

Background: Leishmaniasis is a neglected zoonosis produced by 20 different flagellated parasites of the *Leishmania* genus, a protozoan transmitted to humans and other vertebrates by the bite of dipteran insects of the *Phlebotominae* subfamily. It is endemic in Mediterranean countries and the number of cases is expected to increase due to climate change and migration. Prioritizing public health interventions for prevention and control is essential. The objective was to characterize the epidemiology and temporal trends in the incidence of human leishmaniasis in the city of Barcelona, between the years 1996 and 2019.

Methods: A population-based, analytical observational study among residents in the city of Barcelona was conducted of all the cases of leishmaniasis reported between 1996 and 2019 to the Public Health Agency. The epidemiological survey contains clinical, diagnostic, and epidemiological data, including contact with suspicious mammals or insects. Annual incidence-rates were calculated by sex, age, and country of origin. Chi-square tests were used to assess association between studied risk factors, periods of time and type of leishmaniasis.

Results: During the study period a total of 177 cases of leishmaniasis were reported in Barcelona, being 74.6% (n = 132) of the total cases in Spanish born, although within the foreign-born population the incidence was higher. Median age was 34 years (IQR = 10–48) and 121 (66.8%) were male. The main type was cutaneous (46%) followed by visceral (35.1%). The cumulative incidence was 0.47 per 100,000 inhabitants, with the highest incidence found in 2017 (1.60 per 100,000 inhabitants). A higher incidence was observed in the 0–4-year-old group (1.73 per 100,000 inhabitants), but increased during the study period for all age groups. There was an increase of foreign origin cases, and a decrease in the number of cases associated to any immunosuppression.

Conclusion: In Barcelona, leishmaniasis incidence continues to be higher in people under 5 years of age, and 25–64 years old males, but it has also increased in population from foreign country of birth. There is an increase of the cases since 2016, probably due to the changes in the notification system, increasing the diagnosis of cutaneous leishmaniasis. Improvements in the current surveillance system are needed. Notification of the disease, vector, and reservoir control activities are also essential for the control of the disease.

Keywords: parasitology, leishmania, zoonosis, *Phlebotomus*, surveillance, One Health, public health surveillance, infectious disease

INTRODUCTION

Leishmaniasis is a zoonosis produced by 20 different flagellated parasites of the *Leishmania* genus, a protozoan transmitted to humans and other vertebrates by the bite of dipteran insects of *Phlebotominae* subfamily (1, 2). The parasites that cause leishmaniasis are present in 98 countries around the world, causing between 700,000 and 1 million new cases annually, with an estimated 350 million people at risk of infection worldwide (1–4). There are three main clinical forms visceral leishmaniasis (VL), cutaneous leishmaniasis (CL), and mucocutaneous leishmaniasis (ML) (1, 4). VL is the most serious form of leishmaniasis and causes a systemic disease characterized by irregular episodes of fever, spleen and liver enlargement, weight loss and anemia. CL is the most frequent presentation and causes skin lesions that evolve from nodules to painless ulcers, which can leave long lasting scars. ML is the most uncommon form of leishmaniasis, and leads to the destruction of nasooropharyngeal mucosa, usually after years of the initial skin lesions. Diagnosis is established through direct observation or molecular detection of *Leishmania* parasites in tissue specimens, mainly from skin lesions, for cutaneous leishmaniasis, or from bone marrow, for visceral leishmaniasis, although serological tests could also be used in different situations (2). The wide diversity of *Leishmania* species is associated with a difference in the clinical presentation, routes of transmission (zoonotic vs. anthroponotic) and treatment resistance (2, 5). In this sense, VL is usually caused by *L. donovani* or *L. infantum*, while CL can be caused by *L. infanfum*, *L braziliensis*, or *L. tropica*, between others (2).

In urban, periurban and domestic environments, dogs (*Canis lupus familiaris*) are usually considered main reservoirs of the parasite, although synanthropic rodents (e.g., *Rattus norvegicus*), wild rabbits (*Oryctolagus cuniculus*), hares (*Lepus granatensis*), and cats (*Felis catus domesticus*) can also play a relevant role as reservoir host (6–12).

In endemic developing countries, leishmaniasis mainly affects people of lower socioeconomic status, in rural areas with poor housing conditions, with little or no access to health services (1, 13). Within the risk groups, visceral leishmaniasis can present non-specific symptoms in children, and can be fatal without adequate treatment (14). Although coinfection with HIV is considered a public health problem in various parts of the world (15), the introduction of highly effective antiretroviral treatment in developed countries since 1997 has helped to decrease the HIV coinfection (16), so nowadays it is a pathology more common in immunosuppression non-HIV-related (17).

Incidence of Leishmaniasis in Mediterranean countries and across Europe has been described on the rise (1). Autochthonous cases have been recently described in non-endemic areas, like Southern Germany (18), and the number of imported cases has increased in areas such as Sweden or London (19, 20). In Sweden, an increase in diagnoses has been observed since 2013, especially in those under 18 years of age and migrants, mainly from Syria and Afghanistan (19). In London, most diagnoses occurred in tourists returning from the Mediterranean region and soldiers returning from other territories where the pathogen is endemic (20).

Climate change is expected to extend the geographical distribution and seasonality of phlebotomine vectors (7, 21). In Morocco, the increase in minimum temperatures has increased the survival of the sandfly larvae through the winters, extending their activity season. This combined with the increase in human circulation and tourism is thought to be one of the main causes for dissemination of cutaneous leishmaniasis (22). Spain has also experienced an increase in cases, though this phenomenon has been attributed to multiple factors, including improvements in notification, the seasonality of sandflies (16) and a growing urbanization that favors the contact between reservoirs and humans (23).

Studies in different areas of Spain have reported seroprevalence varying from 4 to 35% in dogs, with a high proportion of them not showing any clinical signs of leishmaniasis (24, 25). *Phlebotomus perniciosus* and *Phlebotomus ariasi* are the main vectors of *Leishmania infantum* in the Iberian Peninsula (23, 26). Moreover, in Spain, leishmaniasis is a hypoendemic, mandatory notifiable disease since 1995 (27), but reporting is compulsory for every Autonomous Region (CCAA) through the National Surveillance Network since 2015 (28). During the 2005–2017 period, Spain had an incidence rate of 0.62 cases per 100,000 inhabitants (16, 25), with a heterogeneous distribution, mainly affecting the Mediterranean region (the Valencian Community, Catalonia, the Balearic Islands and Andalusia), except for the Community of Madrid, where a large community outbreak was identified in 2009 and 2010 linked to a newly identified reservoir (26). The objective of this study is to characterize the epidemiology and temporal trends in the incidence of human leishmaniasis in the city of Barcelona, between the years 1996 and 2019.

METHODOLOGY

Study Design and Population

A population-based, analytical observational study was conducted with all reported leishmaniasis cases between

1996 and 2019. Data were drawn from the registry of notifiable diseases of the Epidemiology Service of the Public Health Agency of Barcelona (ASPB). The registry includes cases individually notified to the Epidemiology Service by healthcare professionals and, since 2016, it also includes laboratory notifications to the Catalan Microbiologic Notification System (SNMC) (29).

Variables

The registry of notifiable diseases contains the information included in the epidemiological surveys of cases carried out by public health nurses from the Epidemiology Service.

The epidemiological survey contains clinical, diagnostic, and epidemiological data, among others (**Annex 1**). The variables of interest included: age, sex, country of birth, date of onset of symptoms (onset, diagnosis, and notification data), type of leishmaniasis, history of immunosuppressive disease or immunosuppressive treatment, as well as history of contact with an infected dog or another animal suspected of infection and travel to an endemic country according to WHO's current guidelines at the time of the survey (30).

Inclusion and Exclusion Criteria

All cases of leishmaniasis from patients who resided in the city of Barcelona and who met the case definition according to local guidelines were included (**Annex 2**). Cases were excluded if the patients resided in another city than Barcelona.

Analysis

Annual incidence-rates and its confidence interval (95%) were calculated by sex, age, and country of birth, in relation to the municipal registry of the city of Barcelona (31). The microbiological confirmation and national surveillance system were modified in 2016 (28). Consequently, to test for temporal changes in the influence of these variables on the incidence of leishmaniasis, the study period was divided into three periods: 1996–2005 ($n = 55$), 2006–2015 ($n = 52$), and 2016–2019 ($n = 70$).

The risk factors obtained from the survey were analyzed by the three proposed periods and the clinical presentation of the leishmaniasis. Cases were classified according to the Available Family Income Index of the municipal district of residence (IRFD for "Index renda familiar disponible"), into disadvantaged (IRFD < 1) or favored (IRFD > 1) neighborhood (32). In 2019, 62.2% of Barcelona's population lived in disadvantaged neighborhoods (31). A chi-squared or a Fisher's exact test were performed, as appropriate, and a $p < 0.05$ was considered significant. All the analyses were done using the program STATA version 15.

RESULTS

Between 1996 and 2019, 177 cases of leishmaniasis were reported in Barcelona (**Table 1**). The median age was 34 years [interquartile range (IQR): 10–48]. 66.8% ($n = 121$) of the diagnoses occurred in men. According to origin, most cases occurred in native population (**Table 1**), however, a sustained increase in cases from foreign-born population were observed since 2003 (**Figure 1**). The main type of leishmaniasis was cutaneous (45.2%, $n = 80$), followed by visceral (34.5%, $n = 61$), and only 2.3% ($n = 4$) was mucocutaneous. 61.6% ($n = 109$) of the cases occurred in people who lived in disadvantaged municipal districts. 68.4% ($n = 121$) of the cases progressed to healing without sequel, 6.21% ($n = 11$) progressed with sequel, and 1.63% ($n = 3$) died (**Table 1**). The diagnosis were made by biopsy in 61% of the cases ($n = 108$), by a serological test in 21.5% ($n = 38$) and by culture in 19.4% ($n = 21$).

TABLE 1 | Descriptive statistics of the leishmaniasis cases reported in Barcelona between 1996 and 2019 ($n = 177$).

	n	%
Sex		
Men	121	68.4%
Women	55	31.1%
Country of origin		
Native	132	74.6%
Foreign	45	25.4%
Type of leishmaniasis		
Visceral	61	34.5%
Cutanous	80	45.2%
Mucocutaneous	4	2.3%
Missing	32	18.1%
Neighborhood's available family income index (AFII)		
Disadvantaged (AFII <1)	109	61.6%
Favored (AFII > 1)	57	32.2%
Missing	11	6.2%
Evolution		
Cured without sequelae (a)	121	68.4%
Cured with sequelae (a)	11	6.2%
Dead	3	1.7%
Lost to follow up (b)	42	23.7%

(a) Sequelae defined by the surveyor's criteria.
(b) Of the 42 lost cases of "Evolution," 9 cases were identified as "lost" by the person who carried out the survey, while the rest of the cases had no information.
In all the missing cases of the Type of leishmaniasis and Neighborhood, the value was not recorded in the epidemiological survey.

The cumulative incidence during the study period was 0.47 per 100,000 inhabitants (**Table 2**), with the highest incidence found in 2017 (1.6 per 100,000 inhabitants) and the lowest in 2012 (**Figure 2**). Incidence was generally higher in men than women (0.68 vs. 0.27 per 100,000 inhabitants) and in foreign-born over Spanish-born population (0.74 vs. 0.41 per 100,000 inhabitants). Slight changes in incidence were observed between the first and second period (0.36–0.32 per 100,000), increasing significantly to 1.08 per 100,000 after 2016. An increase of the incidence was observed in all age groups, especially in the third period, with the higher incidence found in the 0–4-year-old group (1.73 per 100,000 inhabitants) (**Table 2**).

During the three studied periods there was an increase of the cutaneous leishmaniasis in the second and third period (0–51.9 to 75.7%, $p < 0.001$), and a decrease of the visceral leishmaniasis in the final period (54.6 to 46.2% to a 10%, $p < 0.001$) (**Table 3**). Male sex accounted for over 80% of the cases in ages 25–64,

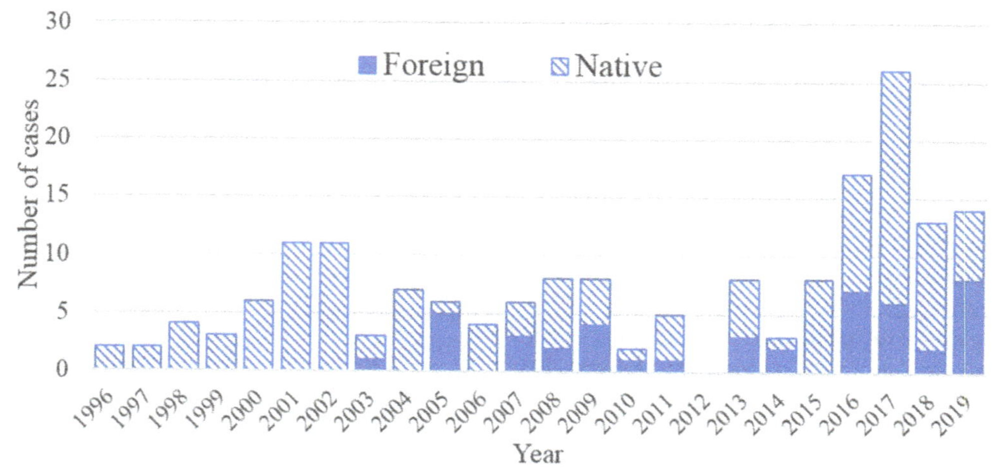

FIGURE 1 | Total number of cases of leishmaniasis, in Spanish born population (native) and foreigner country of birth, in Barcelona between 1996 and 2019 ($n = 177$ cases).

TABLE 2 | Incidence of leishmaniasis per 100,000 inhabitants and confidence interval (95%), by complete study time and periods 1996–2005 ($n = 55$), 2006–2015 ($n = 52$), and 2016–2019 ($n = 70$), Barcelona.

		1996–2005	2006–2015	2016–2019	Total
Sex	Female	0.14 [0.06–0.22]	0.22 [0.12–0.32]	0.73 [0.44–1.02]	0.27 [0.19–0.34]
	Male	0.61 [0.43–0.79]	0.41 [0.27–0.55]	1.47 [1.04–1.89]	0.68 [0.56–0.80]
Age	0–4	2.00 [0.87–3.13]	1.15 [0.35–1.94]	2.59 [0.67–4.51]	1.73 [1.52–1.93]
	5–14	0.17 [0.09–0.24]	0.00	1.64 [0.56–2.71]	0.37 [0.15–0.59]
	15–24	0.16 [0.10–0.22]	0.14 [0.08–0.20]	1.03 [0.21–1.85]	0.28 [0.11–0.45]
	25–44	0.71 [0.47–0.95]	0.44 [0.26–0.62]	0.91 [0.49–1.33]	0.62 [0.48–0.76]
	45–64	0.11 [0.00–0.22]	0.35 [0.17–0.53]	0.70 [0.30–1.09]	0.31 [0.19–0.42]
	65 or more	0.03 [0.01–0.05]	0.15 [0.02–0.28]	1.23 [0.65–1.81]	0.30 [0.18–0.42]
Country of origin	Native	0.34 [0.24–0.44]	0.28 [0.19–0.37]	0.95 [0.68–1.22]	0.41 [0.34–0.48]
	Foreign	0.50 [0.09–0.90]	0.48 [0.24–0.72]	1.48 [0.88–2.08]	0.74 [0.52–0.96]
Total		0.36 [0.27–0.45]	0.32 [0.23–0.41]	1.08 [0.83–1.33]	0.47 [0.40–0.54]

without greater differences during the studied periods. Over 60% of cases occurred in disadvantaged neighborhoods during the three periods ($p = 0.261$). Leishmaniasis in foreign subjects increased over time, but only accounted for a third of the total cases in the last period. A significant decrease in cases related to any immunosuppression (due to disease or treatment) was observed ($p < 0.001$).

All types of leishmaniasis occurred mainly in Spanish born, men, and people from disadvantaged neighborhoods (**Table 4**). Visceral leishmaniasis was present in 40.9% of the cases that referred contact with an animal and 26% of the cases that referred intravenous drug use. A 33.8% of the cases who referred travel to an endemic country presented a cutaneous type of leishmaniasis (endemic country according to WHO's current guidelines at the time of the survey). Most of the visceral leishmaniasis required a hospital admission and it was the only leishmaniasis type related to a fatal outcome.

Even if the current epidemiological survey does not systematically collect information on type of comorbidities, homelessness status, species of *Leishmania* or the type of animals that could have acted as a reservoir, it was possible to extract some of this information from the comments included by interviewers. Regarding comorbidities, it was observed that an 18.4% ($n = 35$) of the studied population had a diagnosis of HIV and two cases were described as Hepatitis C positive. Four cases were informed to be homeless. Seven cases were characterized as *Leishmania donovani*, and one case was described as *Leishmania braziliensis*.

DISCUSSION

The results of this study have shown an increase in the incidence of leishmaniasis in the city of Barcelona from 1996 to 2019. This increase only appears as statistically significant for the period 2016-2019. The establishment of the *Catalan Microbiologic*

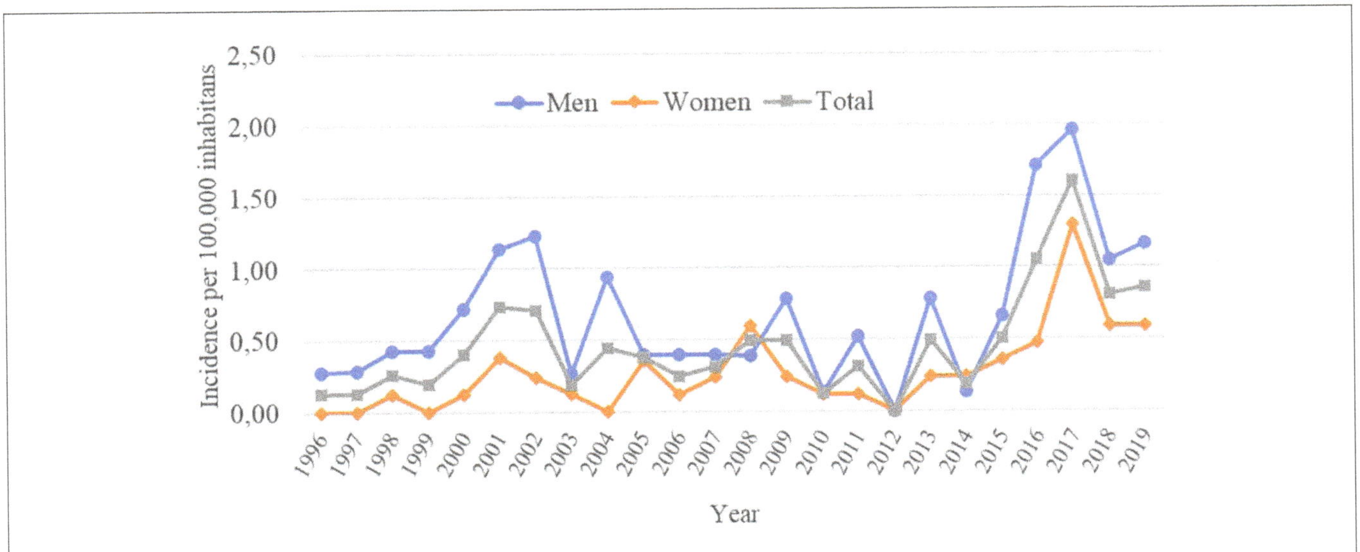

FIGURE 2 | Annual incidence of leishmaniasis per 100,000 inhabitants, by complete sample and sexes. Barcelona, 1996–2019. (n = 177 cases).

TABLE 3 | Cases of leishmaniasis according to type of disease and risk factors, during the three studied periods.

	1996–2005 *N* (%)	2006–2015 *N* (%)	2016–2019 *N* (%)	Total *N* (%)	*p*-value
Type of leishmania					<0.001
Visceral	30 (54.6%)	24 (46.2%)	7 (10%)	61 (34.5%)	
Cutaneous	0	27 (51.9%)	53 (75.7%)	80 (45.2%)	
Mucocutaneus	1 (1.82)	0	3 (4.3%)	4 (2.3%)	
Risk factors					
Male sex by ages					
Male (0–4)	7 (58.3%)	4 (50%)	2 (28.6%)	13 (48.3%)	0.545 *f*
Male (5–14)	2 (100%)	0	5 (55.6%)	7 (63.6%)	0.491 *f*
Male (15–24)	1 (33.3%)	1 (50%)	3 (50%)	5 (45.5%)	1 *f*
Male (25–44)	30 (90.9%)	16 (72.7%)	14 (77.8%)	60 (82.2%)	0.202 *f*
Male (45–64)	4 (100%)	9 (64.3%)	11 (91.7%)	24 (80%)	0.149 *f*
Male (65 or more)	0	2 (40%)	10 (56.6%)	12 (50%)	0.640 *f*
D sadvantaged neighborhood	31 (63.3%)	36 (75%)	42 (60.9%)	109 (65.7%)	0.261
Foreign origin	6 (10.9%)	16 (30.8%)	23 (32.9%)	45 (25.4%)	<0.001
Immunosuppression	25 (45.5%)	18 (34.6%)	7 (10%)	50 (28.5%)	<0.001
Due to disease	24 (61.5%)	17 (32.7%)	6 (8.6%)	47 (29.2%)	<0.001
Due to treatment	12 (30.8%)	6 (11.5%)	5 (7.1%)	23 (14.3%)	0.009
Total cases	55 (100%)	52 (100%)	70 (100%)	177 (100%)	

P-values presented with an italic f (f) when Fisher's exact test is performed.

Notification System as a consequence of the decree 203/2015 (29), which requires mandatory notification of all identified cases by laboratories, is likely to have contributed greatly to the observed trend, together with other factors such as the improvement in diagnostic tools and possibly a real change in disease burden. The increase is observed in all ages, being greater in the younger population and male adults. The number of foreign-born cases has increased since 2003 while the number of cases associated to immunosuppression has decreased. There is also a change in the type of leishmaniasis in the three studied periods, with an increase of cutaneous leishmaniasis.

The cumulative incidence during these 24 years of observation was higher than previously reported in analysis of the same database (0.33 per 100,000 inhabitants between 1997 and 2014) (33) but lower than the reported incidence of Spain (16, 25). After the modification of the confirmation and surveillance system (28, 29), there was a significant increase of the total incidence probably due to an improved reporting, and because a possible increase in the clinical suspicion at primary care level.

Our study has shown that men between 25 and 64 years old present a higher incidence of leishmaniasis in all the studied periods. Previous studies have associated this correlation with the incidence of HIV in this group (33). However, the reasons why men of working age have a higher incidence of leishmaniasis are diverse, and cannot be exclusively related to this comorbidity, even when the data obtained through the epidemiological survey does not allow us to test for further causality. In this population, men accounted for 91.9% of the cases related to alcoholism, 81.3% of cases with a history of intravenous drug use and 70% of traveling to endemic countries. Studies have described a male bias in certain infectious diseases (34), including leishmaniasis (35), proposing physiological and behavioral theories. However, the evidence is not conclusive, and we cannot exclude that man are more exposed to infected vectors because of their social or working activities.

By age groups, there was a consistent high incidence in cases under 5 years of age, but also a rise in the cases over 65 years since 2001. In the younger population, the main causes are associated to a lack of effective immune response (14, 33). In our sample, an 88.9% of the age group 0-4 was from native origin, a 66.7% presented a visceral type of leishmaniasis, and

TABLE 4 | Type of Leishmaniasis according to risk factors and evolution.

	Visceral *N* (%)	Cutaneous *N* (%)	Muco cutaneous *N* (%)	Total *N* (%)	*P*-value (a)
Risk factors					
Foreign origin	12 (19.7%)	26 (32.5%)	0	45 (27.9%)	0.092 *f*
Male sex	43 (71.7%)	52 (65%)	4 (100%)	109 (68.1%)	0.491
Disadvantaged neighborhood	39 (69.6%)	51 (64.6%)	3 (75%)	102 (75%)	0.911
Immunosuppression	31 (50.8%)	8 (10%)	1 (25%)	50 (31.1%)	<0.001 *f*
Contact with animal	25 (40.9%)	9 (11.3%)	1 (25%)	35 (21.8%)	<0.001 *f*
Travel to endemic country	8 (13.1%)	27 (33.8%)	0	35 (20.1%)	<0.001 *f*
History of transplant	1 (1.6%)	1 (1.3%)	0	2 (1.2%)	*
History of alcoholism	8 (13.1%)	3 (3.8%)	1 (25%)	12 (6.9%)	<0.001 *f*
History of transfusion	5 (8.2%)	0	0	5 (2.9%)	*
Intravenous drug use	16 (26.2%)	0	0	16 (9.2%)	*
Evolution					
Hospital admission	57 (93.4%)	1 (1.3%)	1 (25%)	62 (32.6%)	
Cured without sequels	51 (83.6%)	67 (83.8%)	3 (75%)	121 (68.4%)	
Cured with sequels	4 (6.6%)	6 (7.5%)	1 (25%)	11 (6.2%)	
Death	2 (3.3%)	0	0	3 (1.7%)	
Total	61 (34.5%)	80 (45.2%)	4 (2.3%)	177 (100%)	

Barcelona, 1996–2019 (missing values = 32; 18.08%). P-values presented with an italic f (f) when Fisher's exact test is performed, and with an asterisk (*) when not performed due to cases with very low frequency.

85.19% evolved to healing without sequel. Is important to notice that there was no differences between native or foreign-born population in this age group during the three studied periods (Fisher's $p = 0.142$). Moreover, cases in the 0-4 age group during the third studied period (2016–2019), only occurred in Spanish-born population. In the elderly group, there was a rise in the diagnosis of cutaneous leishmaniasis, being 64% of the total cases over 65 years of age. This group only presented a 20% history of immunosuppression and a 24% foreign origin. A 76% of the cases evolved to healing without sequel. The reasons for this increase are unclear and may be related to a change in the diagnosis system and access to dermatological services from primary care, but further investigation is required.

Among population from foreign country of birth, there is a persistent increase of incidence since 2003, consistent with a rise in foreign population migrating to Barcelona (3.8% of the total population in 1996 to 25.7% in 2019) (31), but also to international traveling to endemic areas, due to tourism, visiting relatives and work (22, 36). The difference between autochtonous and imported cases is difficult to establish due to the long incubation period of leishmaniasis (2 weeks to several years), and inconsistencies in the reporting of identified *Leishmania* species. Thus, our data might be overestimating the burden of locally acquired *Leishmania*. The introduction risk supposed by *Leishmania braziliensis* imported cases is thought to be limited due to the reported absence of competent vectors in Europe (7), although a possible competence of *P. perniciosus* to *L. tropica* should be accounted (37–39). Improvements in the registry should allow for the systematic report of the species of *Leishmania* involved in the clinical cases.

In relation to vulnerable populations, there was a decrease in cases related to immunosuppression, due to disease or treatment. This decrease could correspond to the improve of the antiretroviral treatments for HIV population (16), as well as improvements in the care of immunosuppressed patients, like transplanted, who presents a very low incidence of cases. In this study, most of the cases occurred in disadvantaged districts of Barcelona, without changes in time. Homeless cases are at a higher risk to get lost to follow up, facing a challenge to the prevention and surveillance strategy for years to come. Even when we did not have access to information of the individual's socio-economic status, the use of the Available Family Income Index is a good proxy to evaluate inequalities within the city (32).

Leishmaniasis is the most relevant endemic zoonosis in the last years in the Mediterranean basin, due to the coexistence of *Leishmania* protozoa; reservoirs such as hare (11, 40), rabbits (10), rodents and dogs (9, 41), and competent vectors (sandflies from the genus *Phlebotomus*). As a Mediterranean city, Barcelona has the appropriate climatic characteristics for local transmission of *Leishmania* sp. The presence of the two main vectors, *Phlebotomus perniciosus* and *Phlebotomus ariasi*, are known due to the monitoring of the city of Barcelona by the ASPB, the institution responsible for the vector surveillance and control in the city (42). Furthermore, recent research indicates that Norway rat, a synanthropic murid that shows high abundance and deeply distribution in the sewer system of the city (6), could play a relevant role as host reservoir of Leishmaniasis (43). At this point, it is important to emphasize the sewers have been also recorded as suitable breeding site for sandflies in Barcelona (unpublished data).

Climate change is affecting the geographical distribution and seasonality of many species, including sandflies, and increased connectivity has facilitated the expansion of different insect vectors into new geographical areas (7, 21). A climate change induced expansion of vector competent species will at the same time lead to an expansion of the risk area for leishmaniasis. The expansion of the green areas across the city due to the Climate change action plan (44) should consider the potential risk of increase in competent vector distribution and reservoirs. Overall, there is a need to enforce the surveillance system of leishmaniasis. Therefore, we recommend undertaking surveys in the city to characterize the distribution and abundance of different vectors, as a strategy to establish an effective surveillance and control program to reduce the risk of transmission.

Our results show that that autochthonous transmission is occurring in the city of Barcelona and consequently a more in-depth study of the vectors present in the city should be carried out, in order to know their distribution, abundance, and blood feeding behavior and thus have a diagnosis of the risk of transmission and spillover into humans. Epidemiological, vectorial and health surveillance must have in consideration the high risk groups, like homeless and exposed workers, as those who work in sewer systems, together with vector control programs associated to renovation works affecting the underground structure that may facilitate the movement of *Phlebotomus* into inhabited areas (3).

The main limitations of this study are the loss of follow up of some cases, and the lack of information regarding significant variables. There is a regular loss of cases each year, which may be due to cases that occurred in the homeless, or people that were in transit and the clinical history is incomplete. There is a clear need to review the current epidemiological survey to systematically collect information on the detected leishmania species, the type of treatment used and its efficacy, as well as homelessness status, to better characterize the impact of leishmaniasis on vulnerable populations. Identifying the domestic animals that act as reservoirs and ensuring they receive the necessary treatments to reduce the risk of new transmissions to humans should also be a priority to reduce the risk of local outbreaks (45, 46). It is also important to quantify the role that non-domestic animal species may play as reservoirs associated to human infection cases in the city (5, 47). Collaboration at an epidemiological and entomological level is one of the pillars to reduce the risks of transmission, thus trying to work on a One Health concept that integrates the different fields involved in the transmission processes.

Even though leishmaniasis is an endemic disease in Spain, the city of Barcelona will continue to be a highly transited city, with a higher migration rate and tourism, which may favor the occurrence of imported cases. This constitutes an entomological, clinical, and epidemiological challenge, due to the variety of clinical presentations and adaptation to vectors or local reservoirs.

AUTHOR CONTRIBUTIONS

TM, J-PM, and CR worked in the conception and first design of the work. LM, PS, and EM were in charge of the acquisition of the data, and organization of the database. DP performed the statistical analysis and wrote the first draft of the manuscript. DP, LM, and JF worked in the interpretation of data for the work. DP and LM were in charge of drafting the work. RB-M, JF, PS, EM, CR, and TM critically revised the manuscript. All authors provide their final approval of the version to be published and agreed to be accountable for all aspects of the work in ensuring that questions related to the accuracy or integrity of any part of the work are appropriately investigated and resolved.

ACKNOWLEDGMENTS

To the nursing team of the ASPB, for their work in the follow-up of cases that has allowed us to carry out this study.

REFERENCES

1. Inceboz, T. Epidemiology and ecology of leishmaniasis. In: Rodriguez-Morales AJ, editor. *Current Topics in Neglected Tropical Diseases.* IntechOpen (2019). 487 p. doi: 10.5772/intechopen.86359
2. Burza S, Croft SL, Boelaert M. Leishmaniasis. *Lancet.* (2018) 392:951–70. doi: 10.1016/S0140-6736(18)31204-2
3. de Vries HJ, Reedijk SH, Schallig HD. Cutaneous leishmaniasis: recent developments in diagnosis and management. *Am J Clin Dermatol.* (2015) 16:99–109. doi: 10.1007/s40257-015-0114-z
4. World Health Organization. *Leishmaniasis Key Facts.* (2020). Available online at https://www.who.int/news-room/fact-sheets/detail/leishmaniasis (accesed December 23, 2020).
5. World Health Organization. *Control de las leishmaniasis. Serie de Informes Técnicos.* Tech Rep Ser 949:1-186 (2010). 200 p. Available online at: https://apps.who.int/iris/bitstream/handle/10665/82766/WHO_TRS_949_spa.pdf;jsessionid=5D05F70187908572FB89D8C1F49ABEF7?sequence=1 (accesed December 23, 2020).
6. Galán-Puchades MT, Gómez-Samblás M, Suárez-Morán JM, Osuna A, Sanxis-Furió J, Pascual J, et al. Leishmaniasis in Norway Rats in Sewers, Barcelona, Spain. *Emerg Infect Dis.* (2019) 25:1222–4. doi: 10.3201/eid2506.181027
7. Ready PD. Leishmaniasis emergence in Europe. *Euro Surveill.* (2010) 15:19505. doi: 10.2807/ese.15.10.19505-en
8. Velez R, Ballart C, Domenech E, Abras A, Fernández-Arévalo A, Gómez SA, et al. Seroprevalence of canine *Leishmania infantum* infection in the Mediterranean region and identification of risk factors: the example of North-Eastern and Pyrenean areas of Spain. *Prev Vet Med.* (2019) 162:67–75. doi: 10.1016/j.prevetmed.2018.10.015
9. Abbate JM, Arfuso F, Napoli E, Gaglio G, Giannetto S, Latrofa MS, et al. *Leishmania infantum* in wild animals in endemic areas of southern Italy. *Comp Immunol Microbiol Infect Dis.* (2019) 67:101374. doi: 10.1016/j.cimid.2019.101374
10. Jiménez M, González E, Martín-Martín I, Hernández S, Molina R. Could wild rabbits (*Oryctolagus cuniculus*) be reservoirs for Leishmania infantum in the focus of Madrid, Spain? *Vet Parasitol.* (2014) 202:296–300. doi: 10.1016/j.vetpar.2014.03.027
11. Molina R, Jiménez MI, Cruz I, Iriso A, Martín-Martín I, Sevillano O, et al. The hare (*Lepus granatensis*) as potential sylvatic reservoir of Leishmania infantum in Spain. *Vet Parasitol.* (2012) 190:268–71. doi: 10.1016/j.vetpar.2012.05.006
12. Martín-Sánchez J, Acedo C, Muñoz-Pérez M, Pesson B, Marchal O, Morillas-Márquez F. Infection by *Leishmania infantum* in cats: epidemiological study in Spain. *Vet Parasitol.* (2007) 145:267–73. doi: 10.1016/j.vetpar.2006.11.005
13. Okwor I, Uzonna J. Social and economic burden of human leishmaniasis. *Am J Trop Med Hyg.* (2016) 94:489–93. doi: 10.4269/ajtmh.15-0408
14. Ramos JM, Clavijo A, Moral L, Gavilan C, Salvador T, González de Dios J. Epidemiological and clinical features of visceral leishmaniasis in children in Alicante Province, Spain. *Paediatr Int Child Health.* (2018) 38:203–8. doi: 10.1080/20469047.2018.1468585
15. Graepp-Fontoura I, Soeiro Barbosa D, Paes A, Santos FS, Santos Neto M, Fontoura VM, et al. Epidemiological, clinical and laboratory aspects of human visceral leishmaniasis (HVL) associated with human immunodeficiency virus (HIV) coinfection: a systematic review. *Parasitology.* (2018) 145:1801–18. doi: 10.1017/S003118201800080X
16. Fernández Martínez B, Gómez Barroso D, Cano Portero R. La leishmaniasis en España: evolución de los casos notificados a la Red Nacional de Vigilancia Epidemiológica desde 2005 a 2017 y resultados de la vigilancia de 2014 a 2017. *Bol Epidemiol Sem.* (2019) 27:15–27.
17. Horrillo L, Castro A, Matía B, Molina L, García-Martínez J, Jaqueti J, et al. Clinical aspects of visceral leishmaniasis caused by *L. infantum* in adults. Ten years of experience of the largest outbreak in Europe: what have we learned? *Parasit Vectors.* (2019) 12:359. doi: 10.1186/s13071-019-3628-z
18. Haeberlein S, Fischer D, Thomas SM, Schleicher U, Beierkuhnlein C, Bogdan C. First assessment for the presence of phlebotomine vectors in Bavaria, Southern Germany, by combined distribution modeling and field surveys. *PLoS One.* (2013) 8:e81088. doi: 10.1371/journal.pone.0081088
19. Söbirk, SK, Inghammar M, Collin M, Davidsson L. Imported

leishmaniasis in Sweden 1993-2016. *Epidemiol Infect.* (2018) 146:1267–74. doi: 10.1017/S0950268818001309
20. Wall EC, Watson J, Armstrong M, Chiodini PL, Lockwood DN. Epidemiology of imported cutaneous leishmaniasis at the Hospital for Tropical Diseases, London, United Kingdom: use of polymerase chain reaction to identify the species. *Am J Trop Med Hyg.* (2012) 86:115–8. doi: 10.4269/ajtmh.2012.10-0558
21. Chalghaf B, Chemkhi J, Mayala B, Harrabi M, Benie GB, Michael E, et al. Ecological niche modeling predicting the potential distribution of Leishmania vectors in the Mediterranean basin: impact of climate change. *Parasit Vectors.* (2018) 11:461. doi: 10.1186/s13071-018-3019-x
22. Kholoud K, Bounoua L, Sereno D, El Hidan M, Messouli M. Emerging and re-emerging leishmaniases in the mediterranean area: what can be learned from a retrospective review analysis of the situation in Morocco during 1990 to 2010? *Microorganisms.* (2020) 8:1511. doi: 10.3390/microorganisms8101511
23. Arce A, Estirado A, Ordobas M, Sevilla S, García N, Moratilla L, et al. Re-emergence of Leishmaniasis in Spain: community outbreak in Madrid, Spain, 2009 to 2012. *Euro Surveill.* (2013) 18:20546. doi: 10.2807/1560-7917.ES2013.18.30.20546
24. World Health Organization. *Leishmaniasis Country Profiles.* Spain (2020). Available online at: https://www.who.int/leishmaniasis/burden/Leishmaniasis_Spain/en/ (accessed November 23, 2020).
25. Gálvez R, Montoya A, Cruz I, Fernández C, Martín O, Checa R, et al. Latest trends in Leishmania infantum infection in dogs in Spain, Part I: mapped seroprevalence and sand fly distributions. *Parasit Vectors.* (2020) 13:204. doi: 10.1186/s13071-020-04081-7
26. González E, Molina R, Jiménez M. Rabbit trypanosome detection in Phlebotomus perniciosus sand flies from the leishmaniasis outbreak in Madrid, Spain. *Acta Trop.* (2018) 187:201–6. doi: 10.1016/j.actatropica.2018.08.011
27. *Real Decreto 2210/1995, de 28 de diciembre, por el que se crea la red nacional de vigilancia epidemiológica.* Ministerio de Sanidad y Consumo.
28. *Orden SSI/445/2015, de 9 de marzo, por la que se modifican los anexos I, II y III del Real Decreto 2210/1995, de 28 de diciembre, por el que se crea la red nacional de vigilancia epidemiológica, relativos a la lista de enfermedades de declaración obligatoria, modalidades de declaración y enfermedades endémicas de ámbito regional.* Ministerio de Sanidad y Consumo.
29. Generalitat de Catalunya. *Decret 203/2015, de 15 de setembre, pel qual es crea la Xarxa de Vigilància Epidemiològica i es regulen els sistemes de notificació de malalties de declaració obligatòria i brots epidèmics.*
30. World Health Organization. *Status of Endemicity of Cutaneous Leishmaniasis.* (2019). Available online at: https://apps.who.int/neglected_diseases/ntddata/leishmaniasis/leishmaniasis.html (accessed March 24, 2021).
31. Ajuntament de Barcelona. *Xifres Oficials de la Población.* Departament de Estadísticas y Difusió de dades (2020). Available online at: http://www.bcn.cat/estadistica/catala/dades/tpob/pad/ine/index.htm (accessed November 30, 2020).
32. Ajuntament de Barcelona. *Distribució Territorial de la Renda Familiar.* Departament de Estadísticas y Difusió de dades (2020). Available online at: https://www.bcn.cat/estadistica/catala/dades/economia/renda/rdfamiliar/index.htm (accessed November 30, 2020).
33. Riera C, Napp S, Manzanares S. Epidemiología de la leishmaniasis humana en la ciudad de Barcelona (1997-2014). *Rev Enf Emerg.* (2016) 15:68–76.
34. Guerra-Silveira F, Abad-Franch F. Sex Bias in infectious disease epidemiology: patterns and processes. *PLoS One.* (2013) 8:e62390. doi: 10.1371/journal.pone.0062390
35. Cloots K, Burza S, Malaviya P, Hasker E, Kansal S, Mollett G, et al. Male predominance in reported Visceral Leishmaniasis cases: Nature or nurture? A comparison of population-based with health facility-reported data. *PLoS Negl Trop Dis.* (2020) 14:e0007995. doi: 10.1371/journal.pntd.0007995
36. Orduna T, Lloveras S, Gonzalez GD, Falcone CC, Garro SL, Echazarreta SE. Abstract 32.025: new world cutaneous Leishmaniasis in travelers (1994-2008) experience in Argentina. In: *International Congress on Infectious Diseases (ICID) Abstracts.* doi: 10.1016/j.ijid.2010.02.1797
37. Di Muccio T, Scalone A, Bruno A, Marangi M, Grande R, Armignacco O, et al. Epidemiology of imported leishmaniasis in Italy: implications for a European endemic country. *PLoS One.* (2015) 10:e0129418. doi: 10.1371/journal.pone.0129418
38. Bongiorno G, Di Muccio T, Bianchi R, Gramiccia M, Gradoni L. Laboratory transmission of an Asian strain of *Leishmania tropica* by the bite of the southern European sand fly Phlebotomus perniciosus. *Int J Parasitol.* (2019) 49:417–421. doi: 10.1016/j.ijpara.2018.12.009
39. Vaselek S, Volf P. Experimental infection of *Phlebotomus perniciosus* and *Phlebotomus tobbi* with different Leishmania tropica strains. *Int J Parasitol.* (2019) 49:831–5. doi: 10.1016/j.ijpara.2019.05.009
40. Jiménez M, González E, Iriso A, Marco E, Alegret A, Fúster F, et al. Detection of Leishmania infantum and identification of blood meals in *Phlebotomus perniciosus.* from a focus of human leishmaniasis in Madrid, Spain. *Parasitol Res.* (2013) 112:2453–9. doi: 10.1007/s00436-013-3406-3
41. Montoya-Alonso JA, Morchón R, Costa-Rodríguez N, Matos JI, Falcón-Cordón Y, Carretón E. Current distribution of selected Vector-Borne Diseases in dogs in Spain. *Front Vet Sci.* (2020) 7:564429. doi: 10.3389/fvets.2020.564429
42. Agència de Salut Pública de Barcelona. *Memoria d'activitat del Servei de Vigilància i Control de Plagues Urbanes.* (2018). Available online at: https://www.aspb.cat/arees/plagues-urbanes/vigilancia-i-control-de-plagues-ambientals/
43. Pascual J, Franco S, Bueno-Marí R, Peracho V, Montalvo T. Demography and ecology of Norway rats, Rattus norvegicus, in the sewer system of Barcelona (Catalonia, Spain). *J Pest Sci.* (2020) 93:711–22. doi: 10.1007/s10340-019-01178-6
44. Ajuntament de Barcelona. *Plan Clima 2018-2013.* (2020). Available online at: https://ajuntament.barcelona.cat/ecologiaurbana/ca/que-fem-i-per-que/energia-i-canvi-climatic/pla-clima (accessed December 23, 2020).
45. Postigo JA. Leishmaniasis in the World Health Organization Eastern Mediterranean Region. *Int J Antimicrob Agents.* (2010) 36(Suppl 1):S62–5. doi: 10.1016/j.ijantimicag.2010.06.023
46. World Health Organization. *Manual on Case Management and Surveillance of the Leishmaniasis in the WHO European Region.* (2017). Available online at: https://www.euro.who.int/__data/assets/pdf_file/0006/341970/MANUAL-ON-CASE-MANAGEMENT_FINAL_with-cover-and-ISBN.pdf (accessed March 24, 2021).
47. Alemayehu B, Alemayehu M. Leishmaniasis: a review on parasite, vector and reservoir host. *Health Sci J.* (2017) 4:519. doi: 10.21767/1791-809X.1000519

5

Hematological and Biochemical Changes in Dogs Naturally Infected with *Dirofilaria repens*

Magdalena E. Wysmołek[1], Artur Dobrzyński[2], Ewa Długosz[1], Michał Czopowicz[3], Marcin Wiśniewski[1], Piotr Jurka[2] and Maciej Klockiewicz[1]*

[1] Division of Parasitology, Department of Preclinical Sciences, Institute of Veterinary Medicine, Warsaw University of Life Sciences-SGGW, Warsaw, Poland, [2] Department of Small Animal Diseases and Clinic, Institute of Veterinary Medicine, Warsaw University of Life Sciences-SGGW, Warsaw, Poland, [3] Division of Veterinary Epidemiology and Economics, Institute of Veterinary Medicine, Warsaw University of Life Sciences-SGGW, Warsaw, Poland

***Correspondence:**
Magdalena E. Wysmołek
magdalena_wysmolek@sggw.edu.pl

Subcutaneous dirofilariosis is a zoonotic disease emerging throughout Europe caused by the filarial nematode *Dirofilaria repens*. Despite its increasing prevalence, there is a large gap in knowledge of the impact of the parasite on the host. Currently classified as being non-pathogenic, recent evidence suggests that skin dirofilariosis is associated with dermatological conditions including concomitant pruritus, neoplastic processes, inflammation, and even blindness in dogs and humans. The aim of this study was to determine if natural canine *D. repens* infection leads to biological changes in the canine host. In a real-life veterinary clinic setting, animals are often presented to clinicians for unrelated issues, and *D. repens* is incidentally identified during inspection. As such, we compared hematological and biochemical parameters of 218 uninfected and 197 dogs naturally infected with *D. repens*. Interestingly, animals infected with *D. repens* had lower numbers of lymphocytes ($p < 0.001$), red blood cells ($p < 0.001$), and thrombocytes ($p = 0.025$), decreased hematocrit ($p < 0.001$), and increased alkaline phosphatase ($p = 0.016$) and creatinine activity ($p = 0.023$) compared to uninfected dogs. We further selected a subpopulation of 214 dogs having *prima facie* hematological and biochemical results within normal reference ranges to evaluate the effect of *D. repens* infections in seemingly healthy dogs. Among these patients, 93 dogs infected with *D. repens* had lower numbers of lymphocytes ($p = 0.031$), red blood cells ($p = 0.025$), and hematocrit ($p = 0.002$), higher glucose levels ($p = 0.023$), and border line elevated alkaline phosphatase levels ($p = 0.054$) compared to 121 uninfected animals. Despite being categorized as asymptomatic, we have observed hematological and biochemical changes associated with *D. repens* infections in dogs, and our data suggest that dirofilariosis may induce a state of chronic stress. These results link the presence of skin dirofilariosis to biological changes in the canine host, suggesting a mechanism for pathogenicity and shedding new light on the host–parasite relationship.

Keywords: *Dirofilaria repens*, subcutaneous dirofilariosis, dog, hematology, biochemistry

INTRODUCTION

Dirofilaria immitis and *Dirofilaria repens* are both filarial nematodes that have zoonotic potential and cause canine heartworm disease and skin dirofilariosis in dogs, respectively. Despite its predominance throughout Europe and being the primary causative agent of human dirofilariasis, *D. repens* has received much less attention and study than *D. immitis* (1).

Briefly, dirofilariosis is a vector-borne disease transmitted by mosquitos. Mosquitos uptake microfilariae (Mf) circulating in the bloodstream of a definitive host during blood meals. After 2 weeks, Mf develop into infective larvae and are injected into a new host when the mosquito takes another blood meal. In the new host, the L3 larvae penetrate into subcutaneous tissue where they mature into adult skin filarial worms, copulate, and release Mf into the circulating bloodstream. Adult *D. repens* can survive and reproduce in a host for as long as 5–10 years (2) and may actively migrate within the host tissues during this period what considerably hampers their detection (3).

Dirofilaria spp. infections can be divided into microfilaremic and amicrofilaremic (occult). Microfilaremic infections are diagnosed using a modified Knott's test or by examining blood smears; Mf can be differentiated between species by morphology or using multiplex PCR. Although *D. immitis* amicrofilaremic infection may be diagnosed using a standard commercial test for adult female parasite antigens, there is no such rapid test available for the detection of *D. repens* occult infection in dogs (1).

In humans, the adult worms can migrate to subcutaneous tissue of different parts of the body (commonly in the head, mainly the periorbital region and neck), but they can also localize in the epididymis, the spermatic cords, the lungs, the breasts, the visceral cavity, or under the conjunctive tissue, lymph nodes, and muscles (4). In dogs, they are usually incidentally found in the scrotum during castration, but they can reach other locations including the periorbital or ectopic regions, such as mesenteric tissue and pelvic cavity (1). Infection with *D. repens* is usually considered asymptomatic, but a growing body of evidence suggest that it can cause significant morbidity, and increasing cases have been reported of severe disease leading to liver or kidney failure (5). *Dirofilaria repens* infections were also connected to neoplastic, sometimes malignant, processes in dogs (6, 7) and humans (8). Furthermore, the presence of adult *D. repens* and circulating Mf in blood or parenchymal organs can influence the course of coexisting diseases in infected animals (5, 9). General emaciation has been observed during massive *D. repens* infections associated with peritonitis, jaundice, degeneration of the liver, and renal failure (5, 10). In such conditions, numerous Mf were found in histopathology of internal organs (5–7). Microfilariae remaining in capillaries or disseminated into parenchymal tissues may be involved in the pathogenesis of tissue lesions and progress of the ongoing disease (5).

Infections presenting with conspicuous clinical signs and a severe course of disease progression are clear indicators to employ anthelmintic intervention for the welfare of infected host, but those that are asymptomatic should not be neglected. Untreated infection increases the zoonotic risk (1), can lead to the development of predisposition to other diseases, and may cause silent undiagnosed morbidity. Unfortunately, there are currently no biochemical markers to assess the impact of *D. repens* infections.

The aim of this study was to determine if natural *D. repens* infection leads to biological changes, which may be detected in a real-life clinical situation, where animals are presented to clinicians for unrelated issues, and *D. repens* comorbidity is incidentally identified during inspection.

Abbreviations: ALP, alkaline phosphatase; ALT, alanine aminotransferase; AST, aspartate transaminase; EDTA, ethylene diamine tetraacetic acid; MCH, mean corpuscular hemoglobin; MCHC, mean corpuscular hemoglobin concentration; MCV, mean corpuscular volume; PCR, polymerase chain reaction; RBC, red blood cell; PMN, polymorphonuclear leukocytes; WBC, white blood cells: leukocytes; Mf, microfilariae.

MATERIALS AND METHODS

Study Design

The flow chart of the study design is shown in **Figure 1**.

Animals

A total of 415 dogs of different breeds, sexes, body weights, health, and breeding status, aged 1–17 years were admitted to the study. Those patients were presented to veterinary clinics for regular health issues and/or because they used to live with dogs previously infected with *D. repens*. All examined dogs lived in Poland and had never left the country before the study.

Sampling

Patients underwent routine physical examination and blood test. *Dirofilaria repens* infection was diagnosed by direct analysis of blood smears, stained blood smears, adult worm examination (if obtained surgically, $n = 24$), and multiplex PCR.

Five dogs with confirmed *Babesia canis* infections were excluded from the data analysis to obtain the pattern characteristic for only one vector-borne disease.

Dogs were assigned to the infected group if at least one of the three parasitological examinations was positive for *D. repens*, and the rest of animals with negative results were qualified to the uninfected group.

We initially compared the parameters within all 415 dogs; 197 were infected, and 218 were uninfected with *D. repens*. Then, within the entire study population, we selected a subpopulation of 214 (98 infected and 112 uninfected) dogs having hematological and biochemical blood parameters within normal reference ranges. We believe that this group represents the asymptomatic patients diagnosed with *D. repens* incidentally.

Laboratory Analysis

Parasitological Examination

Adult worms isolated during surgical procedures were examined under a light microscope and, based on their morphology, were identified as *D. repens*. Microfilariae were detected by microscopic examination of blood smear. Subsequently, genomic DNA was isolated from blood samples using the Blood Mini kit

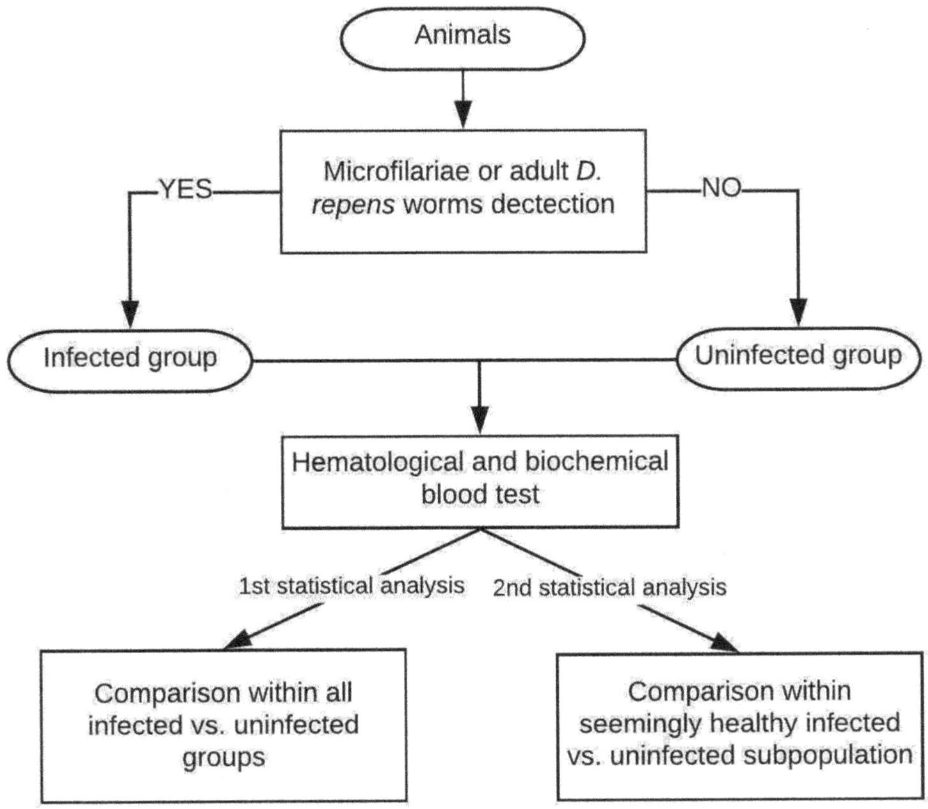

FIGURE 1 | Study design: The examined dogs were classified into the infected group based on the presence of Mf in blood smear/positive result of multiplex PCR/adult *D. repens* parasites found during surgery. Then, blood tests were performed on all individuals. The first statistical analysis included all patients, while the second analysis was performed on a seemingly clinically healthy subpopulation of dogs having blood check-up results within normal reference ranges.

(AA Biotechnology, Poland) and used as a template for multiplex PCR in order to discriminate between *D. immitis* and *D. repens* species according to Gioia et al. (11). PCR results were analyzed by electrophoresis on 2% agarose gels. All infected dogs tested positive for *D. repens* and none for *D. immitis*.

Hematological and Biochemical Analysis

Hematological and biochemical analysis were performed in commercial veterinary diagnostic laboratories. The following standard blood check-up parameters were determined and evaluated according to reference ranges (**Table 1**): white blood cell count (WBC), neutrophil count, lymphocyte count, eosinophil count, red blood cell count (RBC), packed cell volume (hematocrit, HCT), mean corpuscular volume (MCV), platelet count (PLT), enzyme activity [alanine aminotransferase (ALT), aspartate aminotransferase (AST), alkaline phosphatase (ALP)], and metabolite concentration [total protein (TP), glucose, urea, and creatinine].

TABLE 1 | Normal reference values of investigated hematological and biochemical parameters.

	Unit	Reference intervals
RBC	T/L	5–8
HCT	%	35–60
MCV	fL	55–80
PLT	G/L	100–500
WBC	G/L	5–16
AST	U/L	<100
ALT	U/L	<100
ALP	U/L	<200
TP	g/L	50–80
Glucose	mmol/L	3.8–6.7
Urea	mmol/L	3–12
Creatinine	μmol/L	<150

Statistical Analysis

The number of dogs included in both statistical analyses with respect to their hematological and biochemical blood parameters differed due to missing data of some individuals.

Data were presented as a mean ± standard deviation (SD) or a median and interquartile range (IQR) and compared between groups using the unpaired-sample Student's *t*-test or Mann–Whitney U-test depending on the asymmetry of a variable distribution assessed on the basis of histograms. The range was always presented. Categorical variables were presented as the number and proportion of dogs in a given group and compared between groups using the Pearson's chi-square test. Ninety-five percent confidence intervals (95% CI) for proportions were calculated with the Wilson score method (12). A two-tailed significance level (α) was set at 0.05. Total study population analysis was performed in Statistica 12 (StatSoft Inc., Tulsa, OK). The analysis of the subpopulation of dog parameters within normal reference range was performed in TIBCO Statistica 13.3.0 (TIBCO StatSoft Inc., Palo Alto, CA).

The Analysis of Check-Up Parameters Within the Total Study Population

This included 415 dogs: 225 males (54.2%) and 190 females (35.8%). Their age ranged from 8 months to 17 years with the median of 7 years (IQR from 4 to 10 years) and did not differ between sexes ($p = 0.655$). There were 56 castrated dogs (13.5%) and 112 (27.0%) pedigree dogs. Their body weight varied from 1 to 75 kg with the median of 16 kg (IQR from 10 to 25 kg).

Two hundred eighteen dogs (52.5%) were allocated to the infected group and 197 (47.5%) to the uninfected group, respectively. Infected dogs were significantly heavier ($p = 0.041$) and more often belonged to a particular breed ($p < 0.001$).

The Analysis of Parameters Within the Subpopulation Having Results Within Normal Range Values

This included 214 out of 415 dogs with blood check-up within or only slightly (by not more than 25% of the upper limit) deviated from the reference intervals. There were 121 males (56.5%) and 93 females (43.5%). Their age ranged from 1 to 14 years with the arithmetic mean (SD) of 6.8 (3.2) years and did not differ significantly between males and females ($p = 0.190$). There were 171 cross-breed dogs (79.9%) and 43 pedigree dogs (20.1%) belonging to the following breeds: German shepherd ($n = 9$), Yorkshire terrier ($n = 5$), Border collie ($n = 4$), Labrador retriever ($n = 3$), French bulldog ($n = 3$), Chesapeake retriever ($n = 2$), Boxer ($n = 2$), Bavarian mountain dog ($n = 2$), Belgian shepherd ($n = 2$), and Alaskan malamute, Amstaff, Polish hound, Black Russia terrier, Akita Inu, Dachshund, Chinese Crested dog, Bernese Mountain dog, Pug, Poodle, and Welsh terrier ($n = 1$ each).

RESULTS

We first compared blood hematology and biochemistry results within the entire study population. Dogs infected with *D. repens* compared to uninfected individuals had significantly lower lymphocyte count ($p < 0.001$), RBC ($p < 0.001$), Ht ($p = 0.001$), and thrombocyte count ($p = 0.025$) and higher ALP ($p = 0.016$) and creatinine ($p = 0.023$) activity (**Table 2**).

In order to determine if observed changes were present only in patients with abnormal blood test results, we decided to select a subpopulation of dogs having parameters within normal values, which we believe mainly represents the undiagnosed dogs infected with skin dirofilariosis in real-clinical practice. Interestingly, in clinically healthy dogs, animals infected with *D. repens* had significantly reduced RBC ($p = 0.025$), Ht ($p = 0.002$), and lymphocyte ($p = 0.031$) count and significantly elevated glucose concentration ($p = 0.023$). ALP activity was boarder line elevated ($p = 0.054$) (**Table 3**).

DISCUSSION

D. repens is by far the most prevalent causative agent of human and canine dirofilariosis in Europe (1). It is generally believed that *D. repens* infections in dogs are asymptomatic, but several case reports (5–7) and the results of blood parameters in our study suggest that the illness is not non-pathogenic but goes rather undetected.

Underdiagnosis of skin dirofilariosis is mainly due to the lack of diagnostic tools to detect occult infections. Amicrofilaremic infections can occur after previous antiparasitic treatment based on macrocyclic lactones, long prepatent time of the infection or monosex infection. Microfilariae periodicity and low intensity of microfilaremia also contribute to obtaining false negative results while investigating a dog for skin dirofilariosis. In contrast, clinicians are left to their own devices for diagnosing and interpreting importance of *D. repens* infections. Thus, having hematological and biochemical biomarker to suggest the presence and severity of infection might be a supportive tool for managing the disease progression, especially in asymptomatic patients.

Our first analysis of all dogs admitted to the study mirrored the real-clinical scenario of dogs brought for different reasons and showed that dogs additionally infected with *D. repens* compared to those uninfected had significantly lower RBC, thrombocyte, and lymphocyte counts, decreased Ht, and increased ALP activity.

The second analysis included a subpopulation of dogs having parameters within normal reference ranges, and in this group, differences were observed in infected animals, such as lower RBC, Ht, lymphocytes, and higher glucose and elevated boarder line ALP activity comparing to the uninfected group. Despite presenting as clinically healthy dogs, these alterations indicate that *D. repens* infection influenced the functioning of their body.

Statistically significant hematological alterations and ALP increase in dogs infected with *D. repens* are similar to those observed in other filarial disease, especially *D. immitis* infections (13), so the pathogenicity, as claimed by other authors (5, 14), is rather correlated with Mf than the presence of adult parasites.

The lower RBC, hematocrit, and hemoglobin characterize anemia in dogs and may be a result of destructive capability of Mf associated with severe intravascular hemolysis as reported in dogs infected with *Diptelonema reconditum* (15). It also might be connected to inflammation-associated production of pro-inflammatory cytokines resulting in suppression of erythrocytes production and inhibition of iron absorption and utilization (16). Lower thrombocyte count may be due to platelet consumption or presence of antiplatelet antibodies observed in dogs infected with other vector-borne diseases (17) or might be assigned to immune-mediated platelet destruction as reported in dogs infected with *D. immitis* (13). Lymphopenia was not only observed in infected patients in this study but also reported

TABLE 2 | Hematological and biochemical parameters in the total study population.

Parameter	Infected		Uninfected		
Hematology	***n***	**Mean ± SD (range)**	***n***	**Mean ± SD (range)**	***t*-test *p*-value**
WBC (G/L)	206	14.9 ± 9.2 (4.7–84.7)	192	14.5 ± 6.2 (3.5–50.4)	0.640
Neutrophils (G/L)	177	10.4 ± 6.5 (1.6–63.8)	189	10.1 ± 5.4 (1.4–39.8)	0.636
Lymphocytes (G/L)	177	2.4 ± 1.5 (0–9.0)	189	3.1 ± 1.6 (0–9.4)	<0.001
Eosinophils (G/L)	177	0.9 ± 0.9 (0–5.1)	189	0.9 ± 1.0 (0–6.2)	0.904
Erythrocytes (T/L)	206	6.7 ± 1.1 (3.6–10.0)	191	7.1 ± 1.0 (3.7–9.9)	<0.001
Haematocrit (%)	206	43.2 ± 6.8 (22–60)	192	45.5 ± 6.3 (22–65)	0.001
MCV (fl)	206	64.8 ± 4.5 (36–77)	192	64.5 ± 3.5 (53–79)	0.404
PLT (G/L)	206	316 ± 160 (13–1000)	192	351 ± 169 (33–1000)	0.025
Biochemistry	***n***	**Median, IQR (range)**	***n***	**Median, IQR (range)**	**Mann-Whitey *U*-test *p*-value**
AST (U/L)	178	32.1, 25.7–43.1 (2.0–689)	167	33.1, 27.5–40.7 (10.5–178)	0.604
ALT (U/L)	182	41.4, 30.0–73.4 (1.3–3026)	167	41.5, 31.2–56.0 (6.9–765)	0.476
ALP (U/L)	168	48.3, 32.3–84.4 (1.0–2015)	167	42.0, 31.3–59.6 (15.0–1302)	0.016
Total protein (g/L)	143	60, 56–64 (40–99)	166	59, 55–63 (38–88)	0.263
Glucose (mmol/L)[a]	152	4.6, 3.8–5.4 (1.1–19.3)	164	4.5, 3.6–5.3 (1.3–17.2)	0.320
Urea (mmol/L)[b]	184	5.4, 4.2–6.9 (1.2–44.6)	165	5.2, 4.3–6.5 (2.0–39.0)	0.663
Creatinine (μmol/L)[c]	184	88.4, 70.7–106.1 (26.5–539.2)	166	79.6, 70.7–97.2 (44.2–592.3)	0.023

[a] *To convert into mg/dL multiply by 18.*
[b] *To convert into mg/dL multiply by 6.03.*
[c] *To convert into mg/dL multiply by 0.011.*

in another dog infected with *D. repens* (5) and during other canine-borne vector diseases. The mechanism of lymphopenia might be associated to endogenous glucocorticoids release that occurs in response to infectious stimuli or stress, which leads to lymphocyte apoptosis or sequestration of lymphocytes in lymphoid organs (18).

The increase in creatinine was observed in the first analysis in the infected group compared to the uninfected group in our study but was not shown to be statistically significant in dogs infected with *D. immitis.* On the contrary, another parameter suggesting renal damage (urea) was increased in *D. immitis*-infected patients but not in our *D. repens*-infected group (13). A case report describing the most severe course of skin dirofilariosis of a dog coinfected with *D. immitis* suggested that only *D. repens* Mf were involved in kidney damage. However, other reports suggest that microfilaremic (not occult) dogs infected with *D. immitis* show marked signs of kidney damage (14, 19, 20).

ALP was significantly higher in infected dogs. Although not being highly liver specific (21), ALP is a marker having a good sensitivity for liver diseases in dogs, suggesting cholestasic disease or chronic hepatitis/cirrhosis. Other parameters suggesting liver injuries, as ALT and AST were reported to be increased in case reports of dogs infected with *D. repens* (5, 22) and in some dogs in our study. This difference, however, was not statistically significant while comparing the infected and uninfected group, suggesting a rather big variability between infected individuals. Interestingly, the ALP increase was also the only liver parameter changed in *D. immitis*-infected dogs (13). The increase in ALP activity, with AST and ALT activity within normal values, makes a hepatocellular damage unlikely and might be rather due to chronic stress associated with increase in endogenous glucocorticoids (23), although, in patients having elevated AST, ALT, and ALP activity, an injury of the liver was very likely.

A higher level of glucose was observed in dogs infected with *D. repens* having all blood parameters within normal ranges. This also may be the result of higher glucocorticoids levels in these animals, which again suggests a correlation between *D. repens* and development of chronic stress response. Interestingly, glucose level was not significantly changed while the whole population was analyzed, which might suggest that, after development of concomitant disease, the host's body reaction to the infection changes.

TABLE 3 | Hematological and biochemical parameters in clinically healthy dogs with blood check-up results within normal reference ranges.

Parameter	Infected		Uninfected		
	n	mean ± SD (range)	*n*	mean ± SD (range)	*t*-test*p*-value
Hematology					
WBC (G/L)	93	11.89 ± 3.39 (5.1–18.4)	121	12.67 ± 3.65 (5.3–19.6)	0.110
Neutrophils (G/L)	93	8.33 ± 2.98 (1.6–16.2)	121	8.74 ± 3.23 (2.7–16.9)	0.343
Lymphocytes (G/L)	93	2.65 ± 1.46 (0.1–6.4)	121	3.07 ± 1.33 (0.6–7.0)	0.031
		2.3 (1.6–3.4)[a]		2.8 (2.1–4.0)[a]	0.007[b]
Eosinophils (G/L)	93	0.93 ± 0.87 (0–3.5)	121	0.86 ± 0.85 (0–5.6)	0.580
		0.7 (0.3–1.2)[a]		0.7 (0.3–1.1)[a]	0.645[b]
RBC (T/L)	93	7.03 ± 0.78 (5.2–8.9)	121	7.25 ± 0.69 (5.6–9.5)	0.025
Ht (%)	93	45.1 ± 4.5 (35–55)	121	47.0 ± 4.3 (36–56)	0.002
MCV (fl)	93	64.4 ± 3.8 (53–74)	121	65.1 ± 3.3 (58–79)	0.173
PLT (G/L)	93	320 ± 103 (110–598)	121	300 ± 98 (99–565)	0.136
Biochemistry					
AST (U/L)	84	31.9 ± 10.3 (13–66)	101	34.4± 10.1 (11-66)	0.095
ALT (U/L)	84	42.1 ± 19.2 (1–99)	101	42.4 ± 17.2 (14–94)	0.900
ALP (U/L)	82	54.3 ± 35.7 (1–163)	101	45.3 ± 23.5 (15–167)	0.054
		43 (30–63)[a]		40 (31–53)[a]	0.258[b]
Total Protein (g/L)	75	60.3 ± 5.8 (50–76)	100	60.2 ± 6.2 (50–77)	0.902
Glucose (mmol/L)[c]	80	4.76 ± 1.08 (1.6–7.6)	100	4.39 ± 1.07 (2.1–7.6)	0.023
Urea (mmol/L)[d]	85	5.29 ± 1.49 (3.0–12.0)	99	5.42 ± 1.46 (2.1–9.0)	0.537
Creatinine (μmol/L)[e]	85	83.83 ± 19.81 (23.9–130.0)	100	84.33 ± 20.84 (43.3–138.8)	0.868

[a]*Median (IQR).*
[b]*Mann-Whitney U-test.*
[c]*To convert into mg/dL multiply by 18.*
[d]*To convert into mg/dL multiply by 6.03.*
[e]*To convert into mg/dL multiply by 0.011.*

Sometimes parasitological coinfection might positively influence the course of the main disease. For example, it has been reported that coinfection of malaria and hookworms seems to increase malaria incidence but at the same time might protect from malaria severe manifestations in humans (24). Moreover, dogs infected solely with *Babesia canis* compared to those coinfected with *D. repens* displayed more pronounced biochemical changes, implying coinfection with *D. repens* was somehow beneficially counteracting against renal and liver damage characteristic for the course of babesiosis in dogs (9), although in the same study, the authors reported that thrombocytopenia and anemia concomitant with babesiosis in dogs were aggravated in individuals coinfected with *D. repens*. Our results show differences in blood parameters between seemingly asymptomatic *D. repens* patients and uninfected dogs. *D. repens* infection seems to promote glucocorticoids release as chronic stress response associated with lymphopenia, glucose level, and ALP activity increase that may predispose infected individuals to develop other infectious, metabolic, or hormonal diseases in the future. This in turn might explain why dogs presented with different diseases and at the same time coinfected with *D. repens* had more serious alternations in blood parameters than uninfected dogs. We suspect that the chronic stress response observed in seemingly healthy dogs may lead to more deepened alternations of concomitant diseases in the future.

There are several limitations in the presented study, such as no checkups or no final diagnosis of concomitant disease available for all admitted dogs. However, we aimed to show a trend in blood parameter changes related to *D. repens* infection. In dogs with different ailments as well as in asymptomatic dogs, significant differences in blood parameters were noted. Our data suggest that *D. repens* infection indeed induces some biological changes in the host. The length of the infection is not known either, but in naturally infected dogs, it cannot be evaluated. However, this mirrors more adequately the real clinical approach to the problem of increasing spread of *D. repens* parasite.

Our results indicate that *D. repens* infection complicates concomitant diseases, and animals develop more serious and detectable changes such as lower numbers of erythrocytes, lymphocytes, and thrombocytes and higher activity of ALP and creatinine. Even among dogs with blood results within normal reference ranges, individuals infected with *D. repens* showed detectable differences compared to uninfected ones, suggesting that seemingly healthy animals may still have altered biological processes or early indications of disease. The analysis of parameters within dogs having results within normal reference ranges, where the differences between groups are indeed within normal values, suggests a trend and perhaps a predisposition of development of other diseases in the future. Further studies with cortisol level evaluation, the measurements of total but also differentiation between liver ALP (L-ALP) and corticosteroid

ALP (C-ALP) isoforms in infected dogs with full follow-ups could be valuable.

CONCLUSIONS

Our paper describes hematological and biochemical changes in dogs naturally infected with *D. repens*. Alterations such as a decrease in RBC, lymphocytes, thrombocytes, hematocrit, as well as increases in ALP and creatinine could be indicators of coinfection with *D. repens*, especially in endemic regions. Furthermore, the results in clinically healthy dogs suggest that the presence of *D. repens* might lead to development of anemia and a state of chronic stress response, characterized by the combination of lymphopenia and increase in glucose level and ALP activity and, as such, predispose infected dogs to other ailments. This could explain the existence of more serious statistically significant blood parameters alternations in dogs with different ailments simultaneously coinfected with *D. repens*.

Our results strongly indicate that *D. repens* infection has a pejorative influence on the health of the canine host independent of their clinical condition. Finally, the pathogenicity of *D. repens* remains a mystery but needs further investigation in order to comprehend its association with chronic stress response in infected individuals.

ETHICS STATEMENT

Ethical review and approval was not required for the animal study because the blood samples were collected for direct benefit of the patients and the analysis was performed on leftover samples (Act of 15th January 2015 on the protection of animals used for scientific purposes). The director of veterinary services of local dog shelters and the owners of privately owned dogs were informed about the results of Dirofilaria testing of the dogs under their care. Written informed consent for participation was not obtained from the owners because no interventions outside routine care were performed. All blood samples were taken during routine checkups or process of diagnosis in veterinary clinics and only then the results were used to compare the results between *D. repens* infected and uninfected groups of dogs. Multiplex PCR was run on the leftover blood samples. A verbal consent of the owners' to voluntirely test their animals for skin dirofilariosis was present for all dogs admitted in the study. All data were de-indentified before running statistical analysis and the entire anonymity of data has been assured. The director of local dog shelters and the owners of client-owned dogs were informed about the results of Dirofilaria testing of the dogs under their care. Doctors of veterinary medicine were provided with all information that could help them to introduce the best treatment to infected dogs.

AUTHOR CONTRIBUTIONS

AD and MK collected clinical data, parasitic, biological specimens, and performed blood smears. ED and MEW performed PCR. MC performed the statistical analysis of the results. MEW, AD, MK, ED, PJ, and MW planned and discussed the study and the results. MEW wrote the manuscript. All authors read and approved the final version of the manuscript.

ACKNOWLEDGMENTS

The authors are grateful to Bayer Animal Health Poland for supplying reagents to perform laboratory works of the study and providing the possibility to collect the samples and to Mark Kaji for constructive criticism and proofreading the article.

REFERENCES

1. Capelli G, Genchi C, Baneth G, Bourdeau P, Brianti E, Cardoso L, et al. Recent advances on Dirofilaria repens in dogs and humans in Europe. *Parasites Vectors.* (2018) 11:663. doi: 10.1186/s13071-018-3205-x
2. Diaz JH. Increasing risks of human dirofilariasis in travelers. *J Travel Med.* (2015) 22:116–23. doi: 10.1111/jtm.12174
3. Ermakova L, Nagorny S, Pshenichnaya N. Clinical and laboratory features of human dirofilariasis in Russia. *IDCases.* (2017) 9:112–5. doi: 10.1016/j.idcr.2017.07.006
4. Pampiglione S, Rivasi F, Angeli G, Boldorini R, Incensati RM, Pastormerlo M, et al. Dirofilariasis due to *Dirofilaria repens* in Italy, an emergent zoonosis: report of 60 new cases. *Histopathology.* (2001) 38:344–54. doi: 10.1046/j.1365-2559.2001.01099.x
5. Mircean M, Ionică AM, Mircean V, Györke A, Codea AR, Tăbăran FA, et al. Clinical and pathological effects of *Dirofilaria repens* and *Dirofilaria immitis* in a dog with a natural co-infection. *Parasitol Int.* (2017) 66:331–4. doi: 10.1016/j.parint.2017.02.003
6. Pazdzior-Czapula K, Ostrocka-Domagala I, Myrdek P, Mikiewicz M, Gesek M. *Dirofilaria repens* — an etiological factor or an incidental finding in cytologic and histopathologic biopsies from dogs. *Vet Clin Pathol.* (2018) 47:307–11. doi: 10.1111/vcp.12597
7. Harrus S, Harmelin A, Rodrig S, Favia G. *Dirofilaria repens* infection in a dog in Israel. *Am J Trop Med Hyg.* (1999) 61:639–41. doi: 10.4269/ajtmh.1999.61.639
8. Borkowski PK, Rymkiewicz G, Golebiewska J, Nestoros N, Romejko-Jarosinska J, Zarnowska-Prymek H, et al. The first case of human autochtonous subconjunctival dirofilariosis in Poland and MALT lymphoma as possible consequence of this parasitosis. *Infect Agent Cancer.* (2015) 10:1–5. doi: 10.1186/1750-9378-10-1
9. Bajer A, Rodo A, Mierzejewska EJ, Tokasz K, Welc-faleciak R. The prevalence of *Dirofilaria repens* in cats, healthy dogs and dogs with concurrent babesiosis in an expansion zone in central Europe. *BMC Vet Res.* (2016) 12:183. doi: 10.1186/s12917-016-0816-3
10. Schwan EV, Miller DB, De Kock D, Van Heerden A. *Dirofilaria repens* in a cat with acute liver failure. *J S Afr Vet Assoc.* (2000) 71:197–200. doi: 10.4102/jsava.v71i3.713
11. Gioia G, Lecová L, Genchi M, Ferri E, Genchi C, Mortarino M. Highly sensitive multiplex PCR for simultaneous detection and discrimination of *Dirofilaria immitis* and *Dirofilaria repens* in canine peripheral blood. *Vet Parasitol.* (2010) 172:160–3. doi: 10.1016/j.vetpar.2010.04.027
12. Altman DG, Machin D, Bryant TN, Gardner M. *Statistics With Confidence.* 2nd ed. Bristol: BMJ Books (2000).
13. Niwetpathomwat A, Kaewthamasorn M, Tiawsirisup S, Techangamsuwan S, Suvarnvibhaja S. A retrospective study of the clinical hematology and the serum biochemistry tests made on canine dirofilariasis cases in an animal hospital population in Bangkok, Thailand. *Res Vet Sci.* (2007) 82:364–9. doi: 10.1016/j.rvsc.2006.09.002
14. Morchón R, Carretón E, Grandi G, González-Miguel J, Montoya-Alonso JA, Simón F, et al. Anti-*Wolbachia* surface protein antibodies are present in the urine of dogs naturally infected with *Dirofilaria immitis* with circulating

microfilariae but not in dogs with occult infections. *Vector-Borne Zoonotic Dis.* (2012) 12:17–20. doi: 10.1089/vbz.2010.0211
15. Hashem M, Badawy A. Hematological and biochemical studies on filariasis of dogs. *Internet J Vet Med.* (2012) 4:1–7. Available online at: https://ispub.com/IJVM/4/2/3275
16. Sankaran VG, Weiss MJ. Anemia: progress in molecular mechanisms and therapy. *Nat Med.* (2015) 21:221–30. doi: 10.1038/nm.3814
17. Shaw SE, Day MJ, Birtles RJ, Breitschwerdt EB. Tick-borne infectious diseases of dogs. *Trends Parasitol.* (2001) 17:74–80. doi: 10.1016/S1471-4922(00)01856-0
18. Harvey JW. Evaluation of leukocytic disorders. *Vet Hematol.* (2012) 122–76. doi: 10.1016/B978-1-4377-0173-9.00005-1
19. Simón F, Siles-Lucas M, Morchón R, González-Miguel J, Mellado I, Carretón E, et al. Human and animal dirofilariasis: the emergence of a zoonotic mosaic. *Clin Microbiol Rev.* (2012) 25:507–44. doi: 10.1128/CMR.00012-12
20. Abramowsky CR, Powers KG, Aikawa M, Swinehart G. *Dirofilaria immitis.* 5. Immunopathology of filarial nephropathy in dogs. *Am J Pathol.* (1981) 104:1–2.
21. Dirksen K, Burgener IA, Rothuizen J, van den Ingh TSGAM, Penning LC, Spee B, et al. Sensitivity and specificity of plasma ALT, ALP, and bile acids for hepatitis in labrador retrievers. *J Vet Intern Med.* (2017) 31:1017–27. doi: 10.1111/jvim.14716
22. Osińska B, Demiaszkiewicz AW, Pyziel AM, Kuligowska I, Lachowicz J, Dolka I. Prevalence of *Dirofilaria repens* in dogs in central-eastern Poland and histopathological changes caused by this infection. *Bull Vet Inst Pulawy.* (2014) 58:35–9. doi: 10.2478/bvip-2014-0006
23. Fernandez NJ, Kidney BA. Alkaline phosphatase : beyond the liver. *Vet Clin Pathol.* (2007) 36:223-3. doi: 10.1111/j.1939-165X.2007.tb00216.x
24. Nacher M. Interactions between worms and malaria: good worms or bad worms? *Malar J.* (2011) 10:259. doi: 10.1186/1475-2875-10-259

6

Tackling the Threat of Rabies Reintroduction

Santiago Vega [1†], Laura Lorenzo-Rebenaque [1†], Clara Marin [1†], Rosana Domingo [1] and Fernando Fariñas [2†]*

[1] Facultad de Veterinaria, Instituto de Ciencias Biomédicas, Universidad Cardenal Herrera-CEU, CEU Universities, Alfara del Patriarca, Spain, [2] Instituto de Inmunología Clínica y Enfermedades Infecciosas. Grupo One Health, Malaga, Spain

***Correspondence:**
Clara Marin
clara.marin@uchceu.es

† These authors have contributed equally to this work

Rabies is one of the oldest, most important zoonoses worldwide due to its extreme and inevitably lethal nature, causing one death every 9 min worldwide. Recent reports have demonstrated that the *Lyssavirus* continues more alive than ever, despite the control carried out against the virus throughout Europe. In this context, this work reviews the main immunological implications, transmission risk factors and current prevention measures for virus control in Europe, and especially in Spain.

Keywords: rabies, *Lyssavirus*, One Health, zoonosis, dog, bat, Europe

INTRODUCTION

Rabies is one of the oldest and most important zoonoses worldwide, due to its extreme and inevitably lethal outcomes (1, 2). Although the enzootic transmission of rabies is through Carnivora (dogs, jackals, wolves, etc.) and Chiroptera (bats), it can spill over to other mammalian species such as humans, who can end up developing the disease (2). Each year, rabies is estimated to be responsible for 59,000 human cases, mostly in Africa and Asia, and ~99% of human rabies cases are acquired after direct contact with dogs (3–5). The infection usually causes acute progressive encephalitis, and death eventually occurs if it is not treated before symptoms appear (1, 4). Although rabies remains one of the most feared and important threats to public health in the 21st century, it is considered one of the neglected diseases (2, 3).

WHAT HAVE WE LEARNED FROM RABIES DISEASE?

Rabies, a Long Etiological History

Rabies is caused by a group of neurotropic viruses of the genus *Lyssavirus*, belonging to the family *Rhabdoviridae* and order *Mononegavirales* (1, 6). This disease has been known since at least the 23rd century BC (Before Christ) in the Eshuma Code of Babylon (1). Moreover, the Greek ancient world called the disease "lyssa" (after the Greek goddess of madness, rage, and frenzy), due to the clinical signs it presented (6, 7). Since then, rabies has been present worldwide, except in Antarctica (4). The *Lyssavirus* contains a single-stranded RNA genome of negative sense, which encodes five structural proteins: nucleoprotein (N), phosphoprotein (P), matrix protein (M), glycoprotein (G) and the RNA-dependent RNA polymerase (L), in the order 3′-N-P-M-G-L-5′ 7 (6). Currently, the International Committee on Taxonomy of Viruses (ICTV) has delineated the genus into seventeen species, plus one related virus not yet taxonomically assessed, and segregated into three phylogroups (I, II, III-IV) (**Table 1**) (8, 9).

TABLE 1 | Classification of the species of the genus *Lyssavirus* and geographical distribution.

Phylogroup	Specie	Virus name	Distribution
I	*Aravan lyssavirus*	Aravan virus	Central Asia
I	*Australian bat lyssavirus*	Australian bat lyssavirus	Australia
I	*Bokeloh bat lyssavirus*	Bokeloh bat lyssavirus	Europe
I	*Duvenhage lyssavirus*	Duvenhage virus	Southern Africa
I	*European bat 1 lyssavirus*	European bat 1 lyssavirus	Europe
I	*European bat 2 lyssavirus*	European bat 2 lyssavirus	Europe
	Gannoruwa bat lyssavirus	Gannoruwa bat lyssavirus	Asia
III-IV	*Ikoma lyssavirus*	Ikoma lyssavirus	Africa
I	*Irkut lyssavirus*	Irkut virus	East Siberia
I	*Khujand lyssavirus*	Khujand virus	Central Asia
II	*Lagos bat lyssavirus*	Lagos bat virus	Africa
III-IV	*Lleida bat lyssavirus*	Lleida bat lyssavirus	Europe (Spain)
II	*Mokola lyssavirus*	Mokola virus	Sub-Saharan Africa
I	*Rabies lyssavirus*	Rabies virus	Worldwide (except several islands)
II	*Shimoni bat lyssavirus*	Shimoni bat virus	East Africa
I	*Taiwan bat lyssavirus*	Taiwan bat lyssavirus	–
III-IV	*West Caucasian bat lyssavirus*	West Caucasian bat virus	Caucasian region
I	–	Kotalahti bat lyssavirus	–
Unclassified viruses	–	Taiwan bat lyssavirus	–

Fifteen of the seventeen lyssavirus species are hosted by bats (10). Indeed, bats are considered to be the ancestral hosts of lyssaviruses, and although the risk of human exposure is low, sporadic human rabies cases infected through a bat bite have been reported (10–13). Thus, from an epidemiological point of view, there are two epidemiological cycles: terrestrial rabies, maintained by domestic and wild carnivores, and rabies in chiropterans, where the virus is maintained in colonies of bats, both blood-sucking and insectivores or frugivores (14). Furthermore, it is difficult to differentiate the symptoms of the disease caused by any *Lyssavirus* species (10, 11).

Rabies, a Hazardous Disease

The disease has a marked neurotropic character and its action on the nervous system gives rise to a characteristic manifestation of disease with excitatory signs, hallucinations and hydrophobia (furious rabies), or signs of generalised paralysis and coma (paralytic rabies), as a consequence of generally fatal encephalomyelitis (1, 4). As there is no clinical treatment, post-exposure prophylaxis has been demonstrated to be the most effective method to control and prevent human rabies cases worldwide (4). Based on the importance of prevention, the European Union has been focused on the need for the elimination of wildlife rabies in European countries by 2020 (15). Moreover, rabies control under a One Health approach is a top priority for the World Health Organisation (WHO), Food and Agriculture Organisation (FAO), World Organisation for Animal Health (OIE), and Global Alliance for Rabies Control (GARC). These agencies have set the goal of the elimination of dog-mediated human rabies by 2030 (4).

Diagnostic Tools

Rabies diagnosis has been historically based on histopathological methods, such as cytoplasmic inclusion bodies detection (Negri bodies) (16, 17). At present, this methodology has been replaced by immunofluorescence. Also, when virus isolation has been necessary, rabies tissue culture infection or the mouse inoculation test has been used (16, 17). Currently, new techniques are being used for the diagnosis of the virus, such as flow cytometry (18), mass spectrometry (19), immunochromatographic tests and the polymerase chain reaction (PCR) (17).

HISTORICAL OVERVIEW OF RABIES IN EUROPE

Since the earliest descriptions of the disease, the presence of the virus in dogs and wildlife has been reported in European countries (20). In dogs, rabies was endemic until the enforcement of regulations in the keeping of dogs and development of the vaccination progressively eliminated rabies in dogs during the 20th century (20, 21). Although Pasteur developed the earliest effective vaccine against rabies in dogs in 1885, the development and implementation of domestic animal vaccination was carried out from the 1920s (1). With the development of these prevention measures, rabies in dogs was eliminated from European countries, except for the European part of Turkey (22).

However, during the 1940s and thereafter, the disease emerged and became established in the red fox (*Vulpes Vulpes*) population between Russia and Poland, spreading southwards and westwards, and at its maximum extension in the early 1990s reached Southern France (2, 23). At this point, several European governments, with financial support from the European Union, rolled out oral rabies vaccination (**ORV**) campaigns in foxes, laying out the vaccines in baits, which managed to control vulpine rabies (22, 24). The development of ORV was a breakthrough for fox rabies control, and has resulted in the elimination of fox rabies from western Europe, with rapid progress also being made toward elimination in eastern Europe (22). Nevertheless, another rabies wildlife epidemiological cycle, maintained by the racoon dog (*Nyctereutes procyonides*), has been developed in the Baltic countries, many parts of eastern Europe, and Finland (25, 26). The racoon dog was introduced into the European part of Russia by the fur industry from eastern Asia in the first half of the 20th century, and has expanded throughout Europe (25, 26). The potential role of the raccoon dog in rabies transmission has been proven in rabies-free European areas, where the virus re-emerged due to this infected host (27). Therefore, the blueprint for eliminating wildlife-mediated rabies has also been extended to raccoon dogs (21).

Currently, most European countries are considered free of classical rabies, with confirmed rabies cases restricted to bats (1). The first evidence of infected European bat was reported in 1954 in Germany (28). From then on, the cases in bats were regarded as scientific curiosities, until 1985, when the intensive surveillance established after the first human case revealed more than a thousand bat rabies cases in Europe (28, 29).

Six lyssaviruses are reported to circulate in Europe: *European bat 1 lyssavirus* (EBLV-1), *European bat 2 lyssavirus* (EBLV-2), *Bokeloh bat lyssavirus* (BBLV), *West Caucasian bat lyssavirus* (WCBV), *Lleida bat lyssavirus* (LLEBV) and *Kotalahti bat lyssavirus* (KBLV) (30). Four of the viruses, EBLV-1, EBLV-2, BBLV, and KBLV, are associated with European bats of the family *Vespertilionidae* (30). Moreover, the other two lyssaviruses, WCBV and LLEBV, are linked to bats of the family *Miniopteridae* (30). Of these, only EBLV-1 and EBLV-2 have been reported to have caused rabies in humans, and more than 90% of the bat rabies cases have been associated with the bat species *Eptesicus serotinus* ***(E. serotinus)*** infected by EBLV-1 (12). The last European Union One Health 2018 Zoonoses Report confirmed bats as a reservoir for rabies in Europe, as it was present in 2% of the bats sampled (31). In this sense, taking samples from bats is the cornerstone to the knowledge of the dynamics of rabies within their hosts (32). To this end, guidelines on passive and active surveillance programmes were established by a European research consortium, Med-Vet-Net (33). Passive surveillance could include the investigation of sick or dead bats of all indigenous bat species, for testing lyssavirus infections using the detection methods. Moreover, active surveillance comprises the monitoring of free-living indigenous bats for the detection of viral RNA or virus-neutralising antibodies (33, 34). However, in Europe all bat species have been protected, which should be considered in the design and the undertaking of the surveillance initiatives (32). These studies showed that the principal ecological factors for viral persistence have been cross-species mixing and host migration patterns (10). Thus, the public health hazard of bat rabies must not be underestimated in Europe (31).

The Border Between Europe and the African Continent: The Special Situation of Rabies in Spain

Spain is a country located in South-Western Europe on the Iberian Peninsula. At the southern extreme, it is separated from Morocco in Africa by the Strait of Gibraltar sea channel. The two continents are separated by just fourteen kilometres. On the north-eastern border, the Iberian Peninsula is linked to the rest of Europe through the Pyrenees mountain range, which forms a natural border between Spain and France. The Canary Islands at the Atlantic Ocean and the cities of Ceuta and Melilla in the Northern African coast are also part of Spain.

The first evidence of rabies in Spain was reported in the first century AD (*Anno Domini*), in Roman times (35). Over the centuries, attempts to control rabies had been developing through measures such as the control of the movement of dogs and cats in 1786, or washing of bite wounds with soap in an attempt to prevent the disease in 1863 (35). During the 20th century, Spain focused all its efforts on the elimination of rabies with an anti-rabies programme, until 1966, when rabies was eliminated in dogs, and the country was declared free of rabies for the first time (2, 36). The European vulpine rabies never crossed the Pyrenees due to the French ORV programmes (2, 35). However, in 1975, a new outbreak was declared in Malaga, in southern Spain, which might been related to the geographical proximity with Africa and the intense traffic of people, and the most accepted hypothesis was an introduction from Morocco (35). During the epidemic, the disease spread to 133 animals, 76 dogs, 30 cats, two foxes and six of other species with one human fatality (37). To avoid dog-mediated transmission, health measures were established, which included a dogs census, vaccination of susceptible animals, physical confinement and quarantine measures for suspect animals, control and reduction in the number of stray dogs, and the monitoring of dog bite wounds (35). The outbreak continued until 1978, when Spain was considered rabies-free in terrestrial carnivores (36). Nevertheless, every year, the autonomous cities of Ceuta and Melilla report rabies cases, mostly imported from Morocco (36). Infected animals have been also imported into mainland Spanish territories disregarding the official border controls and eventually spreading to other European countries (38).

Since the control of rabies in non-flying mammals, there has been increasing attention to lyssaviruses associated with European bats (39). The first case of rabies in bats was recorded in 1987 in Valencia (eastern Spain), and some sporadic cases in bats have been reported since then (9). A study carried out from 1992 to 2000 showed that EBLV-1, or even other lyssaviruses with cross-reactive antibodies, could have been circulating among bats of different species in several areas of Spain (40). *Lyssavirus* antibodies were detected in four bat species: *Myotis myotis* (*M. myotis*), *Miniopterus schreibersii* (*M. schreibersii*), *Tadarida teniotis* (*T. tenioti*) and *Rhinolophus ferrumequinum* (*R. ferrumequinum*) (40). Moreover, these findings raised the possibility of *M. schreibersii* as a dispersion vector of the disease in southern Europe due to its seasonal migrations, and the possible African origin of the EBLV-1 present in Spain due to the migrations of *T. teniotis* and *M. schreibersii* (40). During 1998–2003, a study of EBLV-1 viruses from *E. isabellinus* in southern Spain revealed the close communities in which EBLV-1 independently circulates, and yet distinct from other EBLV-1 strains circulating in the serotine bats (41). In addition, recent studies have demonstrated the geographical expansion of EBLV-1 in *E. serotinus* and *E. isabellinus* across Iberian Peninsula from Europe (12). In 2011, a new lyssavirus was confirmed in a *M. schreibersii* in the City of Lleida (north-eastern Spain), analysed as part of the rabies surveillance programme in Spain (42). The novel *Lyssavirus* was named LLEBV, and was classified into phylogroup III (42).

According to the previous premises, the emergence of sporadic human cases due to a bat or dog bite would be potentially feasible. Moreover, the dog is the main source responsible for a possible outbreak in Spain, as there is a high risk of importing an infected dog (36, 43). Spain has been officially free of rabies in non-flying mammals since 1978, although two imported cases of human rabies have been recorded in the last 30 years (13). Rabies surveillance data for Spain for the period of 1978–2020 reported 113 cases of rabies in dogs, of which 18 were stray dogs, and two both in cats and horses. However, these cases, except one, were limited to the cities of Ceuta and Melilla, which are located in North Africa (13). Likewise, rabies in wildlife was confirmed in 39 bats, as well as one fox in Ceuta, during this period (13). Thus, rabies remains a public health concern in Spain, and the main risk factors should be considered.

CROSS-IMMUNITY BETWEEN DIFFERENT LYSSAVIRUSES

A certain degree of cross-immunity between different lyssaviruses that can produce rabies has been described. Studies so far seem to show that such cross-immunity is possible between antigenic and genotypically "close" viruses, but not between more "distant" lyssaviruses belonging to different phylogroups (44). Thus, vaccination against classical canine rabies (phylogroup I) appears to confer protection against infection by lyssaviruses belonging to the same phylogroup, but not against European and African lyssaviruses belonging to phylogroups II and III.

New lyssaviruses are being discovered frequently, and although the risk is low, many of these viruses cannot be neutralised by antibodies from the traditional vaccine administered for the prevention of this disease. In view of the goal to end human deaths from dog-mediated rabies from the world by 2030, considering the elimination of dog-mediated rabies from a great part of Europe, consideration should be given to these other viruses that can produce rabies in humans and animals, for which the current vaccine is not protective. Therefore, some experts consider it essential to produce a universal vaccine that covers a broad spectrum of these lyssaviruses (45).

PRINCIPAL RISK FACTORS OF THE DISEASE IN EUROPE

Rabies is widely distributed worldwide, with only a few countries considered free of the disease (1). Since 1977, for rabies information exchange in Europe, the WHO Collaborating Centre for Rabies Surveillance and Research, Friedrich Loeffler Institute in Wusterhausen, Germany, has developed the Rabies Bulletin Europe (46). To date, several European countries have become rabies-free of terrestrial rabies, but rabies remains present in others (38). European rabies risk is based on distinct epidemiological situations: illegal importation of animals, travel to endemic regions, differences in dog vaccination programmes and wildlife rabies.

Illegal Importation of Animals

Although the successful elimination of dog-mediated rabies has been witnessed in the majority of European countries, it remains in certain European countries, as well as on the borders of Europe (47). In this sense, to ensure a sufficient level of safety in rabies, a European regulation establish strict measures on the movement of pet animals into a Member State from another Member State (48). However, illegal importation of pets through failure of border controls remains one of the main risks for rabies in Europe, leading to sporadic cases of rabies in free regions from endemic countries (13, 47, 49). From 2012 to 2020, five illegally imported dogs infected with rabies have been reported in France (2012, 2015, and 2020), Spain (2013) and the Netherlands (2013) from endemic areas (13, 36, 50, 51). These situations have occurred mainly because of importation of animals as pets from North Africa, disregarding the legislation on the movement of pet animals into Europe, and without disclosing the imported animals to the veterinary border control staff and customs officials (38, 43, 52, 53).

Spain presents geographical proximity and a commercial relationship with North Africa, with two cities in North Africa bordering with Morocco (Ceuta and Melilla), and a long-standing historical commercial traffic, fishing activities and labour migration between the Spanish-Moroccan border (54). Currently, rabies is endemic throughout Morocco, with human death reported yearly, remaining a serious public health problem (53). The domestic dog is considered the main reservoir and vector of the virus, and for this reason mass annual vaccination campaigns are conducted (53). However, the concept of responsible dog ownership does not feature in the Moroccan legislation, and vaccination coverage has not exceeded 6% of the total dog population (53). This situation affects Moroccan citizens, and the country has also become a source of rabies for neighbouring European states (43, 53). Every year, imported cases from Morocco are identified in Ceuta and Melilla (36), so compulsory and free of charge rabies vaccination programmes are carried out in these cities, in an attempt to reduce the risk (55). Imported cases pose a threat of rabies reintroduction into rabies-free areas, highlighting the need for reinforcement of border surveillance (38, 56).

Travel to Endemic Regions

Although the risk of a traveller contracting rabies is considered low, no prophylaxis or specific rabies vaccinations are needed for travel to endemic areas (52, 56). In 2019, four imported human rabies case were reported in Latvia, Spain, Italy, and Norway after having contracted the disease through a dog or cat bite while travelling in endemic areas (India, Morocco, Tanzania, and Philippines, respectively) (57). The imported cases of human rabies reflect lack of awareness by travellers visiting rabies-endemic countries, especially in Africa and Asia (43, 52, 57). Travellers to endemic areas should be aware of this, acting with caution and avoiding touching all animals, including puppies, to prevent animal bites (9, 57, 58). Moreover, the recommendations include local wound care, the vaccination, and if indicated, passive immunisation (9).

In addition, the risk increases when travelling with animals. In this sense, recent reports related lack of awareness by travellers of the risk posed by taking their non-vaccinated dogs abroad to an endemic region, or by adopting animals from these areas and taking them back home with them (43, 47).

Differences in Dog Vaccination Programmes

As there is no clinical treatment for this zoonotic disease, and dogs represent a main source of human infection, prevention by vaccination is the mainstay approach to avoid the spread of rabies (1). According to the WHO, vaccination coverage should reach 70% of the dog population to prevent rabies transmission (4). Regular application of the vaccines provides a more cost-effective basic instrument than the post-bite treatment of rabies cases, both short-term and longer-term (1). Indeed, the cost of a post-bite treatment in humans is around US$ 100, while dog vaccination costs are around US$ 0.50 per dog (59).

The WHO Expert Committee on Rabies considered mass vaccination programmes the basis of canine rabies control (46). Moreover, it was recommended that these mass vaccination programmes, which included the primary immunisation of all dogs between 3 months and 1 year old, should be carried out annually, and also emphasised the importance of including cats in these programmes (46).

The threat of rabies requires a constant state of alert, as an immunisation rate of <70% poses a risk to herd immunity in Europe (60). Furthermore, the geographical proximity to territories that are not free of rabies should be of special consideration, as it will pose a risk to the whole of Europe.

In addition to the lack of a coordinated vaccination programme, vaccine failures may occur, due to causes such as failure to administer the vaccine, poor quality rabies vaccine, and poor immune, health and nutritional status of the vaccinated animal (46). In addition, a single shot of vaccine is not enough to achieve long-lasting optimal immunity against rabies, leading to insecure rabies protection rates in a biting animal, despite a history of rabies vaccination (1).

Circulation of the Virus Among Wildlife population

Insectivorous bat species have often been employed as a mosquito biocontrol strategy, and it has been observed that a single bat is able to consume up to 600 mosquitoes per hour (61). Mosquitoes may serve as vectors of mosquito-borne diseases such as Zika virus, West Nile virus, malaria, or dengue (62). This highlights the important role of insectivorous bats in the reduction of mosquito populations and their implication in the protection against mosquito-related disease (63). In fact, in Spain bats are used as a control measure for mosquito populations, although some of the species used have been found positive for the presence of lyssaviruses (30, 64). Even though the risk of possible transmission of bat lyssaviruses to terrestrial mammals are very low in European countries, human and animal rabies cases following a bat bite have been reported (13, 65). Besides, exposure to bats should be regarded as a potential rabies risk in Europe, especially for spelunkers or bat biologists, who have a high risk of contact with rabid bats (38, 66). Recently, Italy has reported a case of WCBV in a cat, which lived near to bat colonies, that could represent the source of the virus (67). Ecological factors such as cross-species mixing and migrations of bat populations could be responsible for the viral persistence in European bats (10).

In Europe, the chiropteran rabies cycle is independent from the terrestrial rabies cycle (24). In 2019, the surveillance data confirmed five cases in animals in Europe, the highest proportion of the cases being in red foxes (two in Romania and one in Poland), followed by one case in a cow and in a wild boar, also in Romania (68). In the early 1960s, red fox rabies emerged in many European countries (13, 25). Over the past three decades, European fox-mediated rabies has been successfully controlled and eliminated in response to the effective implementation of the ORV programmes (13, 69). Countries can be officially declared free of terrestrial rabies when no cases have been detected for a 2-year period (15), a status achieved by European countries such as Finland and The Netherlands in 1991, Italy in 1997, Switzerland in 1998, France in 2000, Belgium and Luxembourg in 2001, the Czech Republic in 2004 and Germany and Austria in 2008 (13). Despite the success achieved, in Italy fox rabies re-emerged in 2009 (13), and a recent emergence and spread of fox rabies into previously rabies-free areas, due to insufficient cross-border cooperation and a false sense of security, highlights the need to stay alert (15, 49).

WILL RABIES EVER BE PREVENTED IN EUROPE?

Although rabies is 100% preventable, one person dies from it every 9 min worldwide (4). Although most of the cases are in Africa and Asia, the public health hazard of rabies must not be underestimated in Europe, because of all the risks their countries present (4, 31). Rabies prevention is based on three cornerstones: (1) improving education and public awareness; (2) access to mass dog vaccination; and (3) increasing the access to treatment medicines and vaccines (4).

Improving Education and Public Awareness

Despite 3 billion people continuing to be at risk of rabies worldwide, rabies continues to be a largely neglected disease (4, 70). In this sense, the European population often overstates the health security of rabies and surveillance should continue (71). Awareness and understanding of how to prevent the disease in animals, when there are reasons to suspect rabies, and what to do in the event of a bite, are crucial to save people (4), not only in endemic areas, but also in rabies-free countries.

In Europe, legislative measures for the control of this zoonosis have been implemented (72). Nevertheless, stricter laws should be enforced to raise awareness of the potential risks of rabies disease and prevent the introduction of rabies into rabies-free European countries (1, 73). These measures should be focused on raising awareness mainly on travel to endemic areas, travelling with pets, and importing and trading in animals from endemic areas (1).

Access to Mass Dog Vaccination

Vaccination of dogs is the key to curtailing rabies transmission between dogs, and from dogs to humans. For ethical, ecological and economic reasons, the slaughtering of rabies vectors should not be considered as a main control and eradication method (74). Prevention of the transmission of rabies at its source through dog vaccination is the most cost-effective strategy to save lives (4). Although rabies control programmes involve a high cost in many countries, the cost of pre-exposure dog vaccination is much lower than the current cost of the emergency post-exposure treatment (74). In fact, just 10% of the financial resources used in post-exposure treatment would able to significantly reduce, or even eliminate, the disease in the canine population, and consequently, the number of human cases (74).

In wildlife, ORV baits have proven to be an effective sophisticated strategy to control and even eliminate fox rabies in European countries, mitigating rabies risks to humans (75). Nevertheless, few eastern European countries and countries bordering Europe are still trying to control it, posing a risk to free-rabies wildlife countries (22). For this reason, the European oral vaccination financing programmes continue to be a necessary strategy, as they are the basis of rabies control in wildlife (22).

Increased Access to Treatment Medicines and Vaccines

The best method of rabies prevention is to avoid bites from mammals, especially high-risk rabies reservoir species (1). However, this is difficult to achieve, as accidental exposures are very common (1). Worldwide, post-bite vaccination incidence has been estimated at 29 million people in a year (9). Appropriate wound management and immediate and adequate post-exposure treatment is almost 100% effective in preventing human rabies deaths (4).

In any case, the severity of the process will mainly depend on the place and type of bite and the speed of the post-exposure prophylaxis (76). Therefore, the importance of knowing the risk to which the population are subjected and the ability to react is the basis for being able to save lives, and because of this, rabies is the only disease where there is a post-exposure immunoprophylaxis protocol in humans (77). Treatment consists of thoroughly washing the bite wound with soap, and if possible with viricidal antiseptic (e.g., povidone iodine or ethanol) for at least 15 min, followed by the administration of passive immunisation with immunoglobulins, and vaccination for active immunity (46).

FINAL COMMENTS AND FUTURE DIRECTIONS

The risk of importing dog rabies cases from North Africa is in increasingly important evidence. Given this situation, the health authorities must increase surveillance, especially at the entry points to the Iberian Peninsula, as motor vehicles entering can illegally transport animals that are sick or in incubation period from North Africa.

Although the risk of importing rabies cases from other territories within Europe is considered to be lower than in the case of North Africa, it should be considered that (1) the free movement of persons and goods in EU countries easily allows the entry of illegally-transported animals from countries that present cases of rabies in domestic animals (mainly dog and cat), and even in wild species (mainly red fox); (2) the lack of specific measures and some relaxation of controls concerning vulpine populations may facilitate outbreaks in countries declared free of this type of rabies; (3) it should not be forgotten that the spread of rabies from sick foxes to dogs is well established, and *vice versa*, as seems to have been in the case of Spain in 1977, when two cases of rabies in foxes were described in the province of Malaga during the 1975 rabies outbreak. These were fortunately isolated cases, unrelated to each other, probably due to the single infection from sick dogs or the consumption of carrion from carcasses.

It is considered necessary to maintain a single criterion throughout Europe regarding compulsory vaccination, which must be annual (depending on the authorised product used for immunisation, which must be applied by authorised veterinarians) to guarantee sufficient protective immunity against rabies, in any case systematically, and which must cover all dogs and cats without exception, as in the case of ferrets or raccoon dogs, which are also particularly susceptible to the rabies virus.

Given the recent cases of bat rabies described in Europe and the considerations set out above concerning the possibility of transmission to terrestrial species, as well as the arrival of animals from other latitudes, whatever the cause, a continuous state of alert of the competent authorities is required. In the same vein, the authorities responsible should encourage and provide adequate funding for specialised research groups to constantly improve the resources available for diagnosis and vaccination, and to search for new vaccine products capable of protecting humans and animal populations from possible exposure to these viruses, which sometimes have insufficient links with classical rabies virus to ensure adequate protection.

AUTHOR CONTRIBUTIONS

All authors wrote the manuscript and performed all the necessary literature searches and data compilation. All authors approved the submitted version.

ACKNOWLEDGMENTS

We wish to thank the members of the microbiology research group Improvement of Food Safety related with the Production System and Final Products (Veterinary Faculty, University CEU-Cardenal Herrera) for their support. English text version revised by N. Macowan English Language Service.

REFERENCES

1. Garg SR. *Rabies in Man and Animals*. 1st ed. Haryana: Springer (2014).
2. Mingo-Casas P, Sandonis V, Vázquez-Morón S, Juste J. Rabies in Spain. A peculiarity in Eurasia The impact on linkage-to-care of an alternative hepatitis C screening method in PWID view project. *Ann Virol Res.* (2017) 3:1030.
3. Fooks AR, Banyard AC, Horton DL, Johnson N, Mcelhinney LM, Jackson AC. Current status of rabies and prospects for elimination. *Lancet.* (2014) 384:1389. doi: 10.1016/S0140-6736(13)62707-5
4. WHO-FAO-OIE. *WHO | Zero by 30: The Global Strategic Plan to End Human Deaths From Dog-Mediated Rabies by 2030.* (2018). Available online at: http://www.who.int/rabies/resources/9789241513838/en/ (accessed May 28, 2020).
5. Fisher CR, Streicker DG, Schnell MJ. The spread and evolution of rabies virus: conquering new frontiers. *Nat Rev Microbiol.* (2019) 16:241–55. doi: 10.1038/nrmicro.2018.11
6. ICTV. *Genus: Lyssavirus - Rhabdoviridae - Mononegavirales - International Committee on Taxonomy of Viruses (ICTV).* (2019). Available online at: https://talk.ictvonline.org/ictv-reports/ictv_online_report/negative-sense-rna-viruses/mononegavirales/w/rhabdoviridae/795/genus-lyssavirus (accessed May 28, 2020).
7. Neville J. Rabies in the Ancient World. In: King A, Fooks AR, Aubert M, Wandeler AI, editors. *Historical Perspective of Rabies in Europe and the Mediterranean Basin.* Paris: OIE (2004). p. 1–12.
8. Shipley R, Wright E, Selden D, Wu G, Aegerter J, Fooks AR, et al. Bats and viruses: emergence of novel lyssaviruses and association of bats with viral zoonoses in the EU. *Trop Med Infect Dis.* (2019) 4:31. doi: 10.3390/tropicalmed4010031
9. WHO. *Classification | Rabies - Bulletin – Europe.* (2020). Available online at: https://www.who-rabies-bulletin.org/site-page/classification (accessed November 2, 2020).
10. Colombi D, Serra-Cobo J, Métras R, Apolloni A, Poletto C, López-Roig M, et al. Mechanisms for lyssavirus persistence in non-synanthropic bats in Europe: insights from a modeling study. *Sci Rep.* (2019) 9:1–11. doi: 10.1038/s41598-018-36485-y
11. Scheffer C, Asano M, Garcia E, Samira M, Fahl DO. Murciélagos hematófagos como reservorios de la rabia. *Rev Peru Med Exp Salud Publica.* (2014) 31:302–9. doi: 10.17843/rpmesp.2014.312.51
12. Mingo-Casas P, Sandonís V, Obón E, Berciano JM, Vázquez-Morón S, Juste J, et al. First cases of European bat lyssavirus type 1 in Iberian serotine bats: implications for the molecular epidemiology of bat rabies in Europe. *PLoS Negl Trop Dis.* (2018) 12:1–9. doi: 10.1371/journal.pntd.0006290
13. WHO. *Rabies.* (2020). Available online at: https://www.who.int/news-room/fact-sheets/detail/rabies (accessed May 28, 2020).
14. Cifuentes JF, Pérez RD, Verjan N. Bat reservoirs for rabies virus and epidemiology of rabies in Colombia: a review. *CES Med Vet Zootec.* (2017) 12:134–50. doi: 10.21615/cesmvz.12.2.5
15. European Commission. *DG Health and Food Safety Overview Report - Rabies Eradication in the EU.* Luxembourg (2017).
16. OIE. *Manual of Diagnostic Tests and Vaccines for Terrestrial Animals.* 6th ed. Vol 1. Paris: OIE (2008).
17. Rupprecht CE, Fooks AR, Abela-Ridder B. *Laboratory Techniques in Rabies.* 5th ed. Vol 1. Geneva: World Health Organization (2018).
18. Bordignon J, Pires Ferreira SC, Medeiros Caporale GM, Carrieri ML, Kotait I, Lima HC, et al. Flow cytometry assay for intracellular rabies virus detection. *J Virol Methods.* (2002) 105:181–6. doi: 10.1016/S0166-0934(02)00064-2
19. Reed M, Stuchlik O, Carson WC, Orciari L, Yager PA, Olson V, et al. Novel mass spectrometry based detection and identification of variants of rabies virus nucleoprotein in infected brain tissues. *PLoS Negl Trop Dis.* (2018) 12:e0006984. doi: 10.1371/journal.pntd.0006984
20. Blancou J. Rabies in Europe and the Mediterranean basin: from antiquity to the 19th Century. In: eds. King A, Fooks AR, Aubert M, Wandeler AI, editors. *Historical Perspective of Rabies in Europe and the Mediterranean Basin.* Paris: OIE (2004). p. 15–23.
21. Müller FT, Freuling CM. Rabies control in Europe: an overview of past, current and future strategies. *Rev Sci Tech.* (2018) 37:409–19. doi: 10.20506/rst.37.2.2811
22. Freuling CM, Hampson K, Selhorst T, Schröder R, Meslin FX, Mettenleiter TC, et al. The elimination of fox rabies from Europe: Determinants of success and lessons for the future. *Philos Trans R Soc B Biol Sci.* (2013) 368:20120142. doi: 10.1098/rstb.2012.0142
23. Westerling B, Andersons Z, Rimeicans J, Lukauskas K, Dranseika A. Rabies in the baltics. In: King A, Fooks AR, Aubert M, Wandeler AI, editors. *Historical Perspective of Rabies in Europe and the Mediterranean Basin.* París: OIE (2004). p. 33–44.
24. European Commission. *The Oral Vaccination of Foxes Against Rabies Report of the Scientific Committee on Animal Health and Animal Welfare* (2002).
25. Mähl P, Cliquet F, Guiot AL, Niin E, Fournials E, Saint-Jean N, et al. Twenty-year experience of the oral rabies vaccine SAG2 in wildlife: A global review. *Vet Res.* (2014) 45:1–17. doi: 10.1186/s13567-014-0077-8
26. Robardet E, Picard-Meyer E, Dobroštana M, Jaceviciene I, Mähar K, MuiŽniece Z, et al. Rabies in the Baltic States: decoding a process of control and elimination. *PLoS Negl Trop Dis.* (2016) 10:1–26. doi: 10.1371/journal.pntd.0004432
27. Sutor A, Schwarz S, Conraths FJ. The biological potential of the raccoon dog (Nyctereutes procyonoides, Gray 1834) as an invasive species in Europe-new risks for disease spread? *Acta Theriol.* (2014) 59:49–59. doi: 10.1007/s13364-013-0138-9
28. Müller W, Cox J, Müller T. Rabies in Germany, Denmark and Austria. In: King A, Fooks AR, Aubert M, Wandeler AI, editors. *Historical Perspective of Rabies in Europe and the Mediterranean Basin.* Paris: OIE (2004).
29. Picard-Meyer E, Robardet E, Arthur L, Larcher G, Harbusch C, Servat A, et al. Bat rabies in France: A 24-year retrospective epidemiological study. *PLoS ONE.* (2014) 9:e98622. doi: 10.1371/journal.pone.0098622
30. Banyard AC, Evans JS, Luo TR, Fooks AR. Lyssaviruses and bats: Emergence and zoonotic threat. *Viruses.* (2014) 6:2974–90. doi: 10.3390/v6082974
31. EFSA. The European Union One Health 2018 zoonoses report. *EFSA J.* (2019) 17:17. doi: 10.2903/j.efsa.2019.5926
32. Leopardi S, Priori P, Zecchin B, Poglayen G, Trevisiol K, Lelli D, et al. Active and passive surveillance for bat lyssaviruses in Italy revealed serological evidence for their circulation in three bat species. *Epidemiol Infect.* (2019) 147:1–6. doi: 10.1017/S0950268818003072
33. Schatz J, Fooks AR, Mcelhinney L, Horton D, Echevarria J, Vázquez-Moron S, et al. Bat rabies surveillance in Europe. *Zoonoses Public Health.* (2013) 60:22–34. doi: 10.1111/zph.12002
34. Schatz J, Freuling CM, Auer E, Goharriz H, Harbusch C, Johnson N, et al. Enhanced passive bat rabies surveillance in indigenous bat species from Germany - a retrospective study. *PLoS Negl Trop Dis.* (2014) 8:2835. doi: 10.1371/journal.pntd.0002835
35. Abellan-Garcia C, Sánchez-Serrano LP, Amador R, Rosinha AJ. Rabies in the Iberian Peninsula. In: King A, Fooks AR, Aubert M, Wandeler AI, editors. *Historical Perspective of Rabies in Europe and the Mediterranean Basin.* Paris: OIE (2004). p. 147–55.
36. Pérez de Diego AC, Vigo M, Monsalve J, Escudero A. The One Health approach for the management of an imported case of rabies in mainland Spain in 2013. *Eurosurveillance.* (2015) 20:1–5.

doi: 10.2807/1560-7917.ES2015.20.6.21033
37. Rodríguez-Ferri E. Estado actual de la rabia animal, con especial referencia a España. *Colección Vet Salud Públ Min Sanidad Consumo.* (1987) 4:1–204.
38. Cliquet F, Picard-Meyer E, Robardet E. Rabies in Europe: what are the risks? *Expert Rev Anti Infect Ther.* (2014) 12:905–8. doi: 10.1586/14787210.2014.921570
39. King AA, Haagsma J, Kappeler A. Lyssavirus infections in European bats In: King AA, Fooks AR, Aubert M, Wandeler AI, editors. *Historical Perspective of Rabies in Europe and the Mediterranean Basin.* Paris: OIE (2004).
40. Serra-Cobo J, Amengual B, Carlos Abellán B, Bourhy H. European bat Lyssavirus infection in Spanish bat populations. *Emerg Infect Dis.* (2002) 8:413–20. doi: 10.3201/eid0804.010263
41. Vázquez-Morón S, Juste J, Ibáñez C, Ruiz-Villamor E, Avellón A, Vera M, et al. Endemic circulation of European bat lyssavirus type 1 in serotine bats, Spain. *Emerg Infect Dis.* (2008) 14:1263–6. doi: 10.3201/1408.080068
42. Aréchiga-Ceballos N, Morón SV, Berciano JM, Nicolás O, López CA, Juste J, et al. Novel lyssavirus in bat, Spain. *Emerg Infect Dis.* (2013) 19:793–5. doi: 10.3201/eid1905.121071
43. Napp S, Casas M, Moset S, Paramio JL, Casal J. Quantitative risk assessment model of canine rabies introduction: Application to the risk to the European Union from Morocco. *Epidemiol Infect.* (2010) 138:1569–80. doi: 10.1017/S0950268810000415
44. Echevarría JE, Banyard AC, McElhinney LM, Fooks AR. Current rabies vaccines do not confer protective immunity against divergent lyssaviruses circulating in Europe. *Viruses.* (2019) 11:892. doi: 10.3390/v11100892
45. Evans JS, Horton DL, Easton AJ, Fooks AR, Banyard AC. Rabies virus vaccines: Is there a need for a pan-lyssavirus vaccine? *Vaccine.* (2012) 30:7447–54. doi: 10.1016/j.vaccine.2012.10.015
46. WHO. *WHO Technical Report Series 931 WHO Expert Consultation on Rabies First Report* (2005).
47. Bourhy H, Dacheux L, Strady C, Mailles A. Rabies in Europe in 2005. *Euro Surveill.* (2005) 10:213–6. doi: 10.2807/esm.10.11.00575-en
48. European Parliament and the Council of the European Union. *Regulation (EC) No. 576/2013 of the European Parliament and of the Council of 12 June 2013 on the Non-commercial Movement of Pet Animals and Repealing Regulation (EC) No 998/2003. J Eur Union L.* (2013) 178:1–26.
49. Müller T, Freuling CM, Wysocki P, Roumiantzeff M, Freney J, Mettenleiter TC, et al. Terrestrial rabies control in the European Union: Historical achievements and challenges ahead. *Vet J.* (2015) 203:10–7. doi: 10.1016/j.tvjl.2014.10.026
50. Berger S. *Rabies: Global Status.* 2018th ed. Los Angeles, CA: GIDEON Informatics Inc. (2018).
51. ECDC. *Rabies Annual Epidemiological Report for 2018.* Stockholm (2018). p. 2000–2.
52. Gautret P, Ribadeau-Dumas F, Parola P, Brouqui P, Bourhy H. Risk for rabies importation from North Africa. *Emerg Infect Dis.* (2011) 17:2187–93. doi: 10.3201/eid1712.110300
53. Darkaoui S, Cliquet F, Wasniewski M, Robardet E, Aboulfidaa N, Bouslikhane M, et al. A century spent combating rabies in Morocco (1911-2015): How much longer? *Front Vet Sci.* (2017) 4:78. doi: 10.3389/fvets.2017.00078
54. Ferrer-Gallardo X. The Spanish-Moroccan border complex: Processes of geopolitical, functional and symbolic rebordering. *Polit Geogr.* (2008) 27:301–21. doi: 10.1016/j.polgeo.2007.12.004
55. WHO. *WHO Rabies Bulletin Europe, No 2.* (2013). p. 1–24. Available online at: http://www.who-rabies-bulletin.org/ (accessed May 29, 2020)
56. Ribadeau-Dumas F, Cliquet F, Gautret P, Robardet E, Le Pen C, Bourhy H. Travel-associated rabies in pets and residual rabies risk, Western Europe. *Emerg Infect Dis.* (2016) 22:1268–71. doi: 10.3201/eid2207.151733
57. ECDC. *Fourth Travel-Related Rabies Case Reported in the EU in 2019.* (2019). Available online at: https://www.ecdc.europa.eu/en/news-events/fourth-travel-related-rabies-case-reported-eu-2019 (accessed June 3, 2020).
58. Malerczyk C, DeTora L, Gniel D. Imported human rabies cases in Europe, the United States, and Japan, 1990 to 2010. *J Travel Med.* (2011) 18:402–7. doi: 10.1111/j.1708-8305.2011.00557.x
59. WHO. *WHO | Vaccinate Dogs to Save Human Lives – World Rabies Day 2012.* WHO (2012).
60. Hampson K, Dushoff J, Cleaveland S, Haydon DT, Kaare M, Packer C, et al. Transmission dynamics and prospects for the elimination of canine rabies. *PLoS Biol.* (2009) 7:e1000053. doi: 10.1371/journal.pbio.1000053
61. Gonsalves L, Bicknell B, Law B, Webb C, Monamy V. Mosquito consumption by insectivorous bats: does size matter? *PLoS ONE.* (2013) 8:1–11. doi: 10.1371/journal.pone.0077183
62. Zeller H, Marrama L, Sudre B, Van Bortel W, Warns-Petit E. Mosquito-borne disease surveillance by the European Centre for Disease Prevention and Control. *Clin Microbiol Infect.* (2013) 19:693–8. doi: 10.1111/1469-0691.12230
63. Reiskind MH, Wund MA. *Bats & Mosquitoes Testing Conventional Wisdom.* Texas: Bat Conservation International. (2010).
64. UCM. *Universidad Complutense de Madrid.* Texas: Bat Conser vation International (2016). Available at: https://www.ucm.es/el-grupo-de-seguimiento-de-fauna-cei-campus-moncloa-aboga-por-el-uso-de-murcielagos-como-control-de-plagas-en-casos-como-el-mosquito-que-trasmite-el-virus-zika-24-de-febrero (accessed June 2, 2020).
65. Racey PA, Hutson AM, Lina PHC. Bat rabies, public health and European bat conservation. *Zoonoses Public Health.* (2013) 60:58–68. doi: 10.1111/j.1863-2378.2012.01533.x
66. Krzowska-Firych J, Tomasiewicz K, Kozøowska A. Post-exposure rabies prophylaxis in humans exposed to animals in Lublin province (Eastern Poland) in 2012–2015–A retrospective study. *Hum Vaccines Immunother.* (2017) 13:1346–51. doi: 10.1080/21645515.2017.1285474
67. Coxon C, McElhinney L, Pacey A, Gauntlett F, Holland S. *Preliminary Outbreak Assessment: Rabies in a Cat in Italy.* (2020). Available online at: https://www.who-rabies-bulletin.org/site-page/classification (accessed November 10, 2020).
68. Gossner CM, Mailles A, Aznar I, Dimina E, Echevarría JE, Feruglio SL, et al. Prevention of human rabies: a challenge for the European Union and the European Economic Area. *Eurosurveillance.* (2020) 25:2000158. doi: 10.2807/1560-7917.ES.2020.25.38.2000158
69. Müller T, Bätza HJ, Freuling C, Kliemt A, Kliemt J, Heuser R, et al. Elimination of terrestrial rabies in Germany using oral vaccination of foxes. *Berl Munch Tierarztl Wochenschr.* (2012) 125:178–90.
70. Wunner WH, Briggs DJ. Rabies in the 21st century. *PLoS Negl Trop Dis.* (2010) 4:591. doi: 10.1371/journal.pntd.0000591
71. Finnegan CJ, Brookes SM, Johnson N, Smith J, Mansfield KL, Keene VL, et al. Rabies in North America and Europe. *J R Soc Med.* (2002) 95:9–13. doi: 10.1177/014107680209500104
72. Directive 2003/99/EC. *Directive 2003/99/EC of the European Parliament and of the Council of 17 November 2003 on the Monitoring of Zoonoses and Zoonotic Agents, Amending Council Decision 90/424/EEC and Repealing Council Directive 92/117/EEC* (2003).
73. Lembo T, Partners for Rabies Prevention. The Blueprint for Rabies Prevention and Control: A Novel Operational Toolkit for Rabies Elimination. *PLoS Negl Trop Dis.* (2012) 6:e1388. doi: 10.1371/journal.pntd.0001388
74. OIE. *OIE's Commitment to Fight Rabies Worldwide.* (2014). Available online at: https://www.oie.int/doc/ged/D14107.PDF (accessed November 14, 2020).
75. Maki J, Guiot AL, Aubert M, Brochier B, Cliquet F, Hanlon CA, et al. Oral vaccination of wildlife using a vaccinia-rabies-glycoprotein recombinant virus vaccine (RABORAL V-RG®): A global review. *Vet Res.* (2017) 48:57. doi: 10.1186/s13567-017-0459-9
76. Andrade BF, Andrade TS, Queiroz LH. Human rabies post-exposure prophylaxis relative to the disease epidemiological status. *Cienc Saude Coletiva.* (2019) 24:315–22. doi: 10.1590/1413-81232018241.32832016
77. Briggs DJ. The role of vaccination in rabies prevention. *Curr Opin Virol.* (2012) 2:309–14. doi: 10.1016/j.coviro.2012.03.007

7

Serological Survey of Canine Vector-Borne Infections

Patricia Pérez Pérez [1,2], *Iván Rodríguez-Escolar* [1], *Elena Carretón* [3*], *José Ángel Sánchez Agudo* [4], *Jacob Lorenzo-Morales* [2,5], *José Alberto Montoya-Alonso* [3] *and Rodrigo Morchón* [1*]

[1] Zoonotic Infections and One Health GIR, Laboratory of Parasitology, Faculty of Pharmacy, University of Salamanca, Salamanca, Spain, [2] Instituto Universitario de Enfermedades Tropicales y Salud Pde Canarias (IUETSPC), Departamento de Obstetricia y Ginecolog, Pediatría, Medicina Preventiva y Salud Pública, Toxicología, Medicina Legal y Forense y Parasitología, Universidad de La Laguna, La Laguna, Tenerife, Spain, [3] Internal Medicine, Faculty of Veterinary Medicine, Research Institute of Biomedical and Health Sciences, University of Las Palmas de Gran Canaria, Las Palmas de Gran Canaria, Spain, [4] Grupo de Investigación en Biodiversidad, Diversidad humana y Biología de la Conservación, Universidad de Salamanca, Salamanca, Spain, [5] CIBER de Enfermedades Infecciosas, Instituto de Salud Carlos III, Madrid, Spain

***Correspondence:**
Elena Carretón
elena.carreton@ulpgc.es
Rodrigo Morchón
rmorgar@usal.es

Various factors are currently causing an increase in vector-borne parasitic diseases at a global scale; among them, some stand out, such as climatic disturbances derived from global change, the increase in movements of reservoir animals, or changes in land made by human activity. In the European continent, there have been an increasing number of epidemiological studies focused on the detection of these diseases, especially in dogs. In Spain, there are few epidemiological studies focused on the evaluation of the biotic and abiotic factors that may influence the distribution, such as climatic zones, orography, or presence of water reservoirs. The aim of this study was to analyze the prevalence and distribution of several canine vector-borne diseases caused by *Dirofilaria immitis*, *Leishmania infantum*, *Anaplasma platys*, and *Ehrlichia canis* in the autonomous community of Castilla y León, the largest region of the Iberian Peninsula, providing a geospatial approach based on a geographic information system (GIS) analysis. Blood from a total of 1,475 domestic dogs from the nine provinces of Castilla y León were analyzed. Also, a GIS analysis of the sample locations was carried out, taking into account the most important predictor variables. The prevalence in dogs infected by *D. immitis* was 7.19%, and the seroprevalence by *L. infantum* was 4.61 and 1.56% for *A. platys* and *E. canis*. Most of the infected animals were located in areas with stagnant water, irrigated agriculture, or riverbanks, always close to forest and woodland vegetation. These results indicate that dogs living in Castilla y León should take prophylactic measures to avoid infections.

Keywords: canine vector borne disease, *D. immitis*, *L. infantum*, GIS, Spain, epidemiology, *E. canis*, *A. platys*.

INTRODUCTION

Canine vector-borne diseases (CVBDs) are caused by several infectious agents, which are transmitted by a wide variety of arthropods, mainly fleas, ticks, mosquitoes, and sandflies. Many of them are zoonotic diseases and are among the most important health problems affecting both domestic dogs and humans worldwide (1). Temperature and humidity are two determining factors that act directly in the establishment and distribution of the vectors and the diseases, as well as other factors derived from human activity such as the increase in the mobility of people and infected animals, or modifications in the landscape, mainly caused by increased irrigated crops or intensive urbanization of new areas. These processes favor the development of some vectors and the infection of the hosts (2–4).

Many of the CVBDs are clinically important, even be fatal, and frequently show unspecific symptoms, which make them difficult to diagnose. These include several zoonotic diseases such as heartworm disease, canine leishmaniasis, and canine anaplasmosis (3–5). In addition, canine ehrlichiosis, although not classified as zoonotic, has been sporadically described in several clinical cases in humans (6, 7).

Nematode *Dirofilaria immitis*, transmitted by culicid mosquitoes, is the causative agent of canine heartworm disease, a chronic disease which can lead to the death of the animal, although many of these animals are asymptomatic and become uncontrolled reservoirs (8). It is a zoonotic parasite which can cause pulmonary dirofilariasis, an asymptomatic infection, but that can be mistaken for lung cancer (2, 9–11). Protozooan *Leishmania infantum*, transmitted by *Phlebotomus* spp., causes canine leishmaniosis and induces a severe disease with serious clinical signs which, if not treated, can lead to the death of the animal. In addition, *L. infantum* can cause cutaneous lesions in humans or visceral leishmaniasis, the latter being a serious condition especially in immunocompromised patients (12). *Anaplasma platys* is the causative agent of canine cyclic thrombocytopenia, while *Ehrlichia canis* is the causative agent of canine monocytic ehrlichiosis. These gram-negative bacteria are mainly transmitted by ticks, and the diseases are characterized by non-specific signs, making diagnosis difficult (13–16). In humans, *E. canis* and *A. platys* have been reported in clinically ill human patients causing from mild, self-limiting febrile illness to fatal infections (6, 7, 17).

In Europe, many epidemiological studies have been published showing a wide variability in the prevalence of the mentioned CVBDs. These differences may be due to the influence exerted by the biotic and abiotic variables of each region as well as the different diagnostic tools used (5, 18). In Spain, few studies have been published on the epidemiological status of these diseases mostly reporting data at a global level without evaluating the influence of environmental factors (i.e., orography, vegetation, climate) of each of the areas studied, especially those focused on *Anaplasma spp.* and *E. canis* (3, 5, 19).

These are CVBDs that are spreading throughout Europe and are considered emerging diseases. Therefore, it is important to evaluate the influence of the possible factors that contribute to this expansion; in this way, more accurate prediction models and measures aimed at stopping this expansion can be studied. The present study is focused on Castilla y León, representing a significant extension of territory, with different orographic and climatic zones depending on the province analyzed, to study the prevalence of the mentioned CVBDs as well as the influence of several biotic and abiotic factors. Also, the implementation of global positioning systems for geolocation of data together with the analysis of the environmental variables of a territory through GIS and spatial correlation models has shown to have a great capacity to understand spatial patterns of distribution of biological events in a territory (20). This ecoinformatic methodology allows the elaboration of predictive models focused on the determination of potential risks of parasitic diseases on a global scope [i.e., (21)] or in specific areas (22, 23).

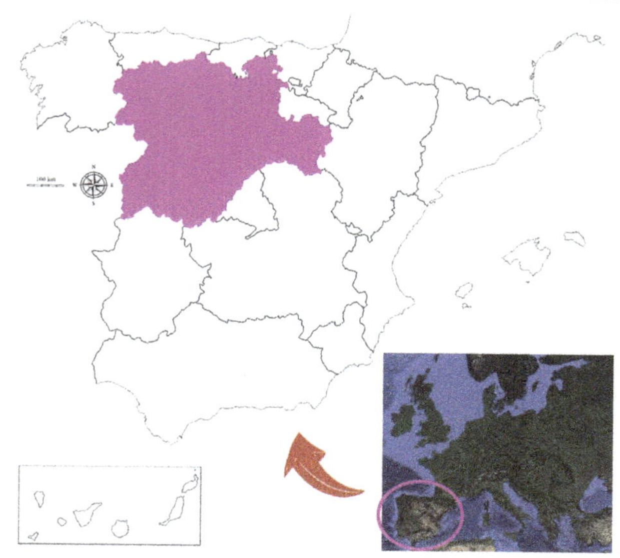

FIGURE 1 | Location of Autonomous Community of Castilla y León, Spain.

Therefore, the aim of this study was to deepen the prevalence as well as the geographic distribution patterns of selected causative agents of CVBDs in the autonomous community of Castilla y León (Spain) by using GIS, to understand the causal relationship between the environmental variables and the prevalence of the infections.

METHODS

Study Area

The Autonomous Community of Castilla y León is located in the northwestern quadrant of the Iberian Peninsula (**Figure 1**). With an area of 94,224 km^2, it is the largest region in Spain and one of the largest of Europe, being greater than seven state members of the European Union (Austria, Belgium, Denmark, Holland, Ireland, Luxembourg, and Portugal). The orography of Castilla y León is mainly formed by a plateau with an average altitude of around 800 m above sea level, surrounded by a belt of mountainous reliefs to the north, east, and south, and bordering the west with Portugal. Administratively, it is divided into nine provinces (León, Zamora, Salamanca, Valladolid, Palencia, Burgos, Soria, Segovia, and Ávila) (**Figure 2**), with León being the largest (15,851 km^2) and Segovia the smallest (6,921 km^2) (24, 25).

According to Köppen's climate classification, Castilla y León falls within the continental's Mediterranean climate, presenting

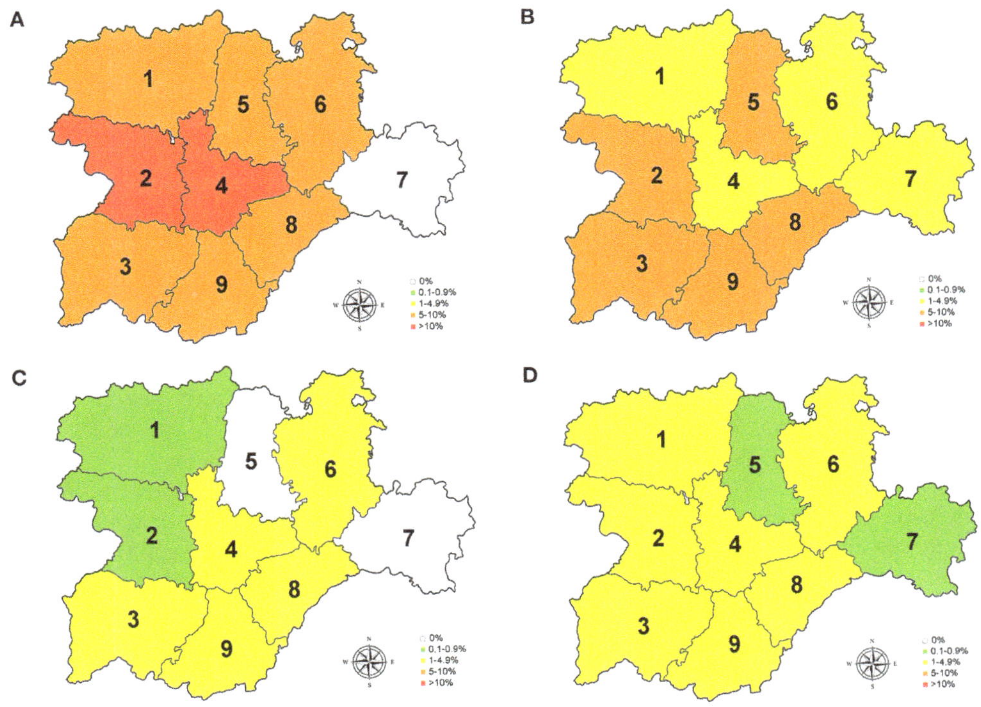

FIGURE 2 | Prevalence for *D. immitis* **(A)**, and seroprevalences for *L. infantum* **(B)**, *A. platys* **(C)**, and *E. canis* **(D)** in the nine provinces of Castilla y León, Spain. 0% (•); 0.1–0.9% (■); 1–4.9% (■); 5–10% (■); >10 (■).1, León; 2, Zamora; 3, Salamanca; 4, Valladolid; 5, Palencia; 6, Burgos; 7, Soria; 8, Segovia; 9, Ávila.

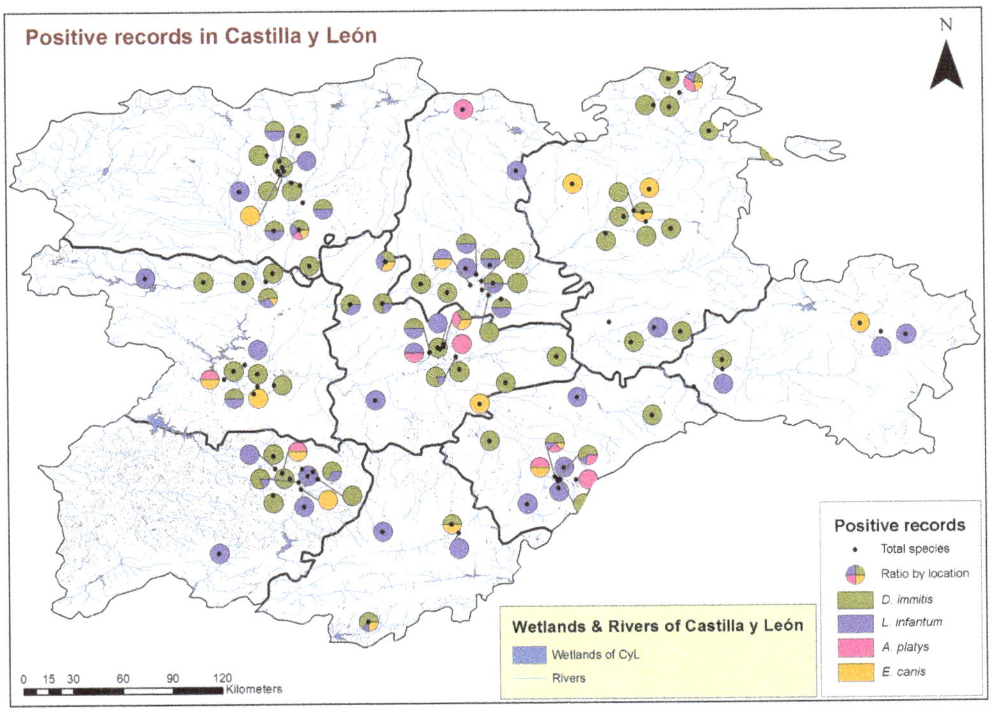

FIGURE 3 | Location of wetlands and rivers and geolocation of dogs infected by *D. immitis* (■), and seroprevalences for *L. infantum* (■), *A. platys* (■), and *E. canis* (■) in the nine provinces of Castilla y León, Spain.

long and cold winters, with average temperatures between 3 and 6°C in January, as well as short, hot summers (average temperatures from 19 to 22°C). The average annual rainfall is about 450–500 mm, accentuated in mountain ranges, but with hardly any rainfall during the summer months. Furthermore, due to the great extension and the orographic diversity of this territory, different sub-climates can be distinguished. A large part falls within the temperate with dry or temperate summer (Csb) or temperate with a dry season and temperate summer (Cfb) sub-climates, the average of the warmest month being below 22°C but above 10°C for ≥5 months. In several areas of the central plateau, the sub-climate is classified as temperate with dry or hot summer (Csa) as it exceeds 22°C during the summer, or cold steppe (BSk), with average annual temperatures below 18°C. At high altitudes in the mountain areas, the climate present is cold temperate with average temperatures below 3°C in the coldest months and dry summers (Dsb or Dsc) (26).

According to the map of phytoclimatic series by Rivas Martínez (27), the vegetation of Castilla y León is mainly included in the Mediterranean region, supra-Mediterranean floor, Carpetano-Iberico-Leonesa biogeographic province. The potential forest formations of quercines are predominant in it: holm oaks (*Quercus ilex* subsp. *ballota*), pyrenean oaks (*Q. pyrenaica*), cork oaks (*Q. suber*), and quejigo oaks (*Q. faginea*), which are planted, managed, and regularly pruned, configuring a manmade ecosystem characterized by a savannah-like physiognomy, locally known as "dehesa systems." These forests cover most of the plains and middle slopes, but some beech (*Fagus sylvatica*) and chestnut forests (*Castanea sativa*) are also present in the mountainous foothills. Sabinas and juniper trees (*Juniperus* sp.) practically complete most of this forest landscape, together with the riverside communities associated with the main rivers and streams that cross the territory.

Sample Collection

The study included a total of 1,475 blood samples from domestic dogs, collected between September 2019 and December 2020 (**Table 1**). Samples were collected from dogs undergoing medical examination in 44 veterinary clinics and hospitals, with at least four veterinary clinics for each province of Castilla y León. The participation of clinics and hospitals was voluntary, and samples were collected throughout the duration of the study. Samples came from both owned and shelter dogs. The criteria for inclusion were (a) no previous history of infection, (b) not receiving regular chemoprophylaxis for the studied vector-borne diseases, and (c) owner consent to participate in the survey. Epidemiological data, such as sex, age at presentation to the clinics, and habitat (indoor, outdoor, or indoor/outdoor: at least 1–50% of the time spent outdoors), were recorded.

Blood samples were collected from the cephalic or jugular vein, placed in 3-ml serum tubes, and centrifuged. Serum samples were kept at −20°C until tests were performed. All samples were tested for the detection of *D. immitis* antigens and for the detection of antibodies against *L. infantum*, *E. canis*, and *A. platys* by using Uranotest Quattro (Uranovet, Barcelona Spain) following the manufacturer's instructions.

Statistical Analysis

Data were analyzed by using SPSS Base 20.0 software (SPSS Inc./IBM, Chicago, IL, USA). A descriptive analysis of the variables considered was carried out considering the proportions of the qualitative variables. Chi-square and Fisher exact tests to compare proportions were performed. Sex, age, and habitat were considered as variables in the analysis for the autonomous community of Castilla y León and for each province. For the statistical analysis, dogs were grouped into five age groups (<1 year, from 1 to 5 years, from 5 to 10 years, from 10 to 15 years,

TABLE 1 | Prevalence and seroprevalences of the studied vector-borne infections by sex, age, and habitat in Castilla y León, Spain.

		D. immitis		***L. infantum***		***A. platys***		***E. canis***	
	n	**+**	**%**	**+**	**%**	**+**	**%**	**+**	**%**
SEX									
Male	748	57	7.62	36	4.81	11	1.47	9	1.20
Female	727	49	6.74	32	4.40	12	1.65	14	1.93
AGE									
<1 year	68	8	11.76	4	5.88	1	1.47	1	1.47
1–5 years	563	34	6.04	28	4.97	8	1.42	7	1.24
>5–10 years	545	44	8.07	23	4.22	10	1.83	13	2.39
>10-15 years	281	19	6.76	11	3.91	4	1.42	2	0.71
>15 years	18	1	5.56	2	11.11	0	0.00	0	0.00
HABITAT									
Indoor	546	24	4.40	22	4.03	6	1.10	2	0.37
Outdoor	646	55	8.51	39	6.04	9	1.39	14	2.17
Indoor/Outdoor	283	27	9.54	7	2.47	8	2.83	7	2.47
TOTAL	1,475	106	7.19	68	4.61	23	1.56	23	1.56

n, number of dogs sampled; +, positive animals; %, percentage of positive animals.

TABLE 2 | Numbers of dogs sampled and prevalence of *D. immitis* by sex, age, and habitat in the nine provinces of Castilla y León, Spain.

	1-León			2-Zamora			3-Salamanca			4-Valladolid			5-Palencia			6-Burgos			7-Soria			8-Segovia			9-Ávila		
	+	*n*	%	+	*n*	%	+	*n*	%	+	*n*	%	+	*n*	%	+	*n*	%	+	*n*	%	+	*n*	%	+	*n*	%
SEX																											
Male	9	121	7.44	10	65	15.38	6	68	8.82	10	88	11.36	4	50	8.00	7	128	5.47	0	61	0.00	5	110	4.55	6	57	10.53
Female	7	101	6.93	3	44	6.82	4	69	5.80	7	78	8.97	4	62	6.45	17	156	10.90	0	57	0.00	6	114	5.26	1	46	2.17
AGE																											
<1 year	2	8	25.00	2	8	25.00	1	9	11.11	0	5	0.00	0	2	0.00	3	22	13.64	0	5	0.00	0	5	0.00	0	4	0.00
1–5 years	5	64	7.81	8	47	17.02	2	41	4.88	4	63	6.35	6	40	15.00	4	97	4.12	0	65	0.00	3	88	3.41	2	58	3.45
>5–10 years	4	82	4.88	3	37	8.11	4	65	6.15	10	55	18.18	1	43	2.33	13	105	12.38	0	37	0.00	4	85	4.71	5	36	13.89
>10–15 years	5	62	8.06	0	16	0.00	3	21	14.29	3	43	6.98	1	25	4.00	4	53	7.55	0	11	0.00	3	45	6.67	0	5	0.00
>15 years	0	6	0.00	0	1	0.00	0	1	0.00	0	0	0.00	0	2	0.00	0	7	0.00	0	0	0.00	1	1	100.00	0	0	0.00
HABITAT																											
Indoor	8	65	12.31	4	50	8.00	1	17	5.88	2	63	3.17	1	21	4.76	4	102	3.92	0	83	0.00	2	117	1.71	2	28	7.14
Outdoor	8	154	5.19	6	46	13.04	7	100	7.00	12	60	20.00	3	65	4.62	14	117	11.97	0	21	0.00	1	20	5.00	4	63	6.35
Indoor/Outdoor	0	3	0.00	3	13	23.08	2	20	10.00	3	43	6.98	4	26	15.38	6	65	9.23	0	14	0.00	8	87	9.20	1	12	8.33
TOTAL	16	222	7.21	13	109	11.93	10	137	7.30	17	166	10.24	8	112	7.14	24	284	8.45	0	118	0.00	11	224	4.91	7	103	6.80

n, number of dogs sampled; +, positive animals; %, percentage of positive animals.

TABLE 3 | Numbers of dogs sampled and seroprevalence of *L. infantum* by sex, age, and habitat in the nine provinces of Castilla y León, Spain.

	1-León			2-Zamora			3-Salamanca			4-Valladolid			5-Palencia			6-Burgos			7-Soria			8-Segovia			9-Ávila		
	+	*n*	%	+	*n*	%	+	*n*	%	+	*n*	%	+	*n*	%	+	*n*	%	+	*n*	%	+	*n*	%	+	*n*	%
SEX																											
Male	5	121	4.13	4	65	6.15	6	68	8.82	5	88	5.68	3	50	6.00	5	128	3.91	1	61	1.64	3	110	2.73	4	57	7.02
Female	4	101	3.96	4	44	9.09	1	69	1.45	2	78	2.56	7	62	11.29	0	156	0.00	2	57	3.51	8	114	7.02	4	46	8.70
AGE																											
<1 year	2	8	25.00	2	8	25.00	0	9	0.00	0	5	0.00	0	2	0.00	0	22	0.00	0	5	0.00	0	5	0.00	0	4	0.00
1–5 years	3	64	4.69	2	47	4.26	2	41	4.88	4	63	6.35	3	40	7.50	2	97	2.06	2	65	3.08	3	88	3.41	7	58	12.07
>5–10 years	1	82	1.22	4	37	10.81	3	65	4.62	3	55	5.45	3	43	6.98	2	105	1.90	1	37	2.70	5	85	5.88	1	36	2.78
>10–15 years	3	62	4.84	0	16	0.00	2	21	9.52	0	43	0.00	3	25	12.00	0	53	0.00	0	11	0.00	3	45	6.67	0	5	0.00
>15 years	0	6	0.00	0	1	0.00	0	1	0.00	0	0	0.00	1	2	50.00	1	7	14.29	0	0	0.00	0	1	0.00	0	0	0.00
HABITAT																											
Indoor	4	65	6.15	2	50	4.00	0	17	0.00	3	63	4.76	3	21	14.29	1	102	0.98	0	83	0.00	8	117	6.84	1	28	3.57
Outdoor	5	154	3.25	6	46	13.04	7	100	7.00	3	60	5.00	5	65	7.69	3	117	2.56	2	21	9.52	1	20	5.00	7	63	11.11
Indoor/Outdoor	0	3	0.00	0	13	0.00	0	20	0.00	1	43	2.33	2	26	7.69	1	65	1.54	1	14	7.14	2	87	2.30	0	12	0.00
TOTAL	0	222	4.05	8	109	7.34	7	137	5.11	7	166	4.22	10	112	8.93	5	284	1.76	3	118	2.54	11	224	4.91	8	103	7.77

n, number of dogs sampled; +, positive animals; %, percentage of positive animals.

TABLE 4 | Numbers of dogs sampled and seroprevalence of *A. platys* by sex, age, and habitat in the nine provinces of Castilla y León, Spain.

	1-León			2-Zamora			3-Salamanca			4-Valladolid			5-Palencia			6-Burgos			7-Soria			8-Segovia			9-Ávila		
	+	*n*	%	+	*n*	%	+	*n*	%	+	*n*	%	+	*n*	%	+	*n*	%	+	*n*	%	+	*n*	%	+	*n*	%
SEX																											
Male	2	121	1.65	1	65	1.54	1	68	1.47	0	88	0.00	0	50	0.00	2	128	1.56	0	61	0.00	2	110	1.82	3	57	5.26
Female	0	101	0.00	0	44	0.00	1	69	1.45	4	78	5.13	0	62	0.00	2	156	1.28	0	57	0.00	4	114	3.51	1	46	2.17
AGE																											
<1 year	0	8	0.00	0	8	0.00	0	9	0.00	0	5	0.00	0	2	0.00	0	22	0.00	0	5	0.00	0	5	0.00	1	4	25.00
1–5 years	1	64	1.56	1	47	2.13	0	41	0.00	1	63	1.59	0	40	0.00	1	97	1.03	0	65	0.00	2	88	2.27	2	58	3.45
>5–10 years	0	82	0.00	0	37	0.00	2	65	3.08	2	55	3.64	0	43	0.00	3	105	2.86	0	37	0.00	2	85	2.35	1	36	2.78
>10–15 years	1	62	1.61	0	16	0.00	0	21	0.00	1	43	2.33	0	25	0.00	0	53	0.00	0	11	0.00	2	45	4.44	0	5	0.00
>15 years	0	6	0.00	0	1	0.00	0	1	0.00	0	0	0.00	0	2	0.00	0	7	0.00	0	0	0.00	0	1	0.00	0	0	0.00
HABITAT																											
Indoor	0	65	0.00	0	50	0.00	0	17	0.00	2	63	3.17	0	21	0.00	0	102	0.00	0	83	0.00	3	117	2.56	1	28	3.57
Outdoor	1	154	0.65	1	46	2.17	0	100	0.00	1	60	1.67	0	65	0.00	3	117	2.56	0	21	0.00	0	20	0.00	3	63	4.76
Indoor/Outdoor	1	3	33.33	0	13	0.00	2	20	10.00	1	43	2.33	0	26	0.00	1	65	1.54	0	14	0.00	3	87	3.45	0	12	0.00
TOTAL	2	222	0.90	1	109	0.92	2	137	1.46	4	166	2.41	0	112	0.00	4	284	1.41	0	118	0.00	6	224	2.68	4	103	3.88

n, number of dogs sampled; +, positive animals; %, percentage of positive animals.

TABLE 5 | Numbers of dogs sampled and seroprevalence of *E. canis* by sex, age, and habitat in the nine provinces of Castilla y León, Spain.

	1-León			2-Zamora			3-Salamanca			4-Valladolid			5-Palencia			6-Burgos			7-Soria			8-Segovia			9-Ávila		
	+	*n*	%	+	*n*	%	+	*n*	%	+	*n*	%	+	*n*	%	+	*n*	%	+	*n*	%	+	*n*	%	+	*n*	%
SEX																											
Male	2	121	1.65	2	65	3.08	1	68	1.47	0	88	0.00	0	50	0.00	0	128	0.00	1	61	1.64	2	110	1.82	1	57	1.75
Female	1	101	0.99	1	44	2.27	1	69	1.45	3	78	3.85	1	62	1.61	4	156	2.56	0	57	0.00	1	114	0.88	2	46	4.35
AGE																											
<1 year	1	8	12.50	0	8	0.00	0	9	0.00	0	5	0.00	0	2	0.00	0	22	0.00	0	5	0.00	0	5	0.00	0	4	0.00
1–5 years	0	64	0.00	1	47	2.13	0	41	0.00	1	63	1.59	0	40	0.00	2	97	2.06	1	65	1.54	1	88	1.14	1	58	1.72
>5–10 years	1	82	1.22	2	37	5.41	2	65	3.08	1	56	1.79	1	43	2.33	2	105	1.90	0	37	0.00	2	85	2.35	2	36	5.56
>10–15 years	1	62	1.61	0	16	0.00	0	21	0.00	1	42	2.38	0	25	0.00	0	53	0.00	0	11	0.00	0	45	0.00	0	5	0.00
>15 years	0	6	0.00	0	1	0.00	0	1	0.00	0	0	0.00	0	2	0.00	0	7	0.00	0	0	#¡DIV/0!	0	1	0.00	0	0	0.00
HABITAT																											
Indoor	0	65	0.00	1	50	2.00	0	17	0.00	0	85	0.00	0	21	0.00	0	102	0.00	0	83	0.00	1	117	0.85	0	28	0.00
Outdoor	2	154	1.30	2	46	4.35	1	100	1.00	2	61	3.28	1	65	1.54	3	117	2.56	0	21	0.00	0	20	0.00	3	63	4.76
Indoor/Outdoor	1	3	33.33	0	13	0.00	1	20	5.00	1	20	5.00	0	26	0.00	1	65	1.54	1	14	7.14	2	87	2.30	0	12	0.00
TOTAL	3	222	1.35	3	109	2.75	2	137	1.46	3	166	1.81	1	112	0.89	4	284	1.41	1	118	0.85	3	224	1.34	3	103	2.91

n, number of dogs sampled; +, positive animals; %, percentage of positive animals.

and >15 years). In all cases, the significance level was established at $p < 0.05$.

GIS Mapping

A map of the sampling area was constructed using ArcMap v.10.8 (ESRI, 2020 Redlands, CA, USA), including the following layers of relevant environmental information that have been considered to be relevant for the dynamics of the analyzed organisms and their transmission vectors: climate, potential vegetation, and surface waters and surface and edaphic humidity (rivers, lakes, lagoons, irrigated croplands, and parks) (28, 29). Thematic symbols were added for easier interpretation of the map. The canine samples were georeferenced by the location of health centers where the veterinary consultations occurred. Therefore, the points shown on the maps correspond to the centroids of the polygons of the postal codes where the analyses of the dogs were carried out. Inferences were drawn from a proximity analysis between the presence points and the environmental characteristics of the layers used. The coordinate system used was gcs_ETRS_1989.

RESULTS

Of the studied dogs, 7.72% were positive for one or several causative agents of CVBDs. The overall prevalence of *D. immitis* was 7.19%, and the seroprevalences of *L. infantum*, *A. platys*, and *E. canis* were 4.61, 1.56, and 1.56%, respectively. Results by sex, age groups, and habitat are shown in **Table 1**. Results for each of the nine provinces of Castilla y León are shown in **Figure 2** and **Tables 2–5**.

No significant differences were found by sex or age in any of the studied causative agents of CVBDs (**Table 1**). However, when habitat was assessed, significant differences were observed in the prevalence of *D. immitis* and seroprevalence of *E. canis* between indoor and outdoor dogs ($p < 0.05$) and between indoor and indoor/outdoor dogs ($p < 0.05$). Significant differences between outdoor and indoor/outdoor were observed in results for *L. infantum* ($p < 0.05$). By provinces, only significant differences were observed in the prevalence of *D. immitis* between indoor and outdoor dogs in Valladolid and between indoor and indoor/outdoor dogs in Segovia ($p < 0.05$) (**Table 2**).

Coinfections were observed in 0.95% of the infected dogs. Of them, 0.34% were infected by *D. immitis* + *L. infantum*, 0.14% by *D. immitis* + *A. platys*, 0.14% by *D. immitis* + *E. canis*, 0.14% by *L. infantum* + *A. platys*, 0.14% by *L. infantum* + *E. canis*, and 0.07% by *A. platys* + *E. canis*. By provinces, coinfections were found in 2.25% of the dogs from León, with 0.9% for *D. immitis* + *L. infantum*, 0.45% for *L. infantum* + *A. platys*, and 0.9% for *L. infantum* + *E. canis*. In Zamora, coinfections were found in 0.73% of the samples, corresponding to *D. immitis* + *A. platys* coinfections. In Valladolid, 0.6% tested positive for *D. immitis* + *E. canis* and 0.6% for *L. infantum* + *A. platys*. In Salamanca, only one dog was infected by *D. immitis* + *A. platys* (0.73%). In Palencia, there were two dogs infected by *D. immitis* + *L. infantum* (1.79%) and in Burgos 0.35% that tested positive for *D. immitis* + *A. platys*, *D. immitis* + *E. canis*, and *A. platys* + *E. canis*. In Soria, Segovia, and Avila, there were no coinfections in any of the samples analyzed.

Regarding *D. immitis*, the highest prevalences were located in the center and west of Castilla y León, where Csb and Cfb climates were present, while no infected dogs were found in Soria (east). Regarding *L. infantum*, the provinces with the highest seroprevalences were located in the south. On the other hand, seroprevalences for *A. platys* and *E. canis* were low but present in the whole region, except for the absence of *A. platys* in Palencia and Soria. According to climate, positive animals for *L. infantum*, *A. platys*, and *E. canis* were found in BSk, Cfb, Csa, and Csf sub-climates.

From a geospatial point of view (**Figures 3, 4**), 94.55% of infected animals were located in areas with high edaphic availability of water, as either stagnant water, irrigated agriculture, or river banks, as well as close to forest and groves vegetation, near holm oak, pyrenean oak groves, quejigo oak forest, or riparian forest, all of them mainly found in wet locations with a great abundance of irrigated arable land in the surrounding area. The remaining 5.45% of the infected animals (12/220) did not usually live in these locations but had been in the same or nearby areas with high soil availability of water and similar vegetation. In fact, 6.6% (7/106) were infected by D. immitis, 5.88% (4/68) by *L. infantum*, 0% (0/23) by *A. platys*, and 4.34% (1/23) by E. canis.

DISCUSSION

This manuscript shows the prevalence and seroprevalence of four causative agents of CVBDs in Castilla y León, the largest region of the Iberian Peninsula and one of the largest territories of the European Union. The highest positivity detected was that of *D. immitis* (7.19%), followed by *L. infantum* (4.61%), *A. platys*, and *E. canis* (1.56%), although these seroprevalences varied according to the geographical location of the provinces and the distribution of the samples tested.

A slight increase in the global prevalence of *D. immitis* was found when compared to a previous study, which reported a prevalence of 6.23% for Castilla y León (3). Although the data should be considered carefully due to the short time between one study and another, it is necessary to keep a constant record of variations in epidemiology to determine if there is an increasing trend in prevalence, which could confirm the expansion of this parasitosis in Spain (8). In Castilla y León, data at the provincial level only had been previously published for Salamanca, where prevalence decreased from 12.3 to 5.8% within 30 years (30–32); furthermore, a hyperendemic zone was previously reported in Salamanca, characterized by irrigated lands near the riverbank and presence of stagnant water, which showed a decreasing prevalence from 33.3 to 16.7% (8, 30–32). The results of the present study showed a slight increase in Salamanca, which may be due to the spread of the disease as well. The occurrence of canine cardiopulmonary dirofilariasis depends mostly on climatic factors such as temperature and humidity, although changes in land use derived from the human activity (e.g., the increase of irrigated crops), and the management of domestic

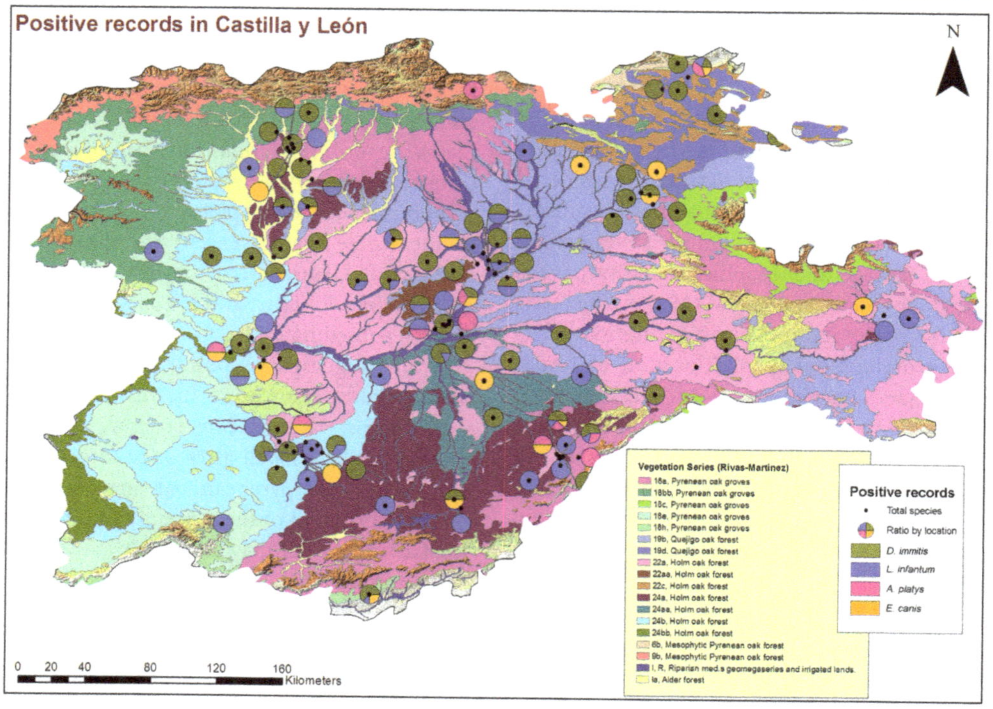

FIGURE 4 | Location of phytoclimatic series and geolocation of dogs infected by *D. immitis* (■), and seroprevalences for *L. infantum* (■), *A. platys* (■), and *E. canis* (■) in the nine provinces of Castilla y León, Spain.

animals also influences on the presence of the parasite and vectors (33). Although initially relegated to south and east of Spain, studies have confirmed the expansion toward northern and colder areas (3, 8). In addition, the presence of *Cx. pipiens*, widely present in Salamanca, has also been demonstrated to transmit the disease in this province (34). The results of this study confirm the risk of transmission specially associated with the presence of stagnant water, irrigated agriculture, crops, riverbanks, forests, and wet vegetation, as was predicted by a geo-environmental model (35), since infected dogs were located in areas with high or very high risk of infection in all provinces of Castilla y León.

Canine leishmaniosis has traditionally been considered as a disease limited to the Mediterranean basin (36), but several studies have reported an incipient increase in the number of cases in some areas of the north and central regions of Spain (3, 5, 37, 38), although the number of published studies is still low (39). Previous studies carried out in Castilla y León are sporadic and with a low number of samples analyzed. One of them showed an overall seroprevalence of 5.74% (3), and at the provincial level, another study carried out in Valladolid showed a seroprevalence of 5.3% (40). Both showed slightly higher prevalences than those reported in the present study, which could be due to the difference in the sampling process (with lower number of samples) rather than a real decrease in the prevalence, since an increase of this disease is being reported in Spain (3, 5, 39). Although from a geographical and climatic point of view, conditions of Castilla y León are very different and less favorable for the development of sandfly vectors from those in Mediterranean regions considered as endemic for *Leishmania*, the disease is well-established since seropositive dogs were found in irrigated areas, with a range of vegetation prone to vector establishment, and, moreover, cases of human leishmaniosis have been reported in Castilla y León (39), so control measures are necessary. It is possible that this expansion found in heartworm and in leishmaniosis is due to the fact that both diseases are considered not present in Castilla y León and, therefore, are not subject to strict prophylactic measures between veterinarians and owners.

Regarding *A. platys* and *E. canis*, few epidemiological data are available in Spain, but those published report the presence of both infectious agents mainly distributed in the provinces along the Mediterranean, although prevalences between 1 and 4.9% have also been reported in inland and isolated areas of the Iberian Peninsula (3, 4). It seems that the presence in the studied territory has decreased, since previous studies reported global prevalences of 19.2% in 1996 and 2% in 2020 for *E. canis* (3, 40, 41). Similar findings have been seen for *Anaplasma spp.*, which previous surveys have reported a global prevalence of 2.74% and prevalence of 19% in Valladolid (3, 40). This decrease is confirmed by the present results. *Ixodes* spp. and *Rhipicephalus sanguineus*, vectors of these diseases, are widely distributed throughout Castilla y León, the Iberian Peninsula, and Europe (42), being mainly located in areas with presence of grass, bushes, or trees. Furthermore, wild animals can act as reservoirs (43, 44), and in those provinces with higher seroprevalences there is a large population of wild animals (wolves, foxes) which in some cases live near houses and villages. In areas bordering the north of the region, where climatic and geographical conditions are much more favorable to vector development, previously reported seroprevalences were notably higher (5.01 and 3.13% to *A. platys* and *E. canis*, respectively) (45). It seems contradictory since climate changes favor the proliferation of ticks, but it could be due to the use of doxycycline for the treatment of several canine infections, as it is known that the dogs in this study did not receive adequate prophylaxis.

No significant differences were found by sex in this study, similar to other previous studies focused on these diseases such as other studies (3, 11, 19, 46). When age was assessed, no significant differences were observed between age groups, although differences have been observed in other epidemiological studies (4, 5, 11, 47–50). Regarding habitat of the animals, significantly higher prevalences were found in outdoor and indoor/outdoor dogs, as described by other authors (3, 5, 11, 51), since outdoor animals are more exposed to vectors. However, the study showed infected dogs living indoors as well. This is because some arthropods, such as mosquitoes, have access to indoors, and because animals living indoors are not fully enclosed and have a certain amount of access to the outdoors. Therefore, prophylactic measures should be applied to all dogs equally.

The preliminary GIS analysis suggests the existence of patterns of appearance of the infections with certain bioclimatic and environmental variables. The presence of areas with stagnant water, irrigation systems, irrigated agriculture, river banks, and different types of climatologies and vegetation favorable for the development of the vectors detected in the same places where positive dogs have been recorded suggests the existence of patterns of occurrence of the reported diseases with certain bioclimatic and environmental variables (35, 52, 53). The establishment of causal circumstances that can serve to predict risk areas requires a more in-depth study both in the resolution of these variables and in the incorporation of others that can explain in a more precise way the interactions between the parasite, its hosts, and the dispersal vectors. Expanding the methodology through the incorporation of spatial correlation analysis is one of the needs in this epidemiological field.

In conclusion, the results of this epidemiological study show a wide distribution of the evaluated causative agents of CVBDs in Castilla y León, which is very significant given the great geographical extension of the territory. The data obtained reveal the influence of the climate, orography, and presence of water, which will allow to comprehend their evolution in Castilla y León. Given the risk of infection or exposure to pathogens, as their presence in humans in Spain has been described, a close relationship between veterinarians, physicians, and public health administrations under the concept of One *Health* is needed. This would allow effective control measures to be carried out on infected animals and vectors, mainly focused on prophylactic measures to be applied routinely on dogs.

AUTHOR CONTRIBUTIONS

EC, RM, and IR-E wrote the manuscript. EC, RM, and JM-A designed the study and obtained funding. PP, IR-E, and JS performed the fieldwork and collected the data. EC, RM, JM-A, and JL-M participated in the revision of the manuscript. All authors participated in the design and production of the figures and have read and agreed to the published version of the manuscript.

ACKNOWLEDGMENTS

The authors would like to thank Marta Ruiz-Somacarrera, degree student in Pharmacy (University of Salamanca), and Xiomara Murcia, masters student in Tropical Diseases (University of Salamanca), for their contribution to the study, and all veterinarians who kindly collaborated and provided samples for this research. Without their collaboration and dedication, this study could not have been carried out. Also, the authors would like to thank CEVA for their help and support throughout all the study.

REFERENCES

1. Springer A, Montenegro VM, Schicht S, Pantchev N, Strube C. Seroprevalence and current infections of canine vector-borne diseases in Nicaragua. *Parasit Vectors.* (2018) 11:585. doi: 10.1186/s13071-018-3173-1
2. Esteban-Mendoza MV, Arcila-Quiceno V, Albarracín-Navas J, Hernández I, Flechas-Alarcón MC, Morchón R. Current situation of the presence of *Dirofilaria immitis* in dogs and humans in Bucaramanga, Colombia. *Front Vet Sci.* (2020) 7:488. doi: 10.3389/fvets.2020.00488
3. Montoya-Alonso JA, Morchón R, Costa-Rodríguez N, Matos JI, Falcón-Cordón Y, Carretón E. Current distribution of selected vector-borne diseases in dogs in Spain. *Front Vet Sci.* (2020) 7:564429. doi: 10.3389/fvets.2020.564429
4. Sainz Á, Roura X, Miró G, Estrada-Peña A, Kohn B, Harrus S, et al. Guideline for veterinary practitioners on canine ehrlichiosis and anaplasmosis in Europe. *Parasit Vectors.* (2015) 8:75. doi: 10.1186/s13071-015-0649-0
5. Montoya A, Checa R, Marino V, Gálvez R, Portero M, De Mari K, et al. Antibodies elicited by the CaniLeish® vaccine: long-term clinical follow-up study of dogs in Spain. *Parasitol Res.* (2021) 120:1471–9. doi: 10.1007/s00436-021-07091-1
6. Perez M, Bodor M, Zhang C, Xiong Q, Rikihisa Y. Human infection with *Ehrlichia canis* accompanied by clinical signs in Venezuela. *Ann N Y Acad Sci.* (2010) 1212:130. doi: 10.1196/annals.1374.016
7. Franco-Zetina M, Adame-Gallegos J, Dzul-Rosado K. Effectivity of diagnostic methods for the detection of human and canine monocytic ehrlichiosis. *Rev Chilena Infectol.* (2019) 36:650–5. doi: 10.4067/S0716-10182019000500650
8. Morchón R, Carretón E, González-Miguel J, Mellado-Hernández I. Heartworm disease (*Dirofilaria immitis*) and their vectors in Europe - new distribution trends. *Front Physiol.* (2012) 3:196. doi: 10.3389/fphys.2012.00196
9. Simón F, Muro A, Cordero M, Martin J. A seroepidemiologic survey of human dirofilariosis in Western Spain. *Trop Med Parasitol.* (1991) 42:106–8.
10. Savić S, Stosic MZ, Marcic D, Hernández I, Potkonjak A, Otasevic S, et al. Seroepidemiological study of canine and human dirofilariasis in the endemic region of Northern Serbia. *Front Vet Sci.* (2020) 7:571. doi: 10.3389/fvets.2020.00571
11. Zumaquero L, Simón F, Carretón E, Hernández I, Sandoval C, Morchón R. Prevalence of canine and human dirofilariosis in Puebla, Mexico. *Vet Parasitol.* (2020) 282:109098. doi: 10.1016/j.vetpar.2020.109098

12. Alvar J, Vélez ID, Bern C, Herrero M, Desjeux P, Cano J, et al. Leishmaniasis Worldwide and global estimates of its incidence. *PLoS ONE.* (2012) 7:e35671. doi: 10.1371/journal.pone.0035671
13. Harrus S. Perspectives on the pathogenesis and treatment of canine monocytic ehrlichiosis (*Ehrlichia canis*). *Vet J.* (2015) 204:239–40. doi: 10.1016/j.tvjl.2015.04.027
14. Cazan CD, Ionică AM, Matei IA, D'Amico G, Muñoz C, Berriatua E, et al. Detection of *Leishmania infantum* DNA and antibodies against *Anaplasma* spp. *Borrelia burgdorferi* sl and *Ehrlichia canis* in a dog kennel in South-Central Romania. *Acta Vet Scand.* (2020) 62:42. doi: 10.1186/s13028-020-00540-4
15. Dyachenko V, Pantchev N, Balzer HJ, Meyersen A, Straubinger RK. First case of Anaplasma platys infection in a dog from Croatia. *Parasit Vect.* (2012) 5:49. doi: 10.1186/1756-3305-5-49
16. Bouzouraa T, René-Martellet M, Chêne J, Attipa C, Lebert I, Chalvet-Monfray K, et al. Clinical and laboratory features of canine *Anaplasma platys* infection in 32 naturally infected dogs in the Mediterranean basin. *Ticks Tick Borne Dis.* (2016) 7:1256–64. doi: 10.1016/j.ttbdis.2016.07.004
17. Zobba R, Schianchi E, Ben Said M, Belkahia H, Messadi L, Piredda R, et al. gltA typing of *Anaplasma* strains related to *A. platys:* taxonomical and one health implications. *Ticks Tick Borne Dis.* (2021) 13:101850. doi: 10.1016/j.ttbdis.2021.101850
18. Panarese R, Iatta R, Mendoza-Roldan JA, Szlosek D, Braff J, Liu J, et al. Comparison of diagnostic tools for the detection of *Dirofilaria immitis* infection in dogs. *Pathogens.* (2020) 9:499. doi: 10.3390/pathogens9060499
19. Díaz-Regañón D, Roura X, Suárez ML, León M, Sainz Á. Serological evaluation of selected vector-borne pathogens in owned dogs from northern Spain based on a multicenter study using a commercial test. *Parasit Vect.* (2020) 13:301. doi: 10.1186/s13071-020-04172-5
20. Pullan RL, Sturrock HJW, Soares Magalhaes RJ, Clements ACA, Brooker SK. Spatial parasite ecology and epidemiology: a review of methods and applications. *Parasitology.* (2012) 139:1870–87. doi: 10.1017/S0031182012000698
21. Weiss DJ, Lucas TCD, Nguyen M, Nandi AK, Bisanzio D, Battle KE, et al. Mapping the global prevalence, incidence, and mortality of *Plasmodium falciparum*, 2000–17: a spatial and temporal modelling study. *Lancet.* (2019) 394:322–31. doi: 10.1016/S0140-6736(19)31097-9
22. Sifaki-Pistola D, Ntais P, Christodoulou V, Mazeris A, Antoniou M. The use of spatial analysis to estimate the prevalence of canine leishmaniasis in Greece and Cyprus to predict its future variation and relate it to human disease. *Am J Trop Med Hyg.* (2014) 91:336–41. doi: 10.4269/ajtmh.13-0459
23. Rinaldi L, Biggeri A, Carbone S, Musella V, Catelan D, Veneziano V, et al. Canine faecal contamination and parasitic risk in the city of Naples (southern Italy). *BMC Vet Res.* (2006) 2:29. doi: 10.1186/1746-6148-2-29
24. European Commission (2021). Available online at: https://ec.europa.eu/growth/tools-databases/regional-innovation-monitor/base-profile/castilla-y-leon (accessed July 6, 2021).
25. *Research and Innovation Strategy for Smart Specialisation (RIS3) of Castilla y León 2014-2020.* (2021). Available online at: https://fuescyl.com/images/03innovacion_conocimiento/Comisionado/RIS3_Castilla_y_Leon_2014-2020_(eng).pdf (accessed September 29, 2021).
26. Agencia Estatal de Meteorología, Ministerio de Agricultura, Alimentación y Medio Ambiente. *Iberian Climate Atlas. Air Temperature and Precipitation (1971-2000)* (2021).
27. Rivas Martínez S. *Memoria del Mapa de Series de Vegetación de España 1: 400000 ICONA Ministerio de Agricultura.* (1987). Available online at: https://www.mitecogobes/es/biodiversidad/servicios/banco-datos-naturaleza/informacion-disponible/memoria_mapa_series_veg_descargasaspx (accessed July 20, 2021).
28. Climate shifts. In: *Worldmaps of Köppen-Geiger Climate Classification.* (2019). Available online at: https://koeppen-geiger.vu-wien.ac.at/shifts.html (accessed July 20, 2021).
29. Ministerio para la Transición Ecológica y el Reto Demográfico (2021). Available online at: https://www.miteco.gob.es/es/biodiversidad/ (accessed July 20, 2021).
30. Diosdado A, Gómez PJ, González-Miguel J, Simón F, Morchón R. Current status of canine dirofilariosis in an endemic area of western Spain. *J Helminthol.* (2018) 92:520–3. doi: 10.1017/S0022149X17000591
31. Morchón R, Mellado I, González-Miguel J, Hernández MV, Hernández L, Simón F. Prevalencia de la dirofilariosis cardiopulmonar canina. *Argos.* (2011) 126:30.
32. Pérez-Sánchez R, Gómez-Bautista M, Grandes AE. Canine filariasis in Salamanca (northwest Spain). *Ann Trop Med Parasitol.* (1989) 83:143–50. doi: 10.1080/00034983.1989.11812322
33. Simón F, Siles-Lucas M, Morchón R, González-Miguel J, Mellado I, Carretón E, et al. Human and animal dirofilariasis: the emergence of a zoonotic mosaic. *Clin Microbiol Rev.* (2012) 25:507–44. doi: 10.1128/CMR.00012-12
34. Morchón R, Bargues MD, Latorre JM, Melero-Alcíbar R, Pou-Barreto C, Mas-Coma S, et al. Haplotype H1 of *Culex pipiens* implicated as natural vector of *Dirofilaria immitis* in an endemic area of Western Spain. *Vector Borne Zoonot Dis.* (2007) 7:653–8. doi: 10.1089/vbz.2007.0124
35. Simón L, Afonin A, López-Díez LI, González-Miguel J, Morchón R, Carretón E, et al. Geo-environmental model for the prediction of potential transmission risk of *Dirofilaria* in an area with dry climate and extensive irrigated crops. The case of Spain. *Vet Parasitol.* (2014) 200:257–64. doi: 10.1016/j.vetpar.2013.12.027
36. Fahrion A, Gasimov E, Joseph S, Grout L, Allan M, Postigo JR. Surveillance of leishmaniasis in the WHO European Region. *Rev Épidémiol Santé Publique.* (2018) 66:S394. doi: 10.1016/j.respe.2018.05.429
37. González E, Jiménez M, Hernández S, Martín-Martín I, Molina R. Phlebotomine sand fly survey in the focus of leishmaniasis in Madrid, Spain (2012-2014): seasonal dynamics, *Leishmania infantum* infection rates and blood meal preferences. *Parasit Vectors.* (2017) 10:368. doi: 10.1186/s13071-017-2309-z
38. Alcover MM, Ribas A, Guillén MC, Berenguer D, Tomás-Pérez M, Riera C, et al. Wild mammals as potential silent reservoirs of *Leishmania infantum* in a Mediterranean area. *Prev Vet Med.* (2020) 175:104874. doi: 10.1016/j.prevetmed.2019.104874
39. Garrote JI, Gutiérrez MP, Izquierdo RL, Dueñas MA, Zarzosa P, Cañavate C, et al. Seroepidemiologic study of *Leishmania infantum* infection in Castilla-Leon, Spain. *Am J Trop Med Hyg.* (2004) 71:403–6. doi: 10.4269/ajtmh.2004.71.403
40. Couto CG, Lorentzen L, Beall MJ, Shields J, Bertolone N, Couto JI, et al. Serological study of selected vector-borne diseases in shelter dogs in central Spain using point-of-care assays. *Vector Borne Zoonotic Dis.* (2010) 10:885–8. doi: 10.1089/vbz.2009.0063
41. Sainz A, Delgado S, Amusátegui I, Tesouro MA. Seroprevalence of canine ehrlichiosis in Castilla-León (northwest of Spain). *Prev Med Vet.* (1996) 29:1–7. doi: 10.1016/S0167-5877(96)01060-4
42. Nicholson WL, Allen KE, McQuiston JH, Breitschwerdt EB, Little SE. The increasing recognition of rickettsial pathogens in dogs and people. *Trends Parasitol.* (2010) 26:205–12. doi: 10.1016/j.pt.2010.01.007
43. Fishman Z, Gonen L, Harrus S, Strauss-Ayali D, King R, Baneth G. A serosurvey of *Hepatozoon canis* and *Ehrlichia canis* antibodies in wild red foxes (*Vulpes vulpes*) from Israel. *Vet Parasitol.* (2004) 119:21–6. doi: 10.1016/j.vetpar.2003.08.012
44. Alkishe A, Raghavan RK, Peterson AT. Likely geographic distributional shifts among medically important tick species and tick-associated diseases under climate change in North America: a review. *Insects.* (2021) 12:225. doi: 10.3390/insects12030225
45. Amusategui I, Tesouro MA, Kakoma I, Sainz A. Serological reactivity to *Ehrlichia canis, Anaplasma phagocytophilum, Neorickettsia risticii, Borrelia burgdorferi* and *Rickettsia conorii* in dogs from northwestern Spain. *Vector Borne Zoonot Dis.* (2008) 8:797–803. doi: 10.1089/vbz.2007.0277
46. Solano-Gallego L, Llull J, Osso M, Hegarty B, Breitschwerdt E. A serological study of exposure to arthropod-borne pathogens in dogs from northeastern Spain. *Vet Res.* (2006) 37:231–44. doi: 10.1051/vetres:2005054
47. Encinas Grandes A, Gómez Bautista M, Martin Novo M, Simón F. Leishmaniasis in the province of Salamanca, Spain. Prevalence in dogs, and seasonal dynamics of vectors. *Ann Parasitol Hum Comp.* (1988) 63:387–97. doi: 10.1051/parasite/1988636387
48. Fisa R, Gállego M, Castillejo S, Aisa MJ, Serra T, Riera C, et al. Epidemiology of canine leishmaniosis in Catalonia (Spain) the example of the Priorat focus. *Vet Parasitol.* (1999) 83:87–97. doi: 10.1016/S0304-4017(99)00074-6
49. Portillo A, Pérez-Martínez L, Santibáñez S, Santibáñez P, Palomar AM, Oteo JA. *Anaplasma* spp. in wild mammals and Ixodes ricinus from the north of Spain. *Vector Borne Zoonot Dis.* (2011) 11:3–8. doi: 10.1089/vbz.2009.0214

50. Vélez R, Ballart C, Domenech E, Abras A, Fernández-Arévalo A, Gómez SA, et al. Seroprevalence of canine *Leishmania infantum* infection in the Mediterranean region and identification of risk factors: the example of North-Eastern and Pyrenean areas of Spain. *Prev Vet Med.* (2019) 162:67–75. doi: 10.1016/j.prevetmed.2018.10.015
51. Morillas F, Sanchez Rabasco F, Ocaña J, Martin-Sanchez J, Ocaña-Wihelmi J, Acedo C. Leishmaniasis in the focus of the Axarquía region, province of Málaga, southern Spain: a survey of humans, dogs, and vector. *Parasitol Res.* (1996) 82:569–70. doi: 10.1007/s0043600 50164
52. Gálvez R, Montoya A, Cruz I, Fernández C, Martín O, Checa R, et al. Latest trends in *Leishmania infantum* infection in dogs in Spain, Part I: mapped seroprevalence and sand fly distributions. *Parasit Vectors.* (2020) 13:204. doi: 10.1186/s13071-020-04081-7
53. Saleh MN, Allen KE, Lineberry MW, Little SE, Reichard MV. Ticks infesting dogs and cats in North America: biology, geographic distribution, and pathogen transmission. *Vet Parasitol.* (2021) 294:109392. doi: 10.1016/j.vetpar.2021.1 09392

Case Studies of Severe Microfilaremia in Four Dogs Naturally Infected with *Dirofilaria repens* as the Primary Disease or a Disease Complicating Factor

Magdalena E. Wysmołek[1]**, *Maciej Klockiewicz*[1]*, *Małgorzata Sobczak-Filipiak*[2]*, *Ewa Długosz*[1] *and Marcin Wiśniewski*[1]

[1] *Division of Parasitology and Parasitic Diseases, Department of Pre-Clinical Sciences, Institute of Veterinary Medicine, Warsaw University of Life Sciences, Warsaw, Poland,* [2] *Department of Pathology and Veterinary Diagnostics, Institute of Veterinary Medicine, Warsaw University of Life Sciences, Warsaw, Poland*

***Correspondence:**
Magdalena E. Wysmołek
magdalena_wysmolek@sggw.edu.pl

Subcutaneous dirofilariosis in dogs, caused by *Dirofilaria repens*, is an underdiagnosed disease, now recognized for its zoonotic potential, and growing distribution and prevalence across Europe and Asia. Our understanding of the pathogenicity in human and canine host remains unclear, but case reports suggest that microfilariae (Mf) as well as adult *D. repens* may directly cause internal organs damage or may be a factor complicating the course of other ailments. The purpose of the study was to report high Mf in dogs and to discuss potential relevance with co-morbidity. Our data from a modified Knott's test performed on 62 infected dogs indicate that the median Mf count in *D. repens* infections is 675 Mf/ml and we consider microfilaremia above 10,000 Mf/ml as high intensity. This collection of case reports discusses 4 cases of high intensity *D. repens* microfilaremia in companion dogs; one presenting pathology from a very high intensity of adult *D. repens* with post-treatment complications, and 3 dogs in which high microfilaremia was detected incidentally during the management of other primary illnesses. To our knowledge this report describes the highest *D. repens* microfilaremia ever detected in a dog, at 178,000 Mf/ml. The issue of high microfilaremic infections in dogs is poorly studied and there is growing need to identify the presentation and understand the mechanisms of associated pathogenesis in the host-parasite relationship.

Keywords: dog, dirofilariosis, microfilaremia, immunology, natural Dirofilaria repens infection

INTRODUCTION

Dirofilaria repens is a zoonotic filarial nematode transmitted to dogs by a mosquito vector and is the principal agent of human dirofilariosis in the Old World (1). Humans are considered a dead-end, accidental host for *D. repens*, but a growing body of case reports suggests that humans may instead be a dual facultative host in which the parasite can achieve maturity and release microfilariae (Mf) into the bloodstream (2, 3). Recently, there has been documentation in Poland of a human patient having microfilaremia (360 Mf/ml) (4). Furthermore, an ocular mucosa associated lymphoid tissue lymphoma (MALT) has been reported in a human patient in Poland as a possible consequence of dirofilariosis (5). The number of human subcutaneous dirofilariosis cases in Europe has increased in recent years and current estimations in some areas is roughly 10 infected out of 100,000 inhabitants (6). True infection prevalence is likely underestimated because of misdiagnosis and under sampling. Additionally, with increasing globalization and climate change (1, 7), these numbers are expected to continue to grow and, therefore, proper diagnosis and treatment in dogs and humans will be increasingly important for managing the spread and disease burden of *D. repens* infections.

Currently, the treatment recommended by the European Society for Dirofilariosis and Angiostrongylosis (ESDA) for *D. repens* infections consists of 2.5 mg/kg moxidectin (in a spot-on formulation containing also 10 mg/kg imidacloprid) given monthly[1]. However, because so few cases of high intensity *D. repens* microfilaremia have been reported (8), there are no guidelines for its management (1), or rationale for its cause.

The gold standard for diagnosis of subcutaneous dirofilariosis is the modified Knott's test which allows visual detection and morphological identification of Mf (9), and was used to evaluate the Mf burden in all cases described in this article. Our data from a modified Knott's tests performed on 62 infected dogs indicate that the median Mf count in *D. repens* infections is 675 Mf/ml (unpublished data), and the authors consider microfilaremia above 10,000 Mf/ml as being high. Dogs presented in this report all tested positive for having high microfilaremia with the highest level ever reported in *D. repens* infection at 178,000 Mf/ml. Helminths are known to suppress the host immune response in order to establish infection. It is therefore possible that patients presenting with high Mf counts may represent a population with pre-existing immunosuppression and are thus, unable to naturally control or respond to infection (9). All dogs in this study were diagnosed with terminal conditions which might be correlated with an underlying immunodeficiency.

CASE #1

Clinical Presentation

A 9-year-old entire male Shepherd dog was admitted to a veterinary clinic on 27/05/2016 due to severe weight loss and two infected purulent wounds in the scrotum area, associated with intensive licking. Physical examination revealed the presence of a chronic bilateral *otitis externa* and an inflammation of the interdigital spaces. Swabs from both ears and interdigital spaces were taken.

Diagnosis

During a blood examination on 03/09/2016 we detected severe leucocytosis [33,64 G/l (reference value 6–12 G/l)] related to the increase in band neutrophils [10% (reference value 0–6%)] with a mild increase in aspartate aminotransferase [91 U/l (reference value 0–45 U/l)], moderate increase in phosphatase kinase [1,160 U/l (reference value 25–467 U/l)], decrease in albumin [1,8 g/dl (reference value 3,3–5,6 g/dl) and the presence of Mf was observed in the blood smear. Identification of *D. repens* was obtained using multiplex PCR performed using primers designed by Genchi et al. (10). The intensity of microfilaremia was evaluated using a modified Knott's test and revealed 14,512 Mf/ml of blood. The ear swab sample tested positive for *Malassezia pachydermatis*, and the swab from interdigital space was positive for *Pseudomonas aeruginosa*.

Treatment

During surgical castration on 7/09/2016, 26 adult *D. repens* worms were found in the spermatic cord, testicles and scrotum tissue. The external canals were treated with nystatin according to the antifungal susceptibility test, and a general antibiotic was administered for the dermatitis of interdigital space according to the antibiogram.

After castration and wound excision, the dog started to gain weight. *Otitis externa* as well as the dermatitis were ameliorating after appropriate treatment. Beginning on 24/10/2016, 6 monthly treatments of topical moxidectin with imidacloprid were administered as efficacious treatment against adult *D. repens* in dogs (11). One week after the first application no Mf were detected in the peripheral blood. The body condition of the dog changed from very thin to normal within 4 months. Despite amelioration of the general condition, a necrosis and pyogranuloma of interdigital spaces associated with severe dermatitis of the abdomen and limbs developed with episodes of amelioration and deteriorations between 10/11/2016 and 28/08/2018. A course of antibiotics was administered according to the antibiogram but no improvement was observed. A generalized demodicosis, caused by *Demodex canis*, was diagnosed and, as the declining clinical state of the dog was progressing and no amelioration could be established, the owner did not wish to pursue further treatment. Finally, the patient became anorexic and expired on 15/09/2018. The cause of death reported after necropsy was a perforated stomach ulcer. Moreover, the histopathological examination of internal organs revealed a chronic cardiac insufficiency and pathological changes indicating a chronic inflammation in the kidneys, liver and spleen.

Discussion

The presence of 26 adult *D. repens* likely caused severe pain and pruritus. It is noteworthy that there were no noticeable behaviors to indicate the extremely high number of Mf circulating in the blood stream. The only obvious clinical and hematological signs were likely associated with presence of a large number of adult worms in the scrotum area. We suspect that the severe dermatitis which appeared post-treatment might have been associated with *Wolbachia* release after *Dirofilaria* spp. adulticide treatment as reported by previous studies in *D. immitis* infections (12–15). Furthermore, German Shepherds are predisposed to primary immunodeficiency (16) and it has been postulated that high microfilaremia might be associated with a state of

[1]https://www.esda.vet/wp-content/uploads/2017/11/GUIDELINES-FOR-CLINICAL-MANAGEMENT-OF-SUBCUTANEOUS-DIROFILARIOSIS-IN-DOGS-AND-CATS.pdf.

immunosuppression (17). The chronic yeast infection (usually secondary to an immune disorder in dogs) as well as the appearance of generalized demodicosis are possible indicators of immunodeficiency in this patient (18, 19).

CASE #2

Clinical Presentation

A 7-year-old male entire Yorkshire Terrier was admitted to the veterinary clinic on 06/08/2019 due to sudden anorexia, apathy and diarrhea. During the clinical examination the dog presented a hypotonic-hyporesponsiveness concomitant with exophthalmos, severe dehydration, hypothermia, bradycardia and pale mucous membranes. A treatment based on dexamethasone, caffeine, atropine, ceftriaxone and fluid therapy was initiated and a blood sample taken for analysis.

Diagnosis

Hematology revealed a severe leukocytosis [58.1 $\times$ $10^3/mm^3$ (reference value 6.0–12.0 $\times$ $10^3/mm^3$)] resulting from neutrophilia [54.2 $\times$ $10^3/mm^3$ (reference value 3.00-10.00 $10^3/mm^3$)], and eosinophilia [23.42 $\times$ $10^3/mm^3$ (reference value 0–0.60 $10^3/mm^3$)] with mild anemia [HCT = 39.5% (reference value 44.0–57.0%)], and a severe increase in alkaline phosphatase [551 U/l (reference value 20–150 U/l)], alanine aminotransferase [131 U/l (reference value 10–118 U/l)] and a decrease in albumin [1.5 g/dL (reference value 2.5–4.4 g/dL)]. The glucose level was 99 mg/dl (reference value 80–120 mg/dl) and the modified Knott's test revealed 11,560 Mf/ml. After testing and excluding Canine Coronavirus (CCV), Canine Parvovirus and *Giardia* spp. infections, and according to anamnesis, a diagnosis of poisoning with taxine alkaloid was decided. On 08/08/2019 the state of the patient continued to deteriorate despite intense care therapy, and a decision of euthanasia was made.

Discussion

It is hard to evaluate the impact of co-infection with *D. repens* in this case, but one can suppose that it may have had a negative influence on the development of the condition, as taxine alkaloids (from yew) can cause lethal poisoning, in particular due to the compound's toxic effect on the cardiovascular apparatus (20). It is certainly possible that the severe microfilaremia might create a blood flow disturbance of capillary circulation by mechanical obstruction. Additionally, it has been observed in other filarial parasitic diseases that dead Mf release toxic products that affect the capillaries (21, 22). Unfortunately, the prognosis in taxine alkaloid poisoning without immediate stomach flushing is usually fatal and the presence of subcutaneous dirofilariosis was not likely influential in the course of the intoxication (20), but may be of concern for chronic anemia.

CASE #3

Clinical Presentation

A 10-year-old entire male mix breed dog was admitted to the clinic due to constipation. During the physical examination a testicular asymmetry, perineal hernia, fecal impaction as well as an anal sac tumor of 2 $\times$ 2 cm were detected.

Diagnosis

The blood test revealed moderate anemia [RBC = 4.98 T/l (reference value 5.5–8.5 T/l), HCT = 32.6% (reference value 37.0–55.0%), HGB = 11,1 g/dl (reference value 12–18 g/dl)], severe leucocytosis [41.04 G/l (reference value 6.0–12.0 G/l)] resulted from: neutrophilia [34.06 G/l (reference value 2.9–13.6 G/l)], monocytosis [2.05 G/l (reference value 0.4–1.6 G/l)], eosinophilia [3.69 G/l (reference value 0–3.1 G/l)], thrombocytopenia [19 G/l (reference value 150–500 G/l)] and 40 150 Mf/ml. In addition, a mild increase in alanine aminotransferase [72 U/l (reference value 0–60.0 U/l)] and a decrease of albumin [3.2 g/dl (reference value 3.3–5.6 g/dl)] were detected, and ultrasonography revealed ascites, which was analyzed. The ascites contained Mf, granulocytes and atypical binucleated cells with many mitotic figures suggesting a neoplastic process. The owner did not wish to pursue any treatment nor euthanize and decided to take the patient home.

Discussion

This is the second report of finding Mf in the body fluid in a dog, the first of which was by Pazdzior-Czapula et al. (23). The issue and association between neoplastic processes and the presence of *D. repens* Mf or adults has been previously observed in cancer of the perianal gland, mast cells, epithelial cells, hemangiopericytoma, and trichoblastoma ribbon in dogs (20), as well as an ocular lymphoma from which the parasite was previously removed from a human patient (5). It has also been reported that parasitic infections or abnormalities of the immune system are at a high risk for developing cancer (5, 24), but the exact relationship between subcutaneous dirofilariosis and neoplastic process is still unknown.

CASE #4

Clinical Presentation

A 10-year-old entire Saint Bernard male was admitted to the clinic due to intolerance of any physical activity and permanent dyspnoea. Four months prior, the dog was pursuing therapy in another clinic and received a treatment of benazepril, spironolactone, theophylline, and nitroglycerin with no diagnosis, but anamnesis of increasing fatigue after physical exercise. During our physical examination, dyspnoea and cyanosis of tongue and mucous membranes (hypoxia) were noted.

Diagnosis

After sedation of the patient, additional diagnostics were performed. Thoracic radiographs revealed a dilation of the esophagus, computed tomography and electrocardiography revealed no alternations. A moderate leucocytosis [16.7 $\times$ $10^3/mm^3$ (reference value 6.0–10.00 x $10^3/mm^3$)], mild neutrophilia [13.90 x $10^3/mm^3$ (3.0–10.00 $\times$ $10^3/mm^3$)], and eosinophilia [1.5 $\times$ $10^3/mm^3$ (reference value 0.0–0.60 $\times$ $10^3/mm^3$)] were observed in the hematology, and the biochemistry parameters were all in normal reference ranges. The echocardiographic measurements were within standard normal age limits. The rapid CANIV-4 commercial test was positive for *D. immitis*, but multiplex PCR revealed only the presence of *D. repens*. A modified Knott's test was performed which detected 178,000 Mf/ml and a double morphological identification of *D. repens*, not *D. immitis* was confirmed. As systolic dysfunction was suspected aspirin was administrated which resulted in mild improvement of clinical signs. A few days later echocardiographic examination was performed and no nematodes were detected in the pulmonary artery. The echocardiographic measurements were within standard normal age limits. Only immobilization brought relief to the dog. A final diagnosis of severe laryngeal paralysis was decided upon, and pharmacological treatment was performed, but with no improvement. Before any surgical interventions could be considered the patient died at home from apparent suffocation. The owners did not permit a necropsy.

Discussion

Laryngeal paralysis is a respiratory disorder that primarily affects older (> 9 years of age), large-breed and giant-breed dogs, such as the Saint Bernard in this case. In many dogs the etiology remains idiopathic, but one possible cause is suggested to involve immune-mediated neuromuscular disease or other immune disorders like systemic lupus erythematosus (25, 26) In humans, a case of a girl treated for systemic lupus erythematosus was diagnosed with concomitant non-human filarial microfilaremic infection. The authors suggested that an immunity disorder might have led to this filarial infection (27). Leucocytosis and eosinophilia are both commonly associated with helminth infections, and neutrophilia can inhibit a Th1 type response, all of which could be expected to be associated with an increased Mf count. However, these numbers alone are very unlikely to facilitate or explain such a high level of microfilaremia. Although it is not possible to come to any conclusions from this case, the incredibly high level of microfilaremia and its co-morbidity with a presentation of symptoms known to be related to compromised immune system function, is highly suggestive of a causal relationship.

FINAL CONCLUSIONS

The goal of this article was to report the details of four cases of high *D. repens* microfilaremia. Hematological and biochemical findings in dogs infected with *Dirofilaria repens* included anemia, thrombocytopenia, leucocytosis, neutrophilia, eosinophilia, monocytosis and increased values of alkaline phosphatase, aspartate transaminase, alanine aminotransferase, blood urea nitrogen, creatinine, bilirubin as well as hypoalbuminemia, which is in keeping with results described by other authors (28, 29).

In the cases presented here, it is difficult to determine how long the animals were infected for or to evaluate the contribution of subcutaneous dirofilariosis to the progression of morbidity in the presence of concomitant conditions. Due to the severity of the underlying diseases and symptoms, anthelmintic treatment was only administered to one dog seen in this collection of case studies. Even in the presence of a high burden of microfilaria, treatment with a standard dose of moxidectin was sufficient to reduce Mf count below detection 6 days after application. It should be noted that there is a 24-h microfilarial periodicity, which makes the time of sampling a factor influencing the result of a Knott test (30).

We suspect that the severe dermatitis that appeared post-treatment might have been associated with *Wolbachia* release after *Dirofilaria* spp. worm death as reported in *Dirofilaria immitis* infections (12). Recently, a case report of *D. repens* microfilaremic infection in a human showed successful treatment with only doxycycline targeting the *Wolbachia* endosymbiont (31).

All of the *D. repens* infections reported here were diagnosed incidentally while investigating concomitant conditions, suggesting that high intensity microfilaremia *per se* may go undiagnosed. This implies that there is a greater reservoir for human infection than previously suspected, and perhaps warrants increased monitoring in endemic areas, such as the regular use of a modified Knott's test. It might be discussed if high microfilaremic dogs represent an epidemiological risk of increased transmission, as most mosquitoes die when feeding on hosts with microfilaremia superior to 7,500 Mf/ml (21). However, the daily microfilarial periodicity permits the possibility that some mosquitoes can survive ingesting blood even from high microfilaremic hosts. Therefore, anthelmintic treatment, even in the absence of parasitic symptoms, should be administrated.

It remains unclear why in some patients, *D. repens* infections appear asymptomatic, and in other cases Mf are suspected to be responsible for severe renal or liver damage (28). Veterinarians should consider dirofilariosis as a primary or co-existing disease that may modify or mask the symptoms or progression of a co-morbidity. Furthermore, high intensity microfilaremia in a blood samples should be taken as a potential indictor of the presence of an underlying serious pathology.

Personal correspondence with veterinary practitioners suggest a beneficial effect of adding to the moxidectin standard treatment an anticoagulant, corticosteroids, and doxycycline, depending on the severity of the clinical state of the patient infected with *D. repens;* this is also recommended in high risk thrombosis development with heartworm disease (12). As reported in lymphatic filariasis, doxycycline treatment against *Wolbachia* provides clinical improvement in patients with lymphedema (32). It has also been noted in loiasis that high microfilarial loads (30,000–50,000 Mf/ml) can lead to capillary obstruction from damaged parasites after anthelmintic treatment, and adding corticosteroids to the anti-parasitic treatment should be taken into consideration by ESDA and veterinary practitioners in high intensity microfilaremia (22).

In human *Loa loa* infections occurring with microfilaremia >10,000 Mf/ml of blood, encephalopathy following ivermectin has been well-documented. Treatment with microfilaricidal agents such as ivermectin and diethylcarbamazine may provoke the passage of L. loa Mf into the cerebrospinal fluid and precipitate an encephalopathy (33, 34). Those reactions were not yet described in filariosis of dogs, but a case of a human *D. repens* infection concomitant with meningoencephalitis was successfully treated by initiation of anti-helminth and anti-inflammatory medicine (35). This could be an interesting issue to follow and explain in further studies.

Adult parasite burden cannot be determined precisely in helminth infections (36), especially in *D. repens* where the worms may reside in any number of tissue locations. In Case #1 we found 26 adult worms during castration. Most case reports present findings of just one or few adult worms, however, we cannot exclude the possibility that these are under representations of total adult numbers localized in different tissues. It has been previously documented that a dog infected with over 300 adult *D. repens* showed a microfilaremia of 7,780 Mf/ml (28). This suggests that the quantity of adult worms may be only one of the factor determining Mf in the blood stream, and it is very likely that the immune system of the host plays a large role in regulating microfilariae burden, as is observed in other helminth infections (28, 37). The mechanism regulating the burden of Mf in the bloodstream is not known. It is suspected that certain aspects of host-helminth relationship may be beneficial to the host given the proper balance parasite load and humoral response in the host (37). This relationship is beginning to be investigated pertaining to autoimmune disease, and could be of future interest in the study of *D. repens* infections.

Density-dependent processes play a key role in the transmission dynamics of vector-borne diseases (36). The relationship between microfilarial density and worm burden in *Onchocerca volvulus* infections in humans has been investigated, yet not fully understood. It has been observed that the microfilariae burden increases with host age, suggesting a development of immunological tolerance, while the density of adult parasites correlating with the microfilariae burden has not been confirmed. Since a purely age-related decline in host responsiveness is not shown, it is likely that immunological responsiveness against Mf diminishes as a consequence of cumulative parasite experience, pointing to immunological habituation or tolerance to the parasite (36).

All four cases presented here feature high microfilaremia in animals with severe co-morbidity and suspected immunodeficiency-related conditions. Helminths are known to suppress the host immune response in order to establish infection. For instance, it has been recently reported that D. repens may influence the host immune response by inducing a state of chronic in the canine host (29). It is possible that patients with high Mf counts may represent a population with pre-existing immunosuppression and are unable to naturally control or respond to the parasites. An improved screening and monitoring to determine the impact of chronic immunodeficiency disease on subcutaneous dirofilariosis and its correlation with neoplastic processes should be taken into consideration by investigators and practitioners for better understanding of *D. repens* pathogenicity.

AUTHOR CONTRIBUTIONS

MW analyzed the data and wrote the manuscript. MS-F performed the histopathological examination of internal organs of the first case. MK, ED, MW, and MS-F critically revised the manuscript. All authors read and approved the final version of the manuscript.

ACKNOWLEDGMENTS

The authors are grateful to Dr. Wojciech Spruch and Dr. Krzysztof Humięcki for providing all clinical data and to Mark Kaji for constructive criticism and proofreading the article.

REFERENCES

1. Capelli G, Genchi C, Baneth G, Bourdeau P, Brianti E, Cardoso L, et al. Recent advances on *Dirofilaria* repens in dogs and humans in Europe. *Parasit Vectors.* (2018) 11:663. doi: 10.1186/s13071-018-3205-x
2. Sulekova LF, Gabrielli S, de Angelis M, Milardi GL, Magnani C, Marco B Di, et al. *Dirofilaria* repens microfilariae from a human node fine-needle aspirate: a case report. *BMC Infect Dis.* (2016) 16:248. doi: 10.1186/s12879-016-1582-3
3. Ermakova L, Nagorny S, Pshenichnaya N, Ambalov Y, Boltachiev K. Clinical and laboratory features of human *Dirofilariasis* in Russia. *IDCases.* (2017) 9:112–5. doi: 10.1016/j.idcr.2017.07.006
4. Kłudkowska M, Pielok L, Frackowiak K, Masny A, Gołab E, Paul M. *Dirofilaria* repens infection as a cause of intensive peripheral microfilariemia in a polish patient: process description and cases review. *Acta Parasitol.* (2018) 63:657–63. doi: 10.1515/ap-2018-0077
5. Borkowski PK, Rymkiewicz G, Golebiewska J, Nestoros N, Romejko-Jarosinska J, Zarnowska-Prymek H, et al. The first case of human autochtonous subconjunctival dirofilariosis in Poland and MALT lymphoma as possible consequence of this parasitosis. *Infect Agent Cancer.* (2015) 10:1–5. doi: 10.1186/1750-9378-10-1
6. Harrus S, Harmelin A, Rodrig S, Favia G. *Dirofilaria* repens infection in a dog in Israel. *Am J Trop Med Hyg.* (1999) 61:639–41. doi: 10.4269/ajtmh.1999.61.639
7. Mazaki-Tovi M, Reich M, Karnieli A, Kuzi S, Aroch I. Marked subcutaneous mast cell and eosinophilic infiltration associated with the presence of multiple *Dirofilaria* repens microfilariae in 4 dogs. *Vet Clin Pathol.* (2016) 4:703–9. doi: 10.1111/vcp.12410
8. Genchi C, Kramer LH. The prevalence of *Dirofilaria immitis* and D. repens in the old world. *Vet Parasitol.* (2020) 280:108995. doi: 10.1016/j.vetpar.2019.108995
9. DŽaja P, Beck A, Kiš G, Kurilj AG, Živičnjak T, Artuković B, et al. *Dirofilaria* repens infection in a dog in croatia - a case report. *Vet Arh.* (2008) 78:521–7.
10. Magnis J, Lorentz S, Guardone L, Grimm F, Magi M, Naucke TJ, et al. Morphometric analyses of canine blood microfilariae isolated by the Knott's test enables *Dirofilaria* immitis and D. repens species-specific and Acanthocheilonema (syn. Dipetalonema) genus-specific diagnosis. *Parasit Vectors.* (2013) 6:48. doi: 10.1186/1756-3305-6-48
11. Gioia G, Lecová L, Genchi M, Ferri E, Genchi C, Mortarino M. Highly sensitive multiplex PCR for simultaneous detection and discrimination of *Dirofilaria immitis* and *Dirofilaria* repens in canine peripheral blood. *Vet Parasitol.* (2010) 172:160–3. doi: 10.1016/j.vetpar.2010.04.027
12. Petry G, Genchi M, Schmidt H, Schaper R, Lawrenz B, Genchi C. Evaluation of the adulticidal efficacy of imidacloprid 10%/moxidectin 2.5 % (w/v) spot-on (advocate®, advantage® multi) against *Dirofilaria* repens in experimentally infected dogs. *Parasitol Res.* (2015) 114:131–44. doi: 10.1007/s00436-015-4519-7

13. Simón F, Siles-Lucas M, Morchón R, González-Miguel J, Mellado I, Carretón E, et al. Human and animal *Dirofilariasis*: the emergence of a zoonotic mosaic. *Clin Microbiol Rev.* (2012) 25:507–44. doi: 10.1128/CMR.00012-12
14. Kramer L, Simón F, Tamarozzi F, Genchi M, Bazzocchi C. Is Wolbachia complicating the pathological effects of *Dirofilaria* immitis infections? *Vet Parasitol.* (2005) 133:133–6. doi: 10.1016/j.vetpar.2005.04.011
15. Kramer L, Grandi G, Leoni M, Passeri B, McCall J, Genchi C, et al. Wolbachia and its influence on the pathology and immunology of *Dirofilaria* immitis infection. *Vet Parasitol.* (2008) 158:191–5. doi: 10.1016/j.vetpar.2008.09.014
16. Grandi G, Morchon R, Kramer L, Kartashev V, Simon F. Wolbachia in *Dirofilaria* repens, an agent causing human subcutaneous *Dirofilariasis*. *J Parasitol.* (2008) 94:1421–3. doi: 10.1645/GE-1575.1
17. Vilson A, Hedhammar A, Reynolds A, Spears J, Satyaraj E, Pelker R, et al. Immunoglobulins in dogs: correspondence and maturation in 15 litters of German shepherd dogs and their dams. *Vet Rec Open.* (2016) 3:e000173. doi: 10.1136/vetreco-2016-000173
18. Paterson S. Discovering the causes of otitis externa. *Pract.* (2016) 38:7–11. doi: 10.1136/inp.i470
19. Jorge MFS, Miguel LMZ, Braghiroli CS, Schmitt JV. Demodicosis as treatment complication of amicrobial pustulosis of the folds. *An Bras Dermatol.* (2018) 93:566–9. doi: 10.1590/abd1806-4841.20187171
20. Vališ M, Kočí J, Tuček D, Lutonský T, Kopová J, Bartoň P, et al. Common yew intoxication: a case report. *J Med Case Rep.* (2014) 8:4. doi: 10.1186/1752-1947-8-4
21. Ibrahim MS, Trpis M. The effect of *Brugia pahangi* infection on survival of susceptible and refractory species of the *Aedes scutellaris* complex. *Med Vet Entomol.* (1987) 1:329–37. doi: 10.1111/j.1365-2915.1987.tb00363.x
22. Placinta IA, Pascual-Camps I, Chiarri-Toumit C, Mata-Moret L, Sanchez-Cañizal J, Barranco-González H. Ocular loiasis affecting a child and its assessment by anterior segment optical coherence tomography. *Rom J Ophthalmol.* (2019) 63:184–7. doi: 10.22336/rjo.2019.28
23. Pazdzior-Czapula K, Otrocka-Domaga I, Myrdek P, Mikiewicz M, Gesek M. *Dirofilaria* repens —an etiological factor or an incidental finding in cytologic and histopathologic biopsies from dogs. (2018) 47:307–11. doi: 10.1111/vcp.12597
24. Mortaz E, Tabarsi P, Mansouri D, Khosravi A, Garssen J, Velayati A, et al. Cancers related to immunodeficiencies: update and perspectives. *Front Immunol.* (2016) 7:365. doi: 10.3389/fimmu.2016.00365
25. MacPhail CM. Laryngeal disease in dogs and cats: an update. *Vet Clin North Am Small Anim Pract.* (2020) 50:295–10. doi: 10.1016/j.cvsm.2019.11.001
26. Kvitko-White H, Balog K, Scott-Moncrieff JC, Johnson A, Lantz GC. Acquired bilateral laryngeal paralysis associated with systemic lupus erythematosus in a dog. *J Am Anim Hosp Assoc.* (2012) 48:60–5. doi: 10.5326/JAAHA-MS-5677
27. Greene BM, Otto GF. Greenough III WB. circulating non-human microfilaria in a patient with systemic lupus erythematosus. *Am J Trop Med Hyg.* (1978) 27:905–9. doi: 10.4269/ajtmh.1978.27.905
28. Mircean M, Ionică AM, Mircean V, Györke A, Codea AR, Tăbăran FA, et al. Clinical and pathological effects of *Dirofilaria* repens and *Dirofilaria* immitis in a dog with a natural co-infection. *Parasitol Int.* (2017) 66:331–4. doi: 10.1016/j.parint.2017.02.003
29. Wysmołek ME, Dobrzyński A, Długosz E, Czopowicz M, Wiśniewski M, Jurka P, et al. Hematological and biochemical changes in dogs naturally infected with *Dirofilaria repens. Front. Vet. Sci.* 7:590. doi: 10.3389/fvets.2020.00590
30. Hawking F. The 24-hour periodicity of microfilariae: biological mechanisms responsible for its production and control. *Proc R Soc London.* (1967) 169:59–76. doi: 10.1098/rspb.1967.0079
31. Lechner AM, Gastager H, Kern JM, Wagner B, Tappe D. Case report: successful treatment of a patient with microfilaremic *Dirofilariasis* using doxycycline. *Am J Trop Med Hyg.* (2020) 102:844–6. doi: 10.4269/ajtmh.19-0744
32. Bennuru S, Nutman TB. Lymphatics in human lymphatic filariasis: *in vitro* models of parasite-induced lymphatic remodeling. *Lymphat Res Biol.* (2009) 7:215–9. doi: 10.1089/lrb.2009.0022
33. Twum-Danso NA. Loa loa encephalopathy temporally related to ivermectin administration reported from onchocerciasis mass treatment programs from 1989 to 2001: implications for the future. *Filaria J.* (2003) 2:S7. doi: 10.1186/1475-2883-2-S1-S7s
34. Gardon J, Gardon-Wendel N, Kamgno J, Chippaux J. Serious reactions after mass treatment of onchocerciasis with ivermectin in an area endemic for Loa loa infection. *Lancet.* (1997) 350:18–22. doi: 10.1016/S0140-6736(96)11094-1
35. Poppert S, Hodapp M, Krueger A, Hegasy G, Niesen W, Kern WV, et al. *Dirofilaria* repens infection and concomitant meningoencephalitis. *Emerg Infect Dis.* (2009) 15:1844–6. doi: 10.3201/eid1511.090936
36. Duerr HP, Dietz K, Schulz-Key H, Büttner DW, Eichner M. The relationships between the burden of adult parasites, host age and the microfilarial density in human onchocerciasis. *Int J Parasitol.* (2004) 34:463–73. doi: 10.1016/j.ijpara.2003.11.008
37. Everts B, Smits HH, Hokke CH, Yazdanbakhsh M. Helminths and dendritic cells: Sensing and regulating via pattern recognition receptors, Th2 and Treg responses. *Eur J Immunol.* (2010) 40:1525–37. doi: 10.1002/eji.200940109

Effectiveness of Fenbendazole and Metronidazole Against *Giardia* Infection in Dogs Monitored for 50-Days in Home-Conditions

Lavinia Ciuca[1], Paola Pepe[1], Antonio Bosco[1], Simone Mario Caccio[2], Maria Paola Maurelli[1], Anna Rosa Sannella[2], Alice Vismarra[3], Giuseppe Cringoli[1], Laura Kramer[3], Laura Rinaldi[1] and Marco Genchi[3]*

[1] Department of Veterinary Medicine and Animal Production, University of Naples Federico II, Naples, Italy, [2] European Union Reference Laboratory for Parasites, Department of Infectious Diseases, Istituto Superiore di Sanità, Rome, Italy, [3] Department of Veterinary Science, University of Parma, Parma, Italy

Correspondence:
Laura Rinaldi
lrinaldi@unina.it

A field trial performed in-home conditions was conducted on 24 dogs naturally infected with *Giardia*, in order to compare the efficacy of fenbendazole and metronidazole. Animals were allocated in groups randomly in order to obtain two groups of 12 dogs each with similar parasitic loads of *Giardia* cysts: dogs in Group A were treated with fenbendazole (Panacur®, Intervet Italia Srl) administered at the dose of 50 mg/kg orally once a day for 5 consecutive days, dogs in Group B were treated with metronidazole (Flagyl®, Zambon Italia Srl) administered orally at the dose of 50 mg/kg, once a day for 5 consecutive days. All the dogs that were shedding *Giardia* cysts after the first treatment (Day 0) were retreated (either at Day 7 or at Day 14 or at Day 21) until a negative result was obtained with the same treatment. Additionally, all the dogs were re-examined at Day 50. All the dogs were tested for the presence of *Giardia* cysts using a fecal flotation method (FLOTAC). The percent efficacy of the treatments (A and B) was calculated at each sampling point (Days 7, 14, 21, and 50) as reduction in mean *Giardia* cysts. After the first therapy, on day 7, 4/12 (33.3%) dogs tested positive for *Giardia* cysts in the Group A and 5/12 (41.7%) in the Group B. Efficacies at (Days 7, 14, 21, and 50) of the treatments against *Giardia* infection were 80.9, 94, 100, and 97% in the Group A and 70.8, 99, 100, and 97.1% in the Group B. Statistically significant differences were not observed between the efficacy of Fenbendazole and Metronidazole against infection by *G. duodenalis* ($P = 0.686$). Molecular analysis revealed full homology (i.e., 100% with JN416550) with the canine specific assemblage D in six positive dogs. Different hypotheses might explain the re-appearance of the *Giardia* cysts in some dogs after treatment, e.g., re-infection from the home environment, the correct medication given by the owners, the diet, as well as treatment failure, but also biological issues related to the intermittent excretion of *Giardia* cysts.

Keywords: *Giardia*, dogs, 50 days post-treatment, fenbendazole, metronidazole, assemblage

INTRODUCTION

Giardia duodenalis (syn. *Giardia lamblia*, *Giardia intestinalis*) is the causative agent of giardiosis and one of the most commonly found parasite in dogs throughout the world (1, 2). Molecular studies have shown that *G. duodenalis* comprises at least eight distinct genetic assemblages (A–H), of which assemblages C and D are found exclusively in dogs, while *Giardia* assemblages A and B have zoonotic potential (3–5).

Infection by *G. duodenalis* in dogs has a worldwide distribution with prevalence rates that vary according to the test population, the diagnostic method used and the geographical area (6, 7). In Italy, prevalence values range between 11.1 and 28.9% in northern (8–10), between 6.4 and 21.4% in central (11–14) and between 7.7 and 14.2% in southern regions (15, 16).

The diagnosis of *Giardia* infection in dogs may pose a challenge, due to a low infectious dose and marked persistence of cysts in the environment as well as a fluctuating excretion of the cysts in the feces that makes the monitoring of this parasite problematic (17, 18). Traditional tools for identification of *Giardia* cysts include fecal smear, zinc sulfate flotation technique (17, 19), immunofluorescence assay (IFA; the gold standard), immunochromatography, enzyme-linked immunosorbent assays (ELISA), and molecular analyses that permit the different *G. duodenalis* assemblages to be distinguished (17, 20, 21). Among the copromicroscopic techniques, a recent study reported a high sensitivity and specificity of FLOTAC technique with zinc sulfate for diagnosis of *Giardia* cysts infection in dogs (19, 22).

Also the control of *Giardia* infection in dogs is prone to a number of issues. Several compounds have been tested against *Giardia* infections in dogs as benzimidazoles, in particular fenbendazole, and metronidazole that poses activity against the parasite (23–28). Other studies reported the efficacy of ronidazole, nitazoxanide, azithromycin, tinidazole, and ipronidazole and other drugs such as quinacrine, furazolidone, in reducing *Giardia* cysts shed by infected dogs (17, 29–32). Another option recommended by the European Scientific Counsel Companion Animal Parasites (ESCAAP) is the combination of febantel (a prodrug metabolized *in vivo* to fenbendazole)/pyrantel/praziquantel at the standard deworming dose (15.0 mg/kg of febantel, 14.4 mg/kg pyrantel, 5.0 mg/kg praziquantel) repeated once daily for 3 days (33). Recently, secnidazole, a molecule that is used for the treatment of giardiosis in humans, has been reported as an effective drug for the treatment of clinical canine giardiosis (34). However, fenbendazole and metronidazole are used routinely to treat giardiosis in dogs and are the only compounds registered in most European countries.

Resistance to antiparasitic drugs has been often suggested to explain treatment failure due to the incomplete parasite removal following treatment or other underlying diseases (e.g., inflammatory bowel diseases, bacterial overgrowth, coinfection with other organisms). Shampooing of dogs (e.g., with a product containing chlorhexidine digluconate) at the beginning and at the end of antiprotozoal treatment is also recommended to reduce re-infections through fecal material on the fur (30). Despite treatment recommendation with fenbendazole for eliminating *Giardia* cysts in dogs, currently, unpublished data from veterinary practices are showing a low efficacy of this drug in eliminating the infection. Taking into account that the ESCCAP Guidelines recommends fenbendazole (1x/d, 50 mg/kg for 3 days) and metronidazole (2x/d, 25 mg/kg for 5-7 days) for the treatment of *Giardia* infections in dogs (33), the purpose of the present study was to reassess the efficacy of these two specific drugs for the treatment of giardiosis in owned dogs, monitored for 50 days in home-conditions.

MATERIALS AND METHODS

Animal Testing and Study Design

A field trial performed in-home conditions was conducted in 2018–2019 on 24 owned dogs naturally infected by *Giardia* spp. and living in the Campania region, southern Italy. The dogs included in the study were referred to the Laboratory of Parasitology and Parasitic Diseases at the Department of Veterinary Medicine and Animal Production, University of Naples Federico II, for coproparasitological analysis. Dog owners were informed about the study protocol and they gave their consent to inclusion of their pets. Animals were allocated in groups randomly in order to obtain two groups of 12 animals each with similar parasitic loads of *Giardia* cysts: group A-fenbendazole (mean cyst per gram of feces-CPG = 20,995) and group B-metronidazole (CPG = 18,580). The cysts were enumerated using a fecal flotation method (Flotation, Translation and Centrifugation) FLOTAC technique (see Laboratory Analysis). In addition, the dogs had the following characteristics: 11 males (five long-haired and six short-haired dogs) and 13 females (six long-haired and seven short-haired dogs), aged between 2 months and 5 years, living indoor but with access to outdoors. All the dogs included in the study did not live in the same household with other animals. Exclusion criteria were animals treated with any antiparasitic drug in the 2 weeks before, animals with any aggressive behavior and animals showing clinical signs of any other diseases. For each animal included in the study, data regarding age, fur length, clinical signs and consistency of fecal samples were recorded and analyzed. For ethical reasons, no untreated control-group of animals was available. Dogs in Group A were treated with fenbendazole tablets (Panacur®, Intervet Italia Srl) administered at the dose of 50 mg/kg orally once a day for 5 consecutive days. Dogs in Group B were treated with metronidazole tablets (Flagyl®, Zambon Italia Srl) administered orally at the dose of 25 mg/kg, orally, twice a day for 5 consecutive days. All the dogs started the first treatment at Day 0. All the dogs that were shedding *Giardia* cysts after the first treatment were retreated (either at Day 7 or at Day 14 or at Day 21) until a negative result was obtained with the same treatment. Additionally, all the dogs were re-examined at Day 50. Treatment efficacy was evaluated based on the mean CPG found in the fecal samples on Day−5 (pre-treatment) and on Days 7, 14, 21, and 50 (post-treatment). Additionally, each dog was subjected to shampooing with chlorhexidine digluconate at the beginning and at the end of each treatment applied. Furthermore, each owner was suggested to follow some basic rules to avoid the reinfection by cleaning and drying the environment, the use of clean utensils for feed and water and proper disposal of feces (33).

Laboratory Analysis

Dogs were initially identified and verified as infected with *Giardia* spp. and then subsequently analyzed at Day−5 (pre-treatment) and at Days 7, 14, 21, and 50 after the first treatment applied (Day 0). The fecal samples analyzed at each sampling point were represented by pools collected on a daily basis for 2 days (prior to the treatment date). Analyses were performed within 24 h of sampling. At each sampling day the feces for all dogs were tested for the presence of *Giardia* cysts using the FLOTAC technique with an analytic sensitivity of 1 cyst per gram (CPG) of feces (19). Each sample was analyzed using zinc sulfate (specific gravity = 1.350).

Fifteen samples collected at Day−5 were fixed in 2.5% potassium bichromate (dilution 1:4) and processed for molecular studies. Briefly, genomic DNA was extracted using the FastDNA SPIN Kit for feces (MP Biomedicals, Solon, Ohio, USA). A nested PCR assay was used to amplify a 511 bp fragment of the beta-giardin gene according to a published protocol (35). DNA from axenic cultures of *Giardia duodenalis* strains of assemblage A (WB, genotype AI) and assemblage B (GS, genotype BIV) was used as positive controls in PCR assays. PCR products were purified using spin columns (QiaQuick PCR Purification kit -Qiagen) and sequenced from both strands.

Treatment Efficacy

The percent efficacy of the treatments (A and B) was calculated at each sampling point from the trial (Days 7, 14, 21, and 50) according to the following formula [adapted from (36)].

$$\%\text{Efficacy} = \frac{\text{Mean CPG day} - 5 - \text{Mean CPG day 7}}{\text{Mean CPG day} \ - 5} \times 100$$

$$\text{CPG} = \text{cysts per gram of feces.}$$

Statistical Analysis

Statistical analysis was performed using Windows SPSS® (version 17.0). The non-parametric Mann-Whitney U test was used to determine the level of significant difference between groups of treatment (A, B).

Assessment Criteria and Clinical Outcome

An arbitrary scoring system (from 1 to 4) was used and a score assigned to each dog, based on fecal consistency and clinical symptoms (lethargic attitude, growth retardation, weight loss, vomiting and flatulence) as follows: (1) formed feces and no clinical symptoms, (2) formed feces and clinical symptoms, (3) soft stools and clinical symptoms, and (4) diarrhea and clinical symptoms.

RESULTS

Table 1 shows dog's data (gender, age, fur length, clinical score), *Giardia* cysts per gram (CPG) of feces (mean, standard deviation) and efficacy (%) of treatment with fenbendazole (Group A) and metronidazole (Group B) at the different study Days (Day−5, Day 7, Day 14, Day 21, and Day 50).

Parasitological results at Day−5 showed mean values of 20,995 *Giardia* CPG (minimum 2,780 CPG, maximum 48,000 CPG) in the Group A (fenbendazole) and 18,580 *Giardia* CPG (minimum 10,848 CPG, maximum 32,178 CPG) in the Group B (metronidazole). On Day 7, cysts of *Giardia* spp. were found in 33.3% (4/12; 95% Confidence Interval (CI) = 11.3–64.5) of the dogs in the Group A and in 41.7% (5/12; 95% CI = 16.5–71.4) of the dogs in the Group B.

The efficacy of fenbendazole was 80.9% at Day 7, 100% at day 14, 97.0% at day 21, and 95.0% at day 50. The efficacy of metronizazole was 70.8% at Day 7, 99.0% at Day 14, 100% at Day 21, and 97.1% at Day 50. Overall, the efficacies of Fenbendazole and Metronidazole against the infection by *G. duodenalis* were not significantly different ($P = 0.686$).

No other co-infections with intestinal parasites were found at copromicroscopic examinations. Briefly, 6 dogs from Group A and 5 dogs from Group B remained negative until Day 50 after they received the first treatment at Day 0. Eight dogs (four from each group), received the second treatment at Day 7 (after the first therapy at Day 0), and two other dogs (one from each group) were retreated for the second time at Day 21 from the Group A and Day 14 from the Group B. Moreover, in the Group B, there was one dog that received three treatments during the study at Days 0, 7 and 14. Finally, two dogs (one from each group), that had received the first treatment at Day 0, were still shedding *Giardia* cysts at the last study Day (Day 50).

Assessment Criteria and Clinical Outcome

At Day−5, feces were unformed to diarrhoeic in dogs belonging to both treatment groups but no adverse responses due to the medications were observed. 33.3% of the dogs had score 1, 25% score 2, 25% score 3, and 16.7% score 4. Regarding the dogs that tested positive for *Giardia* after the treatment (13/24), five belonged to the first category (38.6%), four to the second category (30.8%), one to the third category (7.7%), and three to the fourth (23%).

Molecular Characterization

Giardia DNA could be amplified only from six of the 15 fecal samples tested, three from the Group A (dog's ID numbers = F1, F6, F8) and three from the Group B (dog's ID numbers = M4, M7, M11). The beta-giardin amplification products were sequenced and compared, using BLAST, with all available sequences in the GenBank database. This revealed full homology (e.g., 100% with JN416550) with the canine specific assemblage D in the six positive dogs. The lack of amplification in the remaining samples is likely due to cyst damage resulting from storage conditions.

DISCUSSION

During the last 60 years, a number of chemotherapeutic agents have been introduced and are still in use in the therapy for giardiosis (37). Unfortunately, most drugs used have considerable

TABLE 1 | Groups A-Fenbendazole and B-Metronidazole: dog's data (gender, age, fur length, clinical score), *Giardia* cysts per gram (CPG) of feces (mean, standard deviation), and efficacy (%) of the treatment at the different study days.

Dog ID	Gender (Male/Female)	Age (months/years)	Fur length (Long/Short)	Clinical score	*Giardia* cysts per gram (CPG) of feces				
					Day-5 (Pre-T)	Day 7 (T1)	Day 14 (T2)	Day 21 (T3)	Day 50
GROUP A (FENBENDAZOLE)									
F1	M	2 mos	L	4	22,300	0	0	8,360	0
F2	F	4 yrs	S	3	15,600	0	0	0	0
F3	M	8 mos	L	1	19,200	21,600	0	0	0
F4	M	2 yrs	S	1	7,830	1,230	0	0	0
F5	F	1 yr	S	3	18,894	0	0	0	0
F6	F	3 mos	L	4	24,600	16,828	0	0	0
F7	F	1 yr	L	2	21,080	0	0	0	0
F8	M	9 mos	S	3	31,984	0	0	0	0
F9	F	2 yrs	S	2	22,824	0	0	0	12,576
F10	M	3 yrs	L	1	16,854	0	0	0	0
F11	F	7 mos	S	3	48,000	0	0	0	0
F12	M	3 yrs	L	1	2,780	8,400	0	0	0
				Mean CPG	20,995.5	4,004.8	0.0	696.7	1,048.0
				SD	11390.1	7564.0	0.0	2413.3	3630.4
				%Efficacy	**NA**	**80.9%**	**100%**	**97.0%**	**95.0%**
GROUP B (METRONIDAZOLE)									
M1	F	4 yrs	S	4	19,654	0	0	0	0
M2	F	4 yrs	S	3	11,900	0	0	0	0
M3	F	8 mos	L	1	10,900	0	0	0	0
M4	M	2 yrs	S	1	21,234	0	0	0	0
M5	F	2 yrs	L	2	10,848	0	0	0	0
M6	M	9 mos	S	1	21,280	0	0	0	6,546
M7	M	3 yrs	S	1	18,732	560	156	0	0
M8	F	1 yr	L	2	15,832	17,560	0	0	0
M9	M	6 mos	S	3	17,459	18,981	0	0	0
M10	F	5 yrs	L	2	17,178	17,562	0	0	0
M11	M	5 mos	L	4	32,178	10,400	0	0	0
M12	F	7 mos	S	2	25,765	0	1,987	0	0
				Mean CPG	18,580.0	5,421.9	178.6	0.0	545.5
				SD	6224.6	8161.8	571.3	0.0	1889.7
				%Efficacy	**NA**	**70.8%**	**99.0%**	**100%**	**97.1%**

Pre-T (before treatment); T1 (first treatment); T2 (second treatment) T3 (third treatment). Clinical score: (1) formed feces and no clinical symptoms, (2) formed feces and clinical symptoms, (3) soft stools and clinical symptoms, and (4) diarrhea and clinical symptoms.

adverse effects such as vomiting, bloody diarrhea, abortion, neurological dysfunctions and so they are contraindicated (38). In this context, studies on chemotherapeutic agents play a fundamental role in the rationale for the treatment of giardiosis.

Several benzimidazoles (39, 40), and in particular fenbendazole (23), or the combinations of febantel/fenbendazole with other compounds proved to be effective (24, 25, 41). Metronidazole, a nitroimidazole, and fenbendazole are used routinely to treat giardiosis in dogs (30). Ronidazole showed a good antiprotozoal effect against *Giardia* in dogs (30) and oxfendazole showed a significant decrease in the number of cysts (40).

The findings of the present study did not reveal a significant difference of efficacy between the drugs used (fenbendazole 80.9% vs. metronidazole 70.8% at Day 7). Moreover, after applying the first treatment, both drugs failed to eliminate the *Giardia* cysts in all the dogs. Re-appearance of the cysts in the feces could be attributed to a re-infection, treatment failure, the correct medication given by the owners, the diet, as well as biological issues related to the intermittent excretion of *Giardia* cysts. However, there are no specific information of the dog's environment at home if any attempt was made by the owner to clean up contaminated areas. Faure et al. (42), reported a significant difference of efficacy between fenbendazole and metronidazole (30.3% vs. 91.9%). In our study, fenbendazole showed lower efficacy than that reported by Zajac et al. (26), who obtained 90% efficacy (26). However, it is important to note that in our present study both drugs showed 100% efficacy after two consecutive cycles of treatments, i.e., at Days 14 in the Group A and at Day 21 in the Group B.

Fifteen (62.5%) out of 24 dogs treated from both groups (eight dogs from Group A and seven dogs from Group B) were tested negative for *Giardia* cysts after the first therapy at Day 7. Moreover, there were dogs from both groups A and B, thus showing a persistent infection that has been cleared either at Day 14 or at Day 21 after two or three treatments of 5 days each. It could be possible, that some *Giardia* remained at low abundance in the intestine of these dogs that were still positive after the first treatment applied, or for the dogs that needed to be treated three times until a negative result was obtained, or perhaps we were facing with a treatment failure due to drug resistance. However, future investigations are needed, in order to establish the availability of the drugs in the blood and the capacity of these to eliminate the *Giardia* cysts by *in vitro* methods.

In addition, two dogs from each group (A and B) remained negative after the first therapy (Day 0), until Day 50, when turned positive. In these cases, it was suggested that reinfections from the environment are the most common cause for treatment failure (25, 30) considering that the prepatent period can be as short as 4 days (33). Also, the presence of cysts on the animal's fur, associated with the resistance of the parasite to disinfectants (chlorhexidine gluconate in our study) and environmental conditions and with stress, may explain reinfections (30). Since this is a field trial performed in-home conditions we were not sure about the failure of cleaning and bathing due to the lack of compliance by the owner, thus, the use of hygiene measures such as chlorhexidine digluconate shampoo before and after the treatment might have a considerable influence on our results representing a major issue of this study. Moron-Soto et al. also reported that dogs re-shed cysts following a brief period after antiparasitic treatment when no disinfection or cleaning of their enclosures was performed (31).

Some experimental studies have evaluated also the efficacy of the oral administration of probiotics together with albendazole (38), therefore during the treatment the veterinarian can recommend the administration of probiotics that play a synergistic role with the drug regenerating the intestinal flora. However, in the present study, none of the dogs received a special diet, or probiotics supplements during and after the therapy. Moreover, there are few recent studies that showed that the microbial diversity was not altered by fenbendazole administration, which is in contrast to metronidazole which significantly altered microbial structure and diversity (43–47). Administration of metronidazole to healthy dogs caused significant changes in the microbiome, some of which persist following discontinuation of the drug with unknown clinical effects. Furthermore, some dogs on metronidazole can get neurotoxicity (48, 49). However, in the present study, no adverse responses due to the medications were observed including transient neurological signs due to metronidazole.

There have been two reports examining the effects of secnidazole on *Giardia* in dogs. One, reported 100% efficacy of cyst reduction in two groups of six hospitalized dogs (50). The other one, showed that at 43 days after the first treatment, all 9 dogs were considered to have normal stools, but 4 of the 9 puppies were positive for *Giardia* antigen (34). Bearing these facts in mind, perhaps secnidazole applied twice, 2–3 weeks apart, could be an alternative and easier treatment, with a better compliance as well for treating *Giardia* infection. Further data are needed to prove its efficacy both in field and experimental studies.

Finally, genotyping of *Giardia* demonstrated the host-specific assemblage D in all positive dogs, in agreement with other studies in Italy (12, 35). However, our study presented limitations due to the sample size and due to the poor and inappropriate storage conditions to ensure the effective isolation of DNA from fecal samples. Therefore, further research on distinguish *G. duodenalis* strains, are needed, in order to perform a realistic estimation of zoonotic risk (51).

Based on the findings, as expected in a trial with a small number of individuals in-home conditions, and especially for a parasite with the characteristics of *Giardia* (i.e., having a direct infection and short prepatent period), the authors could only speculate that treatment alone is not sufficient for controlling *Giardia* infection.

A main limitation of our study is based on the small sample size (no. = 12 dogs), the absence of a control group and the allocation of the animals in the two treatment Groups based only on individual *Giardia* CPG assessed at Day−5. However, the limited number of dogs in our study was mainly due to type of study (field trial in-home conditions) that requires a full compliance of both vet practitioners and dog owners. Ethical issues were the main reasons for not including a control group in such a kind of field trial performed in-home conditions. In a similar study, Mirò et al. (52) assessed the efficacy of fenbendazole and mebendazole using 10 per group. As a consequence, in the allocation phase we could not consider other key epidemiological parameters as age, fur length and style of living. Different hypotheses might explain the re-appearance of the *Giardia* cysts in some dogs after treatment, e.g., re-infection from the home environment, the correct medication given by the owners, the diet, as well as treatment failure, but also biological issues related to the intermittent excretion of *Giardia* cysts. Therefore, due to the uncontrolled parameters in this field trial performed in-home conditions, future studies are warranted to produce conclusive evidence for the evaluation of integrated approaches needed for the treatment of dogs naturally infected by *Giardia*.

AUTHOR CONTRIBUTIONS

MG, LR, LC, LK, SMC, ARS, and GC contributed to the conception and design of the study. PP, AB, AV, and MPM organized the database and performed the statistical analysis. MG, LR, and LC wrote the manuscript. All authors contributed to manuscript revision, read, and approved the submitted version.

REFERENCES

1. Ballweber LR, Xiao L, Bowman DD, Kahn G, Cama VA. Giardiasis in dogs and cats: update on epidemiology and public health significance. *Trends Parasitol.* (2010) 26:180–9. doi: 10.1016/j.pt.2010.02.005
2. Thompson RC, Palmer CS, O'Handley R. The public health and clinical significance of *Giardia* and *Cryptosporidium* in domestic animals. *Vet J.* (2008) 177:18–25. doi: 10.1016/j.tvjl.2007.09.022
3. Thompson RCA, Ash A. Molecular epidemiology of *Giardia* and *Cryptosporidium* infections. *Infect Genet Evol.* (2016) 40:315–23. doi: 10.1016/j.meegid.2015.09.028
4. Thompson RC. The zoonotic significance and molecular epidemiology of *Giardia* and giardiasis. *Vet Parasitol.* (2004) 126:15–35. doi: 10.1016/j.vetpar.2004.09.008
5. Ryan U, Zahedi A. Molecular epidemiology of giardiasis from a veterinary perspective. *Adv Parasitol.* (2019) 106:209–54. doi: 10.1016/bs.apar.2019.07.002
6. Bouzid M, Halai K, Jeffreys D, Hunter PR. The prevalence of *Giardia* infection in dogs and cats, a systematic review and meta-analysis of prevalence studies from stool samples. *Vet Parasitol.* (2015) 207:181–202. doi: 10.1016/j.vetpar.2014.12.011
7. Volkmann M, Steiner JM, Fosgate GT, Zentek J, Hartmann S, Kohn B. Chronic diarrhea in dogs - retrospective study in 136 cases. *J Vet Intern Med.* (2017) 31:1043–55. doi: 10.1111/jvim.14739
8. Zanzani SA, Gazzonis AL, Scarpa P, Berrilli F, Manfredi MT. Intestinal parasites of owned dogs and cats from metropolitan and micropolitan areas: prevalence, zoonotic risks, and pet owner awareness in northern Italy. *Biomed Res Int.* (2014) 2014:696508. doi: 10.1155/2014/696508
9. Zanzani SA, Di Cerbo AR, Gazzonis AL, Genchi M, Rinaldi L, Musella V, et al. Canine fecal contamination in a metropolitan area (Milan, north-western Italy): prevalence of intestinal parasites and evaluation of health risks. *Sci World J.* (2014) 2014:132361. doi: 10.1155/2014/132361
10. Simonato G, Frangipane di Regalbono A, Cassini R, Traversa D, Tessarin C, Di Cesare A, et al. Molecular detection of *Giardia duodenalis* and *Cryptosporidium* spp. in canine faecal samples contaminating public areas in Northern Italy. *Parasitol Res.* (2017) 116:3411–18. doi: 10.1007/s00436-017-5671-z
11. Capelli G, Paoletti B, Iorio R, Frangipane Di Regalbono A, Pietrobelli M, Bianciardi P, et al. Prevalence of *Giardia* spp. in dogs and humans in northern and central Italy. *Parasitol Res.* (2003) 90:54–5. doi: 10.1007/s00436-003-0924-4
12. Paoletti B, Traversa D, Iorio R, De Berardinis A, Bartolini R, Salini R, et al. Zoonotic parasites in feces and fur of stray and private dogs from Italy. *Parasitol Res.* (2015) 114:2135–41. doi: 10.1007/s00436-015-4402-6
13. Liberato C, Berrilli F, Odorizi L, Scarcella R, Barni M, Amoruso C, et al. Parasites in stray dogs from Italy: prevalence, risk factors and management concerns. *Acta Parasitol.* (2018) 26:27–32. doi: 10.1515/ap-2018-0003
14. Scaramozzino P, Carvelli A, Iacoponi F, De Liberato C. Endoparasites in household and shelter dogs from Central Italy. *Int J Vet Sci Med.* (2018) 27:45–7. doi: 10.1016/j.ijvsm.2018.04.003
15. Rinaldi L, Maurelli MP, Musella V, Veneziano V, Carbone S, Di Sarno A, et al. *Giardia* and *Cryptosporidium* in canine faecal samples contaminating an urban area. *Res Vet Sci.* (2008) 84:413–5. doi: 10.1016/j.rvsc.2007.05.006
16. Rinaldi L, Pampurini F, Pennacchio S, Ianniello D, Caputo V, Alfano S, et al. *Giardia* in stray dogs in the city of Naples. In: *XXVII Congresso Nazionale della Società Italiana di Parassitologia (SoIPa).* Alghero (2012). p. 289.
17. Tangtrongsup S, Scorza V. Update on the diagnosis and management of *Giardia* spp. infections in dogs and cats top companion. *Anim Med.* (2010) 25:155–62. doi: 10.1053/j.tcam.2010.07.003
18. Uiterwijk M, Nijsse R, Kooyman FNJ, Wagenaar JA, Mughini-Gras L, Koop G, et al. Comparing four diagnostic tests for *Giardia duodenalis* in dogs using latent class analysis. *Parasit Vectors.* (2018) 31:439. doi: 10.1186/s13071-018-3014-2
19. Pepe P, Ianniello D, Alves LC, Morgoglione ME, Maurelli MP, Bosco A, et al. Comparative cost-effectiveness of immunoassays and FLOTAC for diagnosing *Giardia* spp. infection in dogs. *Parasit Vectors.* (2019) 12:158. doi: 10.1186/s13071-019-3425-8
20. Jahan N, Khatoon R, Ahmad S. A comparison of microscopy and enzyme linked immunosorbent assay for diagnosis of *Giardia lamblia* in human faecal specimens. *J Clin Diagn Res.* (2014) 8:4–6. doi: 10.7860/JCDR/2014/9484.5087
21. Uchôa FFM, Sudré AP, Campos SDE, Almosny NRP. Assessment of the diagnostic performance of four methods for the detection of *Giardia duodenalis* in fecal samples from human, canine and feline carriers. *J Microbiol Methods.* (2018) 145:73–8. doi: 10.1016/j.mimet.2018.01.001
22. Cringoli G, Rinaldi L, Maurelli MP, Utzinger J. FLOTAC: new multivalent techniques for qualitative and quantitative copromicroscopic diagnosis of parasites in animals and humans. *Nat Protoc.* (2010) 5:503–15. doi: 10.1038/nprot.2009.235
23. Barr SC, Bowman DD, Heller RL. Efficacy of fenbendazole against giardiasis in dogs. *Am J Vet Res.* (1994) 55:988–90.
24. Barr SC, Bowman DD, Frongillo MF, Joseph SL. Efficacy of a drug combination of praziquantel, pyrantel pamoate, and febantel against giardiasis in dogs. *Am J Vet Res.* (1998) 59:1134–6.
25. Payne PA, Ridley RK, Dryden MW, Bathgate C, Milliken GA, Stewart PW. Efficacy of a combination febantel–praziquantel–pyrantel product, with or without vaccination with a commercial *Giardia* vaccine, for treatment of dogs with naturally occurring giardiasis. *J Am Vet Med Assoc.* (2002) 220:330–3. doi: 10.2460/javma.2002.220.330
26. Zajac AM, Labranche TP, Donoghue AR, Chu TC. Efficacy of fenbendazole in the treatment of experimental *Giardia* infection in dogs. *Am J Vet Res.* (1998) 59:61–3.
27. Barutzki D, Schimmel A, Schaper R. Efficacy of pyrantel embonate, febantel and praziquantel against *Giardia* spp. in naturally infected dogs. In: Olson BE, Olson ME, Wallis PM, editors. *Giardia—The Cosmopolitan Parasite.* Wallingford: CABI (2002). pp. 177–80.
28. Giangaspero A, Traldi G, Paoletti B, Traversa D, Bianciardi P. Efficacy of pyrantel embonate, febantel and praziquantel against *Giardia* species in naturally infected adult dogs. *Vet Rec.* (2002) 150:184–6. doi: 10.1136/vr.150.6.184
29. Zygner W, Jaros D, Gójska-Zygner O, Wedrychowicz H. Azithromycin in the treatment of a dog infected with *Giardia intestinalis*. *Pol J Vet Sci.* (2008) 11:231–4.
30. Fiechter R, Deplazes P, Schnyder M. Control of *Giardia* infections with ronidazole and intensive hygiene management in a dog kennel. *Vet Parasitol.* (2012) 187:93–8. doi: 10.1016/j.vetpar.2011.12.023
31. Moron-Soto M, Gutierrez L, Sumano H, Tapia G, Alcala-Canto Y. Efficacy of nitazoxanide to treat natural *Giardia* infections in dogs. *Parasit Vectors.* (2017) 10:52. doi: 10.1186/s13071-017-1998-7
32. Riches A, Hart CJS, Trenholme KR, Skinner-Adams TS. Anti-*Giardia* drug discovery: current status and gut feelings. *J Med Chem.* (2020) 63:13330–54. doi: 10.1021/acs.jmedchem.0c00910
33. ESCCAP. *Control of Intestinal Protozoa in Dogs and Cats, Guideline 06,* 2nd ed. Malvern (2018).
34. Cheung W, Russo C, Maher S, Malik R, Šlapeta J. Successful use of secnidazole to manage a giardiosis outbreak in a shelter. *Vet Parasitol.* (2019) 274:108911. doi: 10.1016/j.vetpar.2019.08.005
35. Lalle M, Pozio E, Capelli G, Bruschi F, Crotti D, Cacciò SM. Genetic heterogeneity at the beta-giardin locus among human and animal isolates of *Giardia duodenalis* and identification of potentially zoonotic subgenotypes. *Int J Parasitol.* (2005) 35:207–13. doi: 10.1016/j.ijpara.2004.10.022
36. Geurden T, Olson ME, O'Handley RM, Schetters T, Bowman D, Vercruysse J. World Association for the Advancement of Veterinary Parasitology.

(WAAVP): guideline for the evaluation of drug efficacy againstnon-coccidial gastrointestinal protozoa in livestock and companion animals. *Vet Parasitol.* (2014) 204:81–6. doi: 10.1016/j.vetpar.2014.02.050

37. Escobedo AA, Lalle M, Hrastnik NI, Rodríguez-Morales AJ, Castro-Sánchez E, Cimerman S, et al. Combination therapy in the management of giardiasis: What laboratory and clinical studies tell us, so far. *Acta Trop.* (2016) 162:196–205. doi: 10.1016/j.actatropica.2016.06.026
38. Shukla G, Kaur H, Sharma L. Comparative therapeutic effect of probiotic *Lactobacillus casei* alone and in conjunction with antiprotozoal drugs in murine giardiasis. *Parasitol Res.* (2013) 112:2143–9. doi: 10.1007/s00436-013-3394-3
39. Barr SC, Bowman DD, Heller RL, Erb HN. Efficacy of albendazole against giardiasis in dogs. *Am J Vet Res.* (1993) 54:926–8.
40. Villeneuve V, Beugnet F, Bourdoiseau G. Efficacy of oxfendazole for the treatment of giardiosis in dogs. Experiments in dog breeding kennels. *Parasite.* (2000) 7:221–6. doi: 10.1051/parasite/2000073221
41. Bowman DD, Liotta JL, Ulrich M, Charles SD, Heine J, Schaper R. Treatment of naturally occurring, asymptomatic *Giardia* sp. in dogs with Drontal Plus flavour tablets. *Parasitol Res.* (2009) 105:125–34. doi: 10.1007/s00436-009-1503-0
42. Faure L, Fournel S, Nicolas C, Rigaut D. A field clinical study to confirm the efficacy and safety of a metronidazole-based oral suspension in dogs naturally infested by giardiasis: comparison to fenbendazole. *Intern J Appl Res Vet Med Vol.* (2018) 16:110–16.
43. Shmalberg J, Montalbano C, Morelli G, Buckley GJ. A randomized double blinded placebo-controlled clinical trial of a probiotic or metronidazole for acute canine diarrhea. *Front Vet Sci.* (2019) 6:163. doi: 10.3389/fvets.2019.00163
44. Lee NN, Bidot WA, Ericsson AC, Franklin CL. Effects of *Giardia lamblia* colonization and fenbendazole treatment on canine fecal microbiota. *J Am Assoc Lab Anim Sci.* (2020) 59:423–9. doi: 10.30802/AALAS-JAALAS-19-000113
45. Fujishiro MA, Lidbury JA, Pilla R, Steiner JM, Lappin MR, Suchodolski JS. Evaluation of the effects of anthelmintic administration on the fecal microbiome of healthy dogs with and without subclinical *Giardia* spp. and *Cryptosporidium canis* infections. *PLoS ONE.* (2020) 15:e0228145. doi: 10.1371/journal.pone.0228145
46. Suchodolski JS, Markel ME, Garcia-Mazcorro JF, Unterer S, Heilmann RM, Dowd SE, et al. The fecal microbiome in dogs with acute diarrhea and idiopathic inflammatory bowel disease. *PLoS ONE.* (2012) 7:e5190. doi: 10.1371/journal.pone.0051907
47. Scorza V, Lappin MR. Giardiasis. In: Greene CE, editor. *Infectious Diseases of the Dog and Cat.* 4th ed. St. Louis, MO: Elsevier (2012). p. 785–92.
48. Igarashi H, Maeda S, Ohno K, Horigome A, Odamaki T, Tsujimoto H. Effect of oral administration of metronidazole or prednisolone on fecal microbiota in dogs. *PLoS ONE.* (2014) 9:e107909. doi: 10.1371/journal.pone.0107909
49. Dow SW, LeCouteur RA, Poss ML, Beadleston D. Central nervous system toxicosis associated with metronidazole treatment of dogs: five cases. (1984–1987). *J Am Vet Med Assoc.* (1989) 195:365–8.
50. Karahalli C, Ural K. Single dose secnidazol treatment efficacy against naturally occurring Giardia duodenalis in dogs. *Magyar Allat Lapja.* (2017) 139:621–30.
51. Kuk S, Yazar S, Cetinkaya U. Stool sample storage conditions for the preservation of *Giardia intestinalis* DNA. *Mem Inst Oswaldo Cruz.* (2012) 107:965–8. doi: 10.1590/S0074-02762012000800001
52. Miró G, Mateo M, Montoya A, Vela E, Calonge R. Survey of intestinal parasites in stray dogs in the Madrid area and comparison of the efficacy of three anthelmintics in naturally infected dogs. *Parasitol Res.* (2007) 100:317–20. doi: 10.1007/s00436-006-0258-0

10

Seroepidemiological Study of Canine and Human Dirofilariasis in the Endemic Region of Northern Serbia

Sara Savić [1], Marina Zekic Stosic [1], Doroteja Marcic [1], Isabel Hernández [2], Aleksandar Potkonjak [3], Suzana Otasevic [4], Maja Ruzic [5] and Rodrigo Morchón [2*]*

[1] Scientific Veterinary Institute "Novi Sad", Novi Sad, Serbia, [2] Group of Animal and Human Dirofilariasis, Faculty of Pharmacy, Campus Miguel Unamuno, University of Salamanca, Salamanca, Spain, [3] Department of Veterinary Medicine, Faculty of Agriculture, University of Novi Sad, Novi Sad, Serbia, [4] Faculty of Medicine, University of Nis, Nis, Serbia, [5] Clinic for Infectious Diseases, Faculty of Medicine, Clinical Center of Vojvodina, University of Novi Sad, Novi Sad, Serbia

***Correspondence:**
Sara Savić
sara@niv.ns.ac.rs
Rodrigo Morchón
rmorgar@usal.es

Dirofilariasis is a vector-borne zoonotic disease caused mainly by *Dirofilaria immitis* and *Dirofilaria repens* that affect dogs and humans all over the world. Serbia is considered an endemic country to both forms of dirofilariasis, although most of the population is concentrated in the north of the country. The aims of this study were to show the prevalence of *D. immitis* and *D. repens* in dogs and the seroprevalence in humans compared to previous studies in Northern Serbia. In total, 346 dog sera samples and 265 human samples were analyzed. Dog blood samples were analyzed using the modified Knott's method to check whether there were *Dirofilaria* spp. microfilariae and serum samples were checked by a commercial *D. immitis* antigen test. Human serum samples were analyzed with a non-commercial ELISA for detection of specific anti-*D. immitis*, anti-*D. repens,* and anti-*Wolbachia* IgG antibodies, and confirmed by western blotting. The overall prevalence for *Dirofilaria* spp. in dogs was 29.19%. The overall prevalence for *D. immitis* was 26.30%. The percentages of *D. immitis* and *D. repens* microfilaremia in dogs were 25.72 and 1.45%, respectively, while *D. immitis./D. repens* microfilaremia co-infections were also 1.45%. The overall seroprevalence for *Dirofilaria* spp. in humans was 3.77%. The overall seroprevalence for *D. immitis* was 1.51, 1.13% for *D. repens*, and for *D. immitis/D. repens* co-infections was 1.13%. The results indicate that *D. immitis* and *D. repens* are present in dogs and humans in the province of Vojvodina, in the northern part of Serbia. It is most likely associated with the presence of many rivers, the climate, and presence of mosquitoes in the area, so there could be a real public health risk.

Keywords: *Dirofilaria immitis*, *Dirofilaria repens*, Serbia, dogs, humans, prevalence, seroprevalence, Europe

INTRODUCTION

Dirofilariasis is a vector-borne zoonotic disease caused mainly by *Dirofilaria immitis* and *Dirofilaria repens. Dirofilaria immitis* causes heartworm disease in canines and pulmonary dirofilariasis in humans, whereas *D. repens* causes canine subcutaneous dirofilariasis and ocular/subcutaneous dirofilariasis in humans. Both parasites are transmitted by culicid mosquitoes, which inoculate larva 3 into definitive hosts in both animals and humans. For that reason, dirofilariasis is considered a veterinary and public health problem (1, 2).

Canine heartworm disease is a chronic, progressive, and life-threatening disease in which adult worms stay in the pulmonary artery and the heart, in the right ventricle of definitive hosts. In canine subcutaneous dirofilariasis, the adult worms are usually beneath the skin forming a subcutaneous nodule. In both cases, microfilariae circulate in the blood stream and are ingested by several species of mosquito vectors during their blood-feeding (3) and after two successive molts, during the next blood meal (4), stage-3 larvae are inoculated into the definitive host. In humans, *D. immitis* immature worms cause embolization in the pulmonary microarteries, leading to the formation of benign lung nodules (pulmonary dirofilariasis), although most cases are asymptomatic (1). On the other hand, *D. repens* worms do not usually reach the adult stage and immature worms may cause larva migrans syndrome and form subcutaneous nodules, in the ocular region and other organs (1, 3, 5–7). Pulmonary dirofilariasis usually has no clinical symptoms, so most diagnostic tools cannot be used, making it much more difficult to identify. However, subcutaneous/ocular dirofilariasis presents clinical signs that are easier to detect (1, 3). Moreover, *D. immitis* and *D. repens* harbor endosymbiotic bacteria of the genus *Wolbachia*. This bacteria participates in the parasite's life cycle and embryogenesis and plays a key role in the immune and inflammatory response of the organism to the disease (4, 8–10).

Dirofilariasis is on the rise in the European population of dogs and humans (1, 3, 11, 12). It is considered to be an endemic disease in southern European countries and in central and northern countries such as Switzerland, Germany, Netherlands, Lithuania, Slovenia, Czech Republic, Slovakia, and Russia (2, 4, 13–18). In addition, in the last decade, different epidemiological and seroepidemiological studies, alongside clinical reporting, have shown that dirofilariasis has been introduced into the countries of the Balkans peninsula (1, 3, 4, 11, 19). Serbia is considered as an endemic country to both forms of dirofilariasis in dogs (20–24). Few human cases have been reported to be caused by *D. repens* or have had specific antibodies found (25, 26). To explain the rise of dirofilariasis, studies suggest that red foxes and golden jackals may serve as reservoir hosts (27) and *Culex pipiens* and *Aedes vexans* act as vectors of both diseases in Northern Serbia (28).

The aim of this study was to show the prevalence of *D. immitis* and *D. repens* in dogs and the seroprevalence in humans compared to previous studies in Northern Serbia.

MATERIALS AND METHODS

Study Area

The northern part of Serbia (Province of Vojvodina) lies between Hungary, Croatia, and Romania. This northern part of the country is largely plains with a continental climate and a lot of rivers. Summers are hot and have lengthened over time due to climate change, so temperatures over 14°C usually last even through to the end of October. Winters are less and less cold and there has not been much snow during the last several winters. All this means that the mosquito season is prolonged from March to October. The air humidity during the warm period of the year is mostly high, meaning that the conditions for the development of mosquitoes are appropriate. During springtime there is a lot of rain and often in some parts of the country there are floods.

In the province of Vojvodina there is the Danube river, which crosses the country from east to west, while the Tisa river flows from north to south, and there are smaller rivers all around the region (**Figure 2**). There is also an artificial canal system called Danube–Tisa–Danube Canal. It covers the total area in Vojvodina of about 12,700 km^2 and it consists of a number of canals. This Canal is a unique hydro-engineering system for flood control and hydrotechnical management, forestry, water supply, wastewater evacuation, navigation, tourism, fishing, and hunting. Besides these purposes, it also represents a substantial amount of water, convenient for development of mosquitos.

Serum Samples

We analyzed a total of 611 sera samples: 346 dog sera samples (173 male and 173 female) were obtained from dogs analyzed by several veterinary clinics (**Table 1**) and 265 human samples (208 male and 57 female) were provided to the research laboratory from different departments of clinical centers in Northern Serbia (**Table 2**). Human samples were taken from patients with different symptoms, not only those with specific symptoms that could point to dirofilariasis. Variables considered for the analyses were gender, age, and municipality of residence. Samples were collected preserving the privacy of the patients and informing them of how the samples would be used. All samples were collected during the period of 2018 to 2019.

Methods

Dog blood samples were analyzed by applying the modified Knott's technique (29) to check whether there were *Dirofilaria* spp. microfilariae in the blood of the animals included in the study. Morphological characteristics of microfilariae (cephalic and caudal ends) were used in order to differentiate *D. immitis* and *D. repens* microfilariae (30). Dog serum samples were tested for the presence of *D. immitis* adult antigens using a commercial immunochromatographic test kit (VetLine *Dirofilaria* Antigen, NovaTec, Germany) according to the manufacturer's instructions. There is no commercial laboratory test of any kind for *D. repens* in dogs.

Human serum samples were analyzed using a non-commercial ELISA for detection of specific anti-*D. immitis*, anti-*D. repens*, and anti-*Wolbachia* IgG antibodies with some modifications (16, 17, 31, 32). *D. immitis* and *D. repens* adult worm extracts (DiSA and DrSA, respectively) and 1:100 serum dilutions were used to detect the presence of anti-DiSA and DrSA IgG antibodies. Sera samples diluted at 1:40 with a recombinant form of the *Wolbachia* Surface Protein (rWSP) were used to detect the presence of anti-rWSP IgG antibodies. In both cases, goat anti-human IgG (H+L) conjugated to horseradish peroxidase (Sigma-Aldrich, Spain) was used at a 1:4000 dilution. Easy Reader (Bio-Rad laboratories, USA) was used for measuring optical densities (OD) at 492 nm. The cut-off point (OD = 0.8 for DiSA and DrSA and 0.5 for rWSP) was determined by calculating the mean value + 3 standard deviations (3SD) of 50 serum samples obtained from dogs and clinically healthy humans (negative controls) who belonged to an area free of

TABLE 1 | Distribution of prevalence of *D. immitis*, *D. repens*, and co-infections in dogs in Northern Serbia by gender and age.

		D. immitis		*D. repens*		*D. immitis/D. repens*		*Dirofilaria* spp.
	Dog samples n° (%)	Test Positive (%)	Knott Positive (%)	Test Positive (%)	Knott Positive (%)	Test Positive (%)	Knott Positive (%)	TOTAL Positive (%)
Gender								
Male	173 (50.00%)	54 (31.21%)	52 (30.06%)	No test	1 (0.58%)	2 (1.16%)/No test	2 (1.16%)	57 (32.95%)
Female	173 (50.00%)	37 (21.39%)	37 (21.39%)	No test	4 (2.31%)	3 (1.73%)/No test	3 (1.73%)	44 (25.43%)
Age								
<3	162 (46.82%)	44 (27.16%)	44 (27.16%)	No test	1 (0.62%)	0 (0.00%)/No test	0 (0.00%)	45 (27.78%)
3–5	133 (38.44%)	34 (25.56%)	34 (25.56%)	No test	2 (1.50%)	2 (1.50%)/No test	2 (1.50%)	38 (28.57%)
6–8	30 (8.67%)	11(36.66%)	9 (30.00%)	No test	1 (3.33%)	2 (6.67%)/No test	2 (6.67%)	14 (46.66%)
>9	21 (6.07%)	2 (9.52%)	2 (9.52%)	No test	1 (4.76%)	1 (4.76%)/No test	1 (4.76%)	4 (19.05%)
Total	346	91 (26.30%)	89 (25.72%)	No test	5 (1.45%)	5 (1.45%)/No test	5 (1.45%)	101 (29.19%)

TABLE 2 | Distribution of seroprevalence of *D. immitis*, *D. repens*, and co-infections in humans in Northern Serbia by gender and age.

	Human samples n° (%)	*D. immitis*	*D. repens*	*D. immitis/D. repens*	*Dirofilaria* spp.
		ELISA Positive (%)	ELISA Positive (%)	ELISA Positive (%)	TOTAL Positive (%)
Gender					
Male	208 (78.49%)	4 (1.92%)	3 (1.44%)	2 (1.44%)	9 (4.33%)
Female	57 (21.51%)	0	0	1 (1.75%)	1 (1.75%)
Age					
<20	2 (0.75%)	0	0	0	0 (0.00%)
20–40	48 (18.11%)	2 (4.17%)	0	1 (2.08%)	3 (6.25%)
>40	215 (81.13%)	2 (0.93%)	3 (1,40%)	2 (0.93%)	7 (3.25%)
Total	265	4 (1.51%)	3 (1.13 %)	3 (1.13 %)	10 (3.77%)

D. immitis and *D. repens*. When both non-commercial ELISAs gave positive results for the same serum sample, that human sera were considered positive. Additionally, by using western blot analysis performed according to a previously described methodology (16, 33–36), these results were confirmed. Both antigenic extracts were subjected to SDS–PAGE in 12% gels under reduced conditions, and proteins were transferred onto nitrocellulose. Human sera were analyzed at a 1:40 dilution and anti-conjugates at a 1:500 dilution. All samples that were positive with these kits were also analyzed by western blot to determine if they recognized the specific bands for *D. immitis* (17–22 kDa) and for *D. repens* (43–70 kDa).

Geographical Information System

The ArcGIS Pro online software was used for the construction of a map of the sampling area. All layers of relevant environmental information (rivers, irrigated croplands, natural parks, among others) were included and symbolized for a better understanding of the map. All dog and human samples infected with *D. immitis*, *D. repens*, and co-infections were manually georeferenced by GPS at the point of capture. Georeferenced positive data for both hosts are shown in the map.

Statistical Analysis

The SPSS Base 18.0 software for Windows was used for the data analysis. The descriptive analysis of the considered variables was carried out studying the proportions in the qualitative variables. To compare proportions, Chi-square tests were performed. In all the cases, the significance level was established at $p < 0.05$.

RESULTS

The overall prevalence for *Dirofilaria* spp. in dogs was 29.19% (**Table 1**). The overall prevalence for *D. immitis* was 26.30%. The percentage of *D. immitis* microfilaremia in dogs was 25.72% (in all cases with a positive *D. immitis* antigen test), 1.45% for

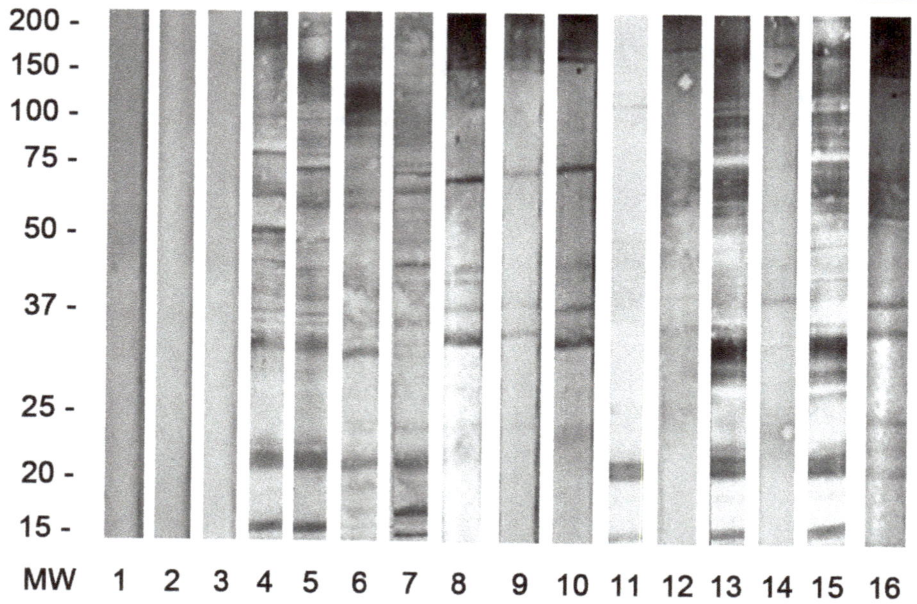

FIGURE 1 | Western blot in all human seropositive cases for *D. immitis* (4–7) with specific bands at 17–22 kDa; for *D. repens* (8–10) with bands at 43–70 kDa; for co-infections *D. immitis/D. repens* (11/12, 13/14, 15/16), and negative sera (1–3).

D. repens microfilaremia, and 1.45% for *D. immitis/D. repens* microfilaremia co-infections (in all cases with a positive *D. immitis* antigen test). There are significant differences between the prevalence for *D. immitis* infected male and female dogs with a higher prevalence in male dogs, whereas the prevalence of *D. repens* was higher in females ($p < 0.05$).

The overall seroprevalence for *Dirofilaria* spp. in humans was 3.77%. These results are shown in **Table 2**. The overall seroprevalence for *D. immitis* was 1.51, 1.13% for *D. repens*, and 1.13% for *D. immitis/D. repens* co-infections. All positive cases were detected in males with significant differences ($p < 0.05$) for *D. immitis* (1.92%) and *D. repens* (1.44%), but not in co-infection (1.44%). All positive samples via western blot analysis are shown in **Figure 1**.

By age, there are significant differences between the seroprevalences of *D. immitis* between the 20–40 range and the other ranges, the seroprevalences of *D. repens* between the over-40 age group and the other ranges and the seroprevalences of co-infections between the 20–40 age group and the other ranges ($p < 0.05$).

Regarding the geolocation of the positive samples of both dogs and people on a map (**Figure 2**), all of them were located in the vicinity of rivers, forest parks, green areas, and even within some cities in northern Serbia. There are only two cases of humans infected with *D. immitis* and *D. repens* in the northeast of the country.

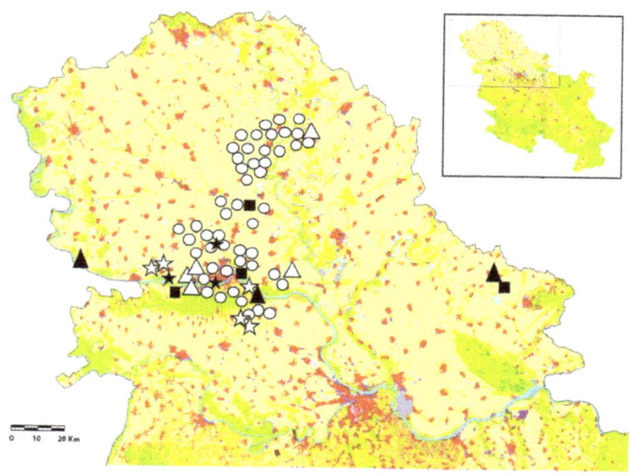

FIGURE 2 | Localization of the *D. immitis* and *D. repens* positive dogs and humans and co-infections in Northern Serbia: *D. immitis* in dogs (○), *D. repens* in dogs (△), *D. immitis/D. repens* in dogs (⋆), and *D. immitis* in humans (■), *D. repens* in humans (▲), and *D. immitis/D. repens* in humans (★). In green (natural grasslands, mixed forest, broad-leaved forest, moors and heathland, parks, forest parks), in red (continuous and discontinuous urban areas) and in blue (rivers, areas of stagnant water, and water bodies).

DISCUSSION

Wherever canine dirofilariasis exists, there is a risk of human infection. The general climatic conditions, local environmental factors, human interventions on the environment, and pet management are also factors that determine the distribution and incidence of illness (36). Humans and *Dirofilaria* spp. species have developed limited mutual adaptation (1). L3s inoculated by mosquitoes are usually eliminated from the host by the immune system. However, an undetermined percentage survives and continues to develop until pre-adult, and in some cases of *D. repens*, until adult, causing pulmonary and subcutaneous nodules or sometimes in the eye area, encapsulated or non-encapsulated. In any case, contact with the infecting larvae and subsequent stages of development stimulates an immune response that can be measured with appropriate techniques (37).

Epidemiological studies of human dirofilariasis, unlike in the dog population, have followed two different approaches. One is reported retrospective reviews and the other is seroepidemiological analyses. Each of these approaches provides information on different yet complementary aspects of human infections. The information obtained through retrospective reviews of reported cases offer only a partial view, since it only includes the part of the affected population that develops some type of clinical manifestation, and regions of endemicity showing vectors with zoo-anthropophilic habits probably have higher frequencies of human infections than reported in the literature. The problem of underreporting may exist due to the fact that symptoms in dirofilariasis patients, especially in pulmonary infections, may be misdiagnosed or unnoticed (1). Seroepidemiological studies compliment this information by detecting contact through the measurement of anti-*Dirofilaria* antibodies, allowing the evaluation of the risk of dirofilariasis infection in a defined geographical region, and constituting an excellent measure of the risk of infection for the human population which resides in an endemic area. Seroepidemiological studies of residents of areas of endemicity reported higher rates of infection in a similar manner to those of canines of the same areas (1, 5, 13, 16, 17, 34).

The aim of the present study was to analyze the prevalence in dogs and the response to anti-*D. immitis* and/or anti-*D. repens* antibodies in the northern region of Serbia (Vojvodina), taking into account that this region has been considered endemic for some time. Furthermore, the aim was to identify the potential risk of infection of the human population in an endemic area.

In Serbia, humidity and temperature conditions during a large proportion of the year allow for the transmission of dirofilariasis, with seroepidemiological data revealing noteworthy prevalence rates in the country's dog populations and human clinical cases caused by both *D. immitis* and *D. repens* (1, 3, 24).

In the current study, a prevalence of 26.30% was observed in dogs infected by *D. immitis*, with 25.72% microfilaremia in the total population, and the presence of *D. repens* larvae in 1 45% of the analyzed dogs. In two regions of Vojvodina (Pancevo and Veliko Gradiste), the previously reported seroprevalence was 22.9% for *D. immitis* and the presence of *D. repens* microfilariae was 39.34% (38). In Bulgaria and Croatia, two neighboring countries, there are studies about the prevalence of *D. immitis* and *D. repens* in dogs (8.1 and 11.1%, respectively) and co-infections (3.2%) (11). Several studies point to an increase in *D. immitis* infections and a decrease of an infection with *D. repens* in recent years (21–23) which is corroborated by results in this study. In addition, infections have also been found to be prevalent in wild canids (39), which could mean there is a risk of *D. immitis* infection between the dog population and the wild canid population. Meanwhile, *D. repens* was found to circulate mostly in golden jackal and red fox populations (27).

With regards to the human population, the seroprevalence for *Dirofilaria* spp. in humans was 3.77, 1.51% for *D. immitis*, 1.13% for *D. repens*, and 1.13% for *D. immitis*/*D. repens* co-infections. This is the first time these tests have been conducted in this region of Serbia. Human cases originating from *D. repens* have only previously been reported in the region of southeastern Serbia (24, 40, 41). In addition, other studies have reported seroprevalences of 9.7% and 8.1% against *D. repens* and D. immitis polyproteins specific antibodies, respectively, and 2.3% in individuals with specific antibodies to both species (26). Similar studies in neighboring countries such as Romania and Moldova have reported seroprevalences of 10.7% for *D. immitis*, 0.2% for *D. repens*, and 0.9% for both parasites (16). In addition, in Croatia there have been human *D. repens* cases reported (3). These seroepidemiological studies are a good tool to measure the risk of infection in a population where there is a high population of infected animals, as well as the presence of vectors, which serve as a vehicle for transmission of the disease (1, 42).

Both animals and infected people were geolocated in the immediate vicinity or in a relatively close environment of potential mosquito breeding areas, which poses a risk to those areas. The two cases of humans infected by *D. immitis* and *D. repens* in the northeast of the country are close to cities where cases of dogs and humans had already been reported (38) and were located in areas near rivers and green areas where mosquitoes breed. The spatial distribution of positive cases has a clear association with different geo-environmental factors, humidity and temperature, the existence of irrigated areas, areas with abundant water, rivers in valleys protected from winds, and proximity to the coast, which are considered risk factors for the transmission of dirofilariasis (43).

In conclusion, the results indicate that *D. immitis* and *D. repens* are present in dogs and humans in the province of Vojvodina, in the northern part of Serbia. It is most probably associated with the presence of many rivers, the climate, and the presence of mosquitoes, so there is a real public health risk. Serology studies in humans can be very useful for indicating the exposure to *Dirofilaria* spp. in a healthy population in order to obtain useful data on the epidemiological scenario of human dirofilariasis in Serbia and in Europe. That exposure was confirmed in the current study. Further studies addressing the control of dirofilariasis in the dog population are needed to reduce the risk of infection in the human population.

ETHICS STATEMENT

Ethical approval was not provided for this study on human participants because People data don't require permission, everyone has verbal consent. Written informed consent to participate in this study was provided by the participants' legal guardian/next of kin. Ethical review and approval was not required for the animal study because the blood samples were taken during a regular blood checkup of the dogs and the consent was gained from the owners so there was no need for the ethical approval. Written informed consent for participation was not obtained from the owners because Verbal consent of client owned dogs.

AUTHOR CONTRIBUTIONS

SS and RM designed the study and wrote the manuscript. MS, DM, IH, AP, SO, and MR performed the fieldwork, collected the data, and performed the experiments. All authors participated in the discussion of the results, corrected, read, and approved the final manuscript.

ACKNOWLEDGMENTS

We would like to thank the staff of veterinary clinics and the different departments of human clinics for their assistance in obtaining blood and serum samples from dogs and humans.

REFERENCES

1. Simón F, Siles-Lucas M, Morchón R, González-Miguel J, Mellado I, Carretón E, et al. Human and animal dirofilariasis: the emergence of a zoonotic mosaic. *Clin Microbiol Rev.* (2012) 25:507–44. doi: 10.1128/CMR.00012-12
2. Genchi C, Kramer L. Subcutaneous dirofilariasis (*Dirofilaria repens*): an infection spreading throughout the old world. *Parasit Vectors.* (2017) 10:517. doi: 10.1186/s13071-017-2434-8
3. Capelli G, Genchi C, Baneth G, Bourdeau P, Brianti E, Cardoso L, et al. Recent advances on *Dirofilaria repens* in dogs and humans in Europe. *Parasit Vectors.* (2018) 11:663. doi: 10.1186/s13071-018-3205-x
4. Morchón R, Carretón E, González-Miguel J, Mellado-Hernández I. Heartworm disease (Dirofilaria immitis) and their vectors in Europe - new distribution trends. *Front Physiol.* (2012) 3:196. doi: 10.3389/fphys.2012.00196
5. Kartashev V, Batashova I, Kartashov S, Ermakov A, Mironova A, Kuleshova Y, et al. Canine and human dirofilariasis in the rostov region (southern Russia). *Vet Med Int.* (2011) 2011:685713. doi: 10.4061/2011/685713
6. Ilyasov B, Kartashev V, Bastrikov N, Morchón R, González-Miguel J, Simón F. Delayed diagnosis of dirofilariasis and complex ocular surgery, Russia. *Emerg Infect Dis.* (2013) 19:326–8. doi: 10.3201/eid1902.121388
7. Ilyasov B, Kartashev V, Bastrikov N, Madjugina L, González-Miguel J, Morchón R, et al. Thirty cases of human subcutaneous dirofilariasis reported in Rostov-on-Don (Southwestern Russian Federation). *Enferm Infecc Microbiol Clin.* (2015) 33:233–7. doi: 10.1016/j.eimc.2014.04.002
8. Kramer LH, Tamarozzi F, Morchón R, López-Belmonte J, Marcos-Atxutegi C, Martín-Pacho R, et al. Immune response to and tissue localization of the Wolbachia surface protein (WSP) in dogs with natural heartworm (*Dirofilaria immitis*) infection. *Vet Immunol Immunopathol.* (2005) 6:303–8. doi: 10.1016/j.vetimm.2005.03.011
9. Grandi G, Morchón R, Kramer L, Kartashev V, Simón F. Wolbachia in *Dirofilaria repens*, an agent causing human subcutaneous dirofilariasis. *J Parasitol.* (2008) 94:1421–3. doi: 10.1645/GE-1575.1
10. Simón F, Kramer LH, Román A, Blasini W, Morchón R, Marcos-Atxutegi C, et al. Immunopathology of *Dirofilaria immitis* infection. *Vet Res Commun.* (2007) 31:161–71. doi: 10.1007/s11259-006-3387-0
11. Farkas R, Mag V, Gyurkovszky M, Takács N, Vörös K, Solymosi N. The current situation of canine dirofilariasis in Hungary. *Parasitol Res.* (2020) 119:129–35. doi: 10.1007/s00436-019-06478-5
12. Velev V, Vutova K, Pelov T, Tsachev I. Human Dirofilariasis in Bulgaria between 2009 and 2018. *Helminthologia.* (2019) 56:247–51. doi: 10.2478/helm-2019-0016
13. Kartashev V, Tverdokhlebova T, Korzan A, Vedenkov A, Simón L, González-Miguel J, et al. Human subcutaneous/ocular dirofilariasis in the Russian Federation and Belarus, 1997-2013. *Int J Infect Dis.* (2015) 33:209–11. doi: 10.1016/j.ijid.2015.02.017
14. Diosdado A, Gómez PJ, González-Miguel J, Simón F, Morchón R. Current status of canine dirofilariasis in an endemic area of western Spain. *J Helminthol.* (2018) 92:520–3. doi: 10.1017/S0022149X17000591
15. Miterpáková M, Valentová D, Cabanová V, Berešíková L. Heartworm on the rise-new insights into *Dirofilaria immitis* epidemiology. *Parasitol Res.* (2018) 117:2347–50. doi: 10.1007/s00436-018-5912-9
16. Ciuca L, Simón F, Rinaldi L, Kramer L, Genchi M, Cringoli G, et al. Seroepidemiological survey of human exposure to *Dirofilaria* spp. in Romania and Moldova. *Acta Trop.* (2018) 187:169–74. doi: 10.1016/j.actatropica.2018.07.012
17. Fontes-Sousa AP, Silvestre-Ferreira AC, Carretón E, Esteves-Guimarães J, Maia-Rocha C, Oliveira P, et al. Exposure of humans to the zoonotic nematode *Dirofilaria immitis* in northern Portugal. *Epidemiol Infect.* (2019) 147:e282. doi: 10.1017/S0950268819001687
18. Sabunas V, Radzijevskaja J, Sakalauskas P, Petkevičius S, Karveliene B, Žiliukiene J, et al. *Dirofilaria repens* in dogs and humans in Lithuania. *Parasit Vectors.* (2019) 12:177. doi: 10.1186/s13071-019-3406-y
19. Ionică AM, Matei IA, D'Amico G, Ababii J, Daskalaki AA, Sándor AD, et al. Filarioid infections in wild carnivores: a multispecies survey in Romania. *Parasit Vectors.* (2017) 10:332. doi: 10.1186/s13071-017-2269-3
20. Savić-Jevdenić S, Vidić B, Grgić Ž, Milovanović A. Brza dijagnostika dirofilarioze pasa u regionu Novog Sada. *Vet Glasnik.* (2004) 58:693–8.
21. Tasić A, Rossi L, Tasic-Otasevic S, Miladinovic-Tasic N, Ilic T, Dimitrijevic S. Survey of canine dirofilariasis in Vojvodina, Serbia. *Parasitol Res.* (2008) 103:1297–302. doi: 10.1007/s00436-008-1132-z
22. Spasojević-Kosić LJ, Lalošević V, Lalošević D, Simin S, Vasić I, Kuruca LJ. Prevalence of dirofilariasis in pet dogs in Novi Sad. *Contemp Agric.* (2012) 61:247–54.
23. Spasojević-Kosić LJ, Lalošević V, Simin, Kuruca LJ. Dirofilariasis and Angiostrongilosis in pet and hunting dogs in Novi Sad, Vojvodina, Serbia. *Arhiv Vet Med.* (2016) 9:53–62. doi: 10.46784/e-avm.v9i2.89
24. Krstić M, Gabrielli S, Ignjatović M, Savić S, Cancrini G, Randelović G, et al. An appraisal of canine and human cases reveals an endemic status of dirofilariasis in parts of Serbia. *Mol. Cell Probes.* (2017) 31:37–41. doi: 10.1016/j.mcp.2016.08.005
25. DŽamić AM, Colović IV, Arsić-Arsenijević VS, Stepanović S, Boričić I, DŽamić Z, et al. Human *Dirofilaria repens* infection in Serbia. *J Helminthol.* (2009) 83:129–37. doi: 10.1017/S0022149X09341346
26. Tasić-Otašević SA, Gabrielli SV, Tasić AV, Miladinović-tasić NL, Kostić JT, Ignjatović AM, et al. Seroreactivity to *Dirofilaria antigens* in people from different areas of Serbia. *BMC Infect Dis.* (2014) 14:68. doi: 10.1186/1471-2334-14-68
27. Potkonjak A, Rojas A, Gutiérrez R, Nachum-Biala Y, Kleinerman G, Savić S, et al. Molecular survey of *Dirofilaria* species in stray dogs, red foxes and golden jackals from Vojvodina, Serbia. *Comp Immunol Microbiol Infect Dis.* (2020) 68:101409. doi: 10.1016/j.cimid.2019.101409
28. Kurucz K, Kepner A, Krtinic B, Zana B, Földes F, Bányai K, et al. First molecular identification of *Dirofilaria* spp. (Onchocercidae) in mosquitoes from Serbia. *Parasitol Res.* (2016) 115:3257–60. doi: 10.1007/s00436-016-5126-y
29. Acevedo RA, Theis JH, Kraus JF, Longhurst WM. Combination of filtration and histochemical stain for detection and differentiation of *Dirofilaria immitis* and *Dipetalonema reconditum* in the dog. *Am J Vet Res.* (1991) 42:537–40.
30. Genchi G, Venco L, Genchi M. Guideline for the laboratory diagnosis of canine and feline *Dirofilaria* infections. In: Genchi C, Rinaldi L, Cringoli G, editors. *Mappe Parassitologighe 8, Dirofilaria immitis* and *Dirofilaria repens* in dog and cat and human infection, eds. Rolando Editore, Salamanca (2007). p. 137–45.
31. Simón F, Muro A, Cordero M, Martin J. A seroepidemiologic survey of human dirofilariasis in Western Spain. *Trop Med. arasitol.* (1991) 42:106–8.
32. Simón F, Prieto G, Morchón R, Bazzocchi C, Bandi C, Genchi C. Immunoglobulin G antibodies against the endosymbionts of filarial nematodes (Wolbachia) in patients with pulmonary dirofilariasis. *Clin Diagn Lab Immunol.* (2003) 10:180–1. doi: 10.1128/CDLI.10.1.180-181.2003
33. Perera L, Muro A, Cordero M, Villar E, Simón F. Evaluation of a 22kDa *Dirofilaria immitis* antigen for the immunodiagnosis of human pulmonary

dirofilariasis. *Trop Med Parasitol.* (1994) 45:249–52.
34. Perera L, Pérez-Arellano JL, Cordero M, Simón F, Muro A. Utility of antibodies against a 22 kD molecule of *Dirofilaria immitis* in the diagnosis of human pulmonary dirofilariasis. *Trop Med Int Health.* (1998) 3:151–5. doi: 10.1046/j.1365-3156.1998.00209.x
35. Santamaría B, Cordero M, Muro A, Simón F. Evaluation of *Dirofilaria immitis* excretory/secretory products for seroepidemiological studies on human dirofilariasis. *Parasite.* (1995) 2:269–73.
36. Simon F, Prieto G, Muro A, Cancrini G, Cordero M, Genchi C. Human humoral immune response to *Dirofilaria* species. *Parassitologia.* (1997) 39:397–400.
37. Carretón E, Morchón R, Montoya-Alonso JA. Chapter 1. Dirofilariasis cardiopulmonar canina. In: Montoya-Alonso JA, Carretón E, editors. *Dirofilariasis. Pautas de Manejo Clínico.* Barcelona: Multimédica Ediciones Veterinarias (2012). p. 1–130.
38. Tasić A, Tasić-Otašević S, Gabrielli S, Miladinović-Tasić N, Ignjatović A, Dordević J, et al. Canine Dirofilaria infections in two uninvestigated areas of Serbia: epidemiological and genetic aspects. *Vector Borne Zoonot Dis.* (2012) 12:1031–5. doi: 10.1089/vbz.2011.0949
39. Cirović D, Penezić A, Pavlović I, Kulišić Z, Cosić N, Burazerović J, et al. First records of Dirofilaria repens in wild canids from the region of central Balkan. *Acta Vet Hung.* (2014) 62:481–8. doi: 10.1556/avet.2014.021
40. Dzamić AM, Arsić-Arsenijević V, Radonjić I, Mitrović S, Marty P, Kranjcić-Zec IF. Subcutaneous *Dirofilaria repens* infection of the eyelid in Serbia and Montenegro. *Parasite.* (2004) 11:239–40.
41. Tasić S, Stoiljković N, Miladinović-Tasić N, Tasić A, Mihailović D, Rossi L, et al. Subcutaneous dirofilariasis in south-east Serbia - case report. *Zoonoses Public Health.* (2011) 58:318–22. doi: 10.1111/j.1863-2378.2010.01379.x
42. Cabrera E, Carretón E, Morchón R, Falcón-Cordón Y, Falcón-Cordón S, Simón F, et al. The Canary Islands as a model of risk of pulmonary dirofilariasis in a hyperendemic area. *Parasitol Res.* (2018) 117:933–6. doi: 10.1007/s00436-018-5774-1
43. Simón L, Afonin A, López-Díez LI, González-Miguel J, Morchón R, Carretón E, et al. Geo-environmental model for the prediction of potential transmission risk of Dirofilaria in an area with dry climate and extensive irrigated crops. The case of Spain. *Vet Parasitol.* (2014) 200:257–4. doi: 10.1016/j.vetpar.2013.12.027

11

Epidemiology of Trypanosomiasis in Wildlife—Implications for Humans at the Wildlife Interface

Keneth Iceland Kasozi[1,2], Gerald Zirintunda[3], Fred Ssempijja[4], Bridget Buyinza[5], Khalid J. Alzahrani[6], Kevin Matama[7], Helen N. Nakimbugwe[3,8], Luay Alkazmi[9], David Onanyang[10], Paul Bogere[11], Juma John Ochieng[4], Saher Islam[12], Wycliff Matovu[5], David Paul Nalumenya[5], Gaber El-Saber Batiha[13], Lawrence Obado Osuwat[14], Mahmoud Abdelhamid[15], Tianren Shen[1,16], Leonard Omadang[3] and Susan Christina Welburn[1,16*]*

[1] *Infection Medicine, Deanery of Biomedical Sciences, College of Medicine and Veterinary Medicine, The University of Edinburgh, Scotland, United Kingdom,* [2] *School of Medicine, Kabale University, Kabale, Uganda,* [3] *Department of Animal Production and Management, Faculty of Agriculture and Animal Sciences, Busitema University Arapai Campus, Soroti, Uganda,* [4] *Faculty of Biomedical Sciences, Kampala International University Western Campus, Bushenyi, Uganda,* [5] *College of Veterinary Medicine Animal Resources and Biosecurity, Makerere University, Kampala, Uganda,* [6] *Department of Clinical Laboratories Sciences, College of Applied Medical Sciences, Taif University, Taif, Saudi Arabia,* [7] *School of Pharmacy, Kampala International University Western Campus, Bushenyi, Uganda,* [8] *Department of Agriculture, Faculty of Vocational Studies, Kyambogo University, Kampala, Uganda,* [9] *Biology Department, Faculty of Applied Sciences, Umm Al-Qura University, Makkah, Saudi Arabia,* [10] *Department of Biology, Faculty of Science, Gulu University, Gulu, Uganda,* [11] *Faculty of Agriculture and Environmental Science, Muni University, Arua, Uganda,* [12] *Department of Biotechnology, Lahore College for Women University, Lahore, Pakistan,* [13] *Department of Pharmacology and Therapeutics, Faculty of Veterinary Medicine, Damanhour University, Damanhour, Egypt,* [14] *School of Medicine and Health Sciences, Soroti University, Soroti, Uganda,* [15] *Department of Parasitology, Faculty of Veterinary Medicine, Aswan University, Aswan, Egypt,* [16] *Zhejiang University-University of Edinburgh Institute, Zhejiang University School of Medicine, Zhejiang University, Haining, China*

***Correspondence:**
Keneth Iceland Kasozi
kicelandy@gmail.com
Susan Christina Welburn
sue.welburn@ed.ac.uk

While both human and animal trypanosomiasis continue to present as major human and animal public health constraints globally, detailed analyses of trypanosome wildlife reservoir hosts remain sparse. African animal trypanosomiasis (AAT) affects both livestock and wildlife carrying a significant risk of spillover and cross-transmission of species and strains between populations. Increased human activity together with pressure on land resources is increasing wildlife–livestock–human infections. Increasing proximity between human settlements and grazing lands to wildlife reserves and game parks only serves to exacerbate zoonotic risk. Communities living and maintaining livestock on the fringes of wildlife-rich ecosystems require to have in place methods of vector control for prevention of AAT transmission and for the treatment of their livestock. Major *Trypanosoma* spp. include *Trypanosoma brucei rhodesiense*, *Trypanosoma brucei gambiense*, *and Trypanosoma cruzi*, *pathogenic for humans*, *and Trypanosoma vivax*, *Trypanosoma congolense*, *Trypanosoma evansi*, *Trypanosoma brucei brucei*, *Trypanosoma dionisii*, *Trypanosoma thomasbancrofti*, *Trypanosma elephantis*, *Trypanosoma vegrandis*, *Trypanosoma copemani*, *Trypanosoma irwini*, *Trypanosoma copemani*, *Trypanosoma gilletti*, *Trypanosoma theileri*, *Trypanosoma godfreyi*, *Trypansoma simiae*, and *Trypanosoma (Megatrypanum) pestanai*. Wildlife hosts for the trypansomatidae include subfamilies of Bovinae, Suidae, Pantherinae, Equidae, Alcephinae, Cercopithecinae, Crocodilinae, Pteropodidae, Peramelidae, Sigmodontidae, and Meliphagidae. Wildlife species are generally considered tolerant to trypanosome infection following centuries of coexistence of vectors and wildlife hosts. Tolerance is influenced by age, sex, species, and physiological condition and parasite challenge. Cyclic transmission through *Glossina* species occurs for *T. congolense*, *T. simiae*, *T. vivax*, *T. brucei*, and *T. b. rhodesiense*, *T. b. gambiense*, and within *Reduviid* bugs for *T. cruzi*. *T. evansi* is mechanically transmitted, and *T. vixax* is also commonly transmitted by biting flies including tsetse. Wildlife animal species serve as long-term reservoirs of infection, but the delicate acquired balance between trypanotolerance and trypanosome challenge can be disrupted by an increase in challenge and/or the introduction of new more virulent species into the ecosystem. There is a need to protect wildlife, animal, and human populations from the infectious consequences of encroachment to preserve and protect these populations. In this review, we explore the ecology and epidemiology of *Trypanosoma* spp. in wildlife.

Keywords: trypanosomes in wildlife, human-wildlife interactions, wildlife-livestock interactions, human African trypanosomiasis, sleeping sickness, *Trypanosoma brucei gambiense*, *Trypanosoma brucei rhodesiense*

INTRODUCTION

The African and American trypanosomiases present significant global health challenge in human, domesticated animal, and wildlife communities. Spillover of parasites from wildlife to domestic livestock and humans and from domestic animal species to wildlife compromises health (1, 2). Most trypanosome infections in wildlife do not cause obvious damage to their host (3, 4), but some wildlife species are highly susceptible to trypanosome infections, including *Rattus nativitatis* and Macleay's rats (*Rattus macleari*) (5).

Trypanosoma are primarily transmitted by vectors (6) within which they undergo complex development cycles. Trypanosomes, which develop in the posterior section of the digestive tract in insects, are called stercorarian, for example, *Trypanosoma cruzi* the causal agent of Chagas disease, common in Latin America (7). Salivarian trypanosomes develop in the anterior part of the insect gut tract and include the causal agents of African animal trypanosomiasis (AAT) or nagana and for human African trypanosomiasis (HAT) caused by *Trypansoma brucei rhodesiense* and *Trypansoma brucei gambiense* that are present across Sub-Saharan Africa (8).

Animal trypanosomiasis is endemic in tropical regions of Africa, parts of Asia, and South America (9). *T. brucei s.l.*, *Trypanosoma congolense*, *Trypanosoma simiae*, and *Trypanosoma uniforme* are transmitted within the tsetse belts of Africa and cannot be transmitted by mechanical vectors (9). *T. vivax* and *Trypansoma evansi* can be transmitted mechanically and occur within and outside tsetse fly-infested zones (10).

EPIDEMIOLOGY OF ANIMAL TRYPANOSOMIASIS

Trypanosomiasis is one of the most important diseases affecting livestock, equines, and dogs within the Sub-Saharan region (11, 12). Cross transmission of parasites between livestock and wildlife hosts has been reported, especially in areas in close proximity to game parks and wildlife reserves. Wildlife species can survive within the tsetse belts across the Sub-Saharan region, despite being reservoir hosts for multiple species of trypanosome. The high prevalence of trypanosomiasis within protected areas traditionally has rendered these areas unattractive for livestock keeping and agricultural production (13).

Phylogenetic analysis shows a remarkable complexity of trypanosome species, subspecies, and strains in tsetse flies, human, domestic, and wildlife hosts. Examining the trypanosome species circulating within an ecosystem is a key to identifying the wildlife reservoirs of infection and transmission parameters to other animal hosts, including livestock within the ecosystem (3). Understanding the various trypanosome species harbored in wildlife hosts can guide preventive and control measures of trypanosomiasis in communities living at the livestock–wildlife interface. A wide variety of trypanosome species are circulating among wildlife hosts including *T. brucei s.l.*, *T. congolense*, *T simiae*, *T. godfreyi*, and *T. theileri* (3).

Hosts and Species of Trypanosomes

Apart from *T. cruzi*, present in South America, and *T. theileri*, present worldwide, trypanosomes infect a large number of wild and domestic ungulate species (6). Infection in the wildlife is influenced by species and habitat (12). Wildlife hosts for trypanosomiasis are numerous and include antelope species, warthogs (*Paecocherus aethiopicus*), elephants (*Loxodanta africana*), hippopotamus (*Hippopotamus amphibius*), lions, hyenas, jackals, caracals, and wild ruminants (14–16). Trypanosome species commonly found in wildlife species include *T. vivax*, *T. brucei s.l.*, *T. congolense*, and *T. evansi* (14). *T. vivax*, a pathogen affecting cattle, has been identified in waterbucks and giraffes, but the strains of *T. vivax* in these two host species were unique (3). Multiple wildlife hosts carry the human-infective zoonotic trypanosome strain *T. b. rhodesiense*, including bushbucks (*Tragelaphus scriptus*), impala (*Aepyceros melampus*), lion (*Panthera leo*), zebra (*Equus *quagga boehma*), warthog (*Phacocoerus africanus*), and duiker (*Sylvicapra grimmia*) (12). *Trypanosoma conglense*, *Trypanosoma simiae*, and *Trypanosoma godfreyi* were identified in Rhinocerus posttranslocation (16).

Infection with trypanosomes can predispose infected animals to other infections (17), and concurrent and opportunistic bacterial infections in wildlife can hasten the onset of clinical trypanosomosis (17).

There are significant associations between taxonomic groups of wildlife hosts and the prevalence of trypanosomiasis. Wildlife hosts from the bovinae group show a high prevalence of trypanosomiasis, especially *T. vivax* and *T. congolense* as well as human infective *T. brucei* (**Table 1**). Infection is attributed to their grazing habits, taking them into contact with tsetse and other biting flies. Wildlife hosts from the Pantherinae group show a very high prevalence of mixed trypanosome infections, as do those from the Suidae (12). A summary of trypanosome species in wildlife hosts and host taxonomy is shown in **Table 1**.

Transmission to Wildlife

Transmission of trypanosome species is generally by biting vectors including *Tsetse flies*, *Tabanids*, *Stomoxys*, *Heamatopota*, and *Hippobosca* (15, 30, 31). Infection in carnivores is additionally from consumption of infected meat as documented in the Felidae and Canidae (31, 32). *Desmodus rotundus* (Vampire bats) also transmit trypanosomiasis (32).

Trypanosomes engage in two patterns of transmissions: Cyclical transmission in which trypanosomes undergo active multiplication within the vectors (tsetse flies) as is common for *T. congolense*, *T. simiae*, *T. vivax*, *T. brucei*, and the human infective trypanosome species (*T. rhodesiense and T. gambiense*); and mechanical transmission through tsetse and alternative vectors including biting flies of the Tabanidae family (horse flies) as well as Stomoxys species. *T. evansi* and *T. vivax* can be mechanically transmitted (33).

Distribution of Reservoir Hosts

Preservation of natural resources including game parks and game reserves has led to an expansion of wildlife populations that serve as reservoirs for AAT and HAT (34). Human encroachment on the game parks and forests has increased AAT transmission between wildlife and domestic livestock, due to increased tsetse-human and tsetse-livestock contacts (34). The distribution of host populations within these areas determine vector and parasite survival. Wildlife hosts including monkeys and warthogs live in less restrictive habitats, unattractive to poachers with limited trophy hunting leading to increased reservoir host multiplication rates. They are widely distributed in the ecological environment and are favorable reservoirs for multiple trypanosome species due to their availability to vectors. Crocodiles and hippopotamus are limited to specific habitats, limiting access of vectors.

Distribution of Tsetse Flies

Trypanosomiasis affects one-third of Africa's land mass (35–37). Tsetse are found across most of West, Eastern, Central, and Southern Africa (38). The different species and subspecies of tsetse are shown in **Table 2**. Tsetse populations require moderate temperatures (23–25°C), high relative humidity (75–90%) with weak saturation deficit and shade (47–49). Temperatures above 34.1°C limit survival of tsetse and trypanosomes (35).

Food Source—Activity and Migration

Differences in wildlife food sources, particularly for wild bovidae, influence their exposure to trypanosomiasis. Among ruminant wildlife hosts, browsers are more at risk of trypanosomiasis compared with grazers; semi-browsers are moderately susceptible. Eland, Waterbuck, Kudu, and Bushbuck are more heavily infected, associated with their preference for inhabiting thickets during tsetse feeding hours, predisposing them to more bites (13, 18).

Diurnal wildlife hosts are more susceptible to trypanosome infection compared with the nocturnal species. Warthogs are most active in the morning and late afternoon and show high infection rates for trypanosomiasis in correlation to vector feeding hours (20). Lions are more infected in areas of high tsetse challenge than low challenge (50). The movement of large numbers of animals within wildlife ecosystems also influences infection. Animals will migrate in the dry season toward water sources that are also tsetse habitats (20).

Pathogenesis of Trypanosomosis

Trypanosome infection leads to erythrophagocytosis and heme catabolism resulting in iron accumulation in tissues and hyperbilirubinemia, liver dysfunction, and multiple organ failure (51). At necropsy, atrophy of body fats, pulmonary edema, hepatomegaly, lymphadenopathy, and hemorrhages are observed. Trypanosomes are found in tissues and body organs, and enlarged periarteriolar sheaths have been observed in wildlife (52).

Clinical Signs

Trypanosomiasis is a chronic progressive disease, and clinical signs may become obvious in advanced stages of the disease (53). Bovines affected by *T. vivax* present with severe anemia, lethargy, photophobia, lacrimation, and inappetence (17, 54, 55); pyrexia fluctuates with the fluctuating parasitemia. Leukopenia, thrombocytopenia, and degenerative and inflammatory lesions are observed in most organs (56). Body condition scores deteriorates gradually, and animals are dehydrated and debilitated before death. Superficial lymph nodes are enlarged and conspicuous. Corneal opacity may be observed with lacrimation (57). Young animals are stunted even with proper feeding, and productivity is impaired by abortions (32, 38). Animals may show localized or generalized edema (58). Except for *T. equiperdum*, other *Trypanosoma* species include similar clinical signs, but variations in intensity may happen in the various species. *Trypanosoma brucei* s.l. infection shows limited clinical signs in bovines of indigenous species but is highly pathogenic in exotic species (59).

Diagnosis of Trypanosomiasis

Trypanosomiasis is characterized by the intermittent presence of parasites in the blood and intermittent fever (54). Parasitological examinations are relatively sensitive during the acute phase

TABLE 1 | Trypanosome species and taxonomy of wildlife hosts.

Taxonomic group	Wildlife host (scientific name)	Trypanosome species	References
Bovidae	Waterbuck *(Kobus ellipsiprymnus)*	*T. vivax, T. congolense, T. brucei, T. evansi*	(12)
Girrafidae	Girraffe (*Giraffa camelopardalis*)	*T. vivax, T. evansi, T. brucei*	(12)
Bovidae	African buffalo (*Syncerus caffer)*	*T. b. rhodesiense, T. congolense, T. brucei*	(12)
	Bushbuck (*Tragelaphus scriptus*)	*T. b. rhodesiense, T. congolense, T. vivax, T. evansi*	(12)
	Greater kudu (*Tragelaphus strepsiceros*)	*T. congolense, T. vivax*	(12)
	Red lechwe (*Kobus leche*)	*T. theileri*	(18)
	Hartebeest (*Alcelaphus buselaphus*)	*T. godfreyi, T. brucei, T. godfreyi*	(18)
	Sable antelope (*Hippotragus niger*)	*T. brucei, T. theileri*	(18)
	African buffalo (*Syncerus caffer*)	*T. theileri, T. godfreyi*	(18)
	Eland (*Taurotragus derbianus)*	*T. vivax, T. congolense, T. brucei*	(12)
	Impala (*Impala impala*)	*T. godfreyi, T. brucei*	(18)
Elephantidae	Elephant (*Loxodanta africana*)	*T. vivax, T. congolense, T. evansi, T. elephantis*	(19)
Hippopotamidae	Hippopotamus (*Hippopotamus amphibius*)	*T. vivax, T. brucei, T. evansi, T. congolense*	(20)
Suidae	Warthog (*Phacocoerus africanus)*	*T. b. rhodesiense, T. vivax, T. congolense, T. evansi*	(20)
	Warthog (*Phacochoerus africanus*)	*T. godfreyi, T. brucei, T. simiae*	(18)
	Feral pig (*Sus scrofa*)	*T. evansi and T. cruzi*	(21)
Pantherinae	Lion (*Panthera leo*)	*T. brucei, T. evansi, T. congolense, T. congolense*	(12, 18)
	Leopard (*Panthera pardus)*	*T. brucei, T. congolense, T. evansi*	(12)
Equidae	Zebra (*Equus quagga boehma*)	*T. b. rhodesiense*	(12)
Cephalophinae	Common duiker (*Sylvicapra grimmia*)	*T. b. rhodesiense, T. vivax, T. congolense*	(12)
Aepycerotinae	Impala (*Aepyceros melampus*)	*T. b. rhodesiense, T. congolense, T. evansi*	(20)
Rhinocerotidae	Rhino (*Diceros bicornis)*	*T. brucei*	(20)
Alcephinae	Wildebeest (*Connochaetes taurinus cooksoni)*	*T. brucei, T. congolense, T. vivax*	(20)
	Hartebeest (*Alcephalus buselaphus*)	*T. evansi, T. brucei*	(20)
Hyaenidae	Hyena (*Hyaena hyaena)*	*T. evansi, T. congolense*	(12)
Cercopithecinae	Vervet monkey *(Cercopithecus species)*	*T. gambiense*	(12)
	Baboon (*Papio cynocephalus)*	*T. congolense*	(12)
Crocodilinae	Crocodile (*Crocodylus niloticus*)	*T. vivax*	(12)
Hippotraginae	Roan antelope (*Hippotraggus equinus)*	*T. vivax, T. congolense*	(12)
Pteropodidae	Megabat/fruit bat (*Chiroptera*)	*Trypanosoma dionisii, T. cruzi*	(22, 23)
Phalangeridae	Brushtail possum (*Trichosurus vulpecula*)	*Trypanosoma* spp.	(17)
Muridae	Brush-tailed rabbit-rat (*Conilurus penicillatus*)	*Trypanosoma* spp.	(5)
Potoroidae	Brush-tailed bettong (*Bettongia penicillata*)	*T. vegrandis, T. copemani*	(24)
Dasyuridae	Northern quoll (*Dasyurus hallucatus*)	*Trypanosoma* spp.	(5)
Peramelidae	Northern brown bandicoot (*Isoodon macrourus*)	*Trypanosoma* spp.	(5)
Phascolarctidae	Koalas (*Phascolarctos cinereus*)	*Trypanosoma irwini, T. copemani*	(25)
	Koalas (*Phascolarctos cinereus*)	*T. gilletti*	(25)
Cervidae	Marsh deer (*Blastocerus dichotomus*)	*Trypanosoma theileri, T. evansi*	(26)
Canidae	African wild dog (*Lycaon pictus*)	*T. godfreyi*	(18)
Potoroidae	Boodie (*Bettongia lesueur*)	*Trypanosoma spp.*	(27)
Tayassuidae	White-lipped peccary (*Tayassu pecari*)	*Trypanosoma evansi and Trypanosoma cruzi*	(21)
Mustelidae	Wild European badger (*Meles meles*)	*Trypanosoma (Megatrypanum) pestanai*	(28)
Meliphagidae	Regent honeyeater (*Anthochaera phrygia*)	*Trypanosoma thomasbancrofti*	(29)

of the disease. Wet blood film examination is used to detect the presence of motile trypomastigotes but has low sensitivity. Blood is taken from the tail or ear veins (55). Fluorescence microscopy can improve sensitivity for thin and thick smears (60). Parasitic concentration by centrifugation and examination of the buffy coat is more sensitive than the wet and thick smears (61). Dark ground or phase-contrast microscopy increases sensitivity at low parasitemia (62). Anion exchange chromatography is also sometimes deployed for detecting low parasitemia (54, 63, 64).

Molecular tests and serological tests are more sensitive than the usual parasitological tests for *Trypanosoma* (3, 63–68). Common serological tests include CFT, ELISA, and IFAT, while the common molecular tests are PCR, LOOP/LAMP, and LFA.

TABLE 2 | Tsetse species, geographical distribution, and wildlife spp. affected by trypanosomiasis.

Subgenus	Glossina species	Glossina subspecies	Country	Wildlife animal spp.	References
Nemorrhina (Palpalis)	*Glossina palpalis*	*G. p. palpalis*	Nigeria, Angola Cameroon,	Bushbuck, primates, warthogs	(36)
	G. tachinoides		Nigeria		(37)
		G. p. gambiesis	Gambia, Senegal, Republic of Guinea	Baboons, monkeys, chimps	(39, 40)
	G. fuscipes	*G. f. fuscipes*	Uganda, Sudan, Ethiopia, Kenya, DRC	Buffaloes, antelopes	(41)
		G. f. martini	Uganda, Tanzania, DRC	Buffaloes	(42)
		G. f. quanzensis	Uganda, Tanzania	Buffaloes, antelopes	(42)
	G. pallicera	*G. p. pallicera*	Cameroon, Ivory coast, Liberia	Antelopes	(43–45)
		G. p. newsteadi	DRC	Lions, leopards	(46)
	G. tachinoides		Nigeria, Ghana, Cameroon	Buffaloes, lions, buffaloes	(46)
	G. caliginea		Nigeria, Congo Brazaville	Cheetah, lions, leopards	(46)
Glossina (morsitans)	*G. morsitans*	*G. m. morsitans*	Nigeria, Uganda, Tanzania, Zambia	Buffaloes, rhinoceros, antelopes	(46)
		G. m. submorsitans	Uganda, Tanzania	Buffaloes, bushbuck, antelopes	(46)
		G. m. centralis	Uganda, Tanzania	Buffaloes, bushbucks, antelopes	(46)
	G. swynnertoni		Nigeria, Congo Brazaville	Lions, cheetahs	(46)
	G. longipalpis		Ivory Coast, Senegal, Mali	Buffaloes, lions	(46)
	G. pallipides		Ethiopia, DRC, Uganda, Kenya, Zambia, Tanzania	Buffaloes, lions, antelopes	(46)
	G. austeni		Kenya, Tanzania, Mozambique	Bushbucks, antelopes, lions	(46)
	G. vanhoofi		DRC	Lions	(46)
	G. tabanformis		Nigeria, DRC	Buffaloes, lions	(46)
	G. severini		DRC	Lions, bushbucks	(46)
	G. schwetzi		Togo. Congo Brazaville	Wild ruminants	(46)
	G. nigrofusca		Ivory Coast, Nigeria, CAR, DRC	Elephants, lions, monkeys	(46)
	G. nashi		Cameroon, Nigeria, Togo	Monkeys, baboons, wild cats	(46)
	G. medicorum		Ghana, Gambia, Nigeria	Lions, buffaloes	(46)
	G. longipennis		Tanzania, Sudan, Kenya	Antelopes, bushbucks, lions	(46)
	G. hanningtoni		Nigeria, Cameroon, Gambia	Bushbucks, buffaloes	(46)
	G. fuscipleuris		CAR, DRC Cameroon	Lions, bushbucks	(46)
	G. brevipalpis		Kenya, DRC, Tanzania	Buffaloes, antelopes	(46)

Low-flow assay (LFA) is cheaper with 96.3% sensitivity and 93.9% specificity (69). Approved tests for AAT are shown in **Table 3**.

TRYPANOSOMES IN WILDLIFE

The majority of trypanosome species require multiple obligatory hosts to complete their life cycles (heteroxenous), and the transmission of the parasites is mainly via hematophagous invertebrate vectors (2, 88). Trypanosomes are found in blood and tissues; blood-borne protozoan trypanosomes (*Trypanosoma vegrandis*) have been identified in wild animals including, but not limited to, the northern brown bandicoot (*Isoodon macrourus*), common brushtail possum (*Trichosurus vulpecula*), northern quoll (*Dasyurus hallucatus*), and brush-tailed rabbit-rat (*Conilurus penicillatus*) (5). *Trypanosoma cruzi, Trypanosoma dionisii*, and an insect trypanosome (*Blastocrithidia*) have been found to infect bats and other mammalian wildlife in Europe and South America (22). Bats, possums, and rats act as reservoirs of trypanosomes for domestic and wild animals, as well as humans (5, 22). *T. cruzi* (Chagas) has been identified in kidney tissue, heart muscle, and blood, urine, and peritoneal fluid of wild spp. including foxes, opossums, raccoons, and striped skunks (89, 90), and parasites can be transmitted from animal-to-animal by contamination of animal wounds with blood, urine, and peritoneal fluid (89, 90).

Trypanosome–Host Relationships

Hosts are classified according to their role as a definitive host [if the mature sexual stage(s) of the parasite occurs within them] or intermediate hosts when the more mature sexual stages of the parasite only aid part of the life cycle (91). Transfer (paratenic) hosts are not vital for the completion of parasitic development cycles but maintain the parasite before it reaches the obligatory/definitive host (92, 93). Invertebrates (vectors) acting as hosts and carriers of parasites facilitate the completion of parasitic life cycles by transmitting parasites (94–96).

Trypanosomes can infect many hosts, transmitted by hematophagous insect vectors mainly the tsetse fly and triatomid kissing bugs (subfamily: Reduviidae) (13, 97). Salivarian trypanosomes, *Trypanosoma brucei, T. rhodesiense*,

TABLE 3 | Approved laboratory tests for trypanosomiasis according to OIE (70).

Test criteria	Objective	Methods	References
Clinical signs	Categorize presentation	Observations	(32, 53, 71)
Microscopy	Direct examination	Wet blood films	(72)
		Thick blood films	(60, 61)
		Thin blood smear films	(72)
	Parasitic concentration	Microhematocrit centrifugation technique	(61)
		Dark ground or phase-contrast buffy coat technique	(62)
		Anion exchange technique	(73–75)
	Cultivation technique	Animal inoculation	(76–78)
Molecular detection	Antigen assays	Trypanosome antigen detection assays	(79)
	Trypanosome DNA	Monospecific PCR	(80)
		Multi-specific PCR	(81, 82)
		LOOP	(68)
		LFA	(69, 83)
Serology	Antibodies	Indirect immunofluorescence test	(84)
		IgG antibody ELISA	(85)
		IgG antibody detection	(86, 87)

T. equiperdum, *T. vivax*, and *T. congolense* are transmitted in tsetse fly (*Glossina* spp.) saliva to the host spp. Hosts are as follows: *T. brucei* s.l. (domestic mammals and humans), *T. vivax* (ruminants, horses, and camels), *T. equiperdum* (equines), *T. simiae* (pigs), and *T. congolense* (dogs and cats) causing *T. evansi* (domestic mammals), and other numerous wildlife hosts such as monkeys, guinea pigs, rabbits, rats, etc., are also affected (91, 98). Stercorian trypanosomes are transmitted through the fecal matter of the insects (*Triatominae*, e.g., *Triatoma infestans*) to host skin where they gain access to tissues. Other vectors of transmission for stercorians include Tabanid flies, stable flies, ticks, and mosquitoes. Stercorians include *Trypanosoma cruzi*, *T. lewisi*, *T. melophagium*, *T. nabiasi*, *T. rangeli*, *T. theileri*, *T. theodori*, *T. lewisi*, *T. cruzi*, bat spp. (*Trypanosoma cruzi marinkellei*, *Trypanosoma dionisii*, *Trypanosoma erneyi*, *Trypanosoma livingstonei*, and *Trypanosoma wauwau*), and others: *Trypanosoma conorhini* and *Trypanosoma rangeli* (94, 95, 98, 99). Among wildlife, *T. cruzi* is found in armadillos, dogs, possums, foxes, bats, raccoons, and striped skunks (5, 22, 89, 90). In addition, *T. melophagum* and *T. theileri* are found in Europe infecting cattle, buffaloes, and antelopes (98).

Trypanotolerance

Trypanotolerant animals show a few clinical signs (96, 97), and trypanosomes are able to evade the host immune responses (100). Trypomastigotes penetrate a variety of host cell types and multiply intracellularly as amastigotes—which eventually infect host cells and differentiate into BFT, which eventually invade the lymphatic and circulatory systems (50, 101). *Trypanosoma* cell membranes are covered with dense variable surface glycoprotein (VSG) homodimers—immunodominant antigens that trigger infected host B- and Th-cell-mediated immune responses. Over 1,000 different VSG genes and pseudogenes are present in the trypanosome genome that can undergo segmental gene recombination to encode an estimated 10,000 different VSG surface coats. High antigenic variability in VSG molecules hinders vaccine development (102).

Wildlife, while generally immunotolerant to trypanosomes (103) can, however, develop clinical trypanosomiasis (104) and show varying levels of trypanotolerance among species (105, 106). Trypanotolerance is influenced by multiple host intrinsic and extrinsic factors and can develop from previous exposure (106). Intrinsic factors include age, sex, species, physiological state, and state of nutrition, while extrinsic factors include temperature, humidity, nature of vegetation, and the nature of wildlife communities (107).

A study in the Serengeti National Park, Tanzania, showed age-dependent infection with *T. congolense* in lions (*Panthera leo*); however, the same animals appeared to have developed cross-immunity following infections to multiple trypanosome species including *T. brucei rhodesiense* (101). Lions are exposed to high challenge from trypanosomes, both from tsetse and also from infected prey, becoming exposed to extremely high numbers of VSGs. This work suggests that animals within a closed exosystem can control infections and, in this case, eliminate the human infective parasite *T. b. rhodesiense* from the infection pool.

Development of Resistance

Trypanotolerance can enable the regulation of parasite levels in the blood (parasitemia) and body tissues. Resistance in wildlife species has been associated with serum xanthine oxidase and catalase and other trypanolytic molecules (108, 109). Stress can affect trypanotolerance in wildlife (71). Trypanotolerance has been investigated in mice and cattle, although these have differences in immune response, i.e., more pronounced B-cell activation in mice than in cattle (50). In cattle, antibody (IgG and IgM) and complement activity against parasitic VSGs leads to protection (110), through antigenic neutralization and IL-4 production (111) (**Figure 1**).

In Cape buffalo, resistance has been associated with non-specific trypanocidal activity in serum, which helps to lower the parasitemia following action of xanthine oxidase (XO), which generates reactive oxygen species (ROS). Since trypanosomes cannot metabolize XO, this cripples parasitic binding and endocytosis (111), trypanosomes are starved of ATP, and death follows (**Figure 1**). An increase in catalase activity is associated with increased parasitemia (112). Some wildlife spp. including the black rhinoceros have significant deficiencies for ATP, catalase, and glycolysis enzymes (conditions that favor trypanosome parasitemia) leading to adaptive evolutionary changes, which help to protect the animals against the parasites (113).

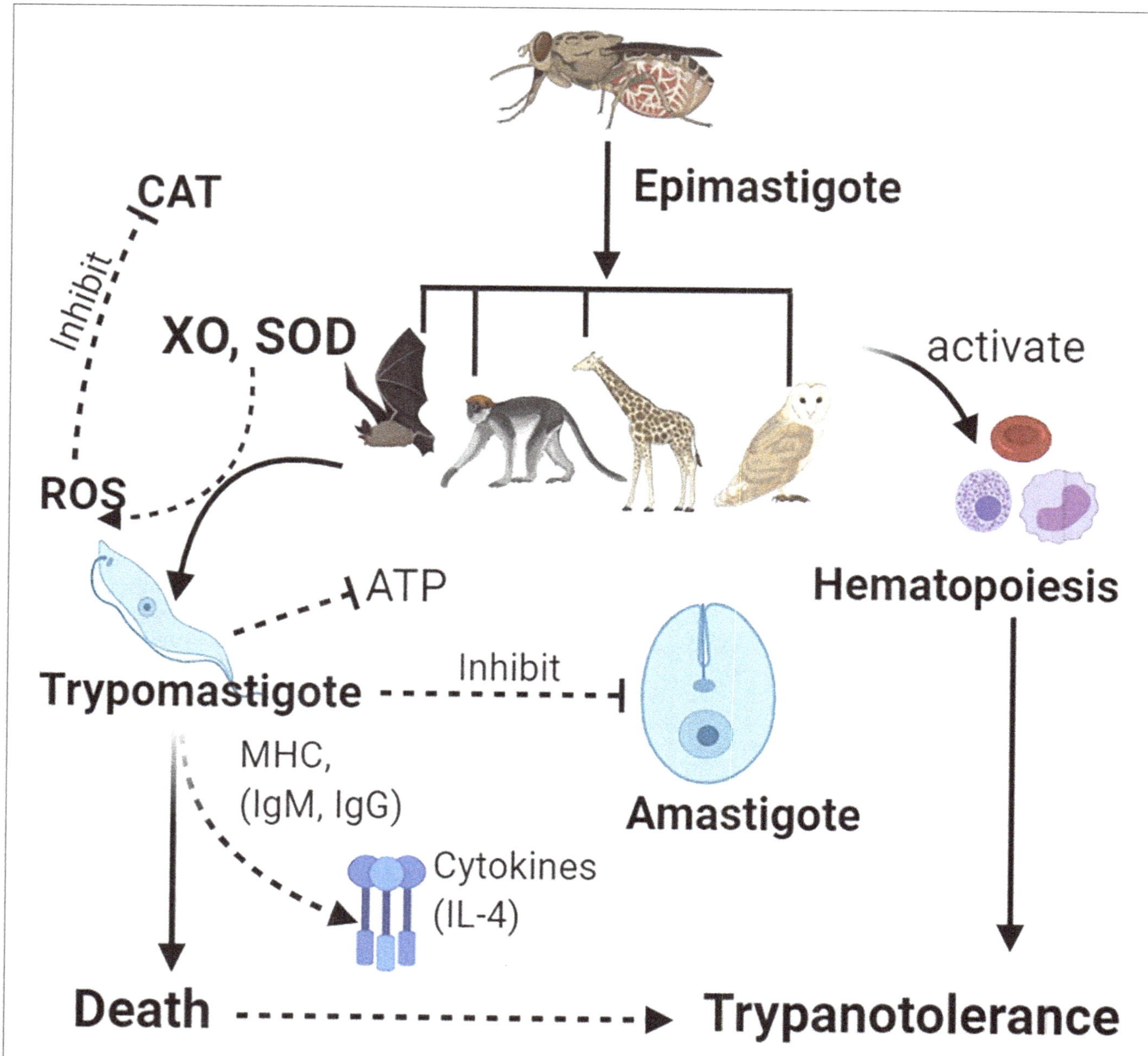

FIGURE 1 | Vectors carrying epimastigotes infect wildlife host species. Epimastigotes transform into trypomastigotes in blood. Host enzymes [e.g., xanthine oxidase (XO) and superoxide dismutase (SOD)] increase production of reactive oxygen species (ROS) such as hydrogen peroxide, which helps clear the parasites, while antioxidant enzymes such as catalase (CAT) lead to increased parasitemia. Immune system activation leads to production of antibodies and cytokines, which neutralize trypanosomes. Inhibition of glycolysis (ATP) leads to deprivation of energy in the parasite for cellular activities. Furthermore, host defenses activate the innate immunity leading to hematopoiesis and an increase in blood cells, thus, leading to trypanotolerance. Wildlife host species subsequently get infected with trypanosomes but rarely succumb to infection.

Wild animals show varying levels of trypanotolerance; the Thomson's gazelle, dikdik, blue forest duiker, jackal, bat-eared fox, ant bear, hyrax, serval, and monkey are all susceptible to *T. rhodesiense* and *T. brucei*, whereas the common duiker, eland, bohor reedbuck, spotted hyena, oribi, bushbuck, impala, warthog, bushpig, porcupine, and baboon are considered resistant (or less susceptible) to *T. b. rhodesiense* and *T. brucei* infection (114, 115). Animals most susceptible are usually found in areas of high tsetse challenge, while those least susceptible (resistant) animals within the population may have acquired resistance through low exposure and challenge over time (116).

The clinical course of trypanosomiasis has been examined in native African buffalo (*Syncerus caffer*), oryxes (*Oryx beisa*), eland (*Taurotragus oryx*), and waterbuck (*Kobus defassa*) following infection with *T. congolense*, *T. vivax*, or *T. brucei*. These animals showed resistance in the form of negligible parasitemia and minimal anemia (115). Wild and domestic animals have been observed to develop resistance to trypanosomiasis after being subjected to prolonged continuous trypanosome infections (117, 118), and as previously mentioned, indigenous bovines are resistant to *T. brucei* within endemic foci in Uganda (114, 115).

TRYPANOSOMIASIS AT THE WILDLIFE, DOMESTIC ANIMAL INTERFACE

Diversity of Trypanosomes in Wildlife

Multiple *Trypanosoma* species and genotypes contribute to a large reservoir of parasite diversity. This presents major problems in the management of trypanosomiasis at the wildlife–domestic animal interface, with the risk of virulent strains emerging that impact both wildlife and domestic populations (5). A review of Australian animal trypanosomes found a huge variety of parasites: *T. pteropi*, *T. thylacis*, *T. hipposideri*, *T. binneyi*, *T. irwini*, *T. copemani*, *T. gilletti*, *T. vegrandis*, *T. lewisi*, *T. melophagium*, *T. theileri*, *T. nabiasi*, *T. evansi*, *T. cruzi*, *T. pteropi*, *T. hipposideri*, *T. binneyi*, *T. thylacis*, *T. copemani*, *T. Irwin*, and *T. gilleti*. Such biodiversity may have negative impacts on the wildlife and national parks, and is associated with biosecurity concerns (88, 119). Newly identified genotypes of wildlife animals include *Trypanosoma vegrandis G6* and *T. vegrandis G3* (5). Furthermore, a study in bats found three *Trypanosoma* spp. (*T. cruzi*, *T. dionisii*, and *Blastocrithidia* spp.) (22) demonstrating the great diversity in several wildlife species.

Infection at the Wildlife, Domestic Animal Interface

Climate change, population pressure, and incentives to end poverty through farming have forced humans to encroach into land previously occupied by wildlife (108, 120). Human encroachment in protected zones runs the risk of parasite transmission from wildlife to domestic animals and zoonotic transmission (108, 109, 121). Synanthropic zoonotic infections are spread from livestock to humans, and exoanthropic infections are spread by wildlife and feral animals to humans—contributing to the increasing gene pool of anthroponoses (98). The cross-species (interspecies) transmission, also known as host jump or spillover, means the potential of an external parasite to invade a new host and infect them to ultimately spread to the whole population of the new host. About 63% of host jumps are responsible for interspecies diseases (109, 122, 123).

Endemic zones are created by encroaching on places of game parks. This has caused a wildlife and livestock interface, and development of the trypanosome parasite reservoirs (117). Wildlife is often implicated as the reservoir of parasites especially trypanosomes (37, 124, 125). It is common for the high incidences of trypanosomiasis in the wildlife to spillover to the domestic cycle in the tsetse fly-infested zones (71). Domestic animals pose a risk to wildlife, particularly the great apes, especially if the domestic carriers are present, for example, cattle and dogs (32).

Infection with *T. b. rhodesiense* is common in communities living proximal to, or that are dependent on, wildlife or eco-tourism (126, 127). In the Luangwa Valley, Zambia, considerable efforts are made to keep domestic animals away from the national park, for biosecurity of livestock keepers, the national parks, and game conservancies (128). In Zambia, HAT infections have been associated with young children attending school and older women demonstrating in the homestead (129, 130).

A study in Australia failed to find *T. cruzi* and *T. evansi* in native domestic and wildlife animals; however, a spillover for exotic *Trypanosoma* spp. was expected that would affect humans, domestic, and wild animals (88). Wildlife (*Clyomys laticeps*, *Thrichomys pachyurus*, and *Oecomys mamorae)* can be reservoir hosts for *Trypanosoma* spp., e.g., *T. evansi* and *T. cruzi* that could infect humans and other wildlife populations without affecting the rodent spp. (131).

Factors That Could Influence Trypanosomiasis Epidemiology in Wildlife Areas

Host species that are widely distributed and with fewer restrictions on habitat have proved to be of more importance to trypanosome diversity due to their unlimited breeding potential and less risk for poaching and trophy hunting. Such hosts include warthogs, bushbucks, kudus, buffaloes, and giraffes (20). More habitat-restricted host species have minimal contribution to the epidemiology of trypanosomiasis in wildlife communities due to their relative safety from trypanosome vectors like Glossina and Tabanids, e.g., crocodiles and hippopotamus.

Differences in feeding patterns of the trypanosome hosts influence the distribution of trypanosomiasis in wildlife areas. Certain preferences maintained by certain hosts like bovines (bushbuck, waterbuck, eland, kudu, etc.) to bushy areas and thickets have predisposed them to higher exposure rates to tsetse and other biting flies, intensifying the spread of trypanosomes (20). Trypanosome diversity among the host species has facilitated the cross-transmission of various trypanosome strains and variants among the hosts, increasing infection rates among wildlife communities at both clinical and subclinical levels. For example, the discovery of three different variants of *T. vivax* in three different host species including a buffalo, a waterbuck, and a giraffe not similar to any published strain, demonstrating genetic diversity, provides insights on pathogen epidemiology (3).

Furthermore, the introduction of new host species from a different geographical location into a wildlife reserve can greatly influence the trypanosome species diversity in a wildlife community. This way, new variants and species of trypanosomes are spread from one host to another by tsetse and other biting flies, resulting in devastating effects on wildlife health and livestock health in the area, for example, the discovery of *T. melophagium*, *T. nabasi*, *T. theieri*, and *T. evansi* in Australia following the introduction of various mammals into their wildlife populations, which had a great impact on the native marsupials (9).

Wildlife Encroachment and the Epidemiology of Trypanosomiasis

Encroachment to wildlife and the increasing human and livestock density as well as the altered patterns in land use are key parameters that govern the transmission of trypanosomes (132). It is expected that understanding how the encroachment to wildlife affects the epidemiology of trypanosomes will inspire practical approaches to improve the understanding of epidemiological characteristics of trypanosome transmission in the context of ecological factors. Encroachment to wilderness areas of Africa increases the epidemiology of trypanosomes, hence, increasing the transmission of HAT. Primarily, wildlife are trypanosome reservoirs; however, growing human and livestock numbers around or in wildlife areas increase the significance of livestock in the transmission cycles thereby increasing the epidemiology of trypanosomes pertinent to human health (132).

Understanding undercurrents associated with the transmission of trypanosomes and in relationship with the encroachment of livestock and humans to wildlife areas are vital to developing robust control measures. This would help identify important parameters on host distributions, tsetse populations, epidemiology of trypanosomes, infection and mortality rates, the significance of livestock, humans, and livestock as hosts in wildlife areas, hence, promoting the progress of models to help in the evaluation and application of control measures (132). Parameters that determine the dynamics in encroachment levels to wildlife areas such as protected area, wildlife density, livestock density, human density, and location according to space and time, would help determine the foci of HAT. This is important since increased human and livestock populations and their distribution may lead to land-use pattern changes in fragmented tsetse habitats, and this inevitably affects the distribution of wildlife species. These ultimately result in increased tsetse abundance and distribution, host selection, and tsetse mortality, which are indicators of increased vector competence (132). Host population density is a key factor in determining the dynamics of tsetse populations, i.e., a decline in host density through encroachment to wildlife areas influences tsetse population changes in space and time. This, in turn, influences the transmission of trypanosomes, and although low host density decreases trypanosome transmission as a consequence of tsetse mortality, the low host density may also be associated with an increased level of trypanosome transmission arising from the hungrier flies that bite humans through increased host-seeking efficiency of tsetse flies (133).

INFECTION CONTROL AT THE WILDLIFE–LIVESTOCK–HUMAN INTERFACE

While communities fail to understand the value of wildlife ecosystems, continued wildlife–human conflict presents an increased risk of infection spillover to humans (18, 118, 134, 135). Game parks, the natural habitats for tsetse species, pose risks to livestock and human populations (136, 137), and parasitic infestations among the livestock and humans equally pose a risk to wildlife. Wildlife reservoirs make approaches of trypanosomosis control at the wildlife–livestock–human interface more complicated (30, 31). There is a need to limit the interaction between livestock and wildlife by preventing encroachment into wildlife-protected zones. Mitigation of risk to prevent trypanosome (and other) infections circulating among livestock and wildlife demands a holistic One Health approach (108, 138, 139). Top–down, approaches, shooting games and radical bush clearing, and insecticide spraying in protected zones are neither practical nor acceptable (140). Stakeholder and community-derived solutions are likely to be sustainable options to explore. Approaches to infection control require to be nuanced in these zones, with communication, education, and interventions embedded within the affected communities. Integrated insect control approaches including the use of insecticide-impregnated targets can protect livestock and game (141). Application of insecticides to cattle, using livestock as live baits, can offer sustainable solutions (138, 142, 143); however, challenges remain on the sustainability of this approach especially in low–middle income countries (LMICs). Insecticides are a reliable method for tsetse control and can be improved by deploying an integrated insecticide approach (139, 141). Routine prophylaxis among livestock can protect livestock and offer collateral benefits for humans and wildlife (144, 145). There is also a need to limit the interaction between livestock and wildlife by stopping encroaching on gazetted wildlife zones to lower the trypanosome prevalence in domesticated livestock (108).

Animal and Human Health for the Environment and Development (AHEAD), launched in 2003, comprises a One Health team of socioeconomic scientists, ecobiologists, veterinarians, agriculturalists, wildlife, and public health specialists that address issues at the wildlife, human, and domestic livestock interface. This includes efforts to monitor parasitic diversity in wildlife species to assist in the strengthening of disease surveillance in LMICs (146). Management and communication with regard to wildlife is key to the One Health approach; in pastoral communities, retaliatory persecution through poisonings of predatory wildlife continues to challenge conservation efforts (147). Conflicts associated with competition for natural resources between livestock-keeping communities and wildlife can be mitigated by a combination of communication and control strategies to promote peaceful coexistence of wildlife and humans as promoted by AHEAD.

Management of Spillover of Trypanosomiasis Among the Human–Wildlife Areas

Communities in the wildlife zones sometimes agree on coexistence with wildlife and the creation of buffer zones (148). However, the coexistence of human communities and wildlife poses risks of outbreaks of various zoonoses (149). In the gazetted wildlife zones, there should be no mixing of domestic animals with wild trypanosomiasis reservoirs. Proper fencing can be used to control the spillover in wildlife borders (150) as part of the integrated trypanosomiasis control strategy. Restrictive models need to be developed by engaging the communities such that they understand these objectives (151). There is a need for legislation on fencing to have restricted movement of livestock and wildlife. The laws need to address the challenges of wildlife biodiversity (152) and penalize encroachers and poachers. This requires an appropriate land tenure system and robust enforcement teams.

Renowned trypanosome hosts like bats need to be removed from urban centers and human dwellings. Bats also live in human dwellings in ceilings and other dark points. African bats are hosts of trypanosomes (153). It is not known whether the African bats are associated with virulent chronic and acute human African trypanosomiasis. However, bats are associated with trypanosomes in central and South America (22, 154, 155).

Research on possible vaccine candidates has not broken through despite emphasis on the VSG pathway (102, 156). This, however, does not translate that research on trypanosome vaccines has reached a dead end since in all the failures, better innovations can transform science to improve understanding in this field (157, 158). This is important since drugs that are used to treat domestic animals have been used to treat wildlife with success (159, 160), although this has not been done against infections with the zoonotic trypanosomes.

Wildlife are usually in contact with insects other than the tsetse flies. It is known that lice can transmit *T. cruzi* (161). The possibility of lice transmitting the zoonotic trypanosomes is not known. Zoonotic trypanosomes have been found in fleas (162), and it is speculated that fleas may transmit trypanosomes among wildlife (163–165). The possible transmission of trypanosomes by other biting arthropods among wildlife needs further investigation. The possibility of transmission along the food chains for carnivores needs further investigation. Wild Canidae that feed on fresh blood from trypanosomiasis reservoirs may acquire infections from the fresh blood. No studies have ever been proposed among at-risk carnivores.

There is a need to study the interactions of trypanosomes with other blood parasites. Trypanosomes interact with babesia especially to worsen the stress conditions of translocation (166–168). The effect of trypanosomes on the immune system likely predisposes the animals to opportunistic infections and tick-borne diseases. The presence of other parasites is possibly a contributing factor to the trypanosomiasis spillover.

CONCLUSION

Trypanosomiasis continues to be a major global challenge, particularly so at the wildlife–domestic livestock interface. Multiple wildlife species serve as maintenance hosts promoting infections at the livestock–wildlife interface. There is a high risk of infection spillover from game parks and conservation areas where parasites and vectors are concentrated in high numbers, and domestic livestock pose risks to wildlife-protected species. The basis of trypanotolerance in wildlife species is not well-understood. The wide genetic diversity exhibited by *Trypanosoma* spp. is a challenge, both exacerbating the risk of increased virulence and making the development of a vaccine unlikely. One Health strategies that are community and environmentally friendly are needed to support stakeholders to mitigate risk. There is a need to strengthen trypanosomiasis research, particularly in LMICs, especially at the human–domestic–wildlife interface to prevent cross-species infection.

AUTHOR CONTRIBUTIONS

KIK and SCW conceptualized the study, designed the study, and analyzed and interpreted the data. KIK, GZ, FS, BB, KJA, KM, HNN, LA, DO, PB, JJO, SI, WM, DPN, GESB, LOO, TS, MA, LO, and SCW collected the data. KIK wrote initial draft while SCW critically reviewed it for intellectual content. All authors approved the manuscript for publication and remain in agreement on all aspects of the work.

REFERENCES

1. World Health Organization. *Tropical Disease Research: Progress 1975-94, Highlights 1993-94, Twelfth Programme Report of the UNDP/World Bank/WHO Special Programme for Research and Training in Tropical Diseases (TDR)*. Geneva: World Health Organization (1995). Available online at: https://www.who.int/tdr/publications/progress-75-94/en/
2. Thompson RCA. Parasite zoonoses and wildlife: one health, spillover and human activity. *Int J Parasitol.* (2013) 43:1079–88. doi: 10.1016/j.ijpara.2013.06.007
3. Auty H, Anderson NE, Picozzi K, Lembo T, Mubanga J, Hoare R, et al. Trypanosome diversity in wildlife species from the serengeti and luangwa valley ecosystems. *PLoS Negl Trop Dis.* (2012) 6:e1828. doi: 10.1371/journal.pntd.0001828
4. Franck SA. Models of parasite virulence. *Q Rev Biol.* (1996) 71:37–78. doi: 10.1086/419267
5. Barbosa A, Reiss A, Jackson B, Warren K, Paparini A, Gillespie G, et al. Prevalence, genetic diversity and potential clinical impact of blood-borne and enteric protozoan parasites in native mammals from northern Australia. *Vet Parasitol.* (2017) 238:94–105. doi: 10.1016/j.vetpar.2017.04.007
6. Desquesnes M, Holzmuller P, Lai D-H, Dargantes A, Lun Z-R, Jittaplapong S. *Trypanosoma evansi* and Surra: a review and perspectives on origin, history, distribution, taxonomy, morphology, hosts, and pathogenic effects. *Biomed Res Int.* (2013) 2013:1–22. doi: 10.1155/2013/194176
7. Barros JHS, Xavier SCC, Bilac D, Lima VS, Dario MA, Jansen AM. Identification of novel mammalian hosts and Brazilian biome geographic distribution of *Trypanosoma cruzi* TcIII and TcIV. *Acta Trop.* (2017) 2017:3. doi: 10.1016/j.actatropica.2017.05.003
8. Osório ALAR, Madruga CR, Desquesnes M, Soares CO, Ribeiro LRR, Costa SCG da. *Trypanosoma (Duttonella) vivax*: its biology, epidemiology, pathogenesis, and introduction in the New World - a review. *Mem Inst Oswaldo Cruz.* (2008) 103:1–13. doi: 10.1590/S0074-02762008000100001
9. Aregawi WG, Agga GE, Abdi RD, Büscher P. Systematic review and meta-analysis on the global distribution, host range, and prevalence of *Trypanosoma evansi*. *Parasites Vectors.* (2019) 12:4. doi: 10.1186/s13071-019-3311-4
10. Büscher P, Gonzatti MI, Hébert L, Inoue N, Pascucci I, Schnaufer A, et al. Equine trypanosomosis: enigmas and diagnostic challenges. *Parasites Vectors.* (2019) 12:19. doi: 10.1186/s13071-019-3484-x
11. Geiger A, Malele I, Abd-Alla AM, Njiokou F. Blood feeding tsetse flies as hosts and vectors of mammals-pre-adapted African Trypanosoma: current and expected research directions. *BMC Microbiol.* (2018) 18:162. doi: 10.1186/s12866-018-1281-x
12. Anderson NE, Mubanga J, Fevre EM, Picozzi K, Eisler MC, Thomas R, et al. Characterisation of the wildlife reservoir community for human and animal trypanosomiasis in the Luangwa Valley, Zambia. *PLoS Negl Trop Dis.* (2011) 5:e1211. doi: 10.1371/journal.pntd.0001211

13. Bengis RG, Kock RA, Fischer J. Infectious animal diseases: the wildlife / livestock interface Wildlife-maintained (indigenous) diseases. *Rev Sci Tech.* (2002) 21:53–65. doi: 10.20506/rst.21.1.1322
14. Mbaya AW, Ahmad T, Igbokwe I. Current survey of trypanosomosis among livestock and wildlife in the arid region of Northeastern, Nigeria. *Bull Anim Hlth Prod Afr.* (2013) 61:323–30. Available online at: https://www.ajol.info/index.php/bahpa/article/view/105265
15. Rahman AH, Ibtisam AG, Rihab AY, Salma AR, Gasmir G. The effect of bovine trypanosomosis and endo-parasitism on milk production of a dairy farm in The White Nile State, Sudan. *Sudan J Vet Res.* (2008) 23:19–27. Available online at: http://sudanjvr.net/journal/11.pdf
16. Obanda V, Kagira JM, Chege S, Okita-Ouma B, Gakuya F. Trypanosomosis and other co-infections in translocated black (*Diceros bicornis michaeli*) and white (*Ceratotherium simum simum*) rhinoceroses in Kenya. *Sci Parasitolo.* (2011) 12:103–7. Available online at: http://www.zooparaz.net/scientia/2011_12_02/sp2011-103-107-vincent.pdf
17. Gupta MP, Kumar H, Singla LD. Trypanosomosis concurrent to tuberculosis in black bucks. *Indian Vet J.* (2009) 86:727–8. Available online at: https://www.cabdirect.org/cabdirect/abstract/20093214671
18. Squarre D, Hayashida K, Gaithuma A, Chambaro H, Kawai N, Moonga L, et al. Diversity of trypanosomes in wildlife of the Kafue ecosystem, Zambia. *Int J Parasitol Parasites Wildl.* (2020) 12:34–41. doi: 10.1016/j.ijppaw.2020.04.005
19. Bruce CD, Hamerton AE, Bateman HR, Mackie FP. A note on the occurrence of a Trypanosome in the African Elephant. *R Soc.* (1908) 12:414–7.
20. Munang'andu HM, Siamudaala V, Munyeme M, Nalubamba KS. A review of ecological factors associated with the epidemiology of wildlife trypanosomiasis in the Luangwa and Zambezi valley ecosystems of Zambia. *Interdiscip Perspect Infect Dis.* (2012) 2012:1–13. doi: 10.1155/2012/372523
21. Herrera HM, Abreu UGP, Keuroghlian A, Freitas TP, Jansen AM. The role played by sympatric collared peccary (*Tayassu tajacu*), white-lipped peccary (*Tayassu pecari*), and feral pig (*Sus scrofa*) as maintenance hosts for *Trypanosoma evansi* and *Trypanosoma cruzi* in a sylvatic area of Brazil. *Parasitol Res.* (2008) 103:619–24. doi: 10.1007/s00436-008-1021-5
22. Hodo CL, Goodwin CC, Mayes BC, Mariscal JA, Waldrup KA, Hamer SA. Trypanosome species, including *Trypanosoma cruzi*, in sylvatic and peridomestic bats of Texas, USA. *Acta Trop.* (2016) 164:259–66. doi: 10.1016/j.actatropica.2016.09.013
23. Clément L, Dietrich M, Markotter W, Fasel NJ, Monadjem A, López-Baucells A, et al. Out of Africa: the origins of the protozoan blood parasites of the *Trypanosoma cruzi* clade found in bats from Africa. *Mol Phylogenet Evol.* (2020) 145:106705. doi: 10.1016/j.ympev.2019.106705
24. Thompson CK, Wayne AF, Godfrey SS, Thompson RCA. Temporal and spatial dynamics of trypanosomes infecting the brush-tailed bettong (*Bettongia penicillata*): a cautionary note of disease-induced population decline. *Parasites Vectors.* (2014) 7:1–11. doi: 10.1186/1756-3305-7-169
25. McInnes LM, Gillett A, Hanger J, Reid SA, Ryan UM. The potential impact of native Australian trypanosome infections on the health of koalas (*Phascolarctos cinereus*). *Parasitology.* (2011) 138:873–83. doi: 10.1017/S0031182011000369
26. Orozco MM, Argibay HD, Minatel L, Guillemi EC, Berra Y, Schapira A, et al. A participatory surveillance of marsh deer (*Blastocerus dichotomus*) morbidity and mortality in Argentina: first results. *BMC Vet Res.* (2020) 16:321. doi: 10.1186/s12917-020-02533-x
27. Averis S, Thompson RCA, Lymbery AJ, Wayne AF, Morris KD, Smith A. The diversity, distribution and host-parasite associations of trypanosomes in Western Australian wildlife. *Parasitology.* (2009) 136:1269–79. doi: 10.1017/S0031182009990801
28. Ideozu EJ, Whiteoak AM, Tomlinson AJ, Robertson A, Delahay RJ, Hide G. High prevalence of trypanosomes in European badgers detected using ITS-PCR. *Parasites Vectors.* (2015) 8:4–9. doi: 10.1186/s13071-015-1088-7
29. Šlapeta J, Morin-Adeline V, Thompson P, McDonell D, Shiels M, Gilchrist K, et al. Intercontinental distribution of a new trypanosome species from Australian endemic Regent Honeyeater (*Anthochaera phrygia*). *Parasitology.* (2016) 143:1012–25. doi: 10.1017/S0031182016000329
30. Diall O, Cecchi G, Wanda G, Argilés-Herrero R, Vreysen MJB, Cattoli G, et al. Developing a progressive control pathway for African animal trypanosomosis. *Trends Parasitol.* (2017) 33:499–509. doi: 10.1016/j.pt.2017.02.005
31. Musinguzi SP, Suganuma K, Asada M, Laohasinnarong D, Sivakumar T, Yokoyama N, et al. A PCR-based survey of animal African trypanosomosis and selected piroplasm parasites of cattle and goats in Zambia. *J Vet Med Sci.* (2016) 78:1819–24. doi: 10.1292/jvms.16-0240
32. Silva R, Barros A, Herrera H. Trypanosomosis outbreaks due to *Trypanosoma evansi* in the Pantanal, Brazil. A preliminary approach on risk factors. *Rev Elev Med Vet Pays Trop.* (1995) 48:315–9. doi: 10.19182/remvt.9432
33. Finelle P. African animal trypanosomiasis. In: *World Animal Review.* Rome: Food and Agriculture Organization of the United Nations (1983). p. 5. Available online at: http://www.fao.org/3/ah809e/AH809E00.htm#Contents
34. Mulenga GM, Henning L, Chilongo K, Mubamba C, Namangala B, Gummow B. Insights into the control and management of human and bovine african trypanosomiasis in Zambia between 2009 and 2019 — a review. *Trop Med Infect Dis.* (2019) 5:115. doi: 10.3390/tropicalmed5030115
35. Geiger A, Ponton F, Simo G. Adult blood-feeding tsetse flies, trypanosomes, microbiota and the fluctuating environment in sub-Saharan Africa. *ISME J.* (2015) 9:1496–507. doi: 10.1038/ismej.2014.236
36. Kaba D, Zacarie T, M'Pondi AM, Njiokou F, Bosson-Vanga H, Kröber T, et al. Standardising visual control devices for tsetse flies: central and west african species *Glossina palpalis palpalis*. *PLoS Negl Trop Dis.* (2014) 8:e2601. doi: 10.1371/journal.pntd.0002601
37. de Gier J, Cecchi G, Paone M, Dede P, Zhao W. The continental atlas of tsetse and African animal trypanosomosis in Nigeria. *Acta Trop.* (2020) 204:105328. doi: 10.1016/j.actatropica.2020.105328
38. Pépin J, Méda H. The epidemiology and control of human African trypanosomiasis. *Adv Parasitol.* (2001) 49:71–132. doi: 10.1016/S0065-308X(01)49038-5
39. Kagbadouno MS, Camara M, Rouamba J, Rayaisse J-B, Traoré IS, Camara O, et al. Epidemiology of sleeping sickness in Boffa (Guinea): where are the trypanosomes? *PLoS Negl Trop Dis.* (2012) 6:e1949. doi: 10.1371/journal.pntd.0001949
40. Rawlings P, Ceesay ML, Wacher TJ, Snow WF. The distribution of the tsetse flies *Glossina morsitans submorsitans* and *G. palpalis gambiensis* (Diptera: Glossinidae) in The Gambia and the application of survey results to tsetse and trypanosomiasis control. *Bull Entomol Res.* (1993) 83:625–32. doi: 10.1017/S0007485300040050
41. Schneider DI, Saarman N, Onyango MG, Hyseni C, Opiro R, Echodu R, et al. Spatio-temporal distribution of Spiroplasma infections in the tsetse fly (*Glossina fuscipes fuscipes*) in northern Uganda. *PLoS Negl Trop Dis.* (2019) 13:e0007340. doi: 10.1371/journal.pntd.0007340
42. Aksoy S, Caccone A, Galvani AP, Okedi LM. Glossina fuscipes populations provide insigths for Human African Trypanosomiasis transmission in Uganda. *Trends Parasitol.* (2013) 29:394–406. doi: 10.1016/j.pt.2013.06.005
43. Kaminsky R. Breeding sites of *Glossina palpalis gambiensis* and *Glossina pallicera pallicera* (Dipt., Glossinidae) in the leaf axils of oilpalms. *Zeitschrift für Angew Entomol.* (1984) 2:257–64.
44. Gouteux JP. Prevalence of enlarged salivary glands in *Glossina palpalis*, *G. pallicera*, and *G. nigrofusca* (Diptera: Glossinidae) from the Vavoua area, Ivory Coast. *J Med Entomol.* (1987) 24:268. doi: 10.1093/jmedent/24.2.268
45. Simo G, Fogue PS, Melachio TTT, Njiokou F, Kuiate JR, Asonganyi T. Population genetics of forest type of Trypanosoma congolense circulating in *Glossina palpalis palpalis* of Fontem in the South-West region of Cameroon. *Parasites Vectors.* (2014) 7:1–10. doi: 10.1186/1756-3305-7-385
46. FAO. *Predicted Distributions of Tsetse in Africa [Internet].* Rome: FAO; AGAH; AHP (2000). Available online at: https://kdna.net/168-2011/african-tryps/pdffilesofpapers/Predicteddistrioftsetse.pdf
47. Ndegwa PN, Irungu LW, Moloo SK. Effect of puparia incubation temperature : increased infection rates of Trypanosoma congolense. *Med Vet Entomol.* (1992) 127–30. doi: 10.1111/j.1365-2915.1992.tb00588.x
48. Courtin F, Rayaissé J, Tamboura I, Serdé O. Updating the Northern Tsetse

Limit in Burkina Faso (1949–2009): impact of global change. *Int J Environ Res Public Health.* (2010) 1708–19. doi: 10.3390/ijerph7041708

49. Bengaly Z, Akoudjin M. Climate, cattle rearing systems and African animal trypanosomosis risk in Burkina Faso. *PLoS ONE.* (2012) 7:49762. doi: 10.1371/journal.pone.0049762
50. Abenga JN, Vuza D. About factors that determine trypanotolerance and prospects for increasing resistance against trypanosomosis. *African J Biotechnol.* (2005) 4:1563–7. Available online at: https://www.ajol.info/index.php/ajb/article/view/71610
51. Stijlemans B, Brys L, Korf H, Bieniasz-Krzywiec P, Sparkes A, Vansintjan L, et al. MIF-mediated hemodilution promotes pathogenic anemia in experimental African trypanosomosis. *PLoS Pathog.* (2016) 12:1005862. doi: 10.1371/journal.ppat.1005862
52. Radcliffe RW, Khairani KO. Health of the forest rhinoceros of southeast Asia: Sumatran and Javan rhinoceros. In: Eric Miller R, Lamberski N, Calle PP, editors. *Fowler's Zoo and Wild Animal Medicine Current Therapy*, Vol. 9, W.B. Saunders (2019). p. 707–15. doi: 10.1016/B978-0-323-55228-8.00100-4
53. Magona JW, Mayende JSP, Olaho-Mukani W, Coleman PG, Jonsson NN, Welburn SC, et al. A comparative study on the clinical, parasitological and molecular diagnosis of bovine trypanosomosis in Uganda. *Onderstepoort J Vet Res.* (2003) 70:213–8.
54. Habila N, Inuwa MH, Aimola IA, Udeh MU, Haruna E. Pathogenic mechanisms of *Trypanosoma evansi* infections. *Res Vet Sci.* (2012) 2011:11. doi: 10.1016/j.rvsc.2011.08.011
55. Das SL, Angad G, Veterinary D. Trypanosomosis (Surra) in livestock. In: Katoch R, Rajesh Godara AY, editors. *Veterinary Parasitology in Indian Perspective.* 1st ed. New Delhi: Satish Serial Publishing House (2015). p. 305–30.
56. Mbaya A, Kumshe H, Okwudiri C. The mechanisms of anaemia in trypanosomosis: a review. *Anemia.* (2012) 2012:29530. doi: 10.5772/29530
57. Silva RAMS, Ramirez L, Souza SS, Ortiz AG, Pereira SR, Dávila AMR. Hematology of natural bovine trypanosomosis in the Brazilian Pantanal and Bolivian wetlands. *Vet Parasitol.* (1999) 85:87–93. doi: 10.1016/S0304-4017(99)00081-3
58. Luckins AG. *Trypanosoma evansi* in Asia. *Parasitol Today.* (1988) 4:137–42. doi: 10.1016/0169-4758(88)90188-3
59. Lisulo M, Sugimoto C, Kajino K, Hayashida K, Mudenda M, Moonga L, et al. Determination of the prevalence of African trypanosome species in indigenous dogs of Mambwe district, eastern Zambia, by loop-mediated isothermal amplification. *Parasites Vectors.* (2014) 7:1–7. doi: 10.1186/1756-3305-7-19
60. Biéler S, Matovu E, Mitashi P, Ssewannyana E, Bi Shamamba SK, Bessell PR, et al. Improved detection of *Trypanosoma brucei* by lysis of red blood cells, concentration and LED fluorescence microscopy. *Acta Trop.* (2012) 121:135–40. doi: 10.1016/j.actatropica.2011.10.016
61. Woo PTK, Rogers D. A statistical study of the sensitivity of the haematocrit centrifuge technique in the detection of trypanosomes in blood. *Trans R Soc Trop Med Hyg.* (1974) 68:319–26. doi: 10.1016/0035-9203(74)90041-8
62. Kirkpatrick CE. Dark-field microscopy for detection of some hemotropic parasites in blood smears of mammals and birds. *Trans Am Microsc Soc.* (1989) 108:190. doi: 10.2307/3226374
63. Marc D. *Compendium of Standard Diagnostic Protocols for Animal Trypanosomoses of African Origin.* Montpellier: CIRAD-OIE (2017). p. 106. Available online at: https://agritrop.cirad.fr/591960/
64. Veer S, Singla LD. Trypanosomosis in cattle and buffaloes from latent carrier status to clinical form of disease: *Indian scenario.* 2005. p. 10–18. Available online at: https://www.researchgate.net/profile/Lachhman-Das-Singla/publication/261361614_Trypanosomosis_in_cattle_and_buffaloes_from_latent_carrier_status_to_clinical_form_of_disease_Indian_scenario/links/5686bb8d08ae1e63f1f5aa17/Trypanosomosis-in-cattle-and-buffaloes-from-latent-carrier-status-to-clinical-form-of-disease-Indian-scenario.pdf
65. Chansiri K, Khuchareontaworn S, Nopporn S. PCR-ELISA for diagnosis of *Trypanosoma evansi* in animals and vector. *Mol Cell Probes.* (2002) 16:173–7. doi: 10.1006/mcpr.2002.0412
66. Claes F, Radwanska M, Urakawa T, Majiwa PAO, Goddeeris B, Büscher P. Variable surface glycoprotein RoTat 1.2 PCR as a specific diagnostic tool for the detection of *Trypanosoma evansi* infections. *Kinetoplastid Biol Dis.* (2004) 3:3. doi: 10.1186/1475-9292-3-3
67. Muraleedharan K. Babesia and babesiosis in livestock of Karnataka State, India- an overview. *Vet Res Int.* (2015) 3:81–8. Available online at: http://jakraya.com/journal/pdf/1002-vriArticle_2.pdf
68. Thekisoe OMM, Kuboki N, Nambota A, Fujisaki K, Sugimoto C, Igarashi I, et al. Species-specific loop-mediated isothermal amplification (LAMP) for diagnosis of trypanosomosis. *Acta Trop.* (2007) 102:182–9. doi: 10.1016/j.actatropica.2007.05.004
69. Kumar R, Dilbaghi N, Kumar S, Gupta AK, Khurana SK, Yadav SC. Development of lateral flow assay for point-of-care diagnosis of trypanosomosis in equines. *J Equine Vet Sci.* (2018) 70:1–6. doi: 10.1016/j.jevs.2018.07.007
70. Oie. *Trypanosomosis (tsetse-transmitted).* (2013). Available online at: www.oie.int/fileadmin/Home/eng/.in./TRYPANO_TSETSE.pdf (accessed May 1–5, 2013).
71. Mbaya AW, Aliyu MM, Ibrahim UI. The clinico-pathology and mechanisms of trypanosomosis in captive and free-living wild animals: a review. *Vet Res Commun.* (2009) 33:793–809. doi: 10.1007/s11259-009-9214-7
72. Pathak KML, Arora JK, Kapoor M. Camel trypanosomosis in Rajasthan, India. *Vet Parasitol.* (1993) 49:319–23. doi: 10.1016/0304-4017(93)90130-F
73. Lejon V, Büscher P, Nzoumbou-Boko R, Bossard G, Jamonneau V, Bucheton B, et al. The separation of trypanosomes from blood by anion exchange chromatography: from Sheila Lanham's discovery 50 years ago to a gold standard for sleeping sickness diagnosis. *PLoS Negl Trop Dis.* (2019) 13:e0007051. doi: 10.1371/journal.pntd.0007051
74. Gutierrez C, Corbera JA, Doreste F, Büscher P. Use of the miniature anion exchange centrifugation technique to isolate *Trypanosoma evansi* from goats. *Ann N Y Acad Sci.* (2004) 1026:149–51. doi: 10.1196/annals.1307.020
75. Lumsden WHR, Kimber CD, Evans DA, Doig SJ. *Trypanosoma brucei*: miniature anion-exchange centrifugation technique for detection of low parasitaemias: adaptation for field use. *Trans R Soc Trop Med Hyg.* (1979) 73:312–7. doi: 10.1016/0035-9203(79)90092-0
76. Ndungu K, Thungu D, Wamwiri F, Mireji P, Ngae G, Gitonga P, et al. Route of inoculation influences *Trypanosoma congolense* and *Trypanosoma brucei brucei* virulence in Swiss white mice. *PLoS ONE.* (2019) 14:e0218441. doi: 10.1371/journal.pone.0218441
77. Ruiz AM, Esteva M, Cabeza Meckert P, Laguens RP, Segura EL. Protective immunity and pathology induced by inoculation of micewith different subcellular fractions of *Trypanosoma cruzi. Acta Trop.* (1985) 42:299–309.
78. Melo RC, Brener Z. Tissue tropism of different *Trypanosoma cruzi* strains. *J Parasitol.* (1978) 64:475–82. doi: 10.2307/3279787
79. Morlais I, Ravel S, Grébaut P, Dumas V, Cuny G. New molecular marker for *Trypanosoma (Duttonella) vivax* identification. *Acta Trop.* (2001) 80:207–13. doi: 10.1016/S0001-706X(01)00160-7
80. Marc D, Ketsarin K, Sarawut Y, Cristina M, Sophie R, Wang MH, et al. Specific primers for PCR amplification of the ITS1 (ribosomal DNA) of *Trypanosoma lewisi. Infect Genet Evol.* (2011) 11:1361–7. doi: 10.1016/j.meegid.2011.04.030
81. Meyer Zum Büschenfelde C, Cramer S, Trumpfheller C, Fleischer B, Frosch S. *Trypanosoma cruzi* induces strong IL-12 and IL-18 gene expression *in vivo* : correlation with interferon-gamma (IFN-γ) production. *Clin Exp Immunol.* (1997) 110:378–85. doi: 10.1046/j.1365-2249.1997.4471463.x
82. Vorraro F, Cabrera WHK, Ribeiro OG, Jensen JR, De Franco M, Ibañez OM, et al. *Trypanosoma cruzi* infection in genetically selected mouse lines: genetic linkage with quantitative trait locus controlling antibody response. *Mediators Inflamm.* (2014) 2014:952857. doi: 10.1155/2014/952857
83. Pinto Torres JE, Goossens J, Ding J, Li Z, Lu S, Vertommen D, et al. Development of a Nanobody-based lateral flow assay to detect active *Trypanosoma congolense* infections. *Sci Rep.* (2018) 8:1–15. doi: 10.1038/s41598-018-26732-7
84. Katende JM, Nantulya VM, Musoke AJ. Comparison between bloodstream and procyclic form trypanosomes for serological diagnosis of African human trypanosomiasis. *Trans R Soc Trop Med Hyg.* (1987) 81:607–8. doi: 10.1016/0035-9203(87)90425-1
85. Ribone ME, Belluzo MS, Pagani D, Marcipar IS, Lagier CM. Amperometric bioelectrode for specific human immunoglobulin G determination: optimization of the method to diagnose American trypanosomiasis. *Anal Biochem.* (2006) 350:61–70. doi: 10.1016/j.ab.2005.11.033
86. Semballa S, Okomo-Assoumou MC, Holzmuller P, Büscher P, Magez S,

Lemesre JL, et al. Identification of a tryptophan-like epitope borne by the variable surface glycoprotein (VSG) of African trypanosomes. *Exp Parasitol.* (2007) 115:173–80. doi: 10.1016/j.exppara.2006.08.008
87. Cappa SMG, Vattuone NH, Menes S, Schmuñis GA. Humoral antibody response and Ig characterization of the specific agglutinins in rabbits during experimental American trypanosomiasis. *Exp Parasitol.* (1973) 34:32–9. doi: 10.1016/0014-4894(73)90059-3
88. Thompson CK, Thompson RCA. Trypanosomes of Australian mammals: knowledge gaps regarding transmission and biosecurity. *Trends Parasitol.* (2015) 31:553–62. doi: 10.1016/j.pt.2015.06.011
89. McKeever S, Gorman GW, Norman L. Occurrence of a *Trypanosoma cruzi*-like organism in some mammals from Southwestern Georgia and Northwestern Florida. *J Parasitol.* (1958) 44:583. doi: 10.2307/3274538
90. Olsen PF, Shoemaker JP, Turner HF, Hays KL. Incidence of *Trypanosoma cruzi* (Chagas) in wild vectors and reservoirs in East-Central Alabama. *J Parasitol.* (1964) 50:599. doi: 10.2307/3276112
91. Lanham SM, Godfrey DG. Isolation of salivarian trypanosomes from man and other mammals using DEAE-cellulose. *Exp Parasitol.* (1970) 28:521–34. doi: 10.1016/0014-4894(70)90120-7
92. Hernández-Orts JS, Montero FE, García NA, Crespo EA, Raga JA, García-Varela M, et al. Transmission of *Corynosoma australe* (Acanthocephala: Polymorphidae) from fishes to South American sea lions *Otaria flavescens* in Patagonia, Argentina. *Parasitol Res.* (2019) 118:433–40. doi: 10.1007/s00436-018-6177-z
93. Hall SR, Lafferty KD, Brown JH, Cáceres CE, Chase JM, Dobson AP, et al. *Chapter Ten Is Infectious Disease Just Another Type of Predator-Prey Interaction? In: Infectious Disease Ecology: Effects of Ecosystems on Disease and of Disease on Ecosystems.* Cambridge: Princeton University Press (2005). p. 223–41. Available online at: https://www.jstor.org/stable/j.ctt7sgg4 (accessed October 19, 2020).
94. Brun R, Hecker H, Lun Z-R. *Trypanosoma evansi* and *T. equiperdum*: distribution, biology, treatment and phylogenetic relationship (a review). *Vet Parasitol.* (1998) 79:95–107. doi: 10.1016/S0304-4017(98)00146-0
95. Haag J. The molecular phylogeny of trypanosomes: evidence for an early divergence of the Salivaria. *Mol Biochem Parasitol.* (1998) 91:37–49. doi: 10.1016/S0166-6851(97)00185-0
96. Geerts S, Osaer S, Goossens B, Faye D. Trypanotolerance in small ruminants of sub-Saharan Africa. *Trends Parasitol.* (2009) 25132–8. doi: 10.1016/j.pt.2008.12.004
97. Giordani F, Morrison LJ, Rowan TG, De Koning HP, Barrett MP. The animal trypanosomiases and their chemotherapy: a review. *Parasitology.* (2016) 143:1862–89. doi: 10.1017/S0031182016001268
98. Shah SS, Khan A. One health and parasites. In: Yasobant S, Saxena D, editors. *Global Applications of One Health Practice and Care.* IGI Global (2019). p. 82–112. doi: 10.4018/978-1-5225-6304-4.ch004
99. Jaffe JJ, McCormack JJ, Gutteridge WE. Dihydrofolate reductases within the genus Trypanosoma. *Exp Parasitol.* (1969) 25:311–8. doi: 10.1016/0014-4894(69)90076-9
100. Radwanska M, Vereecke N, Deleeuw V, Pinto J, Magez S. Salivarian trypanosomosis: a review of parasites involved, their global distribution and their interaction with the innate and adaptive mammalian host immune system. *Front Immunol.* (2018) 9:2253. doi: 10.3389/fimmu.2018.02253
101. Welburn S, Picozzi K, Coleman PG, Packer C. Patterns in age-seroprevalence consistent with acquired immunity against *Trypanosoma brucei* in Serengeti Lions. *PLoS Negl Trop Dis.* (2008) 2:e347. doi: 10.1371/journal.pntd.0000347
102. Black SJ, Mansfield JM. Prospects for vaccination against pathogenic African trypanosomes. *Parasite Immunol.* (2016) 38:735–43. doi: 10.1111/pim.12387
103. Reichard RE. Area-wide biological control of disease vectors and agents affecting wildlife. *OIE Rev Sci Tech.* (2002) 21:179–85. doi: 10.20506/rst.21.1.1325
104. Sudan V, Verma AK, Jaiswal AK. Trypanosomosis of wild animals with emphasis on Indian scenario. *Vet Parasitol.* (2017) 10:25–8. doi: 10.1016/j.vprsr.2017.07.003
105. Begna F, Abebe S, Bekele M. Bovine trypanosomosis in selected villages of Humbo District, Southern Ethiopia. *Glob Vet.* (2011) 7:192–8. Available online at: https://www.idosi.org/gv/GV7(2)11/16.pdf
106. Murray M, Morrison WI, Whitelaw DD. Host susceptibility to african trypanosomiasis: trypanotolerance. *Adv Parasitol.* (1982) 21:1–68. doi: 10.1016/S0065-308X(08)60274-2
107. Kelvin N, Anna BE, Peter JH, Paul SG. Assessing risk factors for trypanosome infections in cattle in wildlife interface areas in Northern Tanzania. *J Infect Dis Epidemiol.* (2019) 5:1510078. doi: 10.23937/2474-3658/1510078
108. Kasozi KI, Namayanja M, Gaithuma AK, Mahero M, Matovu E, Yamagishi J, et al. Prevalence of hemoprotozoan parasites in small ruminants along a human-livestock-wildlife interface in western Uganda. *Vet Parasitol Reg Stud Rep.* (2019) 87:100309. doi: 10.1016/j.vprsr.2019.100309
109. Sarabian C, Curtis V, McMullan R. Evolution of pathogen and parasite avoidance behaviours. *Philos Trans R Soc B Biol Sci.* (2018) 373:20170256. doi: 10.1098/rstb.2017.0256
110. Wang J, Van Praagh A, Hamilton E, Wang Q, Zou B, Muranjan M, et al. Serum xanthine oxidase: origin, regulation, and contribution to control of trypanosome parasitemia. *Antioxid Redox Signal.* (2002) 4:161–78. doi: 10.1089/152308602753625933
111. Naessens J, Grab DJ, Sileghem M. Identifying the mechanisms of trypanotolerance in cattle. In: *The African Trypanosomes.* Boston: Kluwer Academic Publishers (2005). p. 97–111. Available online at: http://link.springer.com/10.1007/0-306-46894-8_8 (accessed October 17, 2020).
112. Wang Q, Murphy N, Black SJ. Infection-associated decline of Cape buffalo blood catalase augments serum trypanocidal activity. *Infect Immun.* (1999) 67:2797–803. doi: 10.1128/IAI.67.6.2797-2803.1999
113. Paglia DE, Miller RE. Red blood cell metabolism in the black rhinoceros (*Diceros bicornis*). *Eur Assoc Zoo Wildl Vet.* (1996) 5:243–5.
114. Estes RD. The comparative behavior of grant's and Thomson's gazelles. *J Mammal.* (1967) 48:189. doi: 10.2307/1378022
115. Mortelmans J, Kageruka P. Trypanotolerant cattle breeds in Zaire. In: Flnelle P, Murray M, Barry JD, Morrison WI, WilliamsRO, Hirum H, Rovis L, Mortelmans J, Kageruka P, Murray M, Morrison WI, Murray PK, Clifford DS, Trail JCM, Maclennan KJR, Letenneur L, editors. *African Animal Trypanosomiasis Selected Articles From the World Animal Review.* Rome: Food and Agriculture Organization of the United Nations (1983). Available online at: http://www.fao.org/3/ah809e/AH809E00.htm#Contents
116. Ashcroft MT, Burtt E, Fairbairn H. Annals of tropical medicine & parasitology the experimental infection of some african wild animals with trypanosoma rhodesiense, *T. Brucei. Ann Trop Med Parasitol.* (1959) 4983:147–61. doi: 10.1080/00034983.1959.11685912
117. Van den Bossche P, Delespaux V. Options for the control of tsetse-transmitted livestock trypanosomosis. an epidemiological perspective. *Vet Parasitol.* (2011) 181:37–42. doi: 10.1016/j.vetpar.2011.04.021
118. Peterson MN, Birckhead JL, Leong K, Peterson MJ, Peterson TR. Rearticulating the myth of human-wildlife conflict. *Conserv Lett.* (2010) 3:74–82. doi: 10.1111/j.1755-263X.2010.00099.x
119. Thompson CK, Godfrey SS, Thompson RCA. Trypanosomes of Australian mammals: a review. *Int J Parasitol Parasites Wildl.* (2014) 3:57–66. doi: 10.1016/j.ijppaw.2014.02.002
120. Barua M, Bhagwat SA, Jadhav S. The hidden dimensions of human-wildlife conflict: health impacts, opportunity and transaction costs. *Biol Conserv.* (2013) 157:309–16. doi: 10.1016/j.biocon.2012.07.014
121. Ohemeng F, Ayivor JS, Lawson ET, Ntiamoa-Baidu Y. Local classifications of fever and treatment sought among populations at risk of zoonotic diseases in Ghana. *PLoS ONE.* (2018) 13:e0201526. doi: 10.1371/journal.pone.0201526
122. Miller RS, Sweeney SJ, Slootmaker C, Grear DA, Di Salvo PA, Kiser D, et al. Cross-species transmission potential between wild pigs, livestock, poultry, wildlife, and humans: implications for disease risk management in North America. *Sci Rep.* (2017) 7:7821. doi: 10.1038/s41598-017-07336-z
123. Borremans B, Faust C, Manlove KR, Sokolow SH, Lloyd-Smith JO. Cross-species pathogen spillover across ecosystem boundaries: mechanisms and theory. *Philos Trans R Soc B Biol Sci.* (2019) 374:20180344. doi: 10.1098/rstb.2018.0344
124. Atuman Y, Kudi CA, Abdu P, Abubakar A. Prevalence of parasites of wildlife in Yankari game reserve and Sumu wildlife park in Bauchi State, Nigeria. *Sokoto J Vet Sci.* (2020) 17:70–9. doi: 10.4314/sokjvs.v17i4.8
125. Gondwe N, Marcotty T, Vanwambeke SO, Pus C De, Mulumba M, Van Den Bossche P. Distribution and density of tsetse flies (glossinidae: Diptera) at the game/people/livestock interface of the nkhotakota game reserve human sleeping sickness focus in malawi. *Ecohealth.* (2009) 6:260–5. doi: 10.1007/s10393-009-0252-y
126. Kaare MT, Picozzi K, Mlengeya T, Fèvre EM, Mellau LS, Mtambo MM, et al. Sleeping sickness—a re-emerging disease in the Serengeti? *Travel Med Infect Dis.* (2007) 5:117–24. doi: 10.1016/j.tmaid.2006.01.014
127. Mwiinde AM, Simuunza M, Namangala B, Chama-Chiliba CM, Machila

N, Anderson N, et al. Estimating the economic and social consequences for patients diagnosed with human African trypanosomiasis in Muchinga, Lusaka and Eastern Provinces of Zambia (2004–2014). *Infect Dis Poverty.* (2017) 6:150. doi: 10.1186/s40249-017-0363-6

128. Anderson NE, Mubanga J, Machila N, Atkinson PM, Dzingirai V, Welburn SC. Sleeping sickness and its relationship with development and biodiversity conservation in the Luangwa Valley, Zambia. *Parasit Vectors.* (2015) 8:224. doi: 10.1186/s13071-015-0827-0
129. Alderton S, Macleod ET, Anderson NE, Machila N, Simuunza M, Welburn SC, et al. Exploring the effect of human and animal population growth on vector-borne disease transmission with an agent-based model of Rhodesian human African trypanosomiasis in eastern province, Zambia. *PLoS Negl Trop Dis.* (2018) 12:e0006905. doi: 10.1371/journal.pntd.0006905
130. Alderton S, Macleod ET, Anderson NE, Palmer G, Machila N, Simuunza M, et al. An agent-based model of tsetse fly response to seasonal climatic drivers: assessing the impact on sleeping sickness transmission rates. *PLoS Negl Trop Dis.* (2018) 12:e0006188. doi: 10.1371/journal.pntd.0006188
131. Rademaker V, Herrera HM, Raffel TR, D'Andrea PS, Freitas TPT, Abreu UGP, et al. What is the role of small rodents in the transmission cycle of *Trypanosoma cruzi* and *Trypanosoma evansi* (Kinetoplastida Trypanosomatidae)? A study case in the Brazilian Pantanal. *Acta Trop.* (2009) 111:102–7. doi: 10.1016/j.actatropica.2009.02.006
132. Auty H, Morrison LJ, Torr SJ, Lord J. Transmission dynamics of rhodesian sleeping sickness at the interface of wildlife and livestock areas. *Trends Parasitol.* (2016) 32:608–21. doi: 10.1016/j.pt.2016.05.003
133. Lord JS, Mthombothi Z, Lagat VK, Atuhaire F, Hargrove JW. Host-seeking efficiency can explain population dynamics of the tsetse fly *Glossina morsitans morsitans* in response to host density decline. *PLoS Negl Trop Dis.* (2017) 11:e0005730. doi: 10.1371/journal.pntd.0005730
134. Dickman AJ. Complexities of conflict: the importance of considering social factors for effectively resolving human-wildlife conflict. *Anim Conserv.* (2010) 13:458–66. doi: 10.1111/j.1469-1795.2010.00368.x
135. Manfredo MJ, Dayer AA. Concepts for exploring the social aspects of Human–Wildlife conflict in a global context. *Hum Dimens Wildl.* (2004) 9:1–20. doi: 10.1080/10871200490505765
136. Van den Bossche P. Some general aspects of the distribution and epidemiology of bovine trypanosomosis in southern Africa. *Int J Parasitol.* (2001) 1:592–8. doi: 10.1016/S0020-7519(01)00146-1
137. Nonga HE, Kambarage DM. Prevalence of Bovine trypanosomosis in Morogoro, Tanzania. *Pakistan J Nutr.* (2009) 8:208–13. doi: 10.3923/pjn.2009.208.213
138. Vreysen MJB, Seck MT, Sall B, Bouyer J. Tsetse flies: their biology and control using area-wide integrated pest management approaches. *J Invertebr Pathol.* (2013) 112(Suppl.1):S15–25. doi: 10.1016/j.jip.2012.07.026
139. Osofsky SA, Kock RA, Kock MD, Kalema-Zikusoka G, Grahn R, Karesh WB. *Building Support for Protected Areas Using a "One Health" Perspective. Friends for Life New Partners in Support of Protected Areas.* (2005). p. 65–79. Available online at: https://vtechworks.lib.vt.edu/handle/10919/65901
140. Kolbe FF, Senekal OFS. The status of the tsetse flies in relation to game conservation and utilization. *South African J Wildl Res.* (1974) 4:43–9.
141. Holmes PH. New approaches to the integrated control of trypanosomosis. *Vet Parasitol.* (1997) 71:121–35. doi: 10.1016/S0304-4017(97)00026-5
142. Allsopp R. Control of tsetse flies (Diptera: Glossinidae) using insecticides: a review and future prospects. *Bull Entomol Res.* (1984) 74:1–23. doi: 10.1017/S0007485300009895
143. Rayaisse JB, Tirados I, Kaba D, Dewhirst SY, Logan JG, Diarrassouba A, et al. Prospects for the development of odour baits to control the tsetse flies *Glossina tachinoidesand G. palpalis* s.l. *PLoS Negl Trop Dis.* (2010) 4:632. doi: 10.1371/journal.pntd.0000632
144. Welburn SC, Coleman P. Human and animal African trypanosomiasis. In: *One Health: The Theory and Practice of Integrated Health Approaches.* Wallingford: CABI (2015). p. 201–21. Available online at: http://www.cabi.org/cabebooks/ebook/20153067417 (accessed October 17, 2020).
145. Eyob E, Matios L. Review on camel trypanosomosis (surra) due to *Trypanosoma evansi*: epidemiology and host response. *J Vet Med Anim Heal.* (2013) 5:334–43. Available online at: https://academicjournals.org/journal/JVMAH/article-full-text-pdf/4BAB67841636
146. Randolph DG, Refisch J, MacMillan S, Wright CY, Bett B, Robinson D, et al. Understanding the linkages between habitat loss, the trade and use of wildlife, and the emergency of novel zoonoses. In: *Zoonotic Diseases and How to Break the Chain of Transmission.* (2020). p. 29–34. Available online at: https://wedocs.unep.org/bitstream/handle/20.500.11822/32316/ZP.pdf?sequence=1&isAllowed=y (accessed October 17, 2020).
147. Weise FJ, Fynn RWS, Stein AB, Tomeletso M, Somers MJ, Périquet S. Seasonal selection of key resources by cattle in a mixed savannah-wetland ecosystem increases the potential for conflict with lions. *Biol Conserv.* (2019) 237:253–66. doi: 10.1016/j.biocon.2019.06.031
148. Ahmad CB, Abdullah J, Jaafar J. Community perspectives on buffer zone for protected areas: a preliminary study. *Procedia Soc Behav Sci.* (2013) 85:198–205. doi: 10.1016/j.sbspro.2013.08.351
149. Kideghesho JR. Co-existence between the traditional societies and wildlife in western Serengeti, Tanzania: its relevancy in contemporary wildlife conservation efforts. *Biodivers Conserv.* (2008) 17:1861–81. doi: 10.1007/s10531-007-9306-z
150. Taylor RD, Martin RB. Effects of veterinary fences on Wildlife conservation in Zimbabwe. *Environ Manage.* (1987) 11:327–34. doi: 10.1007/BF01867160
151. Baral N, Heinen JT. Decentralization and people's participation in conservation: a comparative study from the Western Terai of Nepal. *Int J Sustain Dev World Ecol.* (2007) 14:520–31. doi: 10.1080/13504500709469751
152. Kameri-Mbote P. Land tenure, land use, and sustainability in kenya: toward innovative use of property rights in wildlife management. In: Chalifour NJ, Kameri-Mbote P, Lye LH, Nolon JR, editors. *Land Use Law for Sustainable Development* Cambridge: Cambridge University Press (2006). p. 132–60. doi: 10.1017/CBO9780511511400.012
153. Lima L, Silva FM da, Neves L, Attias M, Takata CSA, Campaner M, et al. Evolutionary insights from bat trypanosomes: morphological, developmental and phylogenetic evidence of a new species, *Trypanosoma (Schizotrypanum) erneyi* sp. nov., in African Bats Closely Related to *Trypanosoma (Schizotrypanum) cruzi* and allied species. *Protist.* (2012) 163:856–72. doi: 10.1016/j.protis.2011.12.003
154. Pinto CM, Ocaña-Mayorga S, Tapia EE, Lobos SE, Zurita AP, Aguirre-Villacís F, et al. Bats, trypanosomes, and triatomines in Ecuador: new insights into the diversity, transmission, and origins of *Trypanosoma cruzi* and Chagas disease. *PLoS ONE.* (2015) 10:e0139999. doi: 10.1371/journal.pone.0139999
155. Cavazzana M, Marcili A, Lima L, da Silva FM, Junqueira ÂCV, Veludo HH, et al. Phylogeographical, ecological and biological patterns shown by nuclear (ssrRNA and gGAPDH) and mitochondrial (Cyt b) genes of trypanosomes of the subgenus *Schizotrypanum parasitic* in Brazilian bats. *Int J Parasitol.* (2010) 40:345–55. doi: 10.1016/j.ijpara.2009.08.015
156. Baral TN. Immunobiology of African trypanosomes: need of alternative interventions. *J Biomed Biotechnol.* (2010) 2010:389153. doi: 10.1155/2010/389153
157. Stijlemans B, Radwanska M, Trez C De, Magez S. African trypanosomes undermine humoral responses and vaccine development: link with inflammatory responses? *Front Immunol.* (2017) 8:1. doi: 10.3389/fimmu.2017.00582
158. La Greca F, Magez S. Vaccination against trypanosomiasis. *Hum Vaccin.* (2011) 7:1225–33. doi: 10.4161/hv.7.11.18203
159. Muhammad G, Saqib M, Sajid MS, Naureen A. *Trypanosoma evansi* infections in Himalayan black bears (*Selenarctos thibetanus*). *J Zoo Wildl Med.* (2007) 38:97–100. doi: 10.1638/06-024.1
160. Botero A, Keatley S, Peacock C, Thompson RCA. *In vitro* drug susceptibility of two strains of the wildlife trypanosome, *Trypanosoma copemani*: a comparison with *Trypanosoma cruzi*. *Int J Parasitol Drugs Drug Resist.* (2017) 7:34–41. doi: 10.1016/j.ijpddr.2016.12.004
161. Argañaraz ER, Hubbard GB, Ramos LA, Ford AL, Nitz N, Leland MM, et al. Blood-sucking lice may disseminate *Trypanosoma cruzi* infection in baboons. *Rev Inst Med Trop São Paulo.* (2001) 43:271–6. doi: 10.1590/S0036-46652001000500007
162. Garcia HA, Rangel CJ, Ortíz PA, Calzadilla CO, Coronado RA, Silva AJ, et al. Zoonotic trypanosomes in rats and fleas of venezuelan slums. *Ecohealth.* (2019) 16:523–33. doi: 10.1007/s10393-019-01440-4
163. Lizundia R, Newman C, Buesching CD, Ngugi D, Blake D, Sin YW, et al. Evidence for a role of the host-specific flea (*Paraceras melis*) in the transmission of *Trypanosoma (Megatrypanum) pestanai* to the European Badger. *PLoS ONE.* (2011) 6:e16977. doi: 10.1371/journal.pone.0016977

164. Schwan TG, Lopez JE, Safronetz D, Anderson JM, Fischer RJ, Maïga O, et al. Fleas and trypanosomes of peridomestic small mammals in sub-Saharan Mali. *Parasit Vectors.* (2016) 9:1–7. doi: 10.1186/s13071-016-1818-5
165. Votýpka J, Suková E, Kraeva N, Ishemgulova A, DuŽí I, Lukeš J, et al. Diversity of Trypanosomatids (Kinetoplastea: Trypanosomatidae) parasitizing fleas (Insecta: Siphonaptera) and description of a New Genus Blechomonas gen. n. *Protist.* (2013) 164:763–81. doi: 10.1016/j.protis.2013.08.002
166. Magona JW, Mayende JSP. Occurrence of concurrent trypanosomosis, theileriosis, anaplasmosis and helminthosis in Friesian, Zebu and Sahiwal cattle in Uganda. *Onderstepoort J Vet Res.* (2002) 140:133–40. Available online at: https://repository.up.ac.za/bitstream/handle/2263/18297/13magona2002.pdf?sequence=1&isAllowed=y
167. Nesbitt ST, Njau BC, Otieno LH. Epizootiology of trypanosomiasis in Lambwe Valley, Kenya, East Africa. *Int J Trop Insect Sci.* (1991) 12:379–84. doi: 10.1017/S1742758400011243
168. Northover AS, Godfrey SS, Keatley S, Lymbery AJ, Wayne AF, Cooper C, et al. Increased *Trypanosoma* spp. richness and prevalence of haemoparasite co-infection following translocation. *Parasit Vectors.* (2019) 12:1–14. doi: 10.1186/s13071-019-3370-6

12

Mosquitoes in an Urban Zoo: Identification of Blood Meals, Flight Distances of Engorged Females and Avian Malaria Infections

Josué Martínez-de la Puente[1,2*], *Ramón Soriguer*[1,2], *Juan Carlos Senar*[3], *Jordi Figuerola*[1,2], *Rubén Bueno-Marí*[4*] *and Tomás Montalvo*[2,5]

[1] Estación Biológica de Doñana (EBD-CSIC), Sevilla, Spain, [2] CIBER Epidemiología y Salud Pública (CIBERESP), Madrid, Spain, [3] Evolutionary and Behavioural Ecology Research Unit, Museu de Ciències Naturals de Barcelona, Barcelona, Spain, [4] Laboratorios Lokímica, Departamento de Investigación y Desarrollo (I+D), Valencia, Spain, [5] Agencia de Salud Pública de Barcelona, Consorci Sanitari de Barcelona, Barcelona, Spain

***Correspondence:**
Josué Martínez-de la Puente
jmp@ebd.csic.es
Rubén Bueno-Marí
rbueno@lokimica.es

Zoological gardens are home to a large number of vertebrate species and as such are suitable sites for both mosquito breeding and maintenance. They are excellent places for entomological studies of mosquito phenology, diversity, and blood-feeding patterns, as well as for xenomonitoring. During 2016, we sampled mosquitoes in Barcelona Zoo and used molecular methods to determine their blood-feeding patterns and the prevalence and diversity of avian malaria parasites. We also estimated the flight distance of engorged mosquitoes in the area. Overall, 1,384 adult *Culex pipiens* s.l., *Culiseta longiareolata*, and *Aedes albopictus* were captured. Birds dominated the diet of *Cx. pipiens* s.l. ($n = 87$) and *Cs. longiareolata* ($n = 6$), while humans were the only blood-meal source of *Ae. albopictus* ($n = 3$). Mosquitoes had a mean flight distance of 95.67 m after feeding on blood (range 38.71–168.51 m). Blood parasites were detected in the abdomen of 13 engorged *Cx. pipiens* s.l., eight of which had fed on magpies. Four *Plasmodium* lineages and a single lineage of the malaria-like parasite *Haemoproteus* were identified. These results suggest that *Cx. pipiens* s.l. is involved in the local transmission of avian *Plasmodium*, which potentially affects the circulation of parasites between and within wildlife and enclosed animals. Vigilance regarding possible mosquito breeding sites in this zoo is thus recommended.

Keywords: ***Aedes albopictus*, avian *Plasmodium*, *Culex pipiens*, malaria, vectors**

INTRODUCTION

Mosquitoes transmit a diversity of vector-borne pathogens affecting humans, livestock, and wildlife (1, 2). In addition to native species, invasive mosquitoes such as alien *Aedes* mosquitoes are involved in the circulation of both imported and locally circulating pathogens (3). This is the case of the invasive Asian tiger mosquito *Aedes albopictus*, which is associated with the local transmission of pathogens such as filarioid worms (e.g., *Dirofilaria* spp.), protozoa (e.g., avian malaria parasites), and viruses (e.g., Dengue virus) (4–6). This species has a broad global distribution and is present in countries outside its native range in America, Europe, Oceania, and Africa (7). In Spain, *Ae. albopictus* was first recorded in 2004 in Catalonia and since then has progressively colonized different parts of this region (8).

Zoos and wildlife parks with non-autochthonous and stabled fauna are excellent sites for studying the ecology and epidemiology of vector-borne pathogens, as studies of sand flies (9, 10), biting midges *Culicoides* (11), and mosquitoes (12–15) have previously shown. Given that captive animals are housed in known locations, the flight distances of captured insect vectors containing blood from these animals can be accurately estimated (10). In addition, these areas are frequented by human visitors and there are often both freely moving animals and animals maintained in captivity, all of which are potentially exposed to the transmission of various pathogens (15). This is especially the case of avian malaria parasites of the genus *Plasmodium*, a group of haemosporidians that naturally circulates between birds and mosquitoes (16) that can severely affect the health and survival of birds in zoos and recovery centers (17–22). However, in spite of their veterinary importance, the transmission dynamics of mosquito-borne avian *Plasmodium* in these particular ecosystems are still poorly understood [e.g., (12, 15, 23, 24)].

Here, we sampled mosquitoes in Barcelona Zoo, a site with a great diversity of mosquito and bird species, many of which are infected by avian malaria parasites (25). We employed a comprehensive approach based on the analysis of mosquito blood-feeding patterns, xenomonitoring (defined as the identification of pathogens in mosquito vectors), and flight distances of engorged females. We used molecular methods to identify the blood-meal sources of both native and alien engorged mosquitoes and to screen for the presence of avian *Plasmodium* in the abdomens of engorged mosquitoes to assess contact rates between potential vectors and parasites in the area.

METHODS

Study Area, Mosquito Sampling, and Species Identification

Mosquitoes were collected in June–November 2016 in Barcelona Zoo using both passive and active trapping techniques (**Figure 1**). BG-Sentinel traps (Biogents GmbH, Regensburg, Germany) were installed for 24 h in three different sites in the zoo, namely, the aviary, the farm, and the terrarium. These sites were selected according to criteria related to host proximity, distance between traps, and cover and protection for the traps. Every 2 weeks, mosquitoes were sampled using BG-Sentinel traps baited with CO_2 during 24 h. In addition, we used entomological aspirators (Improved Prokopack Aspirator, Mod. 1419, John W. Hock Company, FL, USA, and CDC Backpack Aspirator Mod. 2846, BioQuip, CA, USA) to collect mosquitoes resting on vegetation, bins, and animal cages. Aspirations were performed in six pre-established sites distributed throughout the whole zoo (13.5 ha) for 5 min in each area to standardize active adult mosquito sampling and increase the overall number of blood-fed mosquitoes collected. Additionally, 10 standard ovitraps (350 ml water capacity) were installed and monitored weekly to obtain information on mosquito phenology. Larval samplings were conducted occasionally to check for the presence/absence of other species that had not been collected by the above-described methodologies. Mosquitoes were identified using morphological keys (26); females containing any remains of blood meals in their abdomens were stored individually at −80°C until subsequent molecular analyses.

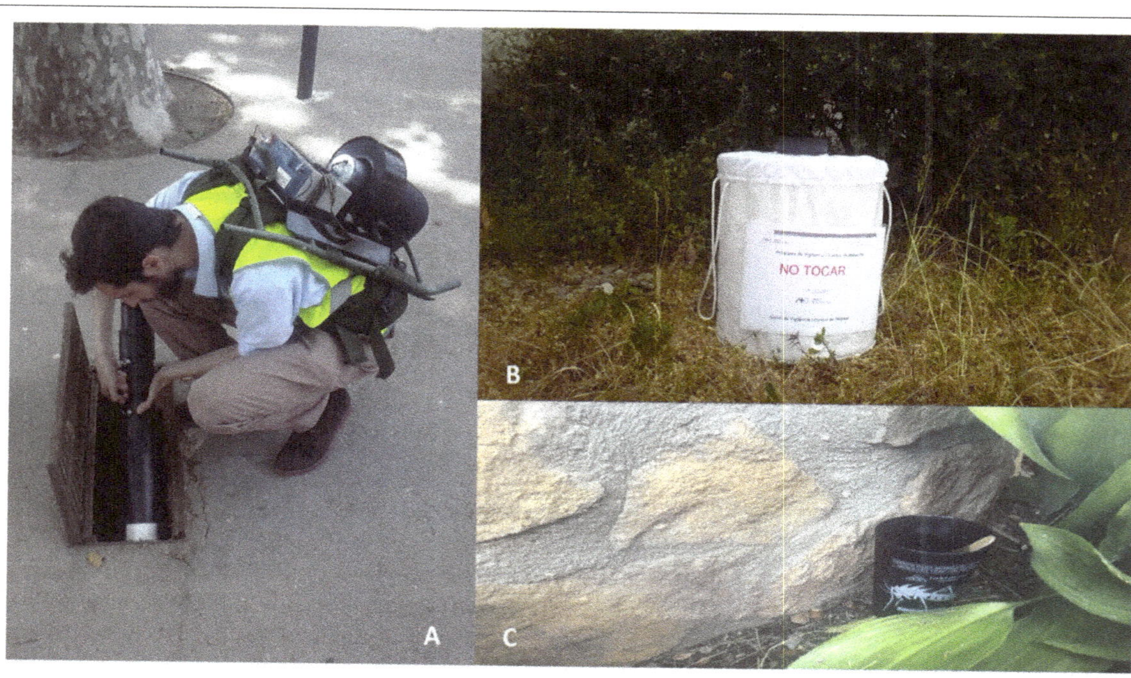

FIGURE 1 | Sampling methods used in this study including direct aspiration in mosquito resting areas **(A)**, BG-Sentinel traps **(B)**, and ovitraps **(C)**.

Molecular Identification of Blood-Meal Sources and Parasites in Engorged Mosquitoes

The abdomen of each engorged mosquito was separated from the head–thorax using sterile tips on Petri dishes. Genomic DNA was isolated from these abdomens using Maxwell® 16 LEV System Research Kit (Promega, Madison, WI). The protocol described by Alcaide et al. (27) involving the amplification of the barcoding region of the cytochrome oxidase subunit 1 (COI) gene was used to identify the blood-meal origin of mosquitoes [see also (28) for the adaptation of the protocol for *Ae. albopictus*]. The presence of avian *Plasmodium*/*Haemoproteus* parasites was screened for following Hellgren et al. (29). Amplified fragments were sequenced using the Macrogen Inc. facilities (Amsterdam, The Netherlands), and the resulting sequences were edited using Sequencher™ v4.9 (Gene Codes Corp.,© 1991–2009, Ann Arbor, MI 48108, USA). Blood-meal sources were identified by comparing sequences obtained with those deposited in public-access databases (GenBank DNA, National Center for Biotechnology Information Blast and the Barcode of Life Data Systems), bearing in mind the species potentially present in the study area. Parasite lineages and, whenever possible, their respective morpho-species were identified by Blast comparison with sequences in GenBank and/or MalAvi (30).

Analyses of Flight Distances of Blood-Fed Female Mosquitoes

We estimated the minimum flight distances of mosquitoes using data concerning where mosquitoes were captured and the locations of caged host species (**Figure 2**). Mosquito trapping areas and enclosures within the zoo of identified vertebrate host species were georeferenced. Only vertebrate species in enclosures in the zoo were considered in the analyses. Freely moving hosts (e.g., humans) were excluded from the analyses. Based on host identification, distances between the centroids of the areas enclosing animals and mosquito sampling points (BG-Sentinel stations or entomological aspiration points) were measured to calculate flight distances. Analyses were carried out with QGIS 3.12 (QGIS Development Team. http://qgis.osgeo.org).

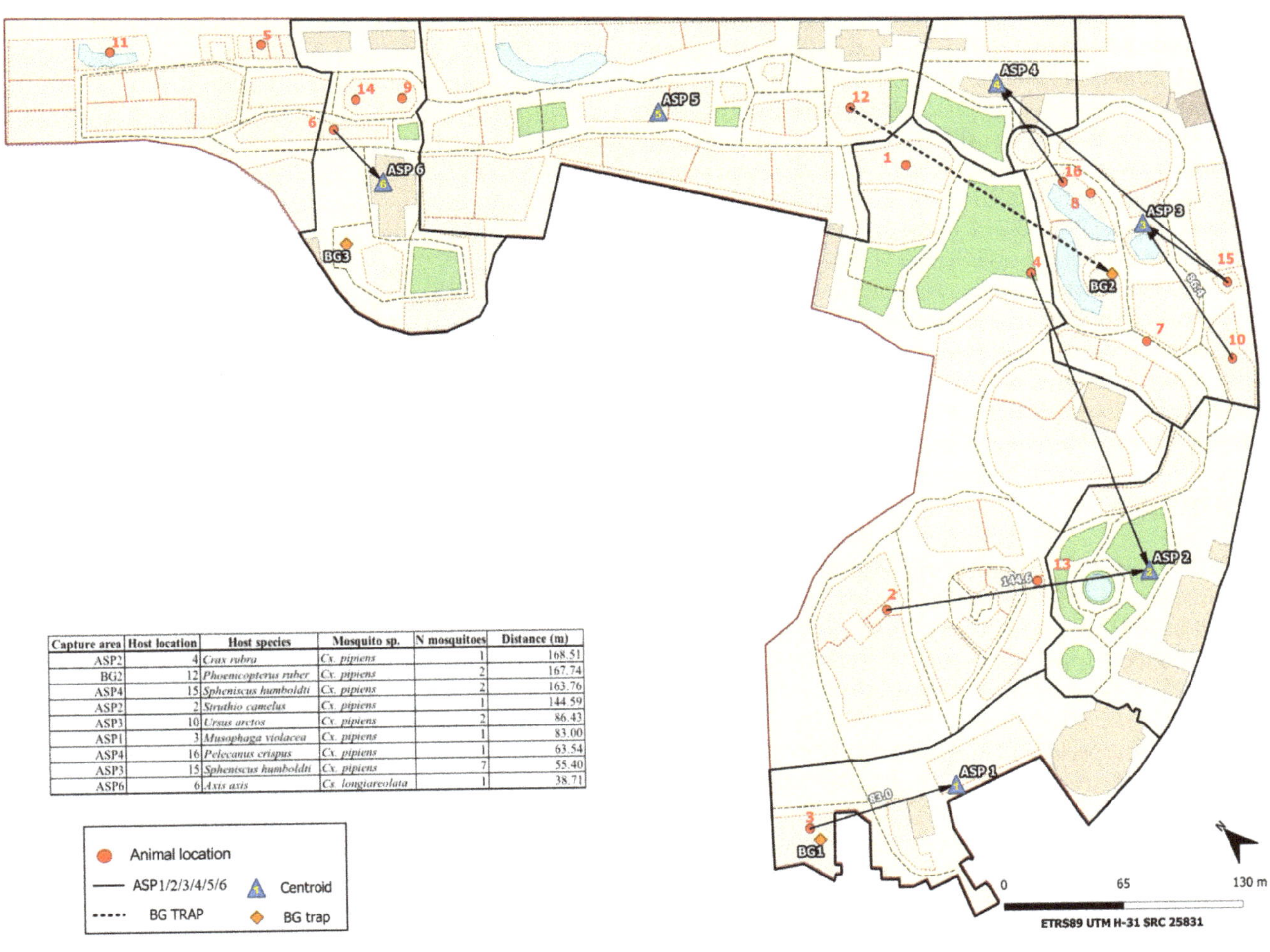

Capture area	Host location	Host species	Mosquito sp.	N mosquitoes	Distance (m)
ASP2	4	*Crax rubra*	*Cx. pipiens*	1	168.51
BG2	12	*Phoenicopterus ruber*	*Cx. pipiens*	2	167.74
ASP4	15	*Spheniscus humboldti*	*Cx. pipiens*	2	163.76
ASP2	2	*Struthio camelus*	*Cx. pipiens*	1	144.59
ASP3	10	*Ursus arctos*	*Cx. pipiens*	2	86.43
ASP1	3	*Musophaga violacea*	*Cx. pipiens*	1	83.00
ASP4	16	*Pelecanus crispus*	*Cx. pipiens*	1	63.54
ASP3	15	*Spheniscus humboldti*	*Cx. pipiens*	7	55.40
ASP6	6	*Axis axis*	*Cs. longiareolata*	1	38.71

FIGURE 2 | Study area and sampling sites of mosquitoes. The post-flight distances of engorged female mosquitoes are shown.

RESULTS

We trapped 1,384 adult *Culex pipiens* s.l. ($n = 733$; 52.96%), *Ae. albopictus* ($n = 490$; 35.40%), and *Culiseta longiareolata* ($n = 161$; 11.63%). In total, 63.29% ($n = 876$) of these mosquitoes were collected using entomological aspirators and the remaining 36.71% ($n = 508$) using BG-Sentinel traps. Catches of *Cx. pipiens* s.l. peaked in June–July, while those of *Ae. albopictus* adults peaked in September–October; these results were supported by both direct collection by entomological aspirators and the BG-Sentinel traps. In addition, we collected 9,658 *Ae. albopictus* eggs, with a maximum in July–October and a peak in August (3,965 eggs).

In all, 137 (9.90%) mosquitoes had some blood remains in their abdomens, of which the vertebrate hosts of 86 (62.32%) were successfully identified (birds and mammals) (**Table 1**). Birds dominated the diet of *Cx. pipiens* s.l. (92.21%; $n = 77$). The three identified *Ae. albopictus* blood meals came from humans, while the six blood meals from *Cs. longiareolata* corresponded to birds. Post-blood-feeding flight distances were calculated for the 18 mosquitoes that had fed on enclosed animals (17 *Cx. pipiens* s.l. and a single *Cs. longiareolata*) (**Figure 2**). For *Cx. pipiens* s.l., the mean post-blood feeding flight distance was 99.02 m, with a maximum of 168.51 m. The only distance measured for *Cs. longiareolata* was 38.71 meters. Overall, 13 (9.49%) out of the 137 engorged mosquitoes analyzed were positive for the presence of parasites (**Table 1**). All the parasite lineages found in this study coincided with *Plasmodium* lineages: Delurb4 ($n = 1$), Delurb5 ($n = 3$), Syat05 ($n = 1$, corresponding to *P. vaughani*), SGS1 ($n = 1$, corresponding to *P. relictum*), and the *Haemoproteus* lineage hCIRCUM04 ($n = 5$, also called BLUTI9). Sequences corresponding to each of the five lineages identified in this study were deposited in GenBank (MT568928–MT568932). In addition, one *Plasmodium* parasite and one *Haemoproteus* parasite were detected in mosquitoes, although the low quality of these sequences did not allow us to accurately identify their parasite lineages. Twelve out of the 13 positive mosquitoes corresponded to *Cx. pipiens* s.l. A single *Cs. longiareolata* was positive for *Haemoproteus* lineage hCIRCUM04.

TABLE 1 | Vertebrate hosts of mosquitoes trapped in the zoological garden of Barcelona during 2016.

Host	*Ae. albopictus*	*Cs. longiareolata*	*Cx. pipiens*	Parasites
Birds				
Ardea cinerea			12	
Ardea sp.		1		
Bubulcus ibis		1	18	
Columba livia			1	*Haemoproteus* sp. (1)
Corvus monedula			1	
Egretta garzetta/sp.			4	
Crax rubra			1	
Musophaga violacea			1	
Myiopsitta monachus			3	
Passer domesticus		1		
Pavo sp.			2	
Pelecanus sp.			1	
Phoenicopterus ruber			2	*P. vaughani* SYAT05 (1)
Pica pica		2	8	*Haemoproteus* hCIRCUM04 (3), *Plasmodium* Delurb5 (3), *Plasmodium* Delurb4 (1), *Plasmodium* sp. (1)
Spheniscus humboldti			9	*P. relictum* SGS1 (1)
Streptopelia decaocto			7	*Haemoproteus* hCIRCUM04 (1)
Struthio camelus			1	
Mammals				
Axis axis		1		
Canis lupus			1	
Homo sapiens	3		3	
Ursus arctos			2	

The parasite lineages identified in mosquitoes fed on each animal are shown. One mosquito with an unidentified blood meal was positive for Haemoproteus (hCIRCUM04).

DISCUSSION

Infections by *Plasmodium* parasites and related haemosporidians are commonly found in birds in zoos (31) and can lead to illness and/or lethal diseases (20–22). These cases usually occur in immunologically naïve species such as penguins originating from areas where the parasites circulating in zoos are not present. These animals are frequently bitten by competent vectors of avian malaria parasites, especially of the genus *Culex* (18), and largely suffer the costs of infections (17, 19). Interestingly, we found that a number of *Cx. pipiens* s.l. had fed on Humboldt penguins (*Spheniscus humboldti*), including mosquitoes with *P. relictum*. Different treatments and prophylactic protocols are applied to penguins to minimize the parasite-induced illness (18), as is also common practice in the study area.

Our results regarding the blood-feeding pattern of mosquitoes support the hypothesis that *Cx. pipiens* s.l. females feed mainly on birds (6, 28, 32). Despite the extremely low sample size, we also found support for the ornithophilic behavior of *Cs. longiareolata*; however, *Ae. albopictus* fed exclusively on humans. This latter species is a nuisance for visitors, especially in summer when it is commonest. These results provide valuable information regarding the blood-feeding sources of these species, which is especially relevant in the case of *Ae. albopictus* as this subject has only to date been investigated at a handful of studies in Europe (6, 25, 28, 33). Identification of the blood-meal sources of mosquitoes in zoos allows researchers to investigate additional aspects of vector ecology such as the flight distances of engorged females. Greenberg et al. (13) recorded an average distance of 106.7 m for mosquitoes of the genus *Aedes* (*Ae. vexans*), *Culex* (*Cx. Quinquefasciatus*, and *Cx. tarsalis*), and *Culiseta* (*Cs. inornata*) in USA. Similar values were reported by Tuten et al. (34) in zoos from USA, where *Anopheles* and *Culex* mosquitoes flew a mean distance of 94.1 m after feeding. Ejiri et al. (12) found that the post-blood-meal flight distance of

Cx. pipiens pallens lay in the range 10–350 m in Japan. Heym et al. (14) estimated the mean post-blood-meal flight distance of *Cx. pipiens* (biotype *pipiens*) in two zoos in Germany as 132.2 and 362.3 m. In this study in a Mediterranean area, engorged *Cx. pipiens* s.l. and *Cs. longiareolata* were captured in average at 95.67 m from their hosts, with a maximum of 168.51 m for *Cx. pipiens* s.l. It is worth highlighting that only a single female of *Cs. longiareolata* was found to have blood from zoo animals and so further studies targeting this species are still required. We were not able to calculate the flight distances of *Ae. albopictus* due to that fact that in this study it fed exclusively on humans.

Our results suggest that encounters between infected birds and competent mosquito vectors frequently occur in the area, which probably facilitates the transmission of avian *Plasmodium* within this zoo (12, 15, 23, 24). Previous studies in the Iberian Peninsula have identified avian *Plasmodium* in mosquitoes of the genera *Culex* and *Aedes* (25, 32, 35, 36), and of them, *Cx. pipiens* probably plays a key role in the transmission of avian *Plasmodium* due to its wide distribution (1), competence for the transmission of different avian *Plasmodium* lineages/species (16, 37), and its ornithophilic behavior (6, 32). A previous study in the same area also identified the presence of avian *Plasmodium* in *Cx. pipiens* s.l. pools (25). Nevertheless, the molecular identification of parasite DNA in mosquitoes does not necessarily imply vector competence (38) and so we were not able to assess the competence of these mosquitoes for avian malaria transmission. This is the case, above all, of *Haemoproteus* parasites, a parasite genus transmitted by *Culicoides* spp. and louse flies (16), that cannot be effectively transmitted by mosquitoes.

CONCLUSION

Barcelona Zoo is a suitable site for the development and maintenance of both native and alien species of mosquitoes. Based on their blood-feeding patterns, *Cx. pipiens* s.l. probably play a role in the local transmission and spread of mosquito-borne pathogens. This ornithophilic mosquito is a well-known vector of avian *Plasmodium* parasites. Thus, *Cx. pipiens* s.l. and the parasites transmitted may have an impact on the health of caged birds and so very likely represent a veterinary concern. In addition, magpies are common hosts of mosquitoes in the area and it is likely that they act as *Plasmodium* spp. reservoirs since high parasite prevalence has been found in the mosquitoes that feed on this bird species.

AUTHOR CONTRIBUTIONS

JM, JF, RB-M, and TM designed the study. JS, RB-M, and TM performed the fieldwork. JM, RS, JF, RB-M, and TM analyzed the samples and data. RS, JF, RB-M, and TM contributed with reagents. JM drafted the first version of the manuscript. All authors read and approved this manuscript.

ACKNOWLEDGMENTS

We thank Isabel Martín and Laura Gómez for their help in the laboratory and Helena Navalpotro for her help collecting mosquitoes. Lokímica contributed assistant workers and logistic support, in particular, Juan López, and Cristina Sesé. The work of the JM and JF was done within the framework of AIM-COST Action CA17108. Two reviewers provided valuable comments on an earlier version of this manuscript.

REFERENCES

1. Farajollahi A, Fonseca DM, Kramer LD, Marm KA. "Bird biting" mosquitoes and human disease: a review of the role of Culex pipiens complex mosquitoes in epidemiology. *Infect Genet Evol.* (2011) 11:1577–85. doi: 10.1016/j.meegid.2011.08.013
2. Folly AJ, Dorey-Robinson D, Hernández-Triana LM, Phipps LP, Johnson N. Emerging threats to animals in the United Kingdom by arthropod-borne diseases. *Front Vet Sci.* (2020) 7:20. doi: 10.3389/fvets.2020.00020
3. Medlock JM, Hansford KM, Schaffner F, Versteirt V, Hendrickx G, Zeller H, et al. A review of the invasive mosquitoes in Europe: ecology, public health risks, control options. *Vector Borne Zoonotic Dis.* (2012) 12:435–47. doi: 10.1089/vbz.2011.0814
4. Cancrini G, Frangipane di Regalbono A, Ricci I, Tessarin C, Gabrielli S, Pietrobelli M, et al. *Aedes albopictus* is a natural vector of *Dirofilaria immitis* in Italy. *Vet Parasitol.* (2003) 118:195–202. doi: 10.1016/j.vetpar.2003.10.011
5. Aranda C, Martínez MJ, Montalvo T, Eritja R, Navero-Castillejos J, Herreros E, et al. Arbovirus surveillance: first dengue virus detection in local *Aedes albopictus* mosquitoes in Europe, Catalonia, Spain, (2015). *Euro Surveill.* (2018) 23:1700837. doi: 10.2807/1560-7917.ES.2018.23.47.1700837
6. Martínez-de la Puente J, Muñoz J, Capelli G, Montarsi F, Soriguer R, Arnoldi D, et al. Avian malaria parasites in the last supper: identifying encounters between parasites and the invasive Asian mosquito tiger and native mosquito species in Italy. *Malar J.* (2015) 14:32. doi: 10.1186/s12936-015-0571-0
7. Kraemer MU, Sinka ME, Duda KA, Mylne AQ, Shearer FM, Barker CM, et al.I. The global distribution of the arbovirus vectors *Aedes aegypti* and *Ae. albopictus*. *Elife.* (2015) 4:e08347. doi: 10.7554/eLife.08347
8. Collantes F, Delacour S, Alarcón-Elbal PM, Ruiz-Arrondo I, Delgado JA, Torrell-Sorio A, et al. Review of ten-years presence of *Aedes albopictus* in Spain 2004-2014: known distribution and public health concerns. *Parasit Vectors.* (2015) 8:655. doi: 10.1186/s13071-015-1262-y
9. Muñoz C, Martínez-de la Puente J, Figuerola J, Pérez-Cutillas P, Navarro R, Ortuño M, et al. Molecular xenomonitoring E, and host identification of *Leishmania* sand fly vectors in a Mediterranean periurban wildlife park. *Transbound Emerg Dis.* (2019) 66:2546–61. doi: 10.1111/tbed.13319
10. Pérez-Cutillas P, Muñoz C, Martínez-de la Puente J, Figuerola J, Navarro R, Ortuño M, et al. A spatial ecology study in a high-diversity host community to understand blood-feeding behaviour in *Phlebotomus* sandfly vectors of *Leishmania*. *Med Vet Entomol.* (2020) 34:164–174. doi: 10.1111/mve.12427
11. England ME, Pearce-Kelly P, Brugman VA, King S, Gubbins S, Sach F, et al. *Culicoides* species composition and molecular identification of host blood meals at two zoos in the UK. *Parasit Vectors.* (2020) 13:139. doi: 10.1186/s13071-020-04018-0
12. Ejiri H, Sato Y, Kim KS, Hara T, Tsuda Y, Imura T, et al. Entomological study on transmission of avian malaria parasites in a zoological garden in Japan: blood meal identification and detection of avian malaria parasite DNA from blood-fed mosquitoes. *J Med Entomol.* (2011) 48:600–7. doi: 10.1603/ME10197
13. Greenberg JA, DiMenna MA, Hanelt B, Hofkin BV. Analysis of post-blood meal flight distances in mosquitoes utilizing zoo animal blood meals. *J Vector Ecol.* (2012) 37:83–9. doi: 10.1111/j.1948-7134.2012.00203.x
14. Heym EC, Kampen H, Schäfer M, Walther D. Mosquito bloodmeal preferences in two zoological gardens in Germany. *Med Vet Entomol.* (2019) 33:203–12. doi: 10.1111/mve.12350
15. Heym EC, Kampen H, Krone O, Schäfer M, Werner D. Molecular detection of vector-borne pathogens from mosquitoes collected

in two zoological gardens in Germany. *Parasitol Res.* (2019) 118:2097–105. doi: 10.1007/s00436-019-06327-5

16. Santiago-Alarcon D, Palinauskas V, Schaefer HM. Diptera vectors of avian *Haemosporidian* parasites: untangling parasite life cycles and their taxonomy. *Biol Rev Camb Philos Soc.* (2012) 87:928–64. doi: 10.1111/j.1469-185X.2012.00234.x
17. Sijbranda DC, Hunter S, Howe L, Lenting B, Argilla L, Gartrell D, et al. Cases of mortality in little penguins (*Eudyptula minor*) in New Zealand associated with avian malaria. *N Z Vet J.* (2017) 65:332–7. doi: 10.1080/00480169.2017.1359124
18. Grilo ML, Vanstreels RE, Wallace R, García-Párraga D, Braga ÉM, Chitty J, et al. Malaria in penguins - current perceptions. *Avian Pathol.* (2016) 45:393–407. doi: 10.1080/03079457.2016.1149145
19. Vanstreels RE, Kolesnikovas CK, Sandri S, Silveira P, Belo NO, Ferreira Junior FC, et al. Outbreak of avian malaria associated to multiple species of *Plasmodium* in magellanic penguins undergoing rehabilitation in southern Brazil. *PLoS ONE.* (2014) 9:e94994. doi: 10.1371/journal.pone.0094994
20. Bueno MG, Lopez RP, de Menezes RM, Costa-Nascimento Mde J, Lima GF, Araújo RA, et al. Identification of *Plasmodium* relictum causing mortality in penguins (*Spheniscus magellanicus*) from São Paulo Zoo, Brazil. *Vet Parasitol.* (2010) 173:123–127. doi: 10.1016/j.vetpar.2010.06.026
21. Jia T, Huang X, Valkiunas G, Yang M, Zheng C, Pu T, et al. Malaria parasites and related *Haemosporidians* cause mortality in cranes: a study on the parasites diversity, prevalence and distribution in Beijing Zoo. *Malar J.* (2018) 17:234. doi: 10.1186/s12936-018-2385-3
22. Olias P, Wegelin M, Zenker W, Freter S, Gruber AD, Klopfleisch R, et al. Avian malaria deaths in parrots, Europe. *Emerg Infect Dis.* (2011) 17:950–2. doi: 10.3201/eid1705.101618
23. Ejiri H, Sato Y, Sawai R, Sasaki E, Matsumoto R, Ueda M, et al. Prevalence of avian malaria parasite in mosquitoes collected at a zoological garden in Japan. *Parasitol Res.* (2009) 105:629–33. doi: 10.1007/s00436-009-1434-9
24. Ejiri H, Sato Y, Kim KS, Tsuda Y, Murata K, Saito K, et al. Blood meal identification and prevalence of avian malaria parasite in mosquitoes collected at Kushiro wetland, a subarctic zone of Japan. *J Med Entomol.* (2011) 48:904–8. doi: 10.1603/ME11053
25. Martínez-de la Puente J, Díez-Fernández A, Montalvo T, Bueno-Marí R, Pangrani Q, Soriguer RC, et al. Do invasive mosquito and bird species alter avian malaria parasite transmission? *Diversity.* (2020) 12:111. doi: 10.3390/d12030111
26. Schaffner E, Angel G, Geoffroy B, Hervy JP, Rhaiem A, Brunhes J. *The Mosquitoes of Europe: An Identification and Training Programme.* Montpellier: IRD Éditions & EID Méditerrannée. (2001).
27. Alcaide M, Rico C, Ruiz S, Soriguer R, Muñoz J, Figuerola J, et al. Disentangling vector-borne transmission networks: a universal DNA barcoding method to identify vertebrate hosts from arthropod bloodmeals. *PLoS ONE.* (2009) 4:e7092. doi: 10.1371/journal.pone.0007092
28. Muñoz J, Eritja R, Alcaide M, Montalvo T, Soriguer RC, Figuerola J, et al. Host-feeding patterns of native *Culex pipiens* and invasive *Aedes albopictus* mosquitoes (*Diptera: Culicidae*) in urban zones from Barcelona, Spain. *J Med Entomol.* (2011) 48:956–60. doi: 10.1603/ME11016
29. Hellgren O, Waldenström J, Bensch S. A new PCR assay for simultaneous studies of *Leucocytozoon, Plasmodium*, and *Haemoproteus* from avian blood. *J Parasitol.* (2004) 90:797–802. doi: 10.1645/GE-184R1
30. Bensch S, Hellgren O, Pérez-Tris J. MalAvi: a public database of malaria parasites and related haemosporidians in avian hosts based on mitochondrial cytochrome b lineages. *Mol Ecol Resour.* (2009) 9:1353–8. doi: 10.1111/j.1755-0998.2009.02692.x
31. Chagas CRF, Valkiunas G, de Oliveira Guimarães L, Monteiro EF, Guida FJ, Simões RF, et al. Diversity and distribution of avian malaria and related haemosporidian parasites in captive birds from a Brazilian megalopolis. *Malar J.* (2017) 16:83. doi: 10.1186/s12936-017-1729-8
32. Martínez-de la Puente J, Ferraguti M, Ruiz S, Roiz D, Soriguer RC, Figuerola J, et al. *Culex pipiens* forms and urbanization: effects on blood feeding sources and transmission of avian *Plasmodium*. *Malar J.* (2016) 15:589. doi: 10.1186/s12936-016-1643-5
33. Valerio L, Marini F, Bongiorno G, Facchinelli L, Pombi M, Caputo B, et al. Host-feeding patterns of *Aedes albopictus* (*Diptera: Culicidae*) in urban and rural contexts within Rome province, Italy. *Vector Borne Zoonotic Dis.* (2010) 10:291–4. doi: 10.1089/vbz.2009.0007
34. Tuten HC, Bridges WC, Paul KS, Adler PH. Blood-feeding ecology of mosquitoes in zoos. *Med Vet Entomol.* (2012) 26:407–16. doi: 10.1111/j.1365-2915.2012.01012.x
35. Ferraguti M, Martínez-de la Puente J, Muñoz J, Roiz D, Ruiz S, Soriguer R, et al. Avian *Plasmodium* in *Culex* and *Ochlerotatus* mosquitoes from southern Spain: effects of season and host-feeding source on parasite dynamics. *PLoS ONE.* (2013) 8:e66237. doi: 10.1371/journal.pone.0066237
36. Ventim R, Ramos JA, Osório H, Lopes RJ, Pérez-Tris J, Mendes L, et al. Avian malaria infections in western European mosquitoes. *Parasitol Res.* (2012) 111:637–45. doi: 10.1007/s00436-012-2880-3
37. Gutiérrez-López R, Martínez-de la Puente J, Gangoso L, Soriguer R, Figuerola J. Plasmodium transmission differs between mosquito species and parasite lineages. *Parasitology.* (2020) 147:441–7. doi: 10.1017/S0031182020000062
38. Valkiunas G. Haemosporidian vector research: marriage of molecular and microscopical approaches is essential. *Mol Ecol.* (2011) 20:3084–6. doi: 10.1111/j.1365-294X.2011.05187.x

13

Survey of Zoonotic and Non-Zoonotic Vector-Borne Pathogens in Military Horses in Lisbon

Hans-Peter Fuehrer[1*], *Ana Margarida Alho*[2], *Feodora Natalie Kayikci*[1], *Bita Shahi Barogh*[1], *Hugo Rosa*[3], *José Tomás*[3], *Hugo Rocha*[3], *Josef Harl*[4] and *Luís Madeira de Carvalho*[2*]

[1] Department of Pathobiology, Institute of Parasitology, University of Veterinary Medicine, Vienna, Austria, [2] CIISA - Centro de Investigação Interdisciplinar em Sanidade Animal, Faculdade de Medicina Veterinária, Universidade de Lisbon, Lisbon, Portugal, [3] Guarda Nacional Republicana, Lisbon, Portugal, [4] Department of Pathobiology, Institute of Pathology, University of Veterinary Medicine, Vienna, Austria

***Correspondence:**
Hans-Peter Fuehrer
hans-peter.fuehrer@vetmeduni.ac.at
Luís Madeira de Carvalho
madeiradecarvalho@fmv.ulisboa.pt

Vector-borne diseases of zoonotic and/or veterinary relevance have been increasingly reported in horses globally, although data regarding working and military horses is lacking. Portuguese military horses may constitute a risk group for these pathogens, as they frequently work outdoors in various regions of the country. This study included 101 apparently healthy horses belonging to the Portuguese National Republican Guard. Blood samples were analyzed to determine the presence and prevalence of piroplasms, *Anaplasmataceae*, *Rickettsia* spp., and filarioid helminths. Overall 32.7% of the horses gave positive results for *Theileria equi*. Two genotypes of *T. equi* were verified. No positive results were recorded for *Anaplasma* spp., *Rickettsia* spp., filarioid helminthes, and *Babesia caballi*. As equine piroplasmosis is a severe infectious tick-borne disease responsible for significant losses in equine production and with numerous impacts in the international movement of horses, adequate treatment, and preventive measures are needed to reduce exposure to vectors and future infections.

Keywords: equine piroplasmosis, military horses, *Theileria equi*, vector-borne diseases, zoonosis, Portugal

INTRODUCTION

Vector-borne diseases (VBDs) have been increasingly reported in horses worldwide (1). Several equine VBDs are of zoonotic relevance and horses potentially serve as sentinels for human infections. The distribution and spread of vector-borne pathogens are limited by the presence of competent arthropod vectors (e.g., ticks, fleas, and mosquitoes) capable of transmitting these pathogens. Military horses may constitute a risk group for VBDs, as they frequently work outdoors in different areas and thus are exposed to vectors present there.

Equine piroplasmosis is a tick-borne disease of equids such as horses, donkeys, mules, and zebras, and is caused by the protozoan parasites *Theileria equi* and *Babesia caballi* (2). Infected animals may carry *B. caballi* for several years and *T. equi* for a whole lifetime (2).

Theileria equi (Laveran, 1901) Mehlhorn, Schein 1998 is one of the most important pathogens of horses in many parts of the world, including Southern Europe. Clinical signs range from asymptomatic to acute, subacute, and chronic cases with fever, anemia, inappetence, and spleno- and hepatomegaly. In severe cases, the infection can lead to death. Transplacental transmission from mares to fetuses can lead to abortion (3), causing significant losses in the equine industry. Additionally, international horse trade facilitates the spread to non-endemic areas (4). Currently, more than 20 potential tick vectors of *T. equi* are known (5, 6). Species of the genera *Dermacentor*, *Rhipicephalus*, and *Hyalomma* are known as competent vectors and several *Ixodes*, *Haemaphysalis*, and *Amblyomma* species are discussed to transmit the parasite as well (2). Various tick species that may act as vectors for equine piroplasms are present in mainland Portugal, namely *Rhipicephalus sanguineus*, *Rhipicephalus annulatus*, *Rhipicephalus bursa*, *Dermacentor marginatus*, *Hyalomma lusitanicum*, and *Hyalomma marginatum* (7, 8). Several genotypes of *T. equi* have been reported in different populations of equids (2, 9). There is evidence that specific genotype assortment occurs within the tick vectors (6). In Portugal, previous studies show different prevalence rates for *T. equi*, which may be associated with the kind of horses/facility involved, the study area and the diagnostic tests used. In horse stud farms in the Ribatejo region, central Portugal, using Complement Fixation (CF), seroprevalence was 45.3%, while using blood smears, the infection was prevalent on 42,6% of the examined horses, with a potential transuterine transmission in 80% of positive mares (10, 11). Further South, in Alentejo region, using CF and IFAT the seroprevalence for *Theileria equi* was 85.1% and recently, using qPCR/nPCR, 56% of the horses examined from the Lisbon and Alentejo areas showed a prevalence of 56% (12, 13).

Members of the family *Anaplasmataceae* (e.g., *Anaplasma*, *Neoehrlichia*, and *Ehrlichia*) are gram-negative, intracellular bacteria infecting domestic and wild animals, but also humans. *Anaplasma phagocytophilum* has been documented in various animals including horses and is the causative agent of equine, canine, and human granulocytic anaplasmosis. Various strains are known and horses can harbor strains of zoonotic potential (14). In Europe, the main vector of this tick-borne pathogen is *Ixodes ricinus*, which is also present in mainland Portugal (7). *Anaplasma phagocytophilum* has previously been detected in *I. ricinus* on Madeira and in *Ixodes ventalloi* in mainland Portugal (Baixa de Palmela, Setubal district) (15, 16). *Anaplasma phagocytophilum* is regularly reported in serology-based studies on horses in Europe including Portugal [e.g., (8, 16, 17)].

Rickettsia species are obligate intracellular, gram-negative bacteria transmitted by various types of arthropods [e.g., ixodid ticks are the main vectors of spotted fever group rickettsiae (18)]. Several studies have documented *Rickettsia* spp. in horses.

Filarioid nematodes are also parasites of horses in Europe. Because of their asymptomatic to minor symptomatic effects, these parasites are neglected and understudied. Adults of *Setaria equina* are located in the peritoneal cavities of horses. Microfilariae of this worldwide distributed helminth can be found in the peripheral blood (19). Mosquitoes of the genera *Culex* and *Aedes* are the vectors of *S. equina*. Another filarioid species parasitizing medial layers or outside layers of tissues within the artery wall of horses is *Onchocerca boehmi* (syn. *Elaeophora boehmi*) (20, 21).

Little is known about the risk of military horses regarding VBDs. In fact, few studies have been conducted so far and no surveillance mechanisms are in place to assess geographical range and prevalence in the country. Considering the emergence of VBDs in Europe, as well as the lack of data on this topic, an epidemiological study was conducted, in order to identify the presence and prevalence of the most significant bacterial and parasitic VBDs of zoonotic and/or non-zoonotic relevance in Portuguese military horses using molecular analysis followed by sequence analysis of positive DNA products.

MATERIALS AND METHODS

Overall 101 military horses (Puro Sangue Lusitano breed) belonging to the Portuguese National Republican Guard (GNR), stabled at guard facilities in metropolitan Lisbon were included in this study. Horses from various job sites were included (55 GNR Lisbon, 46 GNR Lisbon Braço de Prata Expo, 2 GNR Évora, 1 GNR Faro, and 1 GNR Tomar), and information on sex and age were determined. All horses were apparently healthy with no clinical signs compatible with VBDs. Horses were dewormed with moxidectin and praziquantel administered annually (with the exception of sportive horses, which were dewormed twice a year). Horses were not treated against tick infestation. Blood samples were collected at the jugular vein from apparently healthy horses in June ($n = 55$) and July ($n = 46$) in 2017.

A total of 50 μl of blood was spotted on Whatman® filter paper (VWR International GmbH, Vienna, Austria) and dried at room temperature. Afterward, each filter paper was sealed in an envelope separately. Filter papers were shipped to the University of Veterinary Medicine Vienna for molecular analysis. Sections of ~4 mm in diameter were cut out of the center of the blood spots with sterile blades. DNA was extracted with a modified chelex-based technique using InstaGene™ matrix (Bio-Rad Laboratories, Hercules, California) as established previously (22). Extracted DNA was stored at −20°C until further analysis. Samples were screened for the presence of DNA of various vector-borne pathogens of zoonotic and non-zoonotic relevance using specific broad-range PCR assays, under conditions reported previously [(23); **Table 1**] as follows: piroplasms (incl. *Babesia* and *Theileria*) within the *18S* rRNA gene [BTH-1F/BTH-1R; (24)]; *Anaplasmataceae* (incl. *Anaplasma*, *Ehrlichia*, and *Neoehrlichia*) within the *16S* gene [EHR16SD/EHR16SR; (26)]; *Rickettsia* spp. within the *23S/5S* rRNA gene [ITS-F/ITS-R; (27)] and filiarioid helminths targeting a fragment of the mitochondrial *cytochrome c oxidase subunit I gene* [*COI*; H14FilaCOIFw/H14FilaCOIRv; (28)]. Additionally, all samples were further analyzed with a *Babesia* specific PCR analysis [Babfor/Babrev; (25)]. PCR products were analyzed by gel electrophoresis on 2% agarose gels stained with Midori Green Advance DNA stain (Nippon Genetics Europe, Düren, Germany). Positive reaction products were commercially purified and sequenced at LGC Genomics GmbH (Berlin, Germany).

Phylogenetic Analysis of the *T. equi 18S* Sequences

To show the diversity of *18S* lineages of *T. equi*, Bayesian inference (BI) and Maximum likelihood (ML) trees were

TABLE 1 | Primer sequences and PCR protocols used for molecular analysis of vector-borne pathogens in military horses.

Organism	Gene/Locus	Primer sequences (5′→3′)	Amplification protocol	Product size (bp)	References
Piroplasms (*Babesia* spp., *Theileria* spp.)	*18S* rRNA	BTH-1F: CCTGAGAAACGGCTACCACATCT BTH-1R: TTGCGACCATACTCCCCCCA	94°C: 2 min, 40 cycles - 95°C: 30 s, 68°C: 1 min, 72°C: 1 min, 72°C: 10 min	~700	(24)
Babesia spp.	*18S* rRNA	B-For: GACTAGGGATTGGAGGTC B-Rev: GAATAATTCACCGGATCACTC	94°C: 2 min, 30 cycles - 95°C: 1 min, 53°C: 1 min, 72°C: 1 min, 72°C: 7 min	~650	(25)
Anaplasmataceae	*16S* rRNA	EHR16SD: GGTACCYACAGAAGAAGTCC EHR16SR: TAGCACTCATCGTTTACAGC	95°C: 2 min, 35 cycles - 94°C: 1 min, 54°C: 30 s, 72°C: 30 s, 72°C: 5 min	345	(26)
Rickettsia spp.	*23S/5S* rRNA	ITS-F: GATAGGTCGGGTGTGGAAG ITS-R: TCGGGATGGGATCGTGTG	96°C: 4 min, 35 cycles - 94°C: 1 min, 52°C: 1 min, 72°C: 2 min, 72°C: 3 min	350–550	(27)
Filarioid nematodes	mt *COI*	H14FilaCO1Fw: GCCTATTTTGATTGGTGGTTTTGG H14FilaCO1Rv: AGCAATAATCATAGTAGCAGCACTAA	95°C: 2 min, 30–35 cycles - 95°C: 1 min, 53°C: 1 min, 72°C: 1 min, 72°C: 5 min	724	(28)

calculated based on the sequences of the present study, and data was mined from NCBI GenBank. The GenBank sequences were retrieved by performing a BLAST search on a 530 bp *18S* section of *Theileria* spp. To identify the lineages of *T. equi*, the sequences were aligned and sorted with MAFFT v.7 applying the default settings (29). The sequences were visually inspected using BioEdit (30) and all sequences were removed which did not cover the entire length, contained ambiguity characters, and/or obvious sequencing errors, resulting in a total of 220 *T. equi* sequences. The sequences of the present study and NCBI GenBank were combined and a sequence of *Theileria ovis* (AY533144) was added for outgroup comparison. All sequences were re-aligned with MAFFT v.7 applying the option "G-INS-i" and then collapsed to haplotypes using DAMBE (31). The alignment contained 49 unique *T. equi* lineages and 535 sites, of which all 15 gap positions were removed before the phylogenetic analysis. The best-fit substitution model for the 520 bp alignment was inferred using the model search implemented in the W-IQ-TREE web server [http://iqtree.cibiv.univie.ac.at/; (32)], resulting in the model HKY+G. A ML consensus tree was calculated from 1000 bootstrap replicates using W-IQ-TREE. A BI tree was calculated with MrBayes v.3.2.7 (33). The Bayesian analysis was run for 10 million generations (2 runs each with 4 chains, one of which was heated) and every thousandth tree was sampled. The first 25% of trees were discarded as burn-in and a 50% majority-rule consensus tree was calculated from the remaining 7,500 trees.

RESULTS

In this study, 101 military horses were included of which 60 were males and 41 mares. The age ranged between 4 and 24 years ($x = 12.4$ years; $x_{med} = 12$ years). Overall 33 animals (32.7%; CI_{95}: 24.3–42.3%) were infected with a vector-borne pathogen, namely *Theileria equi*. Seventeen males and 16 mares aged between 4 and 18 years ($x = 10.5$) gave positive signals at the molecular analysis for piroplasms. All of the positive horses came from Lisbon (23 at GNR Lisbon Braço de Prata Expo and 10 at GNR Lisbon). Two genotypes of *T. equi* were recorded of which 24 were genotype 1 and seven genotype 2. Both genotypes were present in GNR Lisbon Braço de Prata Expo and GNR Lisbon. The phylogenetic tree of the *18S* sequences shows three main sequence groups or clades, one of which may be divided into two sub-groups (**Figure 1**). The *T. equi* lineages identified in the present study clustered in the first and second clade. Of the 33 *T. equi* positive samples, 24 featured a lineage (genotype 1, 100% match with HM229407), which clustered in the first clade. This lineage and similar ones were isolated from horses in China, Kazakhstan, Russia, Mongolia, Saudi Arabia, South Korea, Spain, Sudan, and Switzerland. Three slightly distinct lineages (KF597077, KF597078, and KF597081) in this clade were isolated from the waterbuck *Kobus ellipsiprymnus* in Kenya. Seven horses sampled in the present study featured a *T. equi* lineage, which clustered in the second clade (**Figure 1**). This lineage (genotype 2, 100% match with EU888906) and similar ones were isolated from horses in Brazil, Croatia, India, Jordan, Egypt, Israel, Saudi Arabia, South Africa, Spain, Turkey, and the USA. The phylogenetic tree (**Figure 1**) features a third clade, which can be subdivided into two subclades (3a and 3b). Subclade 3a contains lineages isolated from horses in Egypt, Israel, Palestine, Turkey, Nigeria, and Sudan. All records come from the Middle East and Northern and Eastern Africa. Two slightly deviating lineages (KF597074 and KF597076) were isolated from the waterbuck *K. ellipsiprymnus* in Kenya. Subclade 3b features lineages isolated from horses in Brazil, China, Cuba, Egypt, Iraq, Israel, South Africa, and the USA.

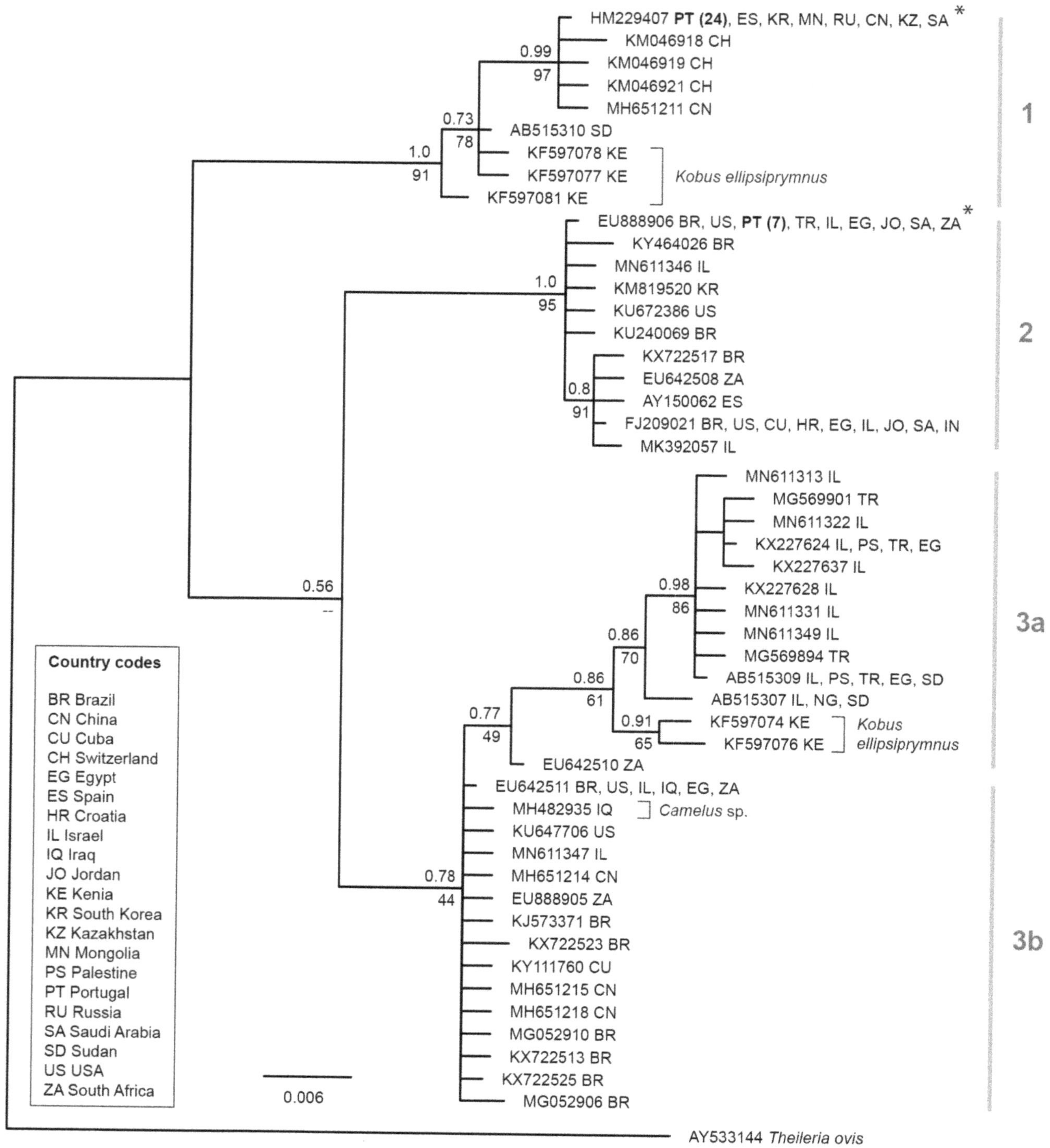

FIGURE 1 | Bayesian inference tree of *T. equi* lineages based on 530 bp sections of the *18S*. The BI posterior probabilities and ML bootstrap values are indicated at most nodes. The scale bar indicates the expected mean number of substitutions per site according to the model of sequence evolution applied. Asterisks mark the lineages isolated from horses in Portugal in the present study. As outgroup a sequence of *Theileria ovis* (AY533144) was included.

Analyses for the presence of DNA of zoonotic agents (e.g., *Anaplasma* spp. and *Rickettsia* spp.) but also other non-zoonotic pathogens (e.g., *Babesia caballi* and filarioid helminths like *Setaria equina* and *Onchocerca boehmi*) gave negative results.

DISCUSSION

Prevalence of equine piroplasmosis vary in endemic regions in Europe for *T. equi* and *B. caballi*, depending on study design and diagnostic techniques used [IFAT, ELISA, PCR; (reviewed in 2)]. The prevalence of *T. equi* is generally higher than that for *B. caballi*. In healthy military horses included in this study, 32.7% (33/101) tested positive for the presence of DNA of *T. equi*. These data confirm a relatively high prevalence of *T. equi* in military horses in Portugal (mainly from the Lisbon area). In the Alentejo region (Southern Portugal) serological analyses with IFAT of 154 horses resulted in 85.1% positive for *T. equi* and 65.6% for *B. caballi* (12). Out of 73 "Puro Sangue Lusitano" horses from Vila Viçosa (Alentejo region, Southern Portugal) 53.4% were positive for *T. equi* using cELISA (34). Ribeiro et al. (8), combining serology and microscopy, reported *T. equi* in 19.1% and *B. caballi* in 11.7% of 162 horses in North of Portugal. Moreover, using PCR techniques, *T. equi* was detected in 56% of horses from central Southern Portugal that presented with clinical or subclinical signs (13). DNA of *T. equi* was found in two out of nine *Rhipicephalus bursa* male ticks collected from horses in the Comunidade Intermunicipal do-Ave (Northern Portugal), but because of the proof of DNA only, the vector capacity of this tick species remains unclear (35).

In the present study, horses between 4 and 18 years were infected with this parasite. It is known that the prevalence of equine piroplasmosis increases with age and that equids infected with *T. equi* remain life-long carriers of this parasite (2). Moreover, it is discussed that male and female horses have different susceptibilities to infection, but the results of various studies are contradictory. Host activity also increases the chance for horses to become infected (2). Grazing was documented to double the risk of becoming infected with *B. caballi* and *T. equi* (36). Outdoor or mixed indoor/outdoor type of housing was also reported as a risk factor for *T. equi* (8). Military horses included in this study are regularly outside, but are also stabled at military facilities. However, regular travel activity to various regions in the country increases the possibility of tick contact. Furthermore, the type of horse breed may also influence the risk of *T. equi* infections (37).

Interestingly we were not able to detect DNA of *B. caballi* in military horses from this study, although an additional *Babesia*-specific PCR was run. Previous studies have shown that horses seropositive for *B. caballi* (but also *T. equi*) are often not positive at PCR analysis (38). However, it is recommended to run cELISA, IFAT, and PCR to assure the identification of acute and chronic equine piroplasm infections (39). Recent research carried out on Lisbon horses, found a 7% prevalence for *Babesia* spp., meaning it may be a residual, but persistent agent, in this area (13).

Anaplasmataceae were not detected in the blood samples of healthy horses analyzed in this study. Using serology, *A. phagocytophilum* has previously been confirmed in nine of 302 horses from mainland Portugal (16) and 13% of 162 horses in Northern Portugal (8). However, it has been shown that seropositivity to *A. phagocytophilum* was significantly higher if compared to PCR results [e.g., (40)]. Therefore, we cannot exclude that horses in this study had previously been in contact with this pathogen. It is discussed that climate change might increase the threat of disease in European horse populations (41).

Although no horses were positive for *Rickettsia* spp. in this study, several *Rickettsia* species have been documented in horses in Europe. Spotted fever-group rickettsiae were reported in 15.03% of 479 horses in Italy using serology (17). Using IFAT, *Rickettsia helvetica* was documented in 36.5% of 63 horses in Sweden (42). In another study, *R. helvetica* and *R. monacensis* were confirmed in ticks collected from ponies in Poland using PCR techniques (43). On Corsica, the presence of *Rickettsia slovaca* and *Rickettsia aeschlimannii* in ticks collected on horses was confirmed (44).

DNA of microfilaria of filarioid helminths was not detected in the present study. However, although infections with these parasites are mainly asymptomatic and neglected, they have been reported in horses in several regions in Europe. In Hungary, microfilariae of *S. equina* were reported in 9.2% (18/195) of horses analyzed, and infection was associated with the presence of still waters nearby (45).

Although only one parasite species was documented, it can be concluded that *T. equi* is among the most important vector-borne transmitted agents infecting horses in Europe. As equine piroplasmosis is a severe infectious tick-borne disease responsible for significant losses in equine reproduction, and with numerous impacts on the international movement of horses, treatment and preventive measures are needed to reduce exposure to future infections.

AUTHOR CONTRIBUTIONS

H-PF, AA, and LM contributed to the conception and design of the study. AA, HRos, JT, and HRoc conducted field and laboratory work. FK and BS conducted the lab work. H-PF and JH analyzed the sequences and performed the phylogenetic analysis. H-PF, AA, JH, and LM wrote and reviewed the manuscript. All authors read and approved the final manuscript.

ACKNOWLEDGMENTS

This study was performed within the framework of the COST action TD1303, EurNegVec.

REFERENCES

1. Brown C, Torres A. *Foreign Animal Diseases*. 7th ed. Boca Raton, FL: Boca Publications (2008) p. 472.
2. Onyiche TE, Suganuma K, Igarashi I, Yokoyama N, Xuan X, Thekisoe O. A review on equine piroplasmosis: epidemiology, vector ecology, risk factors, host immunity, diagnosis and control. *Int J Environ Res Public Health*. (2019) 16:E1736. doi: 10.3390/ijerph16101736
3. Tirosh-Levy S, Gottlieb Y, Mimoun L, Mazuz ML, Steinman A. Transplacental transmission of *Theileria equi* is not a common cause of abortions and infection of foals in Israel. *Animals*. (2020) 10:E341. doi: 10.3390/ani10020341
4. Wise LN, Kappmeyer LS, Mealey RH, Knowles DP. Review of equine piroplasmosis. *J Vet Intern Med*. (2013) 27:1334–46. doi: 10.1111/jvim.12168
5. Scoles GA, Ueti MW. Vector ecology of equine piroplasmosis. *Annu Rev Entomol*. (2015) 60:561–80. doi: 10.1146/annurev-ento-010814-021110
6. Tirosh-Levy S, Steinman A, Einhorn A, Apanaskevich DA, Mumcuoglu KY, Gottlieb Y. Potential tick vectors for *Theileria equi* in Israel. *Med Vet Entomol*. (2020) 34:291–4. doi: 10.1111/mve.12435

7. Caeiro V. General review of tick species present in Portugal. *Parassitologia.* (1999) 41:11–5.
8. Ribeiro AJ, Cardoso L, Maia JM, Coutinho T, Cotovio M. Prevalence of *Theileria equi*, *Babesia caballi*, and *Anaplasma phagocytophilum* in horses from the north of Portugal. *Parasitol Res.* (2013) 112:2611–17. doi: 10.1007/s00436-013-3429-9
9. Qablan MA, Oborník M, PetrŽelková KJ, Sloboda M, Shudiefat MF, Horín P, et al. Infections by *Babesia caballi* and *Theileria equi* in Jordanian equids: epidemiology and genetic diversity. *Parasitology.* (2013) 140:1096–103. doi: 10.1017/S0031182013000486
10. Carvalho-Varela M, Pereira da Fonseca IM, de Carvalho LMM, Sabino-Serra JM, Castelo-Branco A, Afonso-Roque MM, et al. Epidemiogical aspects of horse parasitic diseases in the Ribatejo region (Portugal). In: *VIII International Congress of Parasitology* (Izmir) (1994). p. 321.
11. Rego BMCD. *Study of the natural infection by protozoa of the genus Babesia and Theileria in an equine stud-farm from Ribatejo* (MSc dissertation). Integrated Master in Veterinary Medicine, Faculty of Veterinary Medicine, Technical University of Lisbon, Lisbon, Portugal (2008). p. 69.
12. Malta MJPV. *Diagnosis horse babesiosis and theileriosis in alentejo* (MSc dissertation) Master in Tropical Veterinary Medicine and Animal Production, Faculty of Veterinary Medicine, Technical University of Lisbon, Lisbon, Portugal (2001). p. 89.
13. Barros CJG. *Equine piroplasmosis: molecular diagnosis and evaluation of hematological and inflammatory biomarkers changes in horses with clinical and subclinical disease* (MSc Dissertation) Integrated Master in Veterinary Medicine, Faculty of Veterinary Medicine, University of Lisbon p. 71.
14. Matei IA, Estrada-Peña A, Cutler SJ, Vayssier-Taussat M, Varela-Castro L, Potkonjak A, et al. A review on the eco-epidemiology and clinical management of human granulocytic anaplasmosis and its agent in Europe. *Parasit Vectors.* (2019) 12:599. doi: 10.1186/s13071-019-3852-6
15. Santos AS, Santos-Silva MM, Almeida VC, Bacellar F, Dumler JS. Detection of *Anaplasma phagocytophilum* DNA in *Ixodes* ticks (Acari: Ixodidae) from Madeira Island and Setubal District, mainland Portugal. *Emerg Infect Dis.* (2004) 10:1643–8. doi: 10.3201/eid1009.040276
16. Santos AS, Bacellar F, Dumler JS. A 4-year study of *Anaplasma phagocytophilum* in Portugal. *Clin Microbiol Infect.* (2009) 15(Suppl. 2):46–7. doi: 10.1111/j.1469-0691.2008.02172.x
17. Ebani VV. Serological evidence of *Anaplasma phagocytophilum* and spotted fever group *Rickettsia* spp. exposure in horses from Central Italy. *Pathogens.* (2019) 8:E88. doi: 10.3390/pathogens8030088
18. Parola P, Paddock CD, Socolovschi C, Labruna MB, Mediannikov O, Kernif T, et al. Update on tick-borne rickettsioses around the world: a geographic approach. *Clin Microbiol Rev.* (2013) 26:657–702. doi: 10.1128/CMR.00032-13
19. Coleman SU, Klei TR, French DD. Prevalence of *Setaria equina* (Nematode: Onchocercidae) in southeastern Louisiana horses. *J Parasitol.* (1985) 71:512–3. doi: 10.2307/3281548
20. Supperer R. Filarosen der Pferde in Österreich. *Wiener Tierärztliche Monatsschrift.* (1953) 40:193–220.
21. Lia RP, Mutafchiev Y, Veneziano V, Giannelli A, Abramo F, Santoro M, et al. Filarial infection caused by *Onchocerca boehmi* (Supperer, 1953) in a horse from Italy. *Parasitol Res.* (2017) 116:191–8. doi: 10.1007/s00436-016-5277-x
22. Fuehrer HP, Starzengruber P, Swoboda P, Khan WA, Matt J, Ley B, et al. Indigenous *Plasmodium ovale* malaria in Bangladesh. *Am J Trop Med Hyg.* (2010) 83:75–8. doi: 10.4269/ajtmh.2010.09-0796
23. Cézanne R, Mrowietz N, Eigner B, Duscher GG, Glawischnig W, Fuehrer HP. Molecular analysis of *Anaplasma phagocytophilum* and *Babesia divergens* in red deer (*Cervus elaphus*) in Western Austria. *Mol Cell Probes.* (2017) 31:55–8. doi: 10.1016/j.mcp.2016.07.003
24. Zintl A, Finnerty EJ, Murphy TM, de Waal T, Gray JS. Babesias of red deer (*Cervus elaphus*) in Ireland. *Vet Res.* (2011) 42:7. doi: 10.1186/1297-9716-42-7
25. Blaschitz M, Narodoslavsky-Gföller M, Kanzler M, Stanek G, Walochnik J. *Babesia* species occurring in Austrian *Ixodes ricinus* ticks. *Appl Environ Microbiol.* (2008) 74:4841-6. doi: 10.1128/AEM.00035-08
26. Brown GK, Martin AR, Roberts TK, Aitken RJ. Detection of *Ehrlichia platys* in dogs in Australia. *Aust Vet J.* (2001) 79:554–8. doi: 10.1111/j.1751-0813.2001.tb10747.x
27. Vitorino L, Zé-Zé L, Sousa A, Bacellar F, Tenreiro R. rRNA intergenic spacer regions for phylogenetic analysis of *Rickettsia* species. *Ann N Y Acad Sci.* (2003) 990:726–33. doi: 10.1111/j.1749-6632.2003.tb07451.x
28. HodŽić A, Alić A, Fuehrer HP, Harl J, Wille-Piazzai W, Duscher GG. A molecular survey of vector-borne pathogens in red foxes (*Vulpes vulpes*) from Bosnia and Herzegovina. *Parasit Vectors.* (2015) 8:88. doi: 10.1186/s13071-015-0692-x
29. Katoh K, Standley DM. MAFFT multiple sequence alignment software version 7: improvements in performance and usability. *Mol Biol Evol.* (2013) 30:772–80. doi: 10.1093/molbev/mst010
30. Hall TA. BioEdit: a user-friendly biological sequences alignment editor and analysis program for Windows 95/98/NT. *Nucleic Acids Symp Ser.* (1999) 41:95–8.
31. Xia X, Xie Z. DAMBE: software package for data analysis in molecular biology and evolution. *J Heredity.* (2001) 92:371–3. doi: 10.1093/jhered/92.4.371
32. Trifinopoulos J, Nguyen LT, von Haeseler A, Minh BQ. W-IQ-TREE: a fast online phylogenetic tool for maximum likelihood analysis. *Nucleic Acids Res.* (2016) 44:W232–5. doi: 10.1093/nar/gkw256
33. Ronquist F, Teslenko M, Van Der Mark P, Ayres DL, Darling A, Höhna S, et al. MrBayes 3.2: efficient Bayesian phylogenetic inference and model choice across a large model space. *Syst Biol.* (2012) 61:539–42. doi: 10.1093/sysbio/sys029
34. Sousa S, Almeida A, Simão L, Anastácio S, Madeira de Carvalho LM. *Theleria equi* infection in Puro Sangue Lusitano horses from Vila Viçosa. In: *Proceedings of the II Iberian Congress of Veterinary Epidemiology* (Barcelona) (2010). p. 19.
35. Ferrolho J, Antunes S, Santos AS, Velez R, Padre L, Cabezas-Cruz A, et al. Detection and phylogenetic characterization of *Theileria* spp. and Anaplasma marginale in Rhipicephalus bursa in Portugal. *Ticks Tick Borne Dis.* (2016) 7:443–8. doi: 10.1016/j.ttbdis.2016.01.004
36. Moretti A, Mangili V, Salvatori R, Maresca C, Scoccia E, Torina A, et al. Prevalence and diagnosis of *Babesia* and *Theileria* infections in horses in Italy: a preliminary study. *Vet J.* (2010) 184:346–50. doi: 10.1016/j.tvjl.2009.03.021
37. Montes Cortés MG, Fernández-García JL, Habela Martínez-Estéllez MÁ. Seroprevalence of *Theileria equi* and *Babesia caballi* in horses in Spain. *Parasite.* (2017) 24:14. doi: 10.1051/parasite/2017015
38. Grandi G, Molinari G, Tittarelli M, Sassera D, Kramer LH. Prevalence of *Theileria equi* and *Babesia caballi* infection in horses from northern Italy. *Vector Borne Zoonotic Dis.* (2011) 11:955–956. doi: 10.1089/vbz.2010.0193
39. Mahmoud MS, El-Ezz NT, Abdel-Shafy S, Nassar SA, El Namaky AH, Khalil WK, et al. Assessment of *Theileria equi* and *Babesia caballi* infections in equine populations in Egypt by molecular, serological and hematological approaches. *Parasit Vectors.* (2016) 9:260. doi: 10.1186/s13071-016-1539-9
40. Passamonti F, Veronesi F, Cappelli K, Capomaccio S, Coppola G, Marenzoni ML, et al. *Anaplasma phagocytophilum* in horses and ticks: a preliminary survey of Central Italy. *Comp Immunol Microbiol Infect Dis.* (2010) 33:73–83. doi: 10.1016/j.cimid.2008.08.002
41. Dziegiel B, Adaszek L, Winiarczyk M, García-Bocanegra I, Carbonero A, Debiak P, et al. Comparative analysis of 16S RNA nucleotide sequences of *Anaplasma phagocytophilum* detected in the blood of horses from various parts of Europe. *J Med Microbiol.* (2013) 62:1891–1896. doi: 10.1099/jmm.0.058636-0
42. Elfving K, Malmsten J, Dalin AM, Nilsson K. Serologic and molecular prevalence of *Rickettsia helvetica* and *Anaplasma phagocytophilum* in wild cervids and domestic mammals in the central parts of Sweden. *Vector Borne Zoonotic Dis.* (2015) 15:529–34. doi: 10.1089/vbz.2015.1768
43. Skotarczak B, Wodecka B, Rymaszewska A, Adamska M. Molecular evidence for bacterial pathogens in *Ixodes ricinus* ticks infesting Shetland ponies. *Exp Appl Acarol.* (2016) 69:179–89. doi: 10.1007/s10493-016-0027-4
44. Grech-Angelini S, Stachurski F, Vayssier-Taussat M, Devillers E, Casabianca F, Lancelot R, et al. Tick-borne pathogens in ticks (Acari: Ixodidae) collected from various domestic and wild hosts in Corsica (France), a Mediterranean island environment. *Transbound Emerg Dis.* (2020) 67:745–57. doi: 10.1111/tbed.13393
45. Hornok S, Genchi C, Bazzocchi C, Fok E, Farkas R. Prevalence of *Setaria equina* microfilaraemia in horses in Hungary. *Vet Rec.* (2007) 161:814–6. doi: 10.1136/vr.161.24.814

14

Virulence Plasmids of *Rhodococcus equi* Isolates from Cuban Patients with AIDS

*Daniel Salazar-Rodríguez [1], Yamilé Aleaga-Santiesteban [1], Enrique Iglesias [2], Arturo Plascencia-Hernández [3], Héctor R. Pérez-Gómez [3], Enrique J. Calderón [4], José A. Vázquez-Boland [5] and Yaxsier de Armas [1,6]**

[1] Department of Clinical Microbiology Diagnostic, Hospital Center of Institute of Tropical Medicine "Pedro Kourí," Havana, Cuba, [2] Departamento de Vacunas, Centro de Ingeniería Genética y Biotecnología, Havana, Cuba, [3] Centro Universitario de Ciencias de la Salud de la Universidad de Guadalajara, Guadalajara, Mexico, [4] Instituto de Biomedicina de Sevilla, Hospital Universitario Virgen del Rocío/Consejo Superior de Investigaciones Científicas/Universidad de Sevilla, Centro de Investigación Biomédica en Red de Epidemiología y Salud Pública (CIBERESP), Seville, Spain, [5] Microbial Pathogenesis Group, Edinburgh Medical School (Biomedical Sciences - Infection Medicine), University of Edinburgh, Edinburgh, United Kingdom, [6] Pathology Department, Hospital Center of Institute of Tropical Medicine "Pedro Kourí," Havana, Cuba

***Correspondence:**
Yaxsier de Armas
yaxsier@ipk.sld.cu

Rhodococcus equi is an animal pathogen and zoonotic human opportunistic pathogen associated with immunosuppressive conditions. The pathogenicity of *R. equi* is linked to three animal host-associated virulence plasmids encoding a family of "Virulence Associated Proteins" (VAPs). Here, the PCR-based TRAVAP molecular typing system for the *R. equi* virulence plasmids was applied to 26 *R. equi* strains isolated between 2010 and 2016 at the Institute of Tropical Medicine "Pedro Kourí," Cuba, from individuals living with HIV/AIDS. TRAVAP detects 4 gene markers, *traA* common to the three virulence plasmids, and *vapA*, *vapB*, and *vapN* specific to each of the host-associated plasmid types (equine pVAPA, porcine pVAPB, and ruminant pVAPN). Of the 26 isolates, six were positive to the *vapB* (porcine-type) marker, 4 (15.4%) to the *vapA* (equine-type) marker, and 1 (3.8%) to the *vapN* (ruminant-type) marker. Most of the isolates 14 (53.8%) were negative to all TRAVAP markers, suggesting they lacked a virulence plasmid. To our knowledge, this work is the first to report the molecular characterization of *R. equi* isolates from Cuba. Our findings provide insight into the zoonotic origin of *R. equi* infections in people and the potential dispensability of the virulence plasmid in immunosuppressed patients.

Keywords: *Rhodococcus equi*, aids, human immunodeficiency virus, Cuba, animal host-associated virulence plasmids, TRAVAP virulence plasmid typing, *R. equi* zoonotic infection

INTRODUCTION

Rhodococcus equi is a well-known horse pathogen first described in 1923 by Magnusson as the causative agent of pyogranulomatous pneumonia and lung abscesses in foals aged <6 months (1). *R. equi* also infects other mammals including pigs, cattle, goats, cats, dogs, and humans, in which the infection is believed to be zoonotic (2). The first case of human infection was reported in an adult receiving immunosuppressive therapy in 1966. In the 1980–90's, *R. equi* emerged as an opportunistic pathogen associated with AIDS and other immunosuppresive conditions such as organ transplant chemotherapy and steroid therapy. In humans, *R. equi* causes purulent bronchopneumonia and occasional extrapulmonary pyogenic infections (3, 4).

R. equi is widelspread in nature, inhabits soil and colonizes the intestine of grazing animals and omnivores. The most likely transmission mechanism is inhalation of the bacteria in aerosolized dust particles. In addition, the accidental inoculation of the microorganism in injuries, mucous membranes or ingestion of contaminated food are other possible routes of infection (5). The pathogen is a facultative intracellular parasite capable of replicating within macrophages, thus evading host defense mechanisms (2, 6, 7).

The pathogenicity of *R. equi* is associated with the presence of a virulence plasmid encoding a family of "Virulence Associated Proteins" (VAPs) (2, 6–8). Two different *R. equi* circular virulence plasmid variants were initially characterized: the VapA-encoding pVAPA, found in virulent isolates of equine origin, and the VapB-encoding pVAPB, found in isolates showing intermediate virulence in mice, recovered from submaxillary lymph nodes of slaughtered pigs and human clinical specimens (2, 9–11). Recently, the VapN-encoding linear virulence plasmid, pVAPN, was identified in isolates from bovids and human clinical specimens (12). These *R. equi* virulence plasmids are animal host-specific, with pVAPA being associated with horses, pVAPB with pigs and pVAPN with cattle (ruminants) (2, 8, 11–13). Human isolates, in contrast, can carry any of the three animal host-associated plasmid types. This finding suggested that humans were accidental hosts for *R. equi* and that human infections had a zoonotic origin (2, 8, 13).

Molecular typing of *R. equi* is insufficiently developed and little is known about the epidemiology and transmission of this multihost pathogen (13). Thus far, there has only been one case report of a human *R. equi* infection in Cuba (14). In this study, we used the PCR-based virulence plasmid typing system developed by Ocampo-Sosa et al. (13), complemented with the novel vapN marker for the ruminant-associated virulence plasmid pVAPN (12), to analyze the virulence plasmid carriage of a series of human *R. equi* strains recently isolated from people living with HIV in Cuba.

MATERIALS AND METHODS

A case series study of 26 isolates of *R. equi* from 26 people living with HIV/AIDS was conducted during the period between January 2010 and December 2016. These isolates were obtained from all the patients with *R. equi* / HIV coinfection (one isolate/patient) admitted to the Hospital Center of Institute of Tropical Medicine "Pedro Kourí" (IPK) during this 7-year period. The isolates belong to the collection of the Department of Clinical Microbiology Diagnostic of the Hospital Center of IPK, Havana, Cuba. No data were available in the clinical records of previous contact of patients with farm animals or farm environments.

R. equi isolates were stored at −70°C and revived by incubation in Muller-Hilton broth at 37°C for 24 h. The colonies from the isolates were used for DNA purification using QIAmp kit (Qiagene, Hilden, Germany) following manufacturer's instructions.

The DNA extracted from each isolate (50 ng) was PCR-amplified in a reaction volume of 50 µL, using the *traA*-, *vapA*-, and *vapB*-specific primers of the TRAVAP typing system (13) updated with additional primers for the *vapN* gene marker for the novel pVAPN plasmid (12). The sequences of the primers are shown in **Supplementary Table 1**, PCR reactions were performed using the modifications reported elsewhere (15). Previously, the isolates were confirmed as *R. equi* based on the amplification of a fragment of the *choE* gene encoding cholesterol oxidase (16).

For the detection of each PCR product, 15 µL of the resulting mixture was run on a 1.6% agarose gel containing ethidium bromide. The visualization of the amplicons was carried out by exposing the gel to ultraviolet light in a transilluminator equipment (Macrovue 2011, LKB, Sweden).

The study was approved by the Ethic Committee of Institute of Tropical Medicine "Pedro Kourí" (CEI-IPK 51-18). It was conducted in accordance with national regulations and the Declaration of Helsinki. All participants signed a written informed consent.

RESULTS

The analysis of the 26 isolates of *R. equi* showed that 4 (15.4%) were positive for the *vapA* gene of the equine-associated pVAPA virulence plasmid. The porcine-associated pVAPB plasmid was identified in six isolates (23.1%), as determined by a positive reaction for the *vapB* gene marker. One isolate gave a positive PCR with the *vapN* marker, suggesting it carried the ruminant-associated pVAPN plasmid. The *traA* gene was detected in a total 11 of the 26 cases analyzed (42.3%). Most isolates in this investigation (53.8%) were TRAVAP negative (i.e., negative to the *traA*, *vapA*, *vapB*, and *vapN* PCR markers). The classification of the isolates according to the TRAVAP system is shown in **Supplementary Table 2** and the percentage distribution of each virulence plasmid type in the analyzed sample in **Supplementary Table 3**.

DISCUSSION

In this study, we provide the first molecular characterization of *R. equi* isolates in people living with HIV/AIDS in Cuba, with a focus on the molecular analysis of the animal host-adapted virulence plasmids using the PCR-based TRAVAP typing method (13). These plasmids, designated pVAPA, pVAPB, and pVAPN (2, 11, 12), enable *R. equi* to, respectively, colonize horses, pigs, and ruminants, while they can at the same time be indistinctly found in isolates recovered from non-adapted animal species (i.e., the case of humans) (2, 8). Because these plasmids are associated with specific animal hosts, it is in principle possible to infer the source of zoonotic transmission of human *R. equi* isolates by determining the type of virulence plasmid they carry. The molecular typing of the *R. equi* virulence plasmids has therefore recently emerged as a tool of great epidemiological importance that can provide valuable insight into the possible sources of human rhodococcal infections (2, 12, 13).

A previous survey involving a global collection of *R. equi* isolates showed that about half of human strains carried a pVAPB (porcine type) plasmid (13), suggesting that exposure to pig farms is a major risk factor. This is consistent with our finding that most of the virulence plasmid-positive Cuban isolates carred the pVAPB plasmid type. Our results are comparable to those of previous studies by Takai et al. in Thailand (10), and Ribeiro et al. in Brazil (17, 18), also involving human isolates from HIV-infected patients, which found that the most abundant plasmid type in these isolates was the porcine (*vapB*$^+$) plasmid type, pVAPB. This indicates that the infection by *R. equi* in the sample of Cuban people living with HIV/AIDS involves, like in other countries, the pig as the probable main source of transmission of the microorganism. Pork is one of the main sources of protein intake by Cuban people and many individuals are in close contact with pigs for breeding and meat trade.

The first of the Vap antigen-encoding virulence plasmids to be identified, by Takai et al. in 1991, was the equine-associated pVAPA (9, 19). This plasmid is as an essential virulence determinant of the pathogen in foals and mice (20). In the present work, four human isolates carrying the pVAPA plasmid were identified. This fact suggests that contact with horses might be another significant source of *R. equi* infection in humans in Cuba (transportation by horse-drawn vehicles is a common practice in rural areas), although of comparatively lesser importance than pigs or pig farm environments.

The *traA* gene, used in the TRAVAP typing scheme as an indicator of "presence of a virulence plasmid" (13), encodes a putative conjugative relaxase that is conserved in the three host-associated virulence plasmid types (11, 12). Ocampo et al. demonstrated that of 89 *vapA/B*-negative strains, 40 (44.9%) tested positive for the *traA* gene, indicating that they could also contain a plasmid (13). This *traA*$^+$/*vapAB*$^-$ genotype was later shown to correspond to strains carrying the bovine (ruminant)-associated pVAPN (12). In the study by Ocampo-Sosa et al., as many as 26% of the human isolates analyzed carried the bovine-associated *traA*$^+$/*vapAB*$^-$ (pVAPN) plasmid, suggesting that cattle farm environments are a significant source of human *R. equi* infections. This does not seem to be the case in Cuba, because in the series of 26 isolates analyzed here, only one (3.8%) was positive to the *vapN* marker. Our data are comparable to those of Ribeiro et al. in Brazil, who found that only two out of 74 *R. equi* strains isolated from the lungs of HIV/AIDS patients in the period 1997–2016 carried the *vapN*$^+$ (pVAPN) plasmid (17).

It must be noted that before the introduction of the *traA* marker in 2006 (13), many of the *traA*$^+$/*vapAB*$^-$ (pVAPN) strains—mostly bovine and human clinical isolates—were initially considered to be devoid of a virulence plasmid. This means that all the *R. equi* literature prior to the discovery of the *traA* (13) and *vapN* (12) gene markers, particularly those studies reporting "avirulent/plasmidless" human isolates, must be interpreted with caution. Nevertheless, a significant proportion of *R. equi* human isolates (23 to 43%) actually appear to be devoid of a virulence plasmid, as judged by their negative reaction to the TRAVAP markers (13, 15). This seems to be the case for most of the human strains analyzed in our study, in which the TRAVAP-negative genotype clearly predominated (53.8% of isolates). This high percentage of "avirulent/plasmidless" isolates could be explained by the increased susceptibility of people living with HIV, which may render the virulence plasmid dispensable for *R. equi* to cause an infection. About half of environmental soil isolates of *R. equi* lack a virulence plasmid (13), presumably because it imposes a fitness cost during saprophytic growth in the absence of host selection (2, 8). It is therefore possible to speculate that the *R. equi* strains found in human patients could primarily be non-virulent environmental isolates not directly associated with an animal host. Alternatively, the strains could have lost the plasmid during subculturing in the laboratory. Indeed, spontaneous virulence plasmid curing can be observed during *in vitro* growth of *R. equi* at 37°C (21, 22). However, it cannot be excluded that some of the 14 TRAVAP-negative isolates might harbor some unknown plasmid encoding novel virulent determinants.

Finally, one isolate was positive to *traA* but negative to each of the plasmid type-specific markers *vapA*, *vapB*, and *vapN*. A similar situation was previously observed in a human isolate in a study performed in the United State of America (15), suggesting that there might be microvariability in some of the virulence plasmids' PCR target sequences. An alternative and more interesting possibility is that this may reflect the existence of an additional virulence plasmid type(s) yet to be characterized. It is also worth noting that the *vapN*$^+$ isolate was negative for *traA*, suggesting the existence of microvariability in the *traA* sequence (the *traA* gene is actually a pseudogene in the pVAPN plasmid and is thus theoretically prone to genetic drift) (12). The possibility of TRAVAP gene marker variability may also in part account for the lack of detection of the virulence plasmid in a number of the "avirulent/plasmidless" *R. equi* isolates.

Our study has three limitations: (i) small sample size ($n = 26$), although the isolates were obtained in a period of 7 years and included all cases of *R equi* / HIV coinfection admitted at IPK hospital; (ii) we did not isolate/sequence the virulence plasmids, which would have provided insight into their genetic makeup or the variability underlying the unusual *traA*$^+$/*vapABN*$^-$ and *traA*$^-$/*vapAB*$^-$/*vapN*$^+$ TRAVAP genotypes; and (iii) a history of contact with farm animals, manure or occupational exposure to farm environments was not available from the clinical records. In any case, this study has value in that it is the first, to our knowledge, in reporting the molecular characterization of *R. equi* isolates in people living with HIV/AIDS in Cuba, and indeed in the Caribbean islands.

In summary, our study provides interesting insight into possible animal sources of *R. equi* infection in AIDS patients from Cuba, of value to public health authorities and, more generally, in the interpretation of the epidemiology of *R. equi* infections in people.

AUTHOR CONTRIBUTIONS

YA, EC, and JV-B: conceptualization and supervision. DS-R, YA-S, EI, JV-B, and YA: methodology. AP-H and HP-G: formal analysis. YA, EI, EC, and JV-B: data curation and writing—review and editing. DS-R, YA-S, AP-H, and HP-G: writing—original draft preparation. DS-R and YA-S: visualization. All authors have read and agreed to the published version of the manuscript.

REFERENCES

1. Vázquez-Boland JA, Scortti M, Meijer WG. Conservation of *Rhodococcus equi* (Magnusson 1923) Goodfellow and Alderson 1977 and rejection of *Rhodococcus hoagii* (Morse 1912) Kämpfer et al. 2014. *Int J Syst Evol Microbiol.* (2020) 70:3572–6. doi: 10.1099/ijsem.0.004090
2. Vázquez-Boland JA, Meijer WG. The pathogenic actinobacterium *Rhodococcus equi*: what's in a name? *Mol Microbiol.* (2019) 112:1–15. doi: 10.1111/mmi.14267
3. Takai S, Sawada N, Nakayama Y, Ishizuka S, Nakagawa R, Kawashima G, et al. Reinvestigation of the virulence of *Rhodococcus equi* isolates from patients with and without AIDS. *Lett Appl Microbiol.* (2020) 71:679–83. doi: 10.1111/lam.13386
4. Vergidis P, Ariza-Heredia EJ, Nellore A, Kotton CN, Kaul DR, Morris MI, et al. Rhodococcus infection in solid organ and hematopoietic stem cell transplant recipients. *Emerg Infect Dis.* (2017) 23:510–12. doi: 10.3201/eid2303.160633
5. Muscatello G, Leadon DP, Klay M, Ocampo-Sosa A, Lewis DA, Fogarty U, et al. *Rhodococcus equi* infection in foals: the science of "rattles." *Equine Vet J.* (2007) 39:470–8. doi: 10.2746/042516407X209217
6. von Bargen K, Haas A. Molecular and infection biology of the horse pathogen *Rhodococcus equi*. *FEMS Microbiol Rev.* (2009) 33:870–91. doi: 10.1111/j.1574-6976.2009.00181.x
7. Willingham-Lane JM, Berghaus LJ, Giguère S, Hondalus MK. Influence of plasmid type on the replication of *Rhodococcus equi* in host macrophages. *mSphere.* (2016) 1:e00186-16. doi: 10.1128/mSphere.00186-16
8. MacArthur I, Anastasi E, Alvarez S, Scortti M, Vázquez-Boland JA. Comparative genomics of *Rhodococcus equi* virulence plasmids indicates host-driven evolution of the vap Pathogenicity Island. *Genome Biol Evol.* (2017) 9:1241–7. doi: 10.1093/gbe/evx057
9. Takai S, Hines SA, Sekizaki T, Nicholson VM, Alperin, DA, Osaki M, et al. DNA sequence and comparison of virulence plasmids from *Rhodococcus equi* ATCC 33701 and 103. *Infect Immun.* (2000) 68:6840–7. doi: 10.1128/IAI.68.12.6840-6847.2000
10. Takai S, Tharavichitkul P, Takarn P, Khantawa B, Tamura M, Tsukamoto A, et al. Molecular epidemiology of *Rhodococcus equi* of intermediate virulence isolated from patients with and without acquired immune deficiency syndrome in Chiang Mai, Thailand. *J Infect Dis.* (2003) 188:1717–23. doi: 10.1086/379739
11. Letek M, Ocampo-Sosa AA, Sanders M, Fogarty U, Buckley T, Leadon DP, et al. Evolution of the *Rhodococcus equi* vap pathogenicity island seen through comparison of host-associated *vapA* and *vapB* virulence plasmids. *J Bacteriol.* (2008) 190:5797–805. doi: 10.1128/JB.00468-08

ACKNOWLEDGMENTS

JV-B would like to thank the Horserace Betting Levy Board (UK) for supporting *R. equi* research in his laboratory (grants prj 764/70 and prj 796).

12. Valero-Rello A, Hapeshi A, Anastasi E, Alvarez S, Scortti M, Meijer WG, et al. Invertron-like linear plasmid mediates intracellular survival and virulence in bovine isolates of *Rhodococcus equi*. *Infect Immun.* (2015) 83:2725–37. doi: 10.1128/IAI.00376-15
13. Ocampo-Sosa A, Lewis DA, Navas J, Quigley F, Callejo R, Scortti M, et al. Molecular epidemiology of *Rhodococcus equi* based on *traA*, *vapA*, and *vapB* virulence plasmid markers. *J Infect Dis.* (2007) 196:763–9. doi: 10.1086/519688
14. Salazar Rodríguez D, Migdalia Reyes T, Rodríguez Delgado F, Bandera Tirado F, Reyes Pérez A, Medina Almenares VZ, et al. First molecular detection of *Rhodococcus equi* in a HIV/AIDS patient in Cuba. *Rev Cubana Med Trop.* (2011) 63:253–6.
15. Bryan LK, Alexander ER, Lawhon SD, Cohen ND. Detection of *vapN* in *Rhodococcus equi* isolates cultured from humans. *PLoS ONE.* (2020) 15:e0235719. doi: 10.1371/journal.pone.0235719
16. Ladrón N, Fernández M, Agüero J, González Zörn B, Vázquez-Boland JA, Navas J. Rapid identification of *Rhodococcus equi* by a PCR assay targeting the *choE* gene *J Clin Microbiol.* (2003) 41:3241–5. doi: 10.1128/JCM.41.7.3241-3245.2003
17. Ribeiro MG, Lara GHB, da Silva P, Franco MMJ, de Mattos-Guaraldi AL, de Vargas APC, et al. Novel bovine-associated pVAPN plasmid type in *Rhodococcus equi* identified from lymph nodes of slaughtered cattle and lungs of people living with HIV/AIDS. *Transbound Emerg Dis.* (2018) 65:321–6. doi: 10.1111/tbed.12785
18. Ribeiro MG, Takai S, de Vargas AC, Mattos-Guaraldi AL, Ferreira Camello TC, Ohno R, et al. Identification of virulence-associated plasmids in *Rhodococcus equi* in humans with and without acquired immunodeficiency syndrome in Brazil. *Am J Trop Med Hyg.* (2011) 85:510–3. doi: 10.4269/ajtmh.2011.10-0695
19. Takai S, Koike K, Ohbushi S, Izumi C, Tsubaki S. Identification of 15- to 17-kilodalton antigens associated with virulent *Rhodococcus equi*. *J Clin Microbiol.* (1991) 29:439–43. doi: 10.1128/JCM.29.3.439-443.1991
20. Giguere S, Hondalus MK, Yager JA, Darrah P, Mosser DM, Prescott JF. Role of the 85- kilobase plasmid and plasmid- encoded virulence- associated protein A in intracellular survival and virulence of *Rhodococcus equi*. *Infect Immun.* (1999) 67:3548–57. doi: 10.1128/IAI.67.7.3548-3557.1999
21. Takai S, Sugawara YT, Watanabe Y, Sasaki Y, Tsubaki S, Sekizaki, T. Effect of growth temperature on maintenance of virulent *Rhodococcus equi*. *Vet Microbiol.* (1994) 39:187–92. doi: 10.1016/0378-1135(94)90099-X
22. González-Iglesias P, Scortti M, MacArthur I, Hapeshi A, Rodriguez H, Prescott JF, et al. Mouse lung infection model to assess *Rhodococcus equi* virulence and vaccine protection. *Vet Microbiol.* (2014) 172:256–64. doi: 10.1016/j.vetmic.2014.03.026

15

Chagas Disease in Pregnant Women in the Peruvian Amazon Basin

José-Manuel Ramos-Rincón [1,2†], Sonia Ortiz-Martínez [3†], María-Esteyner Vásquez-Chasnamote [4], Olga-Nohelia Gamboa-Paredes [5], Viviana-Vanessa Pinedo-Cancino [6], Cesar Ramal-Asayag [7,8], Miguel Górgolas-Hernández-Mora [9,10] and Martin Casapía-Morales [7,8,11] on behalf of the Spanish-Peruvian Chagas, HTLV and Strongyloides Network*

[1] Clinical Medicine Department, University Miguel Hernández de Elche, Alicante, Spain, [2] Internal Medicine Service, General University Hospital of Alicante-ISABIAL, Alicante, Spain, [3] Medical Practice El Ballestero, Health Service of Castilla La Mancha, Albacete, Spain, [4] Natural Resources Research Center, Peruvian Amazon National University, Iquitos, Peru, [5] Research Assistant, Amazon Rainforest Civil Association, Iquitos, Peru, [6] Molecular Biology and Immunology Laboratory of the Specialized Unit of LIPNAA-CIRNA, Peruvian Amazon National University, Iquitos, Peru, [7] Infectious Diseases and Tropical Medicine Service, Loreto Regional Hospital, Iquitos, Peru, [8] School of Medicine, National University of the Peruvian Amazon, Iquitos, Peru, [9] Infectious Disease Division, University Hospital Foundation Jiménez Díaz, Madrid, Spain, [10] Medicine Department, Autonomous University of Madrid, Madrid, Spain, [11] Medical Department, Amazon Rainforest Civil Association, Iquitos, Peru

***Correspondence:**
José-Manuel Ramos-Rincón
jose.ramosr@umh.es

† These authors have contributed equally to this work

Aims: To assess the prevalence of Chagas disease in pregnant women in Iquitos City, Peru.

Material and Methods: Cross-sectional survey in 300 pregnant women in Iquitos (Peru) from 1 May 2019 to 15 June 2019. Women were tested using an ELISA serology test.

Results: Serology was positive in one case (prevalence: 0.33%; 95% confidence interval: 7.1–13.9%), of a 25-year-old woman who lived in a wooden house with a leaf roof in a periurban area of Iquitos. She was familiar with kissing bugs and had chronic, asymptomatic Chagas disease.

Conclusion: The prevalence of Chagas disease is low in the urban and peri-urban area of the city of Iquitos.

Keywords: Chagas disease, *Trypanosoma cruzi*, pregnant, Peru, Amazon

INTRODUCTION

Chagas disease is a systemic chronic parasitic infection caused by *Trypanosoma cruzi* that affects 6–7 million people in Central and South America. It is considered a neglected tropical disease and has a high public health impact in the area.

While mainly vector-borne, Chagas disease can also be spread via blood transfusion, transplantation, or from mother to child (1). The latter, congenital route is frequent and especially relevant in areas where there is no vector transmission by insects or blood transfusion. To accelerate the elimination of this transmission route, strategies and methods should be applied to screen, diagnose, and treat all infected pregnant women as well as their newborns and, where appropriate, other children as soon as possible (2).

Chagas disease is endemic throughout the Pacific southwest of Peru, known as the Greater Southern Region, in the departments of Arequipa, Moquegua, Tacna, Ayacucho and Apurimac.

In the past decade, widespread infestation with the vector *Triatoma infestans* and active transmission of Chagas disease to humans have been documented in this area (3, 4). In addition, the northeastern departments of Cajamarca, Amazonas, San Martín, and Ucayali (400–1,000 m above sea level) have also detected the thriving presence of the *Panstrongylus herreri* vector (3). However, there is little knowledge about the prevalence and epidemiology of *Trypanosoma cruzi* in northern Peru (5); the most significant resources have been allocated toward research and control efforts in the south (5).

Iquitos is a city in the Peruvian Amazon Basin, in the Department of Loreto and near the confluence of the Marañon and Ucayali rivers. A few isolated cases of Chagas disease have been documented in the town and surroundings areas (6), but no survey has ever focused on the pregnant population. As these women can unknowingly transmit the disease to their newborns, its detection is highly recommended (2, 7). The aim of this study was to estimate the prevalence of Chagas disease in pregnant women in Iquitos, Peru, in the Peruvian Amazon basin.

METHODS

Setting and Study Period

We performed a cross-sectional survey of Chagas disease, strongyloidiasis, and human T-cell leukemia-lymphoma virus (HTLV) infection in an urban and periurban area of Iquitos (Peruvian Amazon) (**Figure 1**), from 1 May 2019 to 15 June 2019.

Study Population

We included pregnant women attending the health centers in four districts of the greater Iquitos area, located in the Peruvian Amazon. Participants were adults over the age of 18 years and were selected through convenience sampling (i.e., on days when the researcher was at the health center) when they visited the midwife during prenatal check-ups. All participants were informed about the screening and signed informed consent.

Data Collection

On enrollment, participants were asked about sociodemographic variables and their familiarity with Chagas disease. We obtained a blood sample for serological detection of *T. cruzi* antibodies, *S. stercoralis* IgG antibodies, and HTLV antibodies, and a stool sample to test for parasitic infections. Our group published results on the prevalence of strongyloidiasis and other intestinal parasites in a parallel report (8).

Detection of *T. cruzi* IgG antibodies was performed by two different assays: the Chagatest ELISA lysate (Wiener, Rosario, Argentina) and the Chagatest ELISA recombinant v.4.0 (Wiener, Rosario, Argentina). *T. cruzi* infection was considered confirmed if both tests yielded a positive result, while participants were considered seronegative when both tests yielded negative results. Specimens with only one positive test were considered inconclusive. The Chagatests were completed according to manufacturer's instructions and the threshold for positive results was 0.10 optical density (OD) units above the mean absorbance of two negative control specimens included on each plate.

Data Analysis

The collected data were systematically recorded and analyzed using IBM SPSS Statistics, version 22.0. We used the chi-squared test or Fisher's exact test to determine the presence of Chagas disease according to several demographic variables, considering results to be significant where the $P < 0.05$.

RESULTS

The study included 300 pregnant women with a mean age of 26.7 years (standard deviation [SD] 6.4; range 13–38), mean of number of deliveries of 2.9 (SD: 1.7), and a mean gestation period of 172 days (SD: 59). Just under half (44.7%) lived in peri-urban areas, while the rest lived in the city. **Table 1** shows the sociodemographic and epidemiological characteristics of the participants in the study. **Figure 1** Health centers in Iquitos city and surrounding area.

Four participants tested positive on the Chagatest ELISA recombinant v.4.0 with titers > 0.2, but only one had a second positive serology test (Chagatest ELISA lysate) (**Table 2**). Therefore, just one participant (0.33%, 95% CI: 0.02–2.13%) was considered as a definitive positive for Chagas disease. Three other participants had inconclusive results by both ELISAs. Their infection status therefore remained unresolved, and their data were excluded from further analysis. There were no statistically significant differences in the sociodemographic conditions, knowledge of Chagas disease, or housing conditions in cases with positive and negative serology against *T. cruzi*.

The positive case was a 25-year-old woman who lived in a periurban area of Iquitos (**Figure 1**). She had been living in the same house—a wooden construction with a leaf roof—for the last 5 years. She had two other children and was familiar with the "chirimacha" (kissing bugs or triatomines) and reported seeing them at home, but she did not remember being bitten by one. She had not received any blood transfusion and did not have any symptoms of Chagas disease (chest pain, palpitation, dysphagia). Her electrocardiogram was normal, showing a repolarization disorder.

DISCUSSION

Our study demonstrates that the prevalence of asymptomatic Chagas disease in pregnant women is low (0.33%) in the Iquitos area of the Peruvian Amazon Basin. This evidence helps to fill gaps in knowledge arising from the few seroprevalence studies in pregnant women in Peru (7). In 2005, a study performed in Arequipa (southern Peru) in 3,000 pregnant women showed serological positives in 22 (0.7%) participants; only one newborn was IgM positive (9).

The prevalence of Chagas disease in pregnant women, both in our study and the one performed in Arequipa, is low compared to those performed in Bolivia, northern Argentina, or Brazil, which have reported a prevalence of 21, 12.1, and 1.1%, respectively (10–12). In the general population, the literature reports a seroprevalence of Chagas disease in the southern department of Arequipa ranging from 2 to 5.8% (4, 13, 14). In

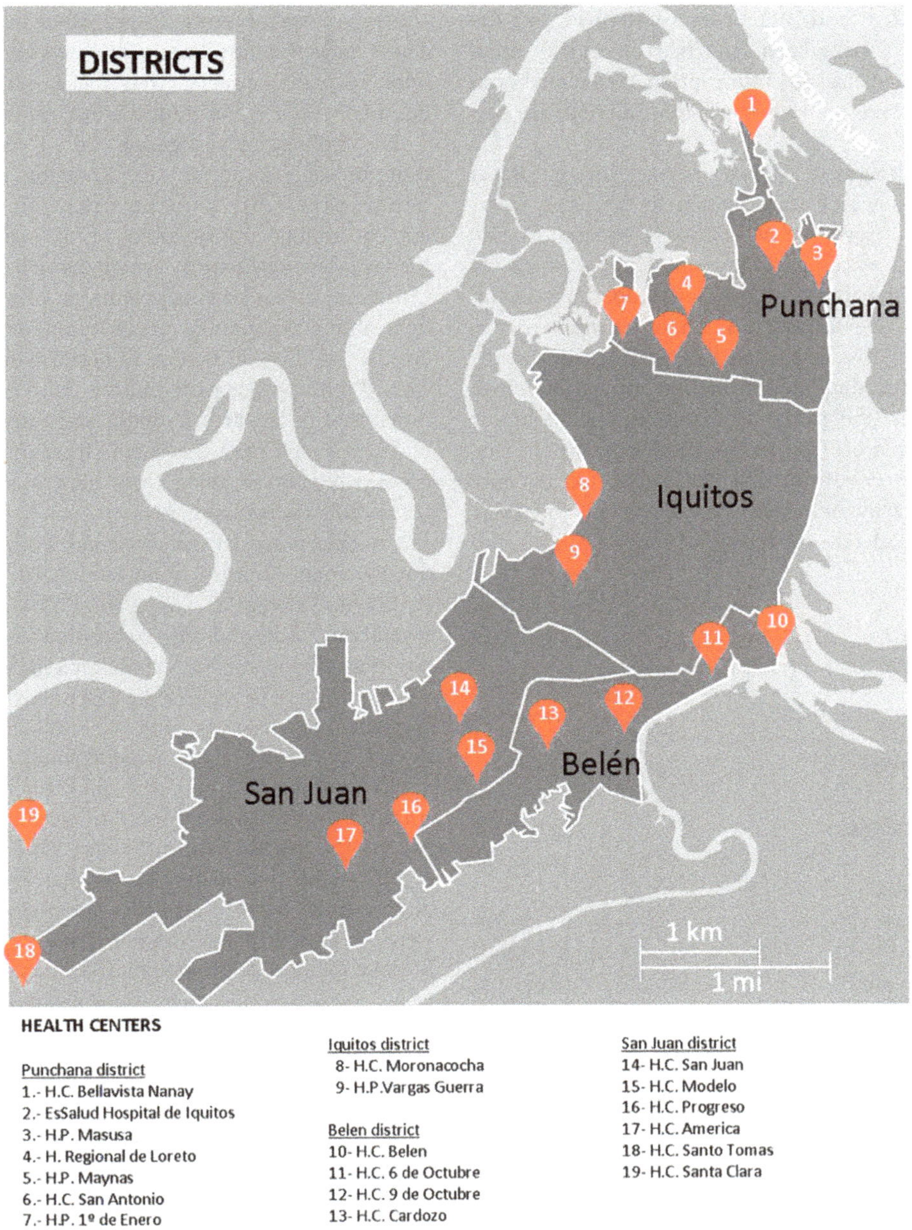

FIGURE 1 | Health centers in Iquitos city and surrounding area.

the north (La Joya and Cajamarca departments), prevalence is slightly higher, between 7.6 and 14.9% (5, 15). Our results from Iquitos are sensibly lower than in these reports from elsewhere in Peru.

However, our results are relevant because they show that Chagas disease, although uncommon, is actually present in the Iquitos area. Asymptomatic Chagas disease cases like the one detected in our survey do occur. Other acute cases have previously been reported in 2006 and 2008 in the Amazon area (6, 16, 17). Therefore, Chagas disease is present not only in the jungle of northern Peru (5) but also in the Amazon basin. That said, seroprevalence of *T. cruzi* in pregnant women appears to be lower than that reported in the endemic areas of Peru (9). There may be small pockets of vector transmission of Chagas disease in Iquitos. Performing small studies around this case could help to uncover more; this adaptive strategy could efficiently identify secondary cases (13).

Chagas disease has been studied elsewhere in the Amazon basin, including in Ecuador [prevalence 3.6% (18)] and in Brazil (seroprevalence 1.5%). Throughout all these areas, Chagas continues to pose a threat to public health, one amplified by deforestation and its associated changes in transmission vectors

(19, 20). Indeed, this region is at risk of transmission due to triatomine-contaminated food (21). Several initiatives, like the Iniciativa Andina (IA), have been launched in priority areas of Latin America to ensure the interruption of vector-borne transmission of Chagas as well as to improve surveillance and disease prevention (22).

The presence of pregnant women in the Amazon Basin who are at risk of congenital transmission to the fetus, along with other reported cases of acute Chagas Diseases (6, 16, 17) should serve as a warning of an (emerging) problem in this area of Peru. While the low prevalence does not justify screening in pregnant or puerperal women, other measures are called for. WHO/PAHO recommends interventions to disrupt vector transmission, including the elimination of the triatomines or other vectors from the study area; another possibility is assessing seroprevalence of *T. cruzi* infection in children 5 or younger (23). Several environmental and social factors may also directly or indirectly influence the biology and behavior of triatomides (24). Spatial clustering of infestation in the urban context may both challenge and inform surveillance and control of vector reemergence after insecticide intervention. These measures have been performed in several departments in Peru, such as Moquegua and Tacna, which were subsequently declared free of vector transmission by the WHO/PAHO (25).

TABLE 1 | Epidemiological characteristics of pregnant women.

Variables	Frequency
Sociodemographic conditions	
Mean age (years)	26 (SD: 6.4)
Mean time living in the place (years)	9.9 (SD: 9.7)
Residence in rural area	134 (44.7%)
Characteristics of pregnancy	
Mean gestational age (days)	172 (SD: 59)
Primiparous	64 (21.3%)
Mean number of pregnancies	2.9 (SD: 1.7)
Mean number of children alive	1.8 (SD: 1.5)
Risk factors for Chagas disease	
History of blood transfusion	15 (5.0%)
Knowledge of Chagas disease	
Any knowledge about Chagas disease	10 (3.3%)
Contact with person with Chagas disease	0 (0.0%)
Characteristics of living houses	
Wood house	286 (95.3%)
Leaf roof	234 (78.0%)
Soil floor	89 (29.7%)

SD, standard deviation.

Entomologic investigation of *T. infentans* and other triatomides is important for knowing the ecology of vector transmission (26). It is important to implement measures for controlling transmission of *T. cruzi* by triatomines in the Amazon basin, with vector surveillance and control with insecticide as has been happening in other parts of Peru (5). In light of our exploratory results and other cases reported in the area, it could be of interest to perform similar studies to those carried out in other parts of Peru (15, 17, 23). Another topic to investigate in the area is dogs, which are important reservoirs of *T. cruzi* and may play a role in reinitiating transmission in previously sprayed areas. Dogs may also serve as indicators of reemerging transmission (24).

Another potential line of research about Chagas disease in the Peruvian Amazon basin is the risk of oral transmission. In Brazil, Venezuela, Colombia, Bolivia, and French Guiana, several outbreaks of orally transmitted Chagas disease have been reported; these have been epidemiologically associated with the consumption of beverages like açai juice (the fruit from a species of palm tree) or sugar cane juice (27). Some cases of Chagas disease have also been described in young indigenous people who drank contaminated juice (17, 26). This line of research should continue in the area, as should health education, in order to prevent the contamination of juice with *T. infestans* excreta (26).

This study has some limitations. First, a complete study of congenital transmission was not performed. Secondly, there were three participants with borderline results according to both ELISAs. As this situation might reflect a window period, it would be necessary to re-test them after 6 months to confirm or rule out infection. Finally, there was no entomologic investigation about species living at the patient's home.

CONCLUSIONS

Although the prevalence of Chagas disease is low in the urban and peri-urban area of the city of Iquitos, it is relevant to advise local authorities that the disease is actually present in the Peruvian Amazon Basin in pregnant women with a risk of congenital transmission. Our results indicate a probable low rate,

TABLE 2 | Results of two serological procedures in positive cases.

Code	Age/health center	Antecedents blood transfusion	Chagatest ELISA recombinant v.4.0 titers	Chagatest ELISA lysate titers	Chagas disease
1	25 years/santa clara	No	1.118	1.416	Yes
2	19 years/san juan	No	0.267	0.011	Inconcusive
3	33 years/san juan	No	0.237	0.029	Inconcusive
4	19 years/San juan	No	0.301	0.038	Inconcusive

but it is necessary to perform more studies and monitor the prevalence of the disease.

AUTHOR CONTRIBUTIONS

J-MR-R: conceptualization, formal analysis, methodology, project administration, supervision, writing—original draft, writing-review and editing, designed the study, analyzed clinical data, prepared, and reviewed the manuscript. SO-M: formal analysis, investigation, project administration, software, supervision, writing—original draft, and writing-review and editing. M-EV-C: methodology and writing-review and editing. O-NG-P: data citation, software, supervision, and writing-review and editing. V-VP-C: data curation, methodology, project administration, and writing-review and editing. CR-A: investigation and writing-review and editing. MG-H-M: conceptualization, writing—original draft, and writing-review and editing. MC-M: conceptualization, project administration, writing—original draft, and writing-review and editing manuscript. All authors contributed to the article and approved the submitted version.

ACKNOWLEDGMENTS

We want to thank all members of the Spanish-Peruvian Chagas, HTLV and Strongyloides Network for their active contribution to the study. We are also grateful to Maria Flores from the Parasitology Service, National Center for Microbiology, Health Institute Carlos III (Madrid, Spain), and Mundo Sano Foundation (Madrid, Spain) for her critical review of the articles and our manuscript. We also express our thanks to Meggan Harris for her assistance in editing this paper and to Jesús Alarcón Utrilla for his assistance in the realization of the figure. **Members of the Spanish-Peruvian Chagas, HTLV and Strongyloides Network**: J.M. Ramos-Rincón & A. Gimeno (Hospital General Universitario Alicante & Universidad Miguel Hernández, Alicante, Spain), J. Llenas-García (Hospital Vega Baja, Orihuela, Spain), M. Górgolas-Hernández-Mora, R. Pérez-Tanoira & L. Prieto (Hospital Universitario Fundación Jiménez-Díaz & Universidad Autónoma de Madrid, Madrid, Spain), S. Ortiz-Martínez (Consultorio El Ballestero, Albacete, Spain) M.E. Vásquez-Chasnamote (Centro de Investigación de Recursos Naturales, Universidad Nacional de la Amazonia Peruana. Iquitos, Peru), O.N. Gamboa-Paredes, J. Parraguez-de-la-Cruz J.J. Alarcón-Baldeón, P. Schillyk-Guerra, J. Bardales-Vásquez, G. Pérez-Bardales, A. Hernández-Vargas, T. Zumaeta Silva, & R.P. Pezo-Flores (Asociación Civil Selva Amazónica, Iquitos, Perú), L.A. Espinoza-Venegas & C. Ramal-Asayag (Hospital Regional de Loreto, Iquitos, Perú), V.V. Pinedo Cancino. Laboratorio de Biología Molecular e Inmunología de la Unidad Especializada, Universidad Nacional de la Amazonia Peruana & Asociación Civil Selva Amazónica, Iquitos, Perú) & Martín Casapía Morales (Hospital Regional de Loreto, & Asociación Civil Selva Amazónica, Universidad Nacional de la Amazonia Peruana, Iquitos, Perú).

REFERENCES

1. Pérez-Molina JA, Molina I. Chagas disease. *Lancet.* (2018) 391:82–94. doi: 10.1016/S0140-6736(17)31612-4
2. Organización Panamericana de la Salud. Nuevas generaciones sin la infección por el VIH, la sífilis, la hepatitis B y la enfermedad de Chagas en las Américas 2018. *ETMI Plus.* Washington, DC: OPS (2019).
3. Cornejo JG, Carpio D. *The Chagasic Endemic Situation in Peru.* (2003). Available online at: http://www.fac.org.ar/tcvc/llave/c296/cornejo.PDF (accessed May 10, 2020).
4. Bowman NM, Kawai V, Levy MZ, Cornejo del Carpio JG, Cabrera L, Delgado F, et al. Chagas disease transmission in periurban communities of arequipa, Peru. *Clin Infect Dis.* (2008) 46:1822–8. doi: 10.1086/588299
5. Alroy KA, Huang C, Gilman RH, Quispe-Machaca VR, Marks MA, Ancca-Juarez J, et al. Prevalence and transmission of trypanosoma cruzi in people of rural communities of the high jungle of Northern Peru. *PLoS Negl Trop Dis.* (2015) 9:e0003779. doi: 10.1371/journal.pntd.0003779
6. Cabrera R, Vega S, Cáceres AG, Ramal AC, Álvarez C., Ladera P, et al. Epidemiological investigation of an acute case of chagas disease in an area of active transmission in Peruvian Amazon region. *Rev Inst Med Trop São Paulo.* (2010) 52:269–72. doi: 10.1590/S0036-46652010000500009
7. Velarde C-N. [Chagas disease in Peru: congenital transmission]. *Rev Soc Bras Med Trop.* (2005) 38(Suppl 2):55–7.
8. Ortiz-Martínez S, Ramos-Rincón JM, Vásquez-Chasnamote ME, Alarcón-Baldeón JJ, Parraguez-De-La-Cruz J, Gamboa-Paredes ON, et al. A cross-sectional study of seroprevalence of strongyloidiasis in pregnant women (Peruvian amazon basin). *Pathogens.* (2020) 9:348. doi: 10.3390/pathogens9050348
9. Mendoza Ticona CA, Córdova Benzaquen E, Ancca Juárez J, Saldaña Díaz J, Torres Choque A, Velásquez Talavera R, et al. Prevalencia de la enfermedad de Chagas en puérperas y transmisión congénita en una zona endémica del Perú. *Rev Panam Salud Pub Pan Am J Public Heal.* (2005) 17:147–53. doi: 10.1590/S1020-49892005000300001
10. Rendell VR, Gilman RH, Valencia E, Galdos-Cardenas G, Verastegui M, Sanchez L, et al. Trypanosoma cruzi-infected pregnant women without vector exposure have higher parasitemia levels: Implications for congenital transmission risk. *PLoS ONE.* (2015) 10:e0119527. doi: 10.1371/journal.pone.0119527
11. Contreras S, Fernandez MR, Agüero F, Desse Desse J, Orduna T, Martino O. Congenital chagas-mazza disease in salta, argentina. *Rev Soc Bras Med Trop.* (1999) 32:633–6. doi: 10.1590/S0037-86821999000600004
12. Martins-Melo FR, da Silveira Lima M, Ramos AN, Alencar CH, Heukelbach J. Systematic review: prevalence of chagas disease in pregnant women and congenital transmission of *Trypanosoma cruzi* in Brazil: a systematic review and meta-analysis. *Trop Med Int Heal.* (2014) 19:943–57. doi: 10.1111/tmi.12328
13. Levy MZ, Kawai V, Bowman NM, Waller LA, Cabrera L, Pinedo-Cancino VV, et al. Targeted screening strategies to detect Trypanosoma cruzi infection in children. *PLoS Negl Trop Dis.* (2007) 1:e103. doi: 10.1371/journal.pntd.0000103
14. Hunter GC, Borrini-Mayorí K, Ancca Juárez J, Castillo Neyra R, Verastegui MR, Malaga Chavez FS, et al. A field trial of alternative targeted screening strategies for chagas disease in Arequipa, Peru. *PLoS Negl Trop Dis.* (2012) 6:e1468. doi: 10.1371/journal.pntd.0001468
15. Delgado S, Neyra RC, Machaca VRQ, Juárez JA, Chu LC, Verastegui MR, et al. A history of Chagas disease transmission, control, and re-emergence in peri-rural La Joya, Peru. *PLoS Negl Trop Dis.* (2011) 5:e970. doi: 10.1371/journal.pntd.0000970
16. Asayag CR, Garay CR, Meza Sanchez G, Angeles C, Jara Baca C, Evans C, et al. Images in clinical tropical medicine eight year old with fever, hepatomegaly, and positive thick smear. *Am J Trop Med Hyg.* (2008) 79:473. doi: 10.4269/ajtmh.2008.79.473
17. Cabrera R, Vega S, Valderrama Y, Cabanillas K, Fernández C, Rodríguez O, et al. New focus of active transmission of Chagas disease in indigenous populations in the Peruvian Amazon basin. *Rev Soc Bras Med Trop.* (2013)

46:367–72. doi: 10.1590/0037-8682-1195-2013

18. Amunarriz M, Quito S, Tandazo V, López M. Seroprevalencia de la enfermedad de chagas en el cantón Aguarico, Amazonia ecuatoriana. *Rev Panam Salud Pub Pan Am J Public Heal.* (2010) 28:25–9. doi: 10.1590/S1020-49892010000700004
19. Magalhães BML, Coelho LIARC, Maciel MG, Ferreira JMBB, Umezawa ES, Coura JR, et al. Inquérito sorológico para doença de chagas em áreas rurais de Manaus, Coari e Tefé na Amazônia Ocidental. *Rev Soc Bras Med Trop.* (2011) 44:697–702. doi: 10.1590/S0037-86822011000600009
20. Castro MCM, Barrett TV, Santos WS, Abad-Franch F, Rafael JA. Attraction of Chagas disease vectors (Triatominae) to artificial light sources in the canopy of primary Amazon rainforest. *Mem Inst Oswaldo Cruz.* (2010) 105:1061–4. doi: 10.1590/S0074-02762010000800019
21. Pinto AYDN, Valente SA, Valente VDC, Ferreira AG, Coura JR. Fase aguda da doença de Chagas na Amazônia brasileira. Estudo de 233 casos do Pará, Amapá e Maranhão observados entre 1988 e 2005. *Rev Soc Bras Med Trop.* (2008) 41:602–14. doi: 10.1590/S0037-86822008000600011
22. Anonimous. X. *Reunión de la Comisión Intergubernamental de la Iniciativa Andina de Control de la Transmisión Vectorial y Transfusional de la Enfermedad de Chagas IPA-y VI Reunón de la Iniciativa Gubernamental de Vigilancia y Prevención de la Enfermedad de Chagas en.* (2020). Available online at: https://www.paho.org/hq/dmdocuments/2012/X-Reunion-AMCHA-2011.pdf (accessed June 2, 2020).
23. Buttenheim AM, Levy MZ, Castillo-Neyra R, McGuire M, Toledo Vizcarra AM, Mollesaca Riveros LM, et al. A behavioral design approach to improving a Chagas disease vector control campaign in Peru. *BMC Pub Health.* (2019) 19:1272. doi: 10.1186/s12889-019-7525-3
24. Castillo-Neyra R, Chou Chu L, Quispe-Machaca V, Ancca-Juarez J, Malaga Chavez FS, Bastos Mazuelos M, et al. The potential of canine sentinels for reemerging *Trypanosoma cruzi* transmission. *Prev Vet Med.* (2015) 120:349–56. doi: 10.1016/j.prevetmed.2015.04.014
25. Náquira C. [Urbanization of Chagas disease in Peru: experiences in prevention and control]. *Rev Peru Med Exp Salud Pub.* (2014) 31:343–7.
26. Cabrera R, Valderrama Y, Meza JR. Perception about chagas disease and the risk of oral transmission in Andoas, Loreto, Peru. *Rev Peru Med Exp Salud Pub.* (2020) 37:174–5. doi: 10.17843/rpmesp.2020.371.4875
27. Andrade DV, Gollob KJ, Dutra WO. Acute Chagas disease: new global challenges for an old neglected disease. *PLoS Negl Trop Dis.* (2014) 8:e3010. doi: 10.1371/journal.pntd.0003010

16

Evidence for Transmission of *Taenia solium* Taeniasis/Cysticercosis in a Rural Area of Northern Rwanda

Lucrecia Acosta Soto[1], *Lucy Anne Parker*[2,3], *María José Irisarri-Gutiérrez*[4,5], *Javier Arturo Bustos*[6,7], *Yesenia Castillo*[7], *Erika Perez*[6], *Carla Muñoz-Antoli*[4], *José Guillermo Esteban*[4], *Héctor Hugo García*[6,7†] and *Fernando Jorge Bornay-Llinares*[1*†]

[1] Área de Parasitología del Departamento de Agroquímica y Medioambiente, Universidad Miguel Hernández de Elche, Alicante, Spain, [2] Departamento de Salud Pública Historia de la Ciencia y Ginecología, Universidad Miguel Hernández de Elche, Alicante, Spain, [3] Centro de Investigación Biomédica en Red de Epidemiología y Salud Pública (CIBERESP), Madrid, Spain, [4] Área de Parasitología, Dpto. Farmacia y Tecnología Farmacéutica y Parasitología, Facultat de Farmàcia, Universitat de València, Valencia, Spain, [5] Dpto. de Ciencias de la Salud, Facultad de Ciencias Biomédicas, Universidad Europea de Madrid, Madrid, Spain, [6] Cysticercosis Unit, Instituto Nacional de Ciencias Neurológicas, Lima, Peru, [7] Center for Global Health, Universidad Peruana Cayetano Heredia, Lima, Peru

***Correspondence:**
Fernando Jorge Bornay-Llinares
f.bornay@umh.es

† These authors have contributed equally to this work and share senior authorship

Cysticercosis is a parasitic infection caused by the metacestode larval stage (cysticercus) of *Taenia solium*. In humans, cysticercosis may infect the central nervous system and cause neurocysticercosis, which is responsible for over 50,000 deaths per year worldwide and is the major cause of preventable epilepsy cases, especially in low-income countries. Cysticercosis infection is endemic in many less developed countries where poor hygiene conditions and free-range pig management favor their transmission. A cross-sectional study was conducted in 680 children from a rural primary school in Gakenke district (Northern province of Rwanda). Stool samples were collected from participants and analyzed using the Kato-Katz method (KK), formol-ether concentration (FEC), and/or copro-antigen enzyme-linked immunosorbent assay (CoAg-ELISA) to detect taeniasis. Blood samples were collected and analyzed using enzyme-linked immunoelectrotransfer blot (EITB) and antigen enzyme-linked immunosorbent assay (Ag-ELISA) to detect human cysticercosis. The overall proportion of taeniasis positivity was 0.3% (2/680), and both cases were also confirmed by CoAg-ELISA. A total of 13.3% (76/572) of the children studied were positive to cysticercosis (*T. solium*-specific serum antibodies detected by EITB), of whom 38.0% (27/71) had viable cysticercus (*T. solium* antigens by Ag-ELISA). This study provides evidence of the highest cysticercosis prevalence reported in Rwanda in children to date. Systematic investigations into porcine and human cysticercosis as well as health education and hygiene measures for *T. solium* control are needed in Gakenke district.

Keywords: ***Taenia solium*, taeniasis, cystcercosis, children, Gakenke, Rwanda**

INTRODUCTION

In *Taenia solium* parasitic infections, humans are the only natural definitive host (taeniasis) while pigs are the intermediate hosts of larval stage (swine cysticercosis) (1). Human cysticercosis results when people become intermediate hosts after ingestion of microscopic viable eggs *via* the fecal-oral route from *T. solium* tapeworm carriers (2). The embryo is released (oncosphere), and it traverses the intestinal mucosa after ingestion. Later, it is transported by the circulatory system and dispersed by the organism producing cysts (cysticerci). The most common locations of cysts are the striated muscle, eyes, or heart tissue and central nervous system (3, 4). The clinical manifestations of cysticercosis are dependent on the number and location of cysticerci within the body (4). Some individuals with cysticercosis will exhibit or develop no symptoms (asymptomatic) or very mild symptoms. Many individuals with cysticercosis have central nervous system involvement (neurocysticercosis) resulting in headache, epileptic seizures, blindness, mental disturbance, and even death (3, 5). Neurocisticercosis (NCC) is the most common parasitic disease in the human nervous system and the most common cause of epilepsy in low-income countries (6).

Currently, cysticercosis is one of the 17 major Neglected Tropical Diseases (NTDs) identified by the WHO as a focus for research and control (7). It is widely prevalent where humans and domestic pig raising coexist. In many developing countries in Central and South America, Africa, and Asia, cysticercosis has major public health implications in humans and pigs (5, 8–11). It is in these places where poverty, poor education, lack of access to diagnosis, and limited management capacity, together with the absence of appropriate prevention measures and control strategies, make it highly endemic (11–13).

The distribution of *T. solium* taeniosis/cysticercosis in Africa is unclear but porcine and human cysticercosis are considered (hyper)-endemic in Central Africa (Rwanda, Burundi, the Democratic Republic of Congo, and Cameroon) (14, 15). In the last 20 years, pig production has increased significantly in the Eastern and Southern Africa (ESA) region, especially in rural, resource-poor, smallholder communities (11, 14). Several studies show a high prevalence of porcine cysticercosis in countries bordering Rwanda. In Uganda, prevalences ranging from 7.1 to 45% have been observed in urban areas in contrast to low percentages of 0.12–10.8% found in rural areas with an observed increment in recent years (9, 16–18). A prevalence of 41.2% has recently been reported in the Democratic Republic of Congo, where the overall prevalence of pigs with active cysticercosis did not significantly differ between the market and the village study sites but was much higher than previously observed by Chartier et al., in 1990 (19, 20). There are no current data for Burundi, but prevalence ranges from 2 to 39% were observed 20 years ago (21). In Tanzania, farm prevalence of porcine cysticercosis was between 17.4 and 18.2% in lingual examination or slaughter-slab prevalence by routine meat inspection respectively, while a maximum of 33.3% has been reported by cysticercal antigens by ELISA (Ag-ELISA) (22–29).

In contrast, Taeniasis has been poorly studied in humans from these countries (30). Eggs of *Taenia* sp. in feces have been reported in Uganda (31). Taeniasis prevalence ranges between 0 and 1.0% have been observed in schoolchildren of Burundi (21). However, prevalence of taeniasis ranging from 0.4 to 5.2% by the Kato-Katz technique or 2.3–5.2% by copro-Ag-ELISA has been estimated in Tanzania (32, 33).

Regarding human cysticercosis, one study estimated 21.6% prevalence of circulating antigen in the Democratic Republic of Congo (34). Several studies in human cysticercosis reveal the strong association between neurocysticercosis and epilepsy in these countries (35, 36). In Burundi, cysticercosis has been observed in 4.9–31.5% of epileptic patients, compared to 4.2% in controls (21, 37–39). On the other hand, a seroprevalence of up to 11.7% has been observed in epileptic patients and in 2.8% of controls (21). Cysticercosis was the cause of seizures in 25% of epileptic patients (38, 40). In Tanzania, cysticercosis prevalence of 16–17% was estimated and it was demonstrated that NCC contributed significantly to epilepsy in adults (32, 41–43). Given these data, it is likely that the situation in Rwanda is similar.

Rwanda has long since been known as a hyperendemic country for Taeniasis/cysticercosis. However, there are few research studies carried out in this country. Already in 1959, 20% of pigs were found to be infected with cysticercosis (44). From 2000 to 2011, pork production in Rwanda increased by 7.8% (45); however, an overall swine cysticercosis prevalence of 3.9% was found in farms, 9.2% in markets, and 4% in butchers (46). In 1956, the first case of human cysticercosis was reported in Rwanda (47). Since then, initial reports have reported isolated cases of disseminated ocular (48) and cutaneous cysticercosis (49, 50). In 1964, the presence of eggs of *Taenia* spp. in populations of the Batwa and Hutu tribes in the Northern and Southern regions of the country was detected (51). Later, *T. solium* cysticerci was detected in 7% of 300 autopsies in Butare (52). In Kigali and Butare, 21 and 21.8% of people with epilepsy are estimated to be seropositive for cysticercosis, respectively (53, 54). To date, there have been no studies in children.

During a coproparasitological study in the school population of Northern Rwanda, eggs from tapeworms were detected in two schoolchildren. After collecting the strobila, the morphology of mature proglottids allowed us to identify the species as *T. solium* in both cases. This observation motivated us to investigate the presence of cysticercosis in the school population of Nemba, with the prospect of introducing control activities.

METHODS

Study Area

Rwanda is a small landlocked country in Central Africa, bordering Uganda to the North, Burundi to the South, Democratic Republic of the Congo to the West, and Tanzania to the East. The estimated population in 2012 was 10.4 million people, thus supporting the densest population in continental Africa, with most of the population engaged in subsistence agriculture (55). A verdant country of fertile and hilly terrain with altitudes varying from 950 m to 4,519 m, the small republic bears the title "Land of a Thousand Hills." The District of Gakenke is one of the five districts of the Northern Province of Rwanda. This

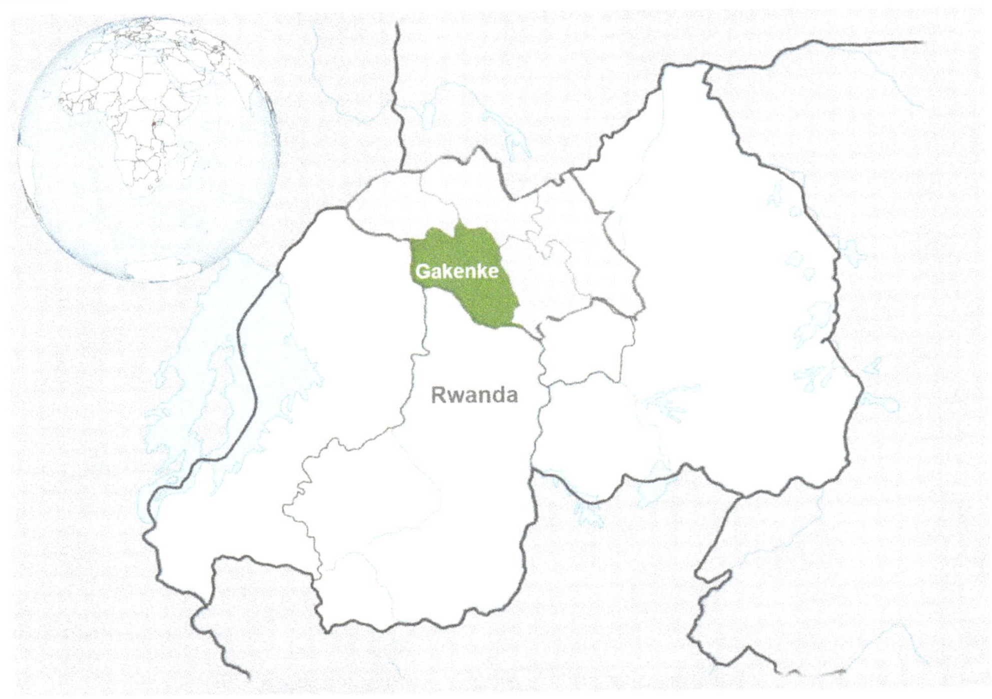

FIGURE 1 | Study location map. District of Gakenke, Northern Province, Rwanda.

district is divided into 19 administrative sectors made of 97 cells, 617 villages, and 345,487 inhabitants living in a total area of 104 km^2 with a population density of 473/km^2 (56). **Figure 1** shows a schematic map of the study area.

Gakenke district is characterized, in general, by high inclined hills separated by rivers and marshlands. The climate in Gakenke district is generally the type of humid climate with the average annual temperature varying between 16.0 and 29.0°C. The rainfalls are relatively abundant with a scale between 1,100 and 1,500 mm per year (56).

Population

Between July and September 2011, the Parasitology Area of University Miguel Hernández de Elche (UMH; Spain) conducted a cross-sectional study in Nemba school I, Gakenke district of Rwanda, as part of an initial phase of a school health program. A total of 771 schoolchildren (371 girls and 400 boys) attended primary education (2nd to 6th grade) and were eligible for inclusion in the study. A total of 708 students (357 boys and 351 girls aged between 6 and 18 years of age; mean $\pm$ SD $=$ 11.00 $\pm$ 2.33 years) were eligible for the study after their parents or guardians provided informed consent. A total of 680 answered the questionnaire and provided stool sample, while 572 provided blood sample (see **Figure 2**).

Sampling and Parasitological Tests

After collection, fresh feces samples were processed and quantified *in situ* (UMH headquarters in Nemba, Rwanda) by the method described by Kato-Katz following WHO recommendations (57). A 41.7-mg sample of fresh feces was used as template according to the Helm teste® manufacturer's recommendations (Bio-Manguinhos/Fiocruz, Brazil). If taeniid eggs were observed, 2 g of Niclosamide and 1 ml of Duphalac® oral solution (667 mg/ml of lactulose) was administered as a laxative to recover the adult where possible.

Additionally, part of each stool sample was preserved in 10% buffered formalin (1:3) (40-ml Falcon tube) and another part was preserved in ethanol 70% (2-ml tube). Sera samples were obtained from whole blood collected of every child by centrifugation and stored at 4°C in Nemba's Hospital until sent to UMH, Spain. Later, all samples were sent to UMH and stored at −20°C until processing. Formalin-embedded samples were sent to the Department of Parasitology of University of Valencia (Spain) where a formol-ether concentration was realized (58). Finally, tree drops of sediment with Lugol's iodine solution were analyzed under a microscope. Sera and fecal samples preserved in ethanol 70% were subsequently sent to the diagnostic laboratory of the Center for Global Health of the Universidad Peruana Cayetano Heredia (UPCH, Lima, Peru) for processing by *T. solium*-specific tests [Coproantigen ELISA, serum antigen detection (Ag-ELISA), and serum antibody detection by enzyme-linked immunoelectrotransfer blot (EITB) assay using lentil lectin-purified parasitic glycoprotein antigens].

Taeniasis: Coproantigen Detection by ELISA (CoAg-ELISA)

In an attempt to find additional carriers of adult *T. solium* worms, a subgroup of 144 fecal samples (~21% of the total) were also screened by coproantigen ELISA (59, 60). Aliquots

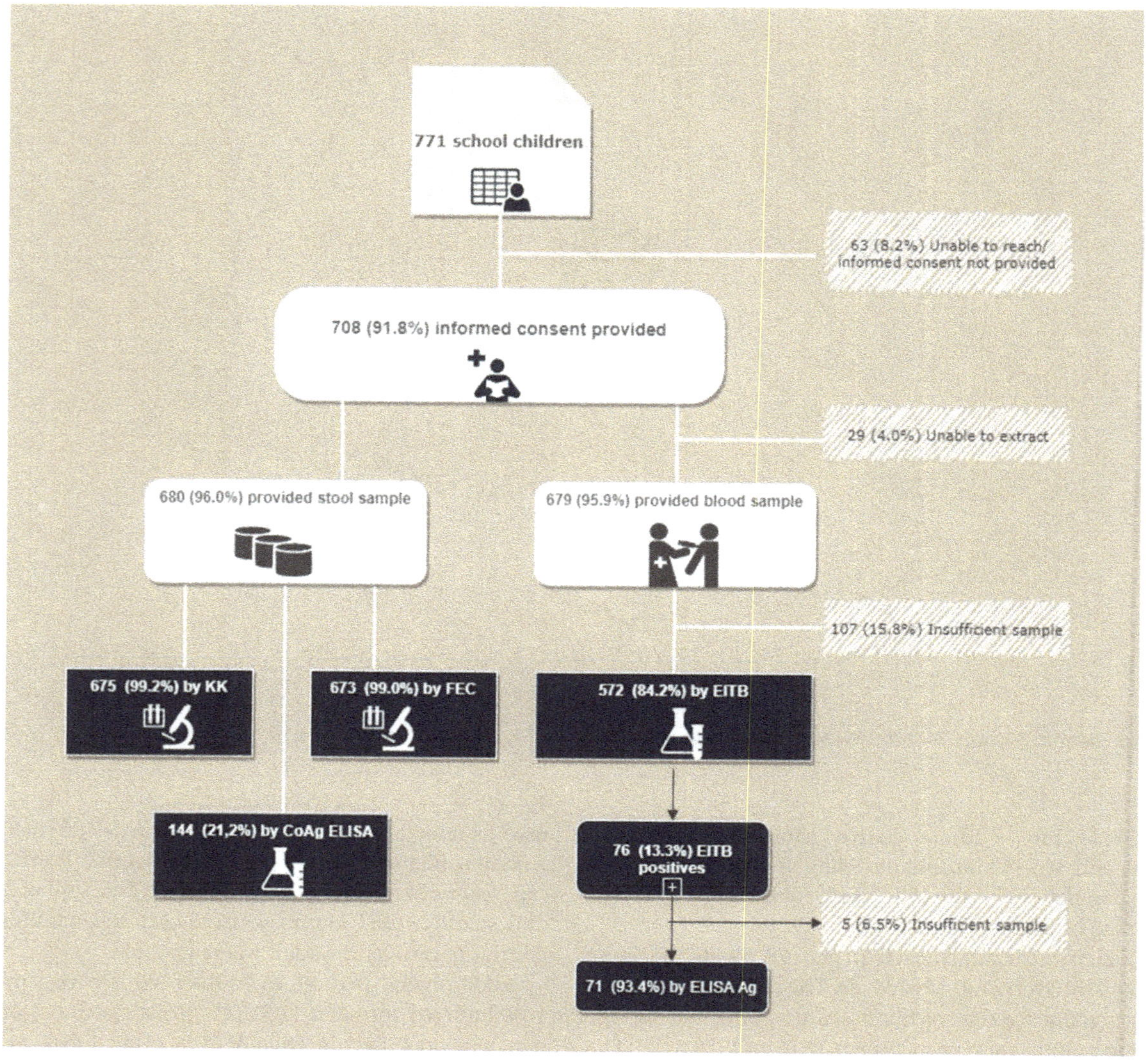

FIGURE 2 | Flow chart for the recruitment of patients.

(1.5 ml) of the stool supernatant were used for CoAg-ELISA after centrifugation at room temperature at 3,200 g for 10 min. The CoAg-ELISA technique was performed as described by Allan et al., by using hyperimmune rabbit anti-*T. solium* IgG as the capture antibody and peroxidase-labeled goat anti-*T. solium* IgG as a conjugate. Processed samples were read with a spectrophotometer (Molecular Devices Inc., Sunnyvale, CA) at 650 nm. Using a known positive pool (P1), we calculated the percentage of positivity (PP) as [optical density (OD) of the sample]/(OD of P1) 100, in order to increase the comparability of the results between plates. A cutoff was determined using a receiver operating characteristic (ROC) curve (61).

Cysticercosis-Specific Tests

Anti-*T. solium* Antibody Detection

A total of 572 sera samples were processed by EITB. The methodology used to perform the test was the same described by Tsang et al. (62) and González et al. (63). An immunoblot of seven cysticercus glycoproteins (GP50, GP42-39, GP24, GP21, GP18, GP14, and GP13), purified by lentil lectin-purified chromatography, gives close to 100% specificity and a sensitivity varying from 70 to 90% (62). This EITB has been widely used for the diagnosis of cysticercosis in human and pig serum samples (64).

T. solium Antigen Detection by ELISA

In order to demonstrate the presence of active infections, an anti-*T. solium* antibody-positive subgroup of children (71 EITB positive samples) were processed in quest by ELISA, to detect circulating cysticercal antigen in the serum (65, 66). A mAb-based ELISA for the detection of circulating antigens was used to detect circulating parasite antigen as described by Brandt et al. in 1992 (67) and later adapted by Van Kerckhoven et al. and Dorny et al. (68, 69). The assay uses Nunc MaxiSorp plates sensitized with a trapping mAb (B158C11A10) in bicarbonate buffer at 5 μg/ml. After blocking, serum samples (pretreated with 5% trichloroacetic acid to break existing immune complexes) are added, followed by the second mAb (B60H8A4-BIOT), streptavidin, o-phenylenediamine (OPD/H2O2) as substrate/chromogen, and incubated in the dark for 15 min. The reaction is stopped with H_2SO_4 and plates are read at 490/650 nm. To minimize inter-plate variation, we used antigen ratio instead of a raw value of optic density (OD). The antigen ratio is estimated by dividing the OD of the tested sample with the mean of eight negative samples plus three standard deviations (70).

Questionnaire and Anthropometric Measurements

A questionnaire was concurrently conducted while blood and stool samples were taken. The children were interviewed, and basic socio-demographic data (age, sex, residence) were recorded as well as specific questions about their living conditions and behaviors. Each child was assigned a unique ID code and removed their shoes so that we could measure their height (in cm) and weight (in kg).

Statistical Analyses

The data were identified and entered into a Microsoft Office Excel 2010 spreadsheet (Microsoft). Statistical analysis was performed using Stata SE 15.0 (StataCorp LLC, USA). We calculated the frequencies of categorical variables and made comparisons using Pearson's Chi-squared-test. Missing values were excluded for the comparisons. Continuous variables were described with means and standard deviations.

RESULTS

Taeniasis Intestinal and Species Identification

The coproparasitological analysis revealed an overall parasitism of 94.9% (639/673) by formol-ether concentration and a helminth parasitism percentage of 31.2% (211/675) by the Kato-Katz technique. In two children [2/680 (0.3%)], eggs of taeniid tapeworm were identified by both methods: Kato-Katz technique [2/675 (0.3%)] and formol-ether concentration [2/673 (0.31%)].

After parental consent, 2 g of Niclosamide and 1 ml of Duphalac® oral solution (667 mg/ml of lactulose) as a laxative were administered and the feces were collected. Two strobiles were recovered from both children and the morphologic study under a magnifying glass after injection with India ink revealed <12 uterine branches compatible with *T. solium*-proglottid demonstrating current tapeworm infection in both children.

Moreover, 144 samples were tested by coproantigen ELISA detection and 2/144 (1.4%) samples had positive results. The positive samples obtained matched the positive samples obtained by Kato-Katz and formol-ether concentration techniques.

Cysticercosis

EITB analysis of a total of 572 sera samples revealed that 13.3% of the students (76/572) presented reactivity to one or more of the specific glycoproteins of *T. solium*, of whom 46.0% (35/76) showed reactivity to three or more bands. A total of 7 of the 76 positive samples showed a single GP 50 band reaction, whereas in 9 of the positive samples, no GP 50 band was observed.

Exposure to *T. solium* was more frequent among girls than boys ($p = 0.014$, **Table 1**) and was especially prevalent in the Mucaca area of Nemba where 21.3% of the children had anti-*T. solium* antibodies ($p < 0.001$). Children of all ages and in all classes had positive EITB results, and there was no obvious relationship with domestic animal rearing. The majority of the children came from homes that used a water pump as their main water source and had a latrine. Consumption of meat was significantly associated with *T. solium* exposure. The highest levels of exposure were among children that reported consuming meat once a month (15.6%) or once a year (19.2%); 13.1% of children who reported that they always washed their hands after going to the toilet had anti-*T. solium* antibodies, and this was not statistically different from children that reported they sometimes or never washed their hands (12.8 and 14.3%, respectively).

Taenia solium antigens were found in 38% (27/71) of children with anti-*T. solium* antibodies suggesting active infection. In addition, 14 of the 27 positive samples for antigen presented more than three bands by EIBT-test. None of the variables considered were associated with antigen presence among seropositive children (**Table 1**).

DISCUSSION

The present study demonstrates a substantial seroprevalence of cysticercosis in children of the Northern Province of Rwanda. The results suggest that more than of 13% of this group of children had been exposed to *T solium*. In addition, among the reactive individuals, 46% had three or more reactive bands by EITB, which is highly suggestive of established cysticercosis infection. Furthermore, of the children with antibodies to cysticercosis, 38% were reactive to the detection of circulating antigen by ELISA, indicating the presence of active cases of neurocysticercosis, as previously demonstrated (65).

In 1982, Fain et al. said that *T. solium* was the most prevalent tapeworm in Rwanda (47). In previous studies in Rwanda, soil-transmitted helminths and schistosomiasis but no tapeworms were found. Since 1964, human taeniosis has not been detected in the country (51). However, analysis based on both microscopy or coproantigen detection of human fecal material cannot identify the species level, and the possibility of *T. saginata* presence cannot be ruled out. Other studies showed high parasitic burden strongly associated with drinking any kind of water (71–73).

The finding of eggs of *Taenia* spp. in two schoolchildren motivated us to deepen the search for associated human cysticercosis. Both children were positive based on microscopy (KK and FEC) and coproantigen detection (copro-Ag-ELISA).

In spite of false positives reported by coproantigen test (74), a high positivity value is highly predictive of a true positive (61). No cross-reactions were observed with other intestinal parasites (protozoa and helminths) present in the children. In this study, the microscopy and coproantigen detection assays had the same sensitivity as has been reported by other authors (59, 75). Our work showed some limitations because we were

TABLE 1 | Results of the cysticercosis-specific tests conducted according to characteristics of the children.

Characteristics	EITB				Ag-ELISA	
	Positive		3 or more bands			
	n/total (%)	*p*-value[a]	*n*/positive EITB (%)	*p*-value[a]	*n*/positive EITB (%)	*p*-value[a]
Sex		0.019		0.598		0.948
Female	48/289 (16.6)		21/48 (43.7)		18/47 (38.3)	
Male	28/282 (9.9)		14/28 (50.0)		9/24 (37.5)	
No data	0/1 (0.0)		0/1 (0.0)		0/0 (0.0)	
Age		0.509		0.606		0.674
6–9 years	20/155 (13.0)		11/20 (55.0)		8/19 (42.1)	
10–14 years	46/363 (12.7)		20/46 (43.5)		15/44 (34.1)	
15–18 years	8/42 (19.0)		3/8 (37.5)		3/6 (50.0)	
No data	2/12 (16.7)		1/2 (50.0)		0/2	
Sector		<0.001		0.711		0.401
Nemba						
Buranga	3/46 (6.5)		2/3 (66.7)		0/3 (0.0)	
Gahinga	7/70 (10.0)		3/7 (42.8)		3/6 (50.0)	
Gisozi	13/202 (6.4)		5/13 (38.5)		3/12 (25.0)	
Mucaca	46/216 (21.3)		24/46 (52.2)		19/43 (45.2)	
Gakenke						
Rusagara	4/25 (16.0)		1/4 (25.0)		11/4 (27.5)	
No data	3/13 (23.1)		0/3 (0.0)		1/3 (33.3)	
School class		0.204		0.545		0.650
P2	15/150 (10.0)		7/15 (46.7)		7/14 (50.0)	
P3	17/114 (14.9)		10/17 (58.8)		6/16 (37.5)	
P4	24/131 (18.2)		8/24 (33.3)		7/23 (30.4)	
P5	15/116 (12.9)		7/15 (46.7)		6/13 (46.1)	
P6	5/61 (8.2)		3/5 (60.0)		1/5 (20.0)	
Domestic animals		0.270		0.299		0.415
Pigs	1/28 (3.6)		0/1 (0.0)		1/1 (100.0)	
Other animals[b]	64/459 (13.9)		31/64 (48.4)		21/59 (35.6)	
None	8/68 (11.8)		2/8 (25.0)		3/8 (37.5)	
Don't know/no answer provided	1/5 (20.0)		1/1 (100.0)		1/1 (100.0)	
No data	2/12 (16.7)		1/2 (50.0)		1/2 (50.0)	
Water source		0.515		0.809		0.077
Piped water	5/58 (8.6)		2/5 (40.0)		0/5 (0.0)	
Water pump/fountain	68/496 (13.7)		31/68 (45.6)		25/63 (39.7)	
Rivers/puddles	0/1 (0.0)		0/0 (0.0)		0/0 (0.0)	
Don't know/no answer provided	1/5 (20.0)		1/1 (100.0)		1/1 (100.0)	
No data	2/12 (16.7)		1/2 (50.0)		1/2 (50.0)	
Toilet		0.432		NA		NA
WC	0/10 (0.0)		0/0 (0.0)		0/0 (0.0)	
Private latrine	72/542 (13.3)		32/72 (44.4)		25/67 (37.3)	
Shared latrine	0/1 (0.0)		0/1 (0.0)		0/0 (0.0)	
Don't know/no answer provided	2/7 (28.6)		2/2 (100.0)		1/2 (50.0)	
No data	2/12 (16.7)		1/2 (50.0)		1/2 (50.0)	
How often do you eat meat?		0.003		0.070		0.818
Once a week	10/159 (6.3)		7/10 (70.0)		2/9 (22.2)	
Once a month	32/205 (15.6)		12/32 (37.5)		11 /30 (36.7)	
Once a year	27/141 (19.2)		11/27 (40.7)		10/25 (40.0)	
Never	3/44 (6.8)		3/3 (100.0)		1/3 (33.3)	
Don't know/no answer provided	2/11 (18.2)		1/2 (50.0)		2/2 (100.0)	

(Continued)

TABLE 1 | Continued

Characteristics	EITB				Ag-ELISA	
	Positive		3 or more bands			
	n/total (%)	*p*-value[a]	*n*/positive EITB (%)	*p*-value[a]	*n*/positive EITB (%)	*p*-value[a]
No data	2/12 (16.7)		1/2 (50.0)		1/2 (50.0)	
How often do you wash your hands after going to the toilet?		0.935		0.367		0.788
Always	26/198 (13.1)		9/26 (34.6)		10/24 (41.7)	
Sometimes	34/266 (12.8)		18/34 (52.9)		12/34 (35.3)	
Never	13/91 (14.3)		6/13 (46.1)		3/10 (30.0)	
Don't know/no answer provided	1/5 (20.0)		1/1 (100.0)		1/1 (100.0)	
No data	2/12 (16.7)		1/2 (50.0)		1/2 (50.0)	
Total	**76/572 (13.3)**		**35/76 (46.0)**		**27/71 (38.0)**	

EITB, Anti-T. solium antibodies detection by enzyme-linked immunoelectrotransfer blot; Ag-ELISA, T. solium antigen detection by ELISA.
[a]p-value from a Chi squared-test comparing answer categories, excluding missing or unknown values.
[b]Other animals: Cows, sheep, goats, rabbits, and chicken.

unable to carry out the coproantigen study on all samples, and the sample of children included came from a single school in the Gakenke district. However, participation was high, and with this study, we can confirm the presence of tapeworm carriers in this area. Additionally, we identified morphologically both adult specimens. Identification to species level in this country or bordering countries except in Tanzania has never been done (33).

To our knowledge, this is the first report of cysticercosis in schoolchildren in Rwanda. In cysticercosis surveys and immunodiagnostic tools applied on humans, serum samples are useful in estimating the prevalence and identifying of *T. solium* infection in the field. *T. solium* antigen in serum could predict the presence of viable brain parasites in patients with apparently calcified cysticercosis only (70). Antibody response in *T. solium* infection in field conditions was found to be a major contributor to the overestimation of the prevalence of cysticercosis in endemic areas (4, 76). The frequency found in these children was higher than prior literature reports in Butare, where 7% of autopsies were positive for cysticercosis (52). Furthermore, 21 and 21.8% of patients with epilepsy in Kigali and southern Rwanda, respectively, are positive for cysticercosis (50, 53, 54). None of the previous studies were performed in children. In our study, it is important to highlight the early age of the population studied, since it is known that the prevalence of cysticercosis in a region increases with the age range studied. We can deduce that the seroprevalence in the adult population is likely to be higher than observed here.

The highest proportion of positive schoolchildren was observed in the same sector where tapeworm carriers were located. We observed small-scale swine production system in Mucaca (personal observation).

The financial losses due to human cysticercosis are very difficult to estimate but are certainly exceeded by the social impact of the disease, especially because of the particular perception of epilepsy in many African communities (14). Conditions like neurocysticercosis are better prevented than treated, because it has the potential to make a healthy person invalid. If the treatment is delayed, there can be irreversible brain damage.

In our study, no association was observed in frequency of hand washing after going to the toilet. However, in our study, close contact with pigs and use of latrines as possible risk factors for cysticercosis were not significantly associated with positive cases as observed in Tanzania (43). The absence of association may be explained by the level of widespread poverty in this area. Interestingly, meat consumption showed a significant association with cysticercosis exposure, but it was not a dose response. It is possible that people with limited resources cannot afford quality meat in these rural areas. Children who reported consuming meat once a month or once a year had higher exposure rates than those who reported consuming meat weekly, but it is possible that here we are seeing the impact of socio-economic status of the children rather than meat consumption itself. It has been shown that vegetarians and other people who do not eat pork can acquire cysticercosis through fecal–oral contamination with *T. solium* eggs from tapeworm carriers (77). Unhygienic sanitary conditions such as limited use or absence of latrines are prevalent in rural areas of Africa where pigs are raised (14, 78, 79). Informally marketed foods, clandestine slaughtering of pigs, lack of trained and qualified meat inspectors, lack of detection and treatment of *T. solium* carriers, and consumption of undercooked or insufficiently cooked pork could be risk factors for taeniosis/cysticercosis among consumers (22, 26, 35).

A nutritional survey and coproparasitological examination was being carried out at the Nemba 1 School, Gakenke district, Rwanda, when two samples harboring *Taenia* spp. eggs were found (unpublished results). It was impossible to obtain more samples or additional information that would allow the analysis of other risk factors or possible variables related to clinical manifestations of the infection. For the reasons stated, we decided to carry out the present study with the sole objective of investigating the presence of infection and transmission of

T. solium in the community. The results obtained confirm the presence and transmission of *T. solium* and support the need to design more extensive future studies.

CONCLUSIONS

Overall, our study shows the presence and transmission of *T. solium* in Gakenke district. The high seroprevalence found in this area allows it to be considered hyperendemic for cysticercosis. To avoid neurological consequences, systematic investigations into porcine and human cysticercosis as well as health education and hygiene measures for *T. solium* control are needed. It is necessary to evaluate the clinical status of schoolchildren involved, carry out a study of contacts, and implement actions for the control and prevention of the disease.

AUTHOR CONTRIBUTIONS

FB-L, HG, and JGE contributed to conception and design of the study. LA, LP, and FB-L supervised and coordinated the field study. LA, MI-G, and FB-L carried out the coproparasitological analysis in the field. CM-A and JGE coordinated the coproparasitological procedures. JB, YC, and EP coordinated and performed the serological and coproantigen tests. LA and LP organized the database-analyzed data, realized formal analysis, and interpretation of data. LA, LP, and HG wrote the first draft of the manuscript. FB-L critically reviewed it and contributed to draft design. All authors contributed to manuscript revision, read, and approved the submitted version.

ACKNOWLEDGMENTS

The authors thank the Laboratory of Nemba Hospital for their technical support and assistance in laboratory and field work duties and Jacinte for her translation. We thank all families for their collaboration and enthusiasm throughout the study.

REFERENCES

1. Flisser A. Taeniasis and cysticercosis due to *Taenia solium*. *Prog Clin Parasitol.* (1994) 4:77–116.
2. García HH, Del Brutto OH. Imaging findings in neurocysticercosis. *Acta Tropica.* (2003) 87:71–8. doi: 10.1016/S0001-706X(03)00057-3
3. White AC. Neurocysticercosis: updates on epidemiology, pathogenesis, diagnosis, and management. *Annu Rev Med.* (2000) 51:187–206. doi: 10.1146/annurev.med.51.1.187
4. Garcia HH, Gonzalez AE, Gilman RH. Taenia solium Cysticercosis and its Impact in Neurological Disease. *Clin Microbiol Rev.* (2020) 33:e00085-19. doi: 10.1128/CMR.00085-19
5. Garcia HH, Del Brutto OH. *Taenia solium* cysticercosis. *Infect Dis Clin North Am.* (2000) 14:97–119. doi: 10.1016/S0891-5520(05)70220-8
6. Preux PM, Druet-Cabanac M. Epidemiology and aetiology of epilepsy in sub-Saharan Africa. *Lancet Neurol.* (2005) 4:21–31. doi: 10.1016/S1474-4422(04)00963-9
7. WHO. *First WHO Report on Neglected Tropical Diseases: Working to Overcome the Global Impact of Neglected Tropical Diseases.* Geneva: World Health Organisation (2010). p. 1–184.
8. Sarti E, Rajshekhar V. Measures for the prevention and control of *Taenia solium* taeniosis and cysticercosis. *Acta Tropica.* (2003) 87:137–43. doi: 10.1016/S0001-706X(03)00034-2
9. Nsadha Z, Thomas LF, Fèvre EM, Nasinyama G, Ojok L, Waiswa C. Prevalence of porcine cysticercosis in the Lake Kyoga Basin, Uganda. *BMC Vet Res.* (2014) 10:239. doi: 10.1186/s12917-014-0239-y
10. Wu HW, Ito A, Ai L, Zhou XN, Acosta LP, Lee Willingham A. Cysticercosis/taeniasis endemicity in Southeast Asia: current status and control measures. *Acta Trop.* (2017) 165:121–32. doi: 10.1016/j.actatropica.2016.01.013
11. Phiri IK, Ngowi H, Afonso S, Matenga E, Boa M, Mukaratirwa S, et al. The emergence of *Taenia solium* cysticercosis in Eastern and Southern Africa as a serious agricultural problem and public health risk. *Acta Tropica.* (2003) 87:13–23. doi: 10.1016/S0001-706X(03)00051-2
12. Willingham AL, Engels D. Control of *Taenia solium* cysticercosis/taeniosis. *Adv Parasitol.* (2006) 61:509–66. doi: 10.1016/S0065-308X(05)61012-3
13. O'Neal SE, Moyano LM, Ayvar V, Gonzalvez G, Diaz A, Rodriguez S, et al. Geographic correlation between tapeworm carriers and heavily infected cysticercotic pigs. *PLoS Negl Trop Dis.* (2012) 12:1953. doi: 10.1371/journal.pntd.0001953
14. Zoli A, Shey-Njila O, Assana E, Nguekam JP, Dorny P, Brandt J, et al. Regional status, epidemiology and impact of *Taenia solium* cysticercosis in Western and Central Africa. *Acta Tropica.* (2003) 87:35–42. doi: 10.1016/S0001-706X(03)00053-6
15. Braae UC, Saarnak CFL, Mukaratirwa S, Devleesschauwer B, Magnussen P, Johansen MV. *Taenia solium* taeniosis/cysticercosis and the co-distribution with schistosomiasis in Africa. *Parasites Vectors.* (2015) 8:323. doi: 10.1186/s13071-015-0938-7
16. Waiswa C, Fèvre EM, Nsadha Z, Sikasunge CS, Willingham AL. Porcine cysticercosis in Southeast Uganda: seroprevalence in Kamuli and Kaliro Districts. *J Parasitol Res.* (2009) 2009:1–5. doi: 10.1155/2009/375493
17. Kisakye J, Mal S. Short communication. Cysticcrcus cclluləsae in pigs slaughtered i~ and around Kampala city. *Uganda J Agric Sci.* (2002) 7:23–4. Available online at: https://www.ajol.info/index.php/ujas/article/view/128878
18. Kungu JM, Dione MM, Ejobi F, Harrison LJS, Poole EJ, Pezo D, et al. Sero-prevalence of *Taenia* spp. cysticercosis in rural and urban smallholder pig production settings in Uganda. *Acta Trop.* (2017) 165:110–5. doi: 10.1016/j.actatropica.2016.01.016
19. Chartier C, Mutesi U, Ndakala NO. Les helminthes du porc domestique en Ituri, Haut-Zaïre. *Ann Soc Belg Med Trop.* (1990) 70:213–25.
20. Praet N, Kanobana K, Kabwe C, Maketa V, Lukanu P, Lutumba P, et al. *Taenia solium* cysticercosis in the democratic Republic of Congo: how does pork trade affect the transmission of the parasite?. *PLoS Negl Trop Dis.* (2010) 4:e817. doi: 10.1371/journal.pntd.0000817
21. Newell E, Vyungimana F, Geerts S, Van Kerckhoven I, Tsang VCW, Engels D. Prevalence of cysticercosis in epileptics and members of their families in Burundi. *Trans R Soc Trop Med Hyg.* (1997) 91:389–91. doi: 10.1016/S0035-9203(97)90251-0
22. Boa ME, Mahundi EA, Kassuku AA, Willingham AL, Kyvsgaard NC. Epidemiological survey of swine cysticercosis using ante-mortem and post-mortem examination tests in the southern highlands of Tanzania. *Vet Parasitol.* (2006) 139:249–55. doi: 10.1016/j.vetpar.2006.02.012
23. Mellau BL, Nonga HE, Karimuribo ED. Slaughter stock abattoir survey of carcasses and organ/offal condemnations in Arusha region, northern Tanzania. *Trop Anim Health Prod.* (2011) 43:857–64. doi: 10.1007/s11250-010-9773-1
24. Mkupasi EM, Ngowi HA, Nonga HE. Prevalence of extra-intestinal porcine helminth infections and assessment of sanitary conditions of pig slaughter slabs in Dar es Salaam city, Tanzania. *Trop Anim Health Prod.* (2011) 43:417–23. doi: 10.1007/s11250-010-9708-x
25. Mkupasi EM, Ngowi HA, Sikasunge CS, Leifsson PS, Johansen MV. Efficacy of ivermectin and oxfendazole against *Taenia solium* cysticercosis and other parasitoses in naturally infected pigs. *Acta Trop.* (2013) 128:48–53. doi: 10.1016/j.actatropica.2013.06.010

26. Komba EVG, Kimbi EC, Ngowi HA, Kimera SI, Mlangwa JE, Lekule FP, et al. Prevalence of porcine cysticercosis and associated risk factors in smallholder pig production systems in Mbeya region, southern highlands of Tanzania. *Vet Parasitol.* (2013) 198:284–91. doi: 10.1016/j.vetpar.2013.09.020
27. Ngowi HA, Kassuku AA, Maeda GEM, Boa ME, Carabin H, Willingham AL. Risk factors for the prevalence of porcine cysticercosis in Mbulu District, Tanzania. *Vet Parasitol.* (2004) 120:275–83. doi: 10.1016/j.vetpar.2004.01.015
28. Yohana C, Mwita C, Nkwengulila G. *The Prevalence of Porcine Cysticercosis and Risk Factors for Taeniasis in Iringa Rural District.* (2013). Available online at: http://repository.udsm.ac.tz:8080/xmlui/handle/123456789/1505 (accessed December 14, 2020).
29. Wilson RT, Swai E. A review of pig pathology in Tanzania. *Trop Anim Health Prod.* (2013) 45:1269–75. doi: 10.1007/s11250-013-0426-z
30. Braae UC, Harrison W, Lekule F, Magnussen P, Johansen MV. Feedstuff and poor latrines may put pigs at risk of cysticercosis—A case-control study. *Vet Parasitol.* (2015) 214:187–91. doi: 10.1016/j.vetpar.2015.08.009
31. Kabatereine NB, Tukahebwa EM, Brooker S, Alderman H, Hall A. Epidemiology of intestinal helminth infestations among schoolchildren in southern Uganda. *East Afr Med J.* (2001) 78:283–6. doi: 10.4314/eamj.v78i6.9019
32. Mwanjali G, Kihamia C, Kakoko DVC, Lekule F, Ngowi H, Johansen MV, et al. Prevalence and risk factors associated with human *Taenia Solium* infections in Mbozi District, Mbeya Region, Tanzania. *PLoS Negl Trop Dis.* (2013) 7:2102. doi: 10.1371/journal.pntd.0002102
33. Eom KS, Chai J-Y, Yong T-S, Min D-Y, Rim H-J, Kihamia C, et al. Morphologic and genetic identification of taenia tapeworms in Tanzania and DNA genotyping of *Taenia solium*. *Korean J Parasitol.* (2011) 49:399. doi: 10.3347/kjp.2011.49.4.399
34. Kanobana K, Praet N, Kabwe C, Dorny P, Lukanu P, Madinga J, et al. High prevalence of *Taenia solium* cysticerosis in a village community of Bas-Congo, Democratic Republic of Congo. *Int J Parasitol.* (2011) 41:1015–8. doi: 10.1016/j.ijpara.2011.06.004
35. Makita K, Fèvre EM, Waiswa C, Kaboyo W, Eisler MC, Welburn SC. Evidence-based identification of the most important livestock related zoonotic diseases in Kampala, Uganda. *J Vet Med Sci.* (2011) 73:49. doi: 10.1292/jvms.11-0049
36. Ngugi AK, Bottomley C, Kleinschmidt I, Wagner RG, Kakooza-Mwesige A, Ae-Ngibise K, et al. Prevalence of active convulsive epilepsy in sub-Saharan Africa and associated risk factors: cross-sectional and case-control studies. *Lancet Neurol.* (2013) 12:253–63. doi: 10.1016/S1474-4422(13)70003-6
37. Nzisabira L, Nsengiyumva G, Bouteille B, Ndayiragije A, Niyongabo T, Bigirimana V, et al. Cysticercosis in the province of Kayanza (Burundi). *Bull Soc Pathol Exot.* (1992) 85:374–7.
38. Nsengiyumva G, Druet-Cabanac M, Ramanankandrasana B, Bouteille B, Nsizabira L, Preux P-MM. Cysticercosis as a major risk factor for epilepsy in Burundi, East Africa. *Epilepsia.* (2003) 44:950–5. doi: 10.1046/j.1528-1157.2003.55302.x
39. Prado-Jean A, Kanobana K, Druet-Cabanac M, Nsengyiumva G, Dorny P, Preux PM, et al. Combined use of an antigen and antibody detection enzyme-linked immunosorbent assay for cysticercosis as tools in an epidemiological study of epilepsy in Burundi. *Trop Med Int Heal.* (2007) 12:895–901. doi: 10.1111/j.1365-3156.2007.01860.x
40. Diagana M, Nsengiyumva G, Tuillas M, Druet-Cabanac M, Bouteille B, Preux PM, et al. Électroencéphalogrammes réalisés chez 250 patients épileptiques dans une zone d'endémie cysticerquienne au Burundi. *Neurophysiol Clin.* (2005) 35:1–10. doi: 10.1016/j.neucli.2004.12.002
41. Mwang'onde BJ, Nkwengulila G, Chacha M. The risk factors for human cysticercosis in Mbulu District, Tanzania. *Onderstepoort J Vet Res.* (2014) 81:5. doi: 10.4102/ojvr.v81i2.719
42. Winkler AS, Willingham AL, Sikasunge CS, Schmutzhard E. Epilepsy and neurocysticercosis in sub-Saharan Africa. *Wiener Klinische Wochenschrift.* (2009) 121:3–12. doi: 10.1007/s00508-009-1242-3
43. Blocher J, Schmutzhard E, Wilkins PP, Gupton PN, Schaffert M, Auer H, et al. A cross-sectional study of people with epilepsy and Neurocysticercosis in Tanzania: clinical characteristics and diagnostic approaches. *PLoS Negl Trop Dis.* (2011) 5:1185. doi: 10.1371/journal.pntd.0001185
44. Thienpont D, De Keyser J, Vandervelden M, Kageruka P. La Cysticercose ce're'brale du porc. *Me'd Trop.* (1959) 39:507–14.
45. Food and Agriculture Organization of the United Nations. *Food Outlook: Biannual Report on Global Food Markets.* Rome: ASHA Lead (2014). p. 18–9. Available online at: http://www.fao.org/3/i4136e/i4136e.pdf
46. Mushonga B, Habarugira G, Birori A, Kandiwa E, Samkange A, Bhebhe E. An epidemiological survey of the magnitude and local perceptions of porcine cysticercosis by two methods in Nyaruguru district, Rwanda. *Vet Parasitol Reg Stud Rep.* (2018) 14:18–24. doi: 10.1016/j.vprsr.2018.07.010
47. Fain A, Musafili I. Verminoses. In: Meheus A, Butera S, Eylenboceh W, Gatera G, Kivits M, Musafili I, editors. *Sante et Maladies au Rwanda.* Bruxelles: Administration Generaale de la Coopération au Développement (1982). p. 314–29.
48. Vanderick F, Fain A, Langi S, Vanbalen H. Deux noveaux cas de c'enurose humaine 'a Taenia brauni au Rwanda, avec une localisation orbitaire du c'enure. *Ann Soc Belg Med Trop.* (1920) 44:1077–9.
49. Gascón J, Corachan M, Ramiréz J. 1989 Gascón_Cysticercosis_5 cases Rwanda. *Med Trop.* (1989) 49:77–80.
50. Tuan J, Kailani L, Ngabitsinze P, Umuganwa S, Munyaneza F, Musoni E, et al. Disseminated cysticercosis in rwanda-case report of a patient presenting with difficulty with walking and skin nodules. *Rwanda Med J.* (2020) 77:30–33. Available online at: https://www.rwandamedicaljournal.org/uploads/1/2/2/1/122149944/cr.19.19.pdf
51. Scaglia M, Gatti S, Malfitano A, Strosselli M, Brusti R. Incidence of intestinal parasitosis among the Batwa and Hutu pygmy tribes of Rwanda. *Bull Soc Pathol Exot Fil.* (1983) 76:818–24.
52. Vanderick FX, Mboryingabo P. La cysticercose humaine au Rwanda [Humain cysticercosis in Rwanda]. *Ann Soc Belg Med Trop.* (1972) 52:153–5.
53. Tsang V, Wilson M. *Taenia solium* cysticercosis: an Unv¡der-recognized but serious public health problem. *Parasitol Today.* (1995) 11:124–6. doi: 10.1016/0169-4758(95)80175-8
54. Rottbeck R, Nshimiyimana JF, Tugirimana P, Düll UE, Sattler J, Hategekimana JC, et al. High prevalence of cysticercosis in people with epilepsy in Southern Rwanda. *PLoS Negl Trop Dis.* (2013) 7:2558. doi: 10.1371/journal.pntd.0002558
55. National Institute of Statistics of Rwanda. *The Third Integrated Household Living Conditions Survey (EICV 3)-Main indicators Report.* (2012). Available online at: https://www.statistics.gov.rw/publication/eicv-3-main-indicators-report
56. Goverment of Rwanda. *Environmental and Management plan (ESMP).* (2019). Available online at: https://gakenke.gov.rw/fileadmin/templates/document/ESMP__GAKENKE.pdf
57. Ash LR, Oriel TC, Savioli L. Bench aids for the diagnosis of intestinal parasites. *World Health Org.* (1996) 54:548. doi: 10.4269/ajtmh.1996.54.5.TM0540050548a
58. Knight WB, Hiatt RA, Cline BL, Ritchie LS. A modification of the formol ether concentration technique for increased sensitivity in detecting *Schistosoma mansoni* eggs. *Am J Trop Med Hyg.* (1976) 25:818–23. doi: 10.4269/ajtmh.1976.25.818
59. Allan JC, Craig PS, Avila G, Flisser A, Noval JG. Immunodiagnosis of taeniasis by coproantigen detection. *Parasitology.* (1990) 101:473–7. doi: 10.1017/S0031182000060686
60. Gonzalez AE, García HH, Gilman RH, Tsang VCW. Control of *Taenia solium*. *Acta Tropica.* (2003) 87:103–9. doi: 10.1016/S0001-706X(03)00025-1
61. Bustos JA, Rodriguez S, Jimenez JA, Moyano LM, Castillo Y, Ayvar V, et al. Detection of *Taenia solium* taeniasis coproantigen is an early indicator of treatment failure for taeniasis. *Clin Vaccine Immunol.* (2012) 19:570–3. doi: 10.1128/CVI.05428-11
62. Tsang VCW, Brand JA, Boyer AE. An enzyme-linked immunoelectrotransfer blot assay and glycoprotein antigens for diagnosing human cysticercosis (*Taenia solium*). *J Infect Dis.* (1989) 159:50–9. doi: 10.1093/infdis/159.1.50
63. Gonzalez AE, Cama V, Gilman RH, Tsang VCW, Pilcher JB, Chavera A, et al. Prevalence and comparison of serologic assays, necropsy, and tongue examination for the diagnosis of porcine cysticercosis in Peru. *Am J Trop Med Hyg.* (1990) 43:194–9. doi: 10.4269/ajtmh.1990.43.194
64. Tsang VCW, Pilcher JA, Zhou W, Boyer AE, Kamango-Sollo EIP, Rhoads ML, et al. Efficacy of the immunoblot assay for cysticercosis in pigs and modulated expression of distinct IgM/ IgG activities to *Taenia solium* antigens in experimental infections. *Vet Immunol Immunopathol.* (1991)

29:69–78. doi: 10.1016/0165-2427(91)90053-F

65. Garcia HH, Harrison LJS, Parkhouse RME, Montenegro T, Martinez SM, Tsang VCW, et al. A specific antigen-detection ELISA for the diagnosis of human neurocysticercosis. *Trans R Soc Trop Med Hyg.* (1998) 92:411–4. doi: 10.1016/S0035-9203(98)91069-0
66. Garcia HH. Serological diagnosis and follow-up of severe neurocysticercosis using HP10 antigen detection: commentary. *Nat Clin Pract Neurol.* (2007) 3:488–9. doi: 10.1038/ncpneuro0563
67. Brandt JRA, Geerts S, Deken R De, Kumar V, Ceulemans F, Brijs L, et al. A monoclonal antibody-based ELISA for the detection of circulating excretory-secretory antigens in *Taenia saginata* cysticercosis. *Int J Parasitol.* (1992) 22:471–7. doi: 10.1016/0020-7519(92)90148-E
68. Van Kerckhoven I, Vansteenkiste W, Claes M, Geerts S, Brandt J. Improved detection of circulating antigen in cattle infected with *Taenia saginata* metacestodes. *Vet Parasitol.* (1998) 76:269–74. doi: 10.1016/S0304-4017(97)00226-4
69. Dorny P, Phiri IK, Vercruysse J, Gabriel S, Willingham AL, Brandt J, et al. A Bayesian approach for estimating values for prevalence and diagnostic test characteristics of porcine cysticercosis. *Int J Parasitol.* (2004) 34:569–76. doi: 10.1016/j.ijpara.2003.11.014
70. Zea-Vera A, Cordova EG, Rodriguez S, Gonzales I, Pretell EJ, Castillo Y, et al. *Parasite Antigen in Serum Predicts the Presence of Viable Brain Parasites in Patients With Apparently Calcified Cysticercosis Only.* (2013). Available online at: https://academic.oup.com/cid/article-abstract/57/7/e154/337081 (accessed December 14, 2020).
71. Mupfasoni D, Karibushi B, Koukounari A, Ruberanziza E, Kaberuka T, Kramer MH, et al. Polyparasite helminth infections and their association to anaemia and undernutrition in Northern Rwanda. *PLoS Negl Trop Dis.* (2009) 3:517. doi: 10.1371/journal.pntd.0000517
72. Emile N, Bosco NJ, Karine B. Prevalence of intestinal parasitic infections and associated risk factors among Kigali Institute of Education students in Kigali, Rwanda. *Trop Biomed.* (2013) 30:718–26. Available online at: http://www.msptm.org/files/718_-_726_Bernard_Karine.pdf
73. Rujeni N, Morona D, Ruberanziza E, Mazigo HD. Schistosomiasis and soil-transmitted helminthiasis in Rwanda: an update on their epidemiology and control. *Infect Dis Poverty.* (2017) 6:8. doi: 10.1186/s40249-016-0212-z
74. Parkhouse RME, Rojas R G, Aguilar CM, Medina C, Ferrer E, Cortez Alcovedes MM. Diagnosis of taeniosis in rural venezuelan communities: preliminary characterization of a *Taenia solium* specific monoclonal (VP-1) coproantigen ELISA. *Acta Trop.* (2020) 207:105445. doi: 10.1016/j.actatropica.2020.105445
75. García HH, González AE, Evans CA, Gilman RH. *Taenia solium Cysticercosis.* (2003). Available online at: www.thelancet.com
76. Jayashi CM, Arroyo G, Lightowlers MW, García HH, Rodríguez S, Gonzalez AE. Seroprevalence and risk factors for *Taenia solium* cysticercosis in rural pigs of Northern Peru. *PLoS Negl Trop Dis.* (2012) 6:1733. doi: 10.1371/journal.pntd.0001733
77. Schantz PM, Moore AC, Muñoz JL, Hartman BJ, Schaefer JA, Aron AM, et al. Neurocysticercosis in an orthodox Jewish community in New York City. *N Engl J Med.* (1992) 327:692–5. doi: 10.1056/NEJM199209033271004
78. Assana E, Lightowlers MW, Zoli AP, Geerts S. *Taenia solium* taeniosis/cysticercosis in Africa: risk factors, epidemiology and prospects for control using vaccination. *Vet Parasitol.* (2013) 195:14–23. doi: 10.1016/j.vetpar.2012.12.022
79. Gweba M, Faleke OO, Junaidu AU, Fabiyi JP, Fajinmi AO. Some risk factors for *Taenia solium* cysticercosis in semi-intensively raised pigs in Zuru, Nigeria. *Vet Ital.* (2010) 46:57–67. Available online at: https://www.izs.it/vet_italiana/2010/46_1/57.htm

17

Donkey Fascioliasis within a One Health Control Action: Transmission Capacity, Field Epidemiology and Reservoir Role in a Human Hyperendemic Area

Santiago Mas-Coma [1], Paola Buchon [2], Ilra R. Funatsu [1], Rene Angles [3], Cristina Mas-Bargues [4], Patricio Artigas [1], M. Adela Valero [1] and M. Dolores Bargues [1]*

[1] Departamento de Parasitología, Facultad de Farmacia, Universidad de Valencia, Valencia, Spain, [2] Unidad de Limnología, Instituto de Ecología, Universidad Mayor de San Andrés (UMSA), La Paz, Bolivia, [3] Cátedra de Parasitología, Facultad de Medicina, Universidad Mayor de San Andrés (UMSA), La Paz, Bolivia, [4] Departamento de Fisiología, Facultad de Medicina, Universidad de Valencia, Valencia, Spain

***Correspondence:**
M. Dolores Bargues
m.d.bargues@uv.es

A One Health initiative has been implemented for fascioliasis control in a human hyperendemic area for the first time. The area selected for this multidisciplinary approach is the Northern Bolivian Altiplano, where the highest prevalences and intensities in humans have been reported. Within the strategic intervention axis of control activities concerning animal reservoirs, complete experimental studies, and field surveys have been performed to assess the fascioliasis transmission capacity and epidemiological role of the donkey for the first time. Laboratory studies with altiplanic donkey-infecting *Fasciola hepatica* and altiplanic *Galba truncatula* snail vector isolates demonstrate that the donkey assures the viability of the whole fasciolid life cycle. Several aspects indicate, however, that *F. hepatica* does not reach, in the donkey, the level of adaptation it shows in sheep and cattle in this high altitude hyperendemic area. This is illustrated by a few-day delay in egg embryonation, longer prepatent period despite similar miracidial infectivity and shorter patent period in the intramolluscan development, lower cercarial production per snail, different cercarial chronobiology, shorter snail survival after shedding end, shorter longevity of shedding snails, and lower metacercarial infectivity in Wistar rats. Thus, the role of the donkey in the disease transmission should be considered secondary. Field survey results proved that liver fluke prevalence and intensity in donkeys are similar to those of the main reservoirs sheep and cattle in this area. Fasciolid egg shedding by a donkey individual contributes to the environment contamination at a rate similar to sheep and cattle. In this endemic area, the pronounced lower number of donkeys when compared to sheep and cattle indicates that the epidemiological reservoir role of the donkey is also secondary. However, the donkey plays an important epidemiological role in the disease spread because of its use by Aymara inhabitants for good transport, movements, and travel from one locality/zone to another, a repercussion to be considered in the present geographical spread of fascioliasis in the Altiplano due to climate change. Donkey transport of parasite and vector, including movements inside the zone under control and potential introduction from outside that zone, poses a problem for the One Health initiative.

Keywords: human fascioliasis hyperendemic, One Health, donkey, *Fasciola hepatica*, *Galba truncatula* experimental transmission, field epidemiology, reservoir role, Bolivia

INTRODUCTION

Human fascioliasis is a parasitic disease to which only secondary public health importance was given until the 1990s (1). The scenario completely changed henceforth, when the number of case reports began to gradually increase in both the Old and New Worlds, but mainly with the description of human endemic areas in many developing countries of Latin America, Africa, and Asia (2), although human infection also occurs in developed countries (3). The public health importance of this emergence was early on recognized by the World Health Organization when including this disease among the group of food-borne trematodiases within the list of Neglected Tropical Diseases (NTDs) (4).

Among the many factors underlying this decision of WHO, the following stand out: (i) the worldwide distribution of this disease caused by two large-sized liver fluke species, *Fasciola hepatica* and *F. gigantica* (5); (ii) its high pathogenicity (6–8), immunological consequences in both the acute (9) and chronic phases (10) of the disease, and its increasing morbidity caused by the immunesuppression-induced very frequent coinfections with other pathogenic microorganisms (11, 12) and parasites (13, 14); (iii) the strong influences of climate change and global change on its transmission and epidemiology (15, 16) because of the lack of a premunition buffer at life cycle end at definitive host level (17, 18); and (iv) its impact on the development of rural communities of low-income countries, including severe clinical pictures (8, 19) and sequelae (8, 20).

The availability of a very efficient drug for human treatment, triclabendazole (21), became crucial in this WHO's decision and subsequent defining of the worldwide strategy of preventive chemotherapy according to different control programs. Such control approaches were adapted to the different transmission patterns and epidemiological situations in the countries presenting human endemic areas and are to be strengthened within the new WHO 2030 road map on NTDs by contributing to sustainable and resilient health systems (22).

South America is the continent presenting the highest number of human fascioliasis endemic areas reported. These areas are characterized for their location at high altitudes in altiplanos and valleys of the Andean region. The main countries affected by this disease because of presenting human endemic areas are Peru (14, 23, 24), Bolivia (13, 25, 26), Argentina (27–29), and Chile (30, 31).

Bolivia stands out because of including the hyperendemic area where the highest prevalences and intensities of fascioliasis have been reported in humans (32) and where children become infected very early in their lives (33). This area is distributed throughout the Northern Bolivian Altiplano, between Lake Titicaca and the valley of the capital city La Paz, at 3,820–4,100 m a.s.l. In 2007–2008, a wide fascioliasis control initiative by yearly mass treatment campaigns was launched by the World Health Organization (WHO) in this area (34, 35) and has been yearly implemented henceforth. Subsequent interannual monitoring assessments indicated infection and reinfection of children by ingestion of metacercariae with freshwater plants or drinking water (36), as a consequence of the high endemicity maintained by the infection rates in livestock (32, 37).

At a PAHO-WHO meeting in La Paz in 2014, it was decided to implement a One Health action to decrease the human risk of liver fluke infection. The One Health is a strategy that encourages interdisciplinary collaboration and communication on health at the human-animal-environmental interface, including multidisciplinary efforts to attain optimal health of people and animals, and the most appropriate measures for the environment (38). This type of approach has been supported by WHO, FAO, and OIE to face the control of zoonotic diseases (39, 40). For the control of fascioliasis in the Bolivian Altiplano, the initiative was planned to include long-term experimental studies, field monitoring assessments and control activities, according to modern standards already analyzed for trematode diseases (41–43).

The wide heterogeneity of transmission patterns and epidemiological scenarios of fascioliasis creates difficulties when applying control activities within a One Health action. Two factors cause these problems:

- Snail vector specificity: Fasciolid species use a wide spectrum of freshwater species of the family Lymnaeidae which present different ecological requirements. These snails are distributed worldwide, but only given species groups are used by the liver flukes, mainly species of *Galba/Fossaria* by *F. hepatica*, species of the *Radix* group by *F. gigantica*, and a singular species *Pseudosuccinea columella* by both fasciolids (44). In South America, *Radix* is absent and fascioliasis transmission is assured by *Galba/Fossaria* species which are malacologically indifferentiable and need DNA marker sequencing for specimen classification (45, 46). Fortunately, only one lymnaeid species has been proved to inhabit the Northern Bolivian Altiplano hyperendemic area, namely *Galba truncatula* imported from Europe by the Spanish "conquistadores" some time ago and which is geographically spreading along the Altiplano at present, due to climate change and human activities (47).
- Mammal host specificity: The adult stage of fasciolids is able to successfully infect and develop in many different domestic and wild species of mainly herbivorous but also

omnivorous mammals. In the Bolivian Altiplano, similarly as throughout all of the Americas, only *F. hepatica* is present, which pronouncedly simplifies the disease characteristics. Wild lagomorphs and rodents, including domestic guinea pigs (*Cavia porcellus*, locally known as "cuyes" or "quwis"), were already proved to play no role in fascioliasis transmission (48). Among domestic animals, only sheep, cattle, pigs, and donkeys have been involved as important reservoirs in that area (32). Other species such as goats, horses, llamas and alpacas, despite being present, play no transmission role due to different reasons (49).

Within the aforementioned One Health initiative, the aim of the present study is to expose the results obtained in experimental studies on *F. hepatica* transmission and field surveys on animal liver fluke infection to assess the role of the donkey in the transmission and epidemiology of the disease in the very high altitude hyperendemic area of the Northern Bolivian Altiplano. To catalog the contribution of the donkey to fascioliasis in this area, results are compared with those of similar studies previously performed on the main altiplanic reservoir species: sheep and cattle (50).

The laboratory studies included the experimental follow-up of the development stages of egg, miracidium, lymnaeid snail vector infection, intramolluscan larval development, cercarial production, chronobiology of the cercarial shedding, vector survival to infection, metacercarial infectivity of mammal host, and adult stage development of altiplanic donkey isolates through altiplanic *G. truncatula* isolates. This is the first time that such experimental fascioliasis studies focus on the donkey. The field studies included the assessment of prevalence, intensity, egg measurements, and egg shedding rates in nature. This is the first time that the epidemiological role of the donkey as animal reservoir is assessed in a human endemic area.

MATERIALS AND METHODS

Experimental Studies

Fasciolid Materials

Fecal samples from naturally infected donkey individuals from the Altiplanic locality of Ancocagua were used for the experimental study of the embryonation of the eggs of *F. hepatica* (**Figure 1**). Eggs isolated by filtration were conserved in natural water under complete darkness at 4°C until starting of the embryogenesis follow up study.

For the experimental infection of lymnaeid snails, *F. hepatica* eggs were similarly obtained from donkeys from Ancocagua (**Figure 1**). Eggs were similarly isolated by filtration and conserved until used for snail infection in the laboratory.

For the experimental infection of Wistar rats, *F. hepatica* metacercariae were obtained from the aforementioned experimentally infected lymnaeid snails. These metacercariae were stored in natural water in total darkness until required. The storage temperature was 4°C, according to the usual standards in liver fluke studies (51).

Eggs of *F. hepatica* were also collected from sheep, cattle, and pigs of the same Northern Bolivian Altiplano human hyperendemic area, although the studies of the isolates of these three definitive reservoir hosts are the focus of other articles to avoid excessive text length and reference number.

Study of the Egg Embryogenesis

The egg embryogenesis was experimentally followed at constant 20°C, at microscopic study intervals of 4 days. Egg development was made by differentiation of (i) eggs including an early developing morula (E.E.D.M.), (ii) eggs in the phase of advanced morula, showing vitelline granules and/or spheroidal cells (E.A.M.), (iii) eggs in the phase of outlined miracidium, in which a miracidial form begins to be observed (E.O.M.), and (iv) eggs in the phase of developed miracidium, in which a fully developed miracidium is observed inside (E.D.M.). For each 4-day study, a total of 33 eggs from each of four host individuals were analyzed between slip and coverslip. Counting did not only include E.E.D.M., E.A.M., E.O.M., and E.D.M., but also (i) degenerated eggs, (ii) empty eggs, and (iii) broken eggs (**Figure 2**). Degenerated, empty, and broken eggs (eggs easily break when open and empty after miracidial release) are very few at the beginning but of course increase with time and are the marked majority in the last days of the follow-up study. Egg counts were noted in percentages per observational day. Percentages of degenerated, empty and broken eggs are not included in the graph of follow-up curves because they do intervene in the transmission.

Experimental Infection of Snails

Fully embryonated eggs were put under light to force the hatching of developed miracidia which were afterwards used for the experimental infection of snails (52). Only laboratory-borne snails were used. Lymnaeid snails of a size of 4.0–5.0 mm were used to assess infection susceptibility, by exposing each snail to miracidia for 4 h in a small Petri dish containing 2 ml of fresh water. The disappearance of the miracidium was taken as verification of its successful penetration into the snail.

The donkey *F. hepatica* isolate was used for individual infection assays of lymnaeid snails under the experimental conditions of a monomiracidial dose and 20/20°C day/night temperature according to a photoperiod of 12 h light/12 h darkness in climatic chambers (HPS-1500, VB-0714, and HPS-500 models of Heraeus-Vötsch) (46). The characteristics, conditions, and number of snails in these snail infection experiments are detailed in **Table 1**. After the infection, snails were returned to 2,000 ml containers, at 90% relative humidity (r.h.), 20/20°C day/night temperature according to 12/12 h light/darkness, and dry lettuce *ad libitum*, until day 30 post-infection, in which they were again isolated in Petri dishes to allow daily monitoring of cercarial shedding by individual snails. Lettuce was provided *ad libitum* to each snail in a Petri dish during both shedding and post-shedding periods until death of the snail. The cercarial shedding was followed by daily counting of metacercariae in each Petri dish.

Laboratory Cultures of the Snail Vector

Galba truncatula has recently been proved to be the only lymnaeid species inhabiting the Northern Bolivian Altiplano

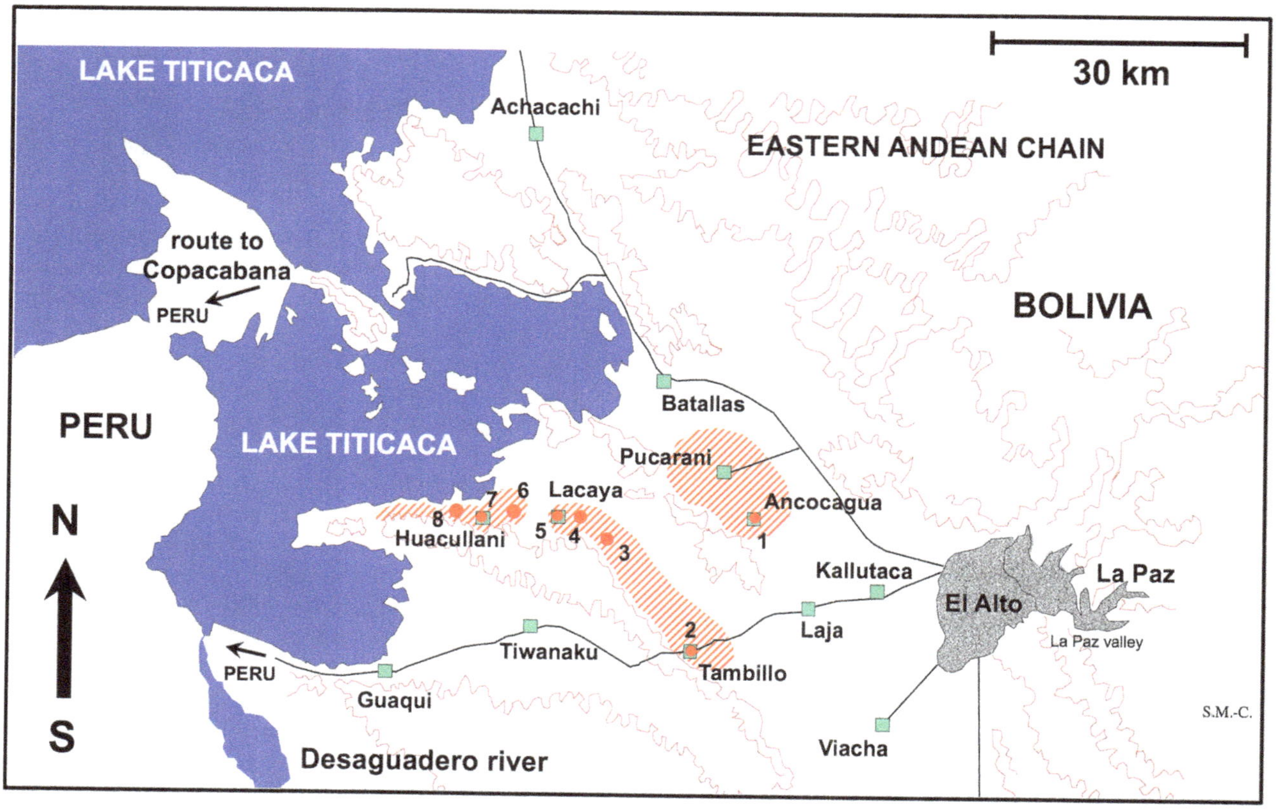

FIGURE 1 | Map showing the Northern Bolivian Altiplano human fascioliasis hyperendemic area, at 3,820–4,100 m altitude, including zones where donkeys were surveyed and localities where lymnaeid snail vector specimens of *Galba truncatula* were collected. Localities: (1) Ancocagua; (2) Tambillo; (3) Korila; (4) Chiripujo; (5) Lacaya Baja; (6) Chojasihui; (7) Huacullani; (8) Queroni.

hyperendemic area, by the sequencing of complete nuclear ribosomal DNA and mitochondrial DNA markers (47). This species is of European origin and differs from the Neotropical species of the *Galba/Fossaria* group of lymnaeids which also act as vectors of fascioliasis in South America (45). Living specimens of *G. truncatula* were collected in the locality of Tambillo (**Figure 1**) and transported under isothermal conditions for their laboratory adaptation to standardized controlled conditions of 20°C, 90% r.h. and a 12/12 h light/darkness photoperiod in the aforementioned precision climatic chambers. The possible natural infection by fasciolids was always individually verified prior to the launch of laboratory cultures. This was performed by keeping each lymnaeid specimen isolated in a Petri dish containing a small amount of natural water. After 24 h, the presence or absence of motionless metacercarial cysts or moving cercariae was verified in each Petri dish. Non-infected lymnaeids were arranged in standard breeding boxes containing 2,000 ml fresh water, to assure locality-pure cultures. The water was changed weekly and lettuce added *ad libitum*.

Laboratory Infections of Wistar Rats

A total of 18 male Wistar rats (Iffa Credo, Barcelona, Spain) aged 4–5 weeks were used throughout. A balanced commercial rodent diet (Panlab Chow A04) and water were provided *ad libitum*, according to standards previously reported (53).

Wistar rats were infected according to methods previously described (54). A dose of 20 *F. hepatica* metacercariae per rat was used (**Table 2**). Animal care, animal health, body condition, and well-being were assessed on a weekly basis by means of checking their body weight and the appearance of the fur. Infected animals presented a lower body weight than negative controls at the end of the experiment. No mortality occurred. Infection prevalence and intensity (number of worms successfully developed in each rat) were established by necropsy 12 weeks after infection. Metacercariae were inoculated orally by means of a gastric tube. The number of Wistar rats in each infection experiment are noted in **Table 2**. Finally, animals were euthanized with an overdose of an anesthetic (IsoFlo; Dr Esteve SA, Barcelona, Spain), and *F. hepatica* worms were collected under a dissecting microscope, according to methods already outlined before (55). The bile duct was initially examined for the presence of flukes, followed by the whole liver, although the rest of the organs were also evaluated. The thoracic and abdominal viscera and cavities were examined and thoroughly rinsed with water to assure the recovery of all worms.

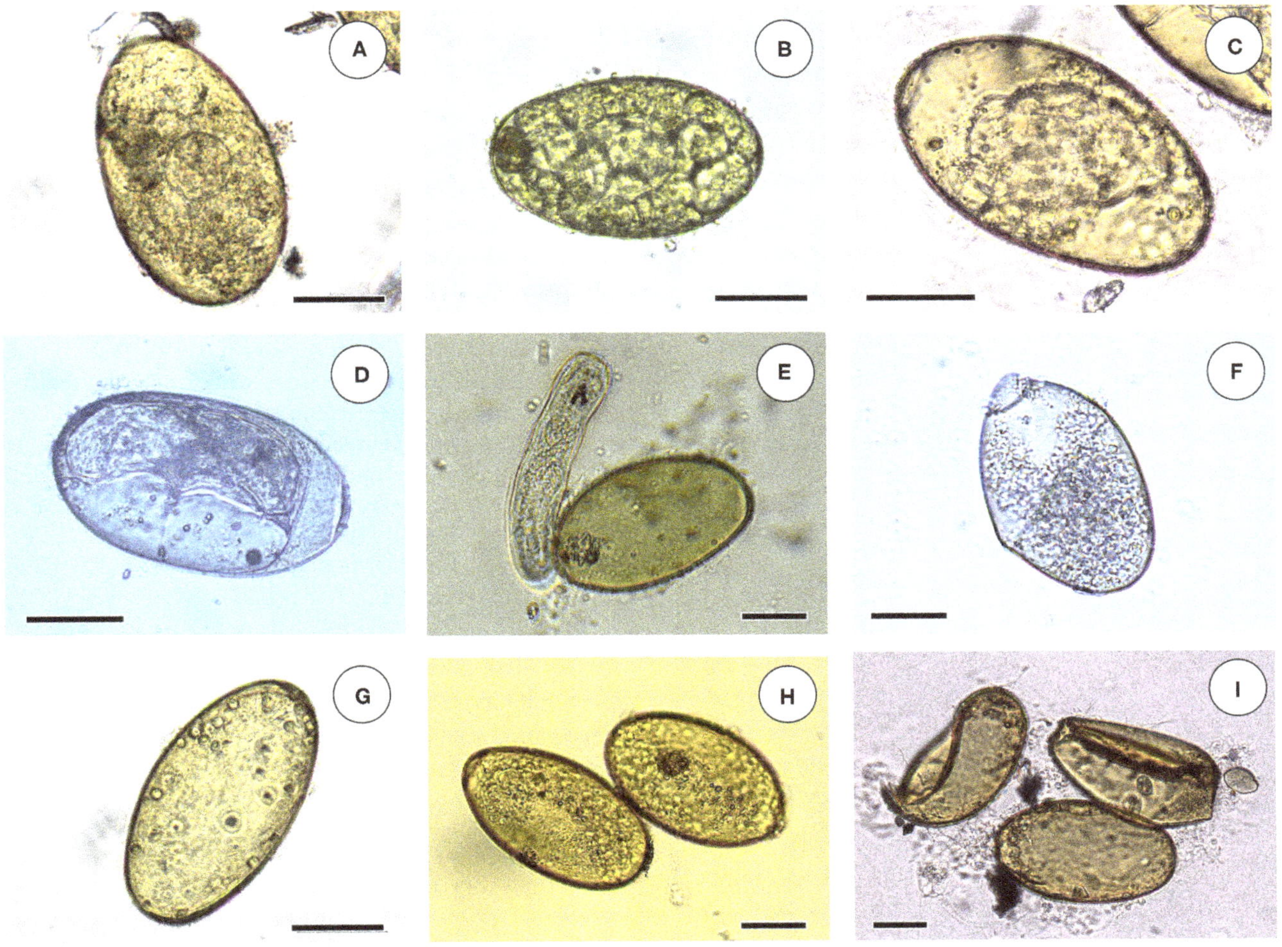

FIGURE 2 | Embryonation stages in liver fluke eggs: **(A)** egg including an early developing morula (E.E.D.M.); **(B)** egg in the phase of advanced morula, showing vitelline granules and spheroidal cells (E.A.M.); **(C)** egg in the phase of outlined miracidium, in which a miracidial form begins to be observed (E.O.M.); **(D)** egg in the phase of developed miracidium, in which a fully developed miracidium is observed inside (E.D.M.); **(E)** empty egg immediately after miracidium hatching; **(F)** broken open egg after miracidial release; **(G)** empty egg; **(H)** two degenerated eggs; **(I)** two broken eggs and an empty egg. Scale bar = 40 µm.

Field Surveys of Donkeys

Host Animals Studied

Fecal samples from a total of 84 donkeys were collected from different zones of the Northern Bolivian Altiplano hyperendemic area (**Table 3**). The geographical distribution of the localities and zones surveyed is shown in **Figure 1**.

In the Altiplano, donkeys are usually found isolated, only rarely more than one specimen accompanying grazing herds of sheep and/or cattle. The surveys were made to assure that a fecal sample of all donkeys found during the survey days could be obtained. Unfortunately, stool sample collection could not be made following the different annual seasons in a zone and, thus, no data are available to analyze the variations of prevalence throughout the different months of the year. In the Altiplano hyperendemic area, donkeys are not treated against liver fluke infection.

Stool Sample Preparation and Study

Only coprological methods for qualitative and quantitative analyses were carried out. Fecal samples were placed in numbered plastic bags, transported to the laboratory within the following 5 h, and maintained at 4°C until examination. From each stool sample a quantity of 4 g was sedimented twice, first with 50 ml of detergent solution (1 ml/1,000 cm^3) after filtration and second with 50 ml water, and stained with methyl green according to a standard method (58), before examination under light microscope for *F. hepatica* eggs. A host individual was considered negative when no eggs were found in its respective stool sample after studying 3 slides. The number of eggs shed by a donkey was used to estimate the infection intensity and was expressed in eggs per gram of stools (epg).

Egg measurements were carried out using a computer image analysis system (CIAS) on the basis of standardized measurements known to be useful for fasciolid species (59). Standardized measurements were taken using a microscope and images captured by a digital camera (3CCD color videocamera Sony DXC-930P), which were then analyzed by image analysis software (ImagePro plus version 5.0 for Windows, Media Cybernetics, Silver Spring, Maryland, USA). Egg characteristics studied were: (a) linear measurements: egg length (EL), egg width

TABLE 1 | Experimental infections of altiplanic lymnaeid snails with *Fasciola hepatica* donkey isolate from the Northern Bolivian Altiplano human hyperendemic area.

Host isolate	Donkey	Sheep[a]	Cattle[a]
F. hepatica geogr. origin	Ancocagua	Batallas	Batallas
Lymnaeid geogr. origin	Tambillo	Huacullani	Huacullani
Miracidial dose	Mono-miracidial	Mono-miracidial	Mono-miracidial
Temperature (12 day/12 h night)	20/20°C	20/20°C	20/20°C
No. lymnaeids infected	35	62	55
No. survivor snails at beginning of shedding (%)	25 (71.4%)	54 (87.1%)	48 (87.3%)
No. shedding snails (%)	7 (28.0%)	28 (51.8%)	12 (25.0%)
Prepatent period in dpi (mean)	52–69 (60.5)	48–92 (55.6)	49–76 (55.5)
Shedding end in dpi (mean)	52–117 (86.1)	52–136 (89.4)	58–135 (101.6)
Shedding length in days	1–49 (26.6)	1–88 (34.7)	1–85 (47.1)
No. total cercariae shed	333	5,542	3,672
No. cercariae/snail (mean)	2–92 (47.6)	8–562 (197.9)	8–581 (306.0)
Snail survival after shedding end in days	1–43 (14.8)	1–132 (24.5)	1–133 (42.3)
Longevity of shedding snails in dpi	77–126 (101.0)	53–192 (113.8)	76–268 (143.9)
Longevity of non-shedding snails in dpi	34–183 (60.7)	49–196 (139.1)	31–209 (105.4)

dpi, days post-infection.
[a]*Data from Mas-Coma et al. (50).*

(EW), and egg perimeter (EPe); (b) areas: egg area (EA); (c) ratios: EL/EW ratio. For each measure, minimum and maximum values, mean, and standard deviation were determined.

Statistical Analyses

To assess the transmission capacity and epidemiological role of the donkey isolate, each characteristic studied was compared with that of the sheep and cattle isolates of *F. hepatica* from the same Northern Bolivian Altiplano, which have been proved to be the main animal reservoir species in this human hyperendemic area. This comparative assessment is feasible because based on data obtained following the same methods and techniques both in the laboratory experiments and in the field work and which have been reported in another study (50).

Statistical analyses were performed using SPSS Statistics 26. Development egg data (E.E.D.M., E.A.M., E.O.M., E.D.M.) were compared by ANOVA test. Statistical comparison of categorical variables was carried out with the Chi-square test and Yates continuity corrected Chi-square test. Means obtained in data from experimental infections of lymnaeid snails and from experimental infections of Wistar rats were compared by non-parametric Kruskal-Wallis test. Fasciolid egg size measurements (EL, EW, EPe, and EL/EW) were compared by *post-hoc* tests (L.S.D., Student–Newman–Keuls and Duncan's tests). Results were considered statistically significant when $p < 0.05$.

RESULTS

Egg Embryonation

The egg embryonation of the donkey isolate of altiplanic *F. hepatica* could be experimentally followed at 20°C until complete development of all eggs (**Figure 3**). An outlined miracidium form begins to be observed inside eggs at day 24. The first fully developed miracidium appears at day 28. Eggs including a fully developed miracidium were henceforth observed in each observational day. The percentage of fully developed miracidia follows an increasing curve until a peak on day 60, after which it gradually decreases until day 127. No statistically significant differences in the average egg embryonation (E.O.M., E.D.M.) of the donkey isolate (36.63%) in the 60 days were detected when compared to the sheep isolate (38.93%) and cattle isolate (26.63%) from the Altiplano ($p > 0.05$).

Snail Infectivity and Intramolluscan Development

Snail vector infection assays performed with the altiplanic donkey isolate furnished results which are shown in **Table 1**, including their comparison with the altiplanic sheep and cattle isolates. The donkey isolate (28.0%) was even slightly more efficient than the cattle isolate (25.0%), although both at distance from the sheep isolate (51.8%). Nevertheless, no statistically significant differences in the percentage of snails successfully infected by a monomiracidial dose at 20/20°C (= the snail infectivity) between the donkey isolate and the two main reservoirs ($p > 0.05$) were detected.

The donkey isolate prepatent period (60.5 days) showed a slightly higher mean value than the sheep isolate (55.6 days) and the cattle isolate (55.5 days). However, no statistically significant differences in prepatent period between the donkey isolate and the two main reservoirs ($p > 0.05$) were detected. The donkey isolate cercarial shedding period (average: 26.6 days) showed a shorter mean value than the sheep isolate (average: 34.7 days) and the cattle isolate (average: 47.1 days). No statistically significant differences in the cercarial shedding period were anyway detected between the donkey isolate and the two main reservoirs ($p > 0.05$).

Significant differences were observed when comparing the smaller production of cercariae per infected snail of the donkey isolate (average: 47.6 cercariae/snail) with that of the sheep (average: 197.9 cercariae/snail) and cattle (average: 306 cercariae/snail) isolates ($p < 0.05$).

The assessment of the infection impact on snails was measured by the snail survival after shedding end in days, as well as by the comparison of the longevity of shedding and non-shedding snails. These three characteristics in the donkey isolate showed mean and maximum dpi values clearly shorter than in sheep and cattle isolates, all of them proving to be statistically different ($p < 0.05$).

TABLE 2 | Experimental infections of Wistar rats with experimentally obtained metacercariae from donkey isolate and comparison with sheep and cattle isolates from the Northern Bolivian Altiplano human hyperendemic area.

Host isolate	**Donkey**		**Sheep**[a]		**Cattle**[a]	
F. hepatica geographical origin	Ancocagua	Ancocagua	Batallas	Ancocagua	Kallutaca	Batallas
Age of metacercariae	6 weeks	10 weeks	1 week	2 weeks	6 weeks	8 weeks
No. metacercariae inoculated per rat	20	20	20	20	20	20
No. inoculated rats	8	10	14	23	4	4
No. rats infected (%)	3 (37.5%)	4 (40.0%)	11 (78.6%)	18 (78.3%)	4 (100%)	2 (50.0%)
No. flukes recovered per rat (mean)	1–6 (3.3)	2–3 (2.7)	1–8 (3.6)	1–10 (3.7)	1–2 (1.7)	1–2 (1.5)
Intensity[b]	6.2%	5.5%	14.3%	14.6%	8.8%	3.7%
Mean % flukes recovered/rat[c]	16.7%	11.2%	18.2%	18.6%	8.8%	7.5%

[a] *Data from Mas-Coma et al. (50).*
[b] *Intensity = total % of flukes recovered = (total No. of flukes recovered/total No. of metacercariae administered in all rats) × 100.*
[c] *Mean % flukes recovered/rat = Mean % of flukes recovered per infected rat = (flukes recovered/metacercariae administered per infected rat) × 100.*

TABLE 3 | Prevalence and intensity of *Fasciola hepatica* infection found by coprological analyses in donkeys of different zones of the Northern Bolivian Altiplano human hyperendemic area and comparison with local prevalences in sheep and cattle from the same zones.

Locality	**Endemic zone**	**Donkey**				**Sheep**[a]	**Cattle**[a]
		Prevalence		**Intensity**		**Prevalence**	**Prevalence**
		No. analyzed/ infected	**%**	**Range (epg)**	**Mean (epg)**	**No. analyzed/infected (%)**	**No. analyzed/infected (%)**
Ancocagua	Pucarani	35/3	8.6[b]	3–43	22.3	170/97 (57.1)	195/22 (11.3)
Tambillo	Tambillo-Lacaya	2/0	0[c]	–	–	230/113 (49.1)	50/2 (4.0)
Korila	Tambillo-Lacaya	1/0	0[c]	–	–	100/87 (87.0)	–
Chiripujo	Tambillo-Lacaya	2/0	0[c]	–	–	–	141/17 (12.0)
Lacaya Baja	Tambillo-Lacaya	10/3	30.0[b]	11–58	32.7	100/64 (64.0)	43/3 (47.0)
Chojasihui	Huacullani	6/3	50.0	14–101	50.7	100/70 (70.0)	29/9 (31.0)
Huacullani	Huacullani	21/11	52.4	4–90	74.0	120/81 (67.5)	210/95 (45.2)
Queroni	Huacullani	7/0	0[c]	–	–	100/70 (70.0)	–
Total		84/20	23.8[b]	3–101	28.1	920/582 (63.7)	768/148 (19.3)

[a] *Data from Buchon et al. (56), Grock et al. (57), Mas-Coma et al. (32, 50).*
[b] *Significantly different vs. sheep and cattle, determined by Chi-square/test Chi-square with Yates' correction ($p < 0.05$).*
[c] *Statistical comparison could not be made.*

Chronobiology of Cercarial Shedding

The chronobiological patterns of cercarial emergence in the donkey isolate are shown in **Figures 4A–D**. The shedding period analyzed according to the mean amounts of cercariae shed daily and weekly from the day of the emergence of the first cercaria by each snail is shown in **Figures 4A,B**, The total length of the shedding period lasted up to 49 days (**Figure 4A**) or 7 weeks (**Figure 4B**), with a mean of 26.6 days (**Table 1**). The daily shedding process appears as an irregular succession of waves in which up to seven peaks may be distinguished. Among them, the first peak is the highest and corresponds to the first day of shedding. The weekly analysis of the curve shows that the highest numbers of cercariae are shed during the first 2 weeks. Interestingly, a gradual increase of the weekly cercarial number from week 3 gives rise to a late peaks on week 6.

When the analysis is made from the day of the miracidial infection, the shedding period shows completely different daily and weekly curves (**Figures 4C,D**). When compared with the aforementioned chronobiological patterns from the day of the

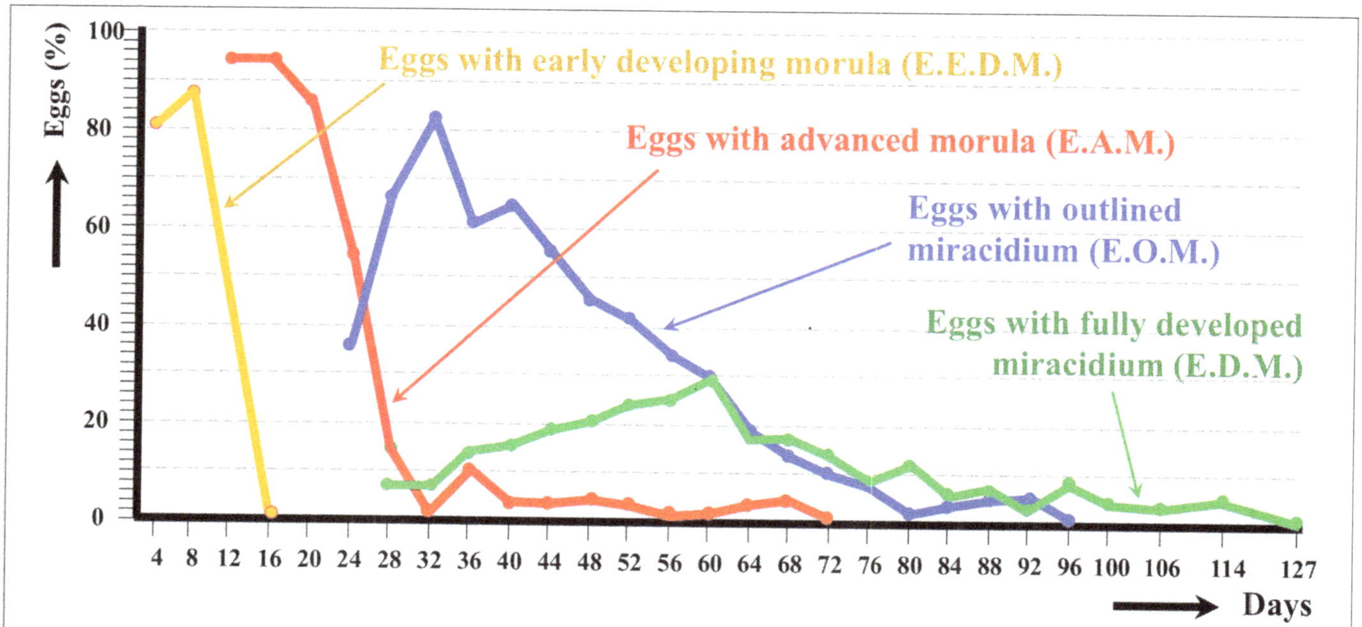

FIGURE 3 | Graph showing the results of the experimental follow-up study of the egg embryonation of the altiplanic donkey isolate of *Fasciola hepatica*, at 4-day study intervals and constant temperature of 20°C. Curves of the percentages of degenerated, empty, and broken eggs are not included.

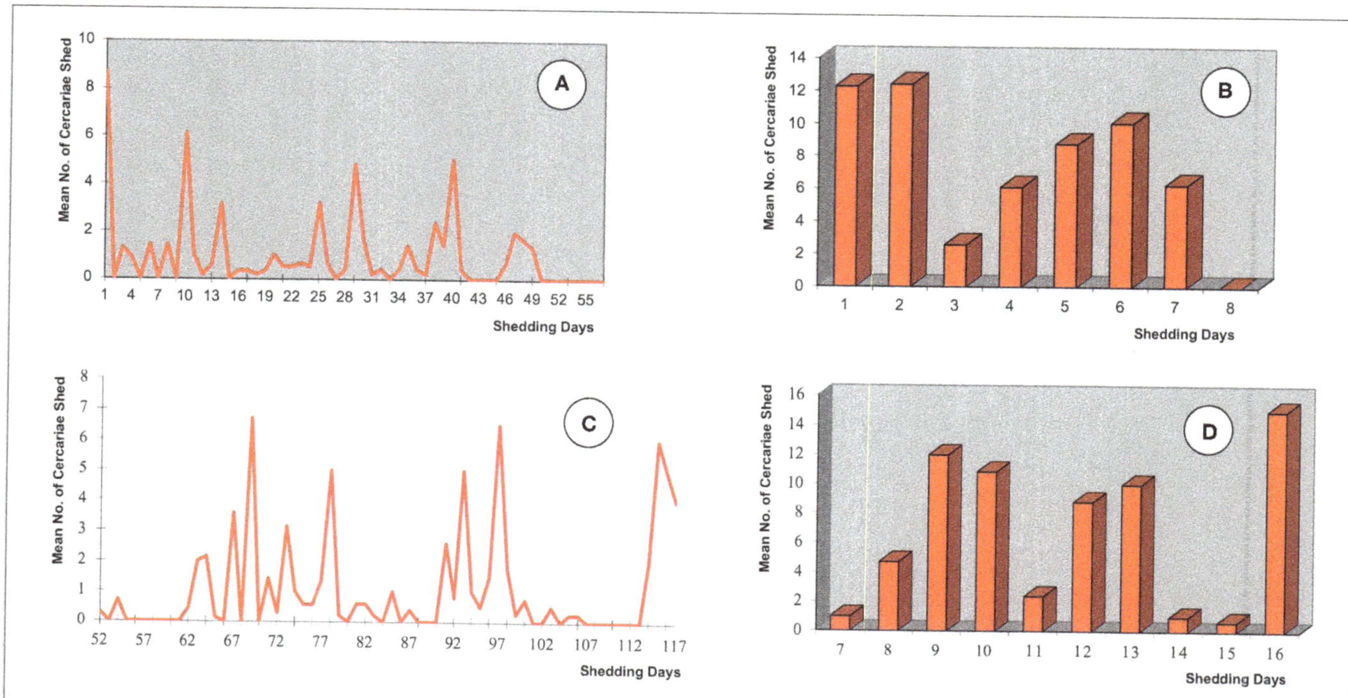

FIGURE 4 | Chronobiological patterns of cercarial emergence by altiplanic *Galba truncatula* monomiracidially infected with the donkey isolate of *Fasciola hepatica* from the Northern Bolivian Altiplano human fascioliasis hyperendemic area: **(A,B)** shedding period analyzed according to the mean amounts of cercariae shed daily and weekly from the day of the emergence of the first cercaria by each snail; **(C,D)** shedding period analyzed according to the mean amounts of cercariae shed daily and weekly from the day of the miracidial infection; prepatent period not shown.

emergence of the first cercaria by each snail (**Figures 4A,B**), several similar peaks appear but two main differences may be distinguished, namely the complete disappearance of the initial peak and the appearance of an evident final peak. These initial and final differences are well-evident in both the daily and the weekly curves. Different delays in the beginning of the cercarial shedding according to different snail specimens, due to individual differences in the prepatent period (**Table 1**), explain the longer daily and weekly curves obtained in this analysis.

Mammal Host Infectivity

Results of the experimental infection of Wistar rats with experimentally obtained metacercariae of the altiplanic donkey isolate are shown in **Table 2**. No statistically significant differences appeared in the infectivity between the donkey isolate and the sheep and cattle isolates regarding the percentage of rats successfully infected (donkey: 38.9%; sheep: 78.4%; cattle: 75.0%; $p > 0.05$). Furthermore, the intensity of infection, measured by the number of flukes recovered per metacercariae inoculated and also per rat, did not show significant differences when comparing the donkey isolate with the sheep and cattle isolates ($p > 0.05$).

Prevalence, Intensity, Egg Measurements, and Shedding Rates

Results obtained in the coprological surveys on donkeys inhabiting selected zones of the fascioliasis hyperendemic area (**Figure 1**) are shown in **Table 3**. However, in the Altiplano the distribution of donkeys is unfortunately very dispersed because of their reduced number when compared to other domestic animals as sheep, cattle, or pigs. So, this equine most frequently appears as individuals isolated throughout large tracts of land and consequently the donkey prevalence data should be considered with the appropriate caution.

A total of 161 eggs from donkey stools were measured. Results and the comparative analysis with fasciolid eggs shed by altiplanic sheep and cattle are shown in **Table 4**. The statistical analysis by *post-hoc* tests (L.S.D., Student–Newman–Keuls and Duncan's tests) showed that, in the Altiplano, EL, EW, EPe, and EL/EW of the fasciolid eggs shed by donkeys are significantly different from the same parameters in the sheep and cattle isolates ($p < 0.05$).

Intensity of infection in donkeys, measured by eggs shed by gram of feces, varied between 3 and 101 epg, with a mean of 28.1 epg (**Table 3**). When considering the amount of stools defecated by each domestic animal species per day, the total number of *F. hepatica* eggs shed with feces by each domestic animal species per day in the Bolivian Altiplano could be estimated (**Table 4**). The daily egg output per donkey per day proved to fit well with the same estimations for sheep and cattle.

DISCUSSION

Donkey Participation in Fascioliasis Transmission

In the life cycle of digenean trematodes, the infection and development of the adult stage in a definitive host species does not mean that this species participates in the transmission of the parasite. This definitive host species may only represent a dead end for the digenean life cycle. In several trematode species, there may even be differences in the viability of the same definitive host species, with geographical populations playing a transmission role whereas others being a blind alley. This occurs in trematode species which show different local adaptations which may be interpreted as long-term repetitive infection events evolving locally. *Schistosoma haematobium*, a human-specific species in nature, is an illustrative example. Although natural infections by *S. haematobium* have also been reported in non-human primates (60), this does not appear to have an epidemiological importance regarding the human disease. A genetically pure strain, i.e., not an hybrid, of this schistosomatid species can be experimentally forced to adapt to a laboratory rat model after long-term reinfection passages (61).

When dealing with a trematode species with a low definitive host species specificity, as is the case of *F. hepatica* or *F. gigantica*, results of surveys on animals in nature may give rise to misinterpretations. The finding of natural infections of a mammal species allows to include this host species among the list of animals affected by the disease caused by the trematode, but does a priori not enable to epidemiologically consider it as a reservoir because it may indeed only be a dead end. This is the case of the donkey in fascioliasis. There have been several surveys on naturally-infected donkeys, but there is still no experimental study demonstrating that it is not a dead end.

To prove that a definitive host species participates in the transmission of a trematode, there is the need to (i) experimentally assess that the life cycle of the parasite is not blocked at any of the subsequent life cycle larval stages until the infection of another definitive host individual, and (ii) demonstrate that the rates of development in all these life cycle phases is sufficient as to estimate a successful transmission in nature. In *Fasciola*, this implies appropriate laboratory research on definitive host egg shedding, egg embryonation, miracidial hatching and snail vector infection, complete intramolluscan larval development until cercarial production, cercarial shedding and its characteristics, metacercarial production and definitive host infection, and final adult stage development until mature stage. The present study has included all these aspects.

Egg Embryonation in Altiplanic Donkey Isolate

Egg embryonation is a key aspect in the assessment of the viability of a definitive host species isolate in the life cycle of fasciolids. Even despite the maturation of the adult stage of the liver fluke, eggs shed with feces of given host species, or local geographical strain of that species, fail to reach complete embryonation of the miracidium. When successful, this process is temperature-dependent.

It should be noted that storage time can influence the development of the egg. This influence was kept to a minimum by reducing the storage period to only 1 month, that is the time from the day of collection in the field until the day after arrival to the laboratory of Valencia where the experimental study was performed taking advantage of the availability of the appropriate high accuracy climate chambers.

In ruminants, the following hatching times were found in southern Europe: 56 days at 15°C, 50 days at 18°C, 27 days at 20°C, 17 days at 25°C, 22 days at 27°C, and 17.5 days at 30°C (62). Results on first hatching times proved to be different In the southern part of Chile: 101 days at 9.1°C, 80 days at 10°C, 57 days at 12.4°C, 44 days at 12.6°C, 42 days at 13.8°C, 34 days at 15.1°C, 28 days at 16°C, 30 days at 16.4°C, and 20 days at 17°C (63). A hatching time of 19–20 days was obtained for 20°C when analyzing the linear correlation between egg development and

TABLE 4 | Comparison of egg measurements **(A)** and egg shedding **(B)** between the *Fasciola hepatica* donkey isolate and the sheep and cattle isolates in the Northern Bolivian Altiplano hyperendemic area.

Host	**Donkey**		**Sheep**		**Cattle**	
No. of eggs studied	**161**		**104**		**168**	
Measurements in μm	**Range**	**Mean ± SD**	**Range**	**Mean ± SD**	**Range**	**Mean ± SD**
(A) Egg Measurements						
EL	96.4–140.8	125.4 ± 8.3	114.8–151.2	130.8 ± 7.1	105.3–155.9	132.0 ± 10.5
EW	63.3–84.7	75.0 ± 3.7	65.5–81.4	72.6 ± 3.9	61.7–82.5	71.1 ± 4.4
EPe	272.1–350.4	318.8 ± 16.3	294.2–368.2	327.6 ± 15.0	270.6–422.9	340.0 ± 33.4
EA	5,562.6–8,686.2	7,177.4 ± 646.1	5,998.2–8,608.4	7,238.0 ± 532.8	5,286.5–9,676.8	7,170.2 ± 802.5
EL/EW	1.3–2.0	1.7 ± 0.1	1.5–2.1	1.8 ± 0.1	1.6–2.3	1.8 ± 0.2
(B) Egg Shedding						
Intensity range (epg)	3–101		3–241[a]		1–96[b]	
Stools/day (kg)	3–8[c]		1–3[d]		15–35[d]	
No.eggs/animal/day[e]	9,000–808,000		3,000–723,000		15,000–3,360,000	

EL, egg length; EW, egg width; EPe, egg perimeter; EA, egg area; EL/EW, egg length/egg width. Measurement values shown as range and mean ± standard deviation (SD).
[a]According to Mas-Coma et al. (49).
[b]After Buchon et al. (56).
[c]Deduced for altiplanic donkeys from their weight.
[d]According to various sources.
[e]Estimations of the range of the number of F. hepatica eggs faecally shed by an animal per day in the Bolivian Altiplano.

temperature (64). At this temperature, the first fully developed miracidium in eggs shed by sheep and cattle from the Northern Bolivian Altiplano appeared at day 24 (50), that is in agreement with the 19–27 day range from the data of the aforementioned studies. In the altiplanic donkey isolate, the first fully developed miracidium appears at day 28. A similar few-day delay is also observed in the curve peak of the percentage of fully developed miracidia, at day 60 in the donkey isolate whereas at day 56 in the altiplanic sheep isolate. However, fully developed miracidia continue to appear until day 127 in the donkey isolate, which is close to day 143 in the sheep isolate. Summing up, results indicate a slightly delayed embryonation but even so a similar complete egg embryonation in length.

Miracidial Infectivity, Intramolluscan Development, and Cercarial Chronobiology

Numerous studies on *F. hepatica*/*G. truncatula* interactions have demonstrated that the processes, including from snail infection up to cercarial shedding and related lymnaeid infection survival, are highly complex and involve many different factors which underlie a large variability (65). The monomiracidial infectivity of 28.0% at 20/20°C of 12 day/12 h night photoperiod in the altiplanic donkey isolate agrees with the range of 14.0–56.8% experimentally found in different *G. truncatula* populations in France (66, 67), as well as with that of 25.0–51.8% detected in altiplanic sheep and cattle isolates (50).

At the aforementioned miracidial dose and experimental temperature, the prepatent period (from infection up to the shedding of the first cercaria) in the altiplanic sheep and cattle isolates (50) proved to be slightly longer than in *F. hepatica*/*G. truncatula* of the lowlands (64, 68, 69). The altiplanic donkey isolate shows an even longer mean prepatent period, despite its range entering within the ranges found in the ruminants.

Under the same conditions, the patent period (length of the cercarial shedding period) in the altiplanic sheep and cattle isolates (50) agreed with the respective knowledge in ruminants of the lowlands (66, 70), but its length in the altiplanic donkey isolate proved to be shorter (**Table 1**).

The chronobiology of the cercarial shedding of the donkey isolate follows a pattern in which a gradual progressive decrease after an initial acrophase as observed in the altiplanic sheep and cattle isolates (71) is not observed. However, the donkey isolate shedding pattern fit well to the 1–14-wave pattern, with a 4–5-wave pattern folllowed by the majority, observed in *F. hepatica*/*G. truncatula* of the lowlands under constant conditions of temperature and photoperiod (72). Despite the shorter length of the shedding process in the donkey isolate, in the curve analyzed from the day of the miracidial infection (**Figure 4C**) two intervals appear in which daily shedding is completely or almost completely arrested, namely in days 80–90 and 102–113. These pauses coincide with days 90, 102, and 111 and days 84 and 121 in which cercarial shedding completely stopped by all shedding snails in the sheep and cattle isolates, respectively (71). These pauses have been linked to the redial generation replication processes.

Cercarial Production, Lymnaeid Survival, and Metacercarial Infectivity

The shorter patent period is related to the lower range and mean of the cercarial productions per snail obtained in the altiplanic donkey isolate when compared to those of not only both altiplanic sheep and cattle isolates (**Table 1**) (50), but also to the low productions found in *F. hepatica*/*G. truncatula* in given lowland populations, such as 120.0 cercariae/snail (73) or 91.7 cercariae/snail (74).

The snail survival after shedding end and the longevity of shedding snails in infections by the altiplanic donkey isolate are also shorter than in those obtained when infecting with the altiplanic sheep and cattle isolates (**Table 1**) (50), although the results confirm that this longevity is longer in infected lymnaeids from high altitude areas than the same survival period known in *F. hepatica*/*G. truncatula* in the lowlands and that this phenomenon is independent on the host isolate of *F. hepatica* (75).

The experimental infections of Wistar rats with metacercariae of the altiplanic donkey isolate allowed to verify its definitive host infectivity (**Table 2**). Although the prevalences were lower, the intensities fitted well in the results obtained with the altiplanic sheep and cattle isolates (50), and also in the present knowledge when dealing with short-aged metacercariae of ruminant origin (51, 76).

Epidemiological Role of the Donkey

The local prevalence of liver fluke infection in donkeys varied pronouncedly according to localities, with values which fit in the prevalence ranges shown by sheep and cattle in the same zones (32, 50, 56, 57). Donkeys in the more remote areas, i.e., in localities of the Tambillo-Huacullani flatland corridor distant from El Alto and La Paz, showed the highest prevalence rates. A few donkeys are usually part of the livestock of Aymara families, although their numbers vary in the different zones. Donkeys are relatively numerous in all zones of the endemic area, although in numbers markedly lower than the populations of cattle, sheep, and pigs. In the Bolivian Altiplano, donkeys are frequently found in pastures besides water collections presenting *G. truncatula* populations. The aforementioned great variability of the liver fluke infection prevalences in donkeys according to localities may be due to the local environmental conditions, mainly linked to the number of freshwater collections inhabited by lymnaeid snails.

Fasciolid infection of donkeys has been reported in many countries of Asia, Africa and the Americas, usually with low prevalence although a few exceptions of high prevalence have been published. In Asia, a local prevalence of 6.6% and an intensity of 7–17 flukes/donkey and another higher 16.6% prevalence have been reported in Iran (77). A lower prevalence of 4.1% was detected in Irak (78). A 16.13% prevalence was found in donkeys of the Central Black Sea region of Turkey (79) and another of 2.6% in Ankara city (80). In Africa, low prevalences were found in several places of Egypt, including 0.37% in Assiut, 3.03% in Gharbia, 6.7% in Al-Fayoum, and 3.08% in Giza, and mid infection rates were also found in that country, such as 14.19% in Kafr El-Sheik, 17.05% in Giza, and 17.6% in Giza and Zagazig area, as previously reviewed (81). However, markedly higher prevalences have been reported in working donkeys from Ethiopia, such as 44.4% (82) and even 80.0% (83). Anyway, low prevalences of 1.5% (84) and 5.73% (85) have also been found in this country. So, the prevalence range of 8.6–52.4% in donkeys according to local zones of the Bolivian Altiplano fit well within the aforementioned data.

In the Americas, besides Bolivia, individual donkeys have been reported to be infected by the liver fluke in Mexico (86) and Argentina (87).

Intensities, measured by individual epg amount per donkey, do not differ from the ones in altiplanic sheep and cattle. The egg outputs ranged between 3 and 145 epg (mean 44.7 epg) in altiplanic sheep (49), whereas in highly infected sheep it reached an amount of 241 epg (= 1,203 eggs per 5 g) in another previous survey performed in the same endemic area (88). In altiplanic cattle, fascioliasis intensity was between 1 and 96 epg (mean 6.8 epg) (49).

Eggs of *F. hepatica* shed by naturally infected donkeys of the Bolivian Altiplano prove to be shorter but thicker than those found in naturally infected altiplanic sheep and cattle (**Table 4**). This agrees with present knowledge about the influence of the definitive host species on the size of fasciolid eggs (89). Interestingly, *F. hepatica* eggs found in palaeoparasitological studies of old donkeys (onagers) in the former Fertile Crescent area, at present Iran, during the Sassanid period, 224-651 AD, also fit in the egg size ranges found in present day donkeys (81).

The total number of liver fluke eggs expelled with feces by a donkey per day in the Northern Bolivian Altiplano, according to the amount of stools defecated by a donkey per day, may be estimated to be between 9,000 and 808,000 eggs/donkey/day. This range overlaps with similar estimates made for sheep and cattle in the same Northern Altiplano hyperendemic area (**Table 4**).

Finally, the susceptibility of the mammal host species to liver fluke infection is an important additional aspect to be considered in a One Health control initiative. If the animal is only able to survive a given period after the infection, its contribution to the disease transmission may be only for a short time and thus negligible when compared with other mammals able to transmit for the rest of their life, as is the case of sheep. If presenting a high immunological refractory response, liver flukes will survive less time inside that host and the contribution to transmission will consequently be restricted in quantity and time, as is the case of several cattle races. Fascioliasis is known to be different in equines and ruminants from the pathogenicity point of view, with the horse as the most resistant, the donkey as the most susceptible, and the mule showing intermediate profile although closer to those of the horse (90). Indeed, *F. hepatica* infection has been reported to be fatal for donkeys (86), and the pathology caused by a *F. gigantica* infection in donkeys has already been analyzed post-mortem in Egypt (91).

The lower adaptation of *F. hepatica* to the donkey is reflected in the longer prepatent period and mainly in the significantly lower number of cercariae produced by infected snails (**Table 1**). This is a priori not surprising, considering the phylogenetic distance between equines and ruminants. Indeed, the origin of *F. hepatica* is known to be linked to mid-sized ovicaprines (5). However, similar studies would be appropriate to assess whether the liver fluke may locally increase its adaptability to the donkey in other regions of the world, mainly eastern Africa and near-eastern Asia.

In mules, it was observed that a massive infection by 97 adult flukes was highly pathogenic and finally fatal, and that the maximum daily output was 794,500 eggs/mule/day (90).

By extrapolation from mule data, the maximum of 808,000 eggs/donkey/day estimated in the Altiplano would mean a massive infection of a donkey by 99 flukes. However, amounts higher than 70 epg were only found in three donkeys, that is the 15.0% of the infected donkeys and 3.6% of the total of donkeys analyzed. Hence, massive infections representing death risk may be only sporadically reached in altiplanic donkeys and probably only in old specimens kept in a highly contaminated place for long periods.

The donkey played a crucial role in human history (92). Of African origin, it was initially domesticated in East-North Africa and the Near East Asian region (93) and was introduced into the Americas by the Spanish "conquistadores" (5). Donkeys have a range of physiological and behavioral adaptations providing them with advantages to survive extreme conditions such as those of drought and high altitude environments. They spend less energy while foraging for food which results in a lower dry matter intake requirement. Low-quality diets are digested by donkeys very efficiently because of a highly selective feeding strategy. The lower energy costs of walking, the longer foraging times per day, and their ability to tolerate thirst, allow donkeys to access more remote, under-utilized sources of forage that are inaccessible to ruminants (94). Thus, although the main introduction purpose was the *in-situ* production of mules, donkeys easily adapted to the hypoxic conditions of the high altitude environments of the Andean valleys and altiplanos, where they were increasingly used by the high altitude communities because of the lower adaptation capacity of horses (95). The biochemical and hematological parameters in mules at high altitude have recently been assessed (90), and in donkeys the respective reference intervals have also been established (96), including the Creole donkey in South America (97). However, the analysis of these parameters in high altitude for Andean donkeys is still pending. Donkeys with ligated bile ducts exhibited the biochemical, pathological, and clinical features including motor coordination impairment, constipation, oedema, dermatitis, and jaundice, together with serum increased levels of total bilirubin and ammonia and decreased levels of total protein and calcium (98).

The donkey, as equines in general, lacks a gallbladder. This means that the bile produced by the liver goes directly to the small intestine, and it is not stored. Animals lacking a gallbladder tend to eat small amounts of food several times a day. Furthermore, the natural diet of grasses that donkeys ingest while grazing is not particularly high in fat, and consequently they digest and absorb it well. Thus, from the point of view of the liver fluke transmission, the eggs cannot be stored in the gallbladder and their faecally excretion should be more regular and constant than in animals having a gallbladder.

Infection by the liver fluke may underlie severe pathogenicity in donkeys. Indeed, the high efficiency of donkeys for energy storage and mobilization has also made them prone to pathological conditions associated with negative energy balance. Pathological consequences mainly concern excessive lipolysis, excessive hepatic triglyceride synthesis, and release into systemic circulation (dyslipidemia), with severe systemic damage. Mortality rates up to 80% have been reported. Dyslipidemias in donkeys occur secondary to physiological dysfunctions and pathological processes, among which mainly liver disease (99). Donkeys are particularly susceptible to hyperlipaemia, a disease caused by too much fat in the blood. When a donkey stops eating enough it goes into a state of negative energy balance. In this state, the body begins to use energy stored as fat deposits and consequently free fatty acids are converted to glucose in the liver under a system controlled by complex hormonal events. Donkeys are not able to appropriately turn off this fat release and blood circulation soon fills up with excess fat. Large amounts of fat trigger liver and kidney failure. Subsequently, all organs may fail leading to irreversible organ damage and death (99). Detection of an increase of plasma triglyceride levels (hyperlipemia) is crucial to assess fat circulation. Measuring the levels of other serum markers indicating liver dysfunction may additionally help. The alterations of serum biochemical and hematological parameters have recently been studied in the infection by fasciolids in both the acute and chronic phase of the disease (7) and may be used for donkey control within a One Health action.

CONCLUDING REMARKS

The experimental studies performed demonstrate that the donkey is a definitive host which assures the viability of the whole life cycle of *F. hepatica* in the Northern Bolivian Altiplano human hyperendemic area. Several aspects indicate, however, that *F. hepatica* does not reach in the donkey the level of adaptation it shows in sheep and cattle in this very high altitude area. This is illustrated by a few-day delay in egg embryonation, longer prepatent period despite similar miracidial infectivity and shorter patent period in the intramolluscan development, lower cercarial production per snail, different cercarial chronobiology, shorter snail survival after shedding end, shorter longevity of shedding snails, and lower metacercarial infectivity in Wistar rats. Thus, the role of the donkey in the transmission of the disease should be considered secondary.

Results of the field surveys proved that liver fluke prevalence and intensity in donkeys are similar to those of the main reservoirs sheep and cattle in this hyperendemic area. Worth mentioning, moreover, fasciolid egg shedding by a donkey individual proved to contribute to the environment contamination at a rate similar to sheep and cattle in that area. The very low percentage of donkeys with high infection burdens suggests a negligible liver fluke pathological impact on donkey survival and hence a long-term contribution of infected donkeys to fascioliasis transmission. In this endemic area, nevertheless, the pronounced lower number of donkeys when compared to sheep and cattle populations indicate that the epidemiological reservoir role of the donkey is also secondary when compared to these ruminants.

There is, however, an aspect of the donkey related to its management by the Aymara inhabitants which has a crucial repercussion in the transmission and epidemiology of the disease in the human hyperendemic area of the Bolivian Altiplano. Aymaras use the donkeys for the transport of goods and merchandises and for movements and travel from one locality/zone to another (**Figure 5**). Thus, this equine host

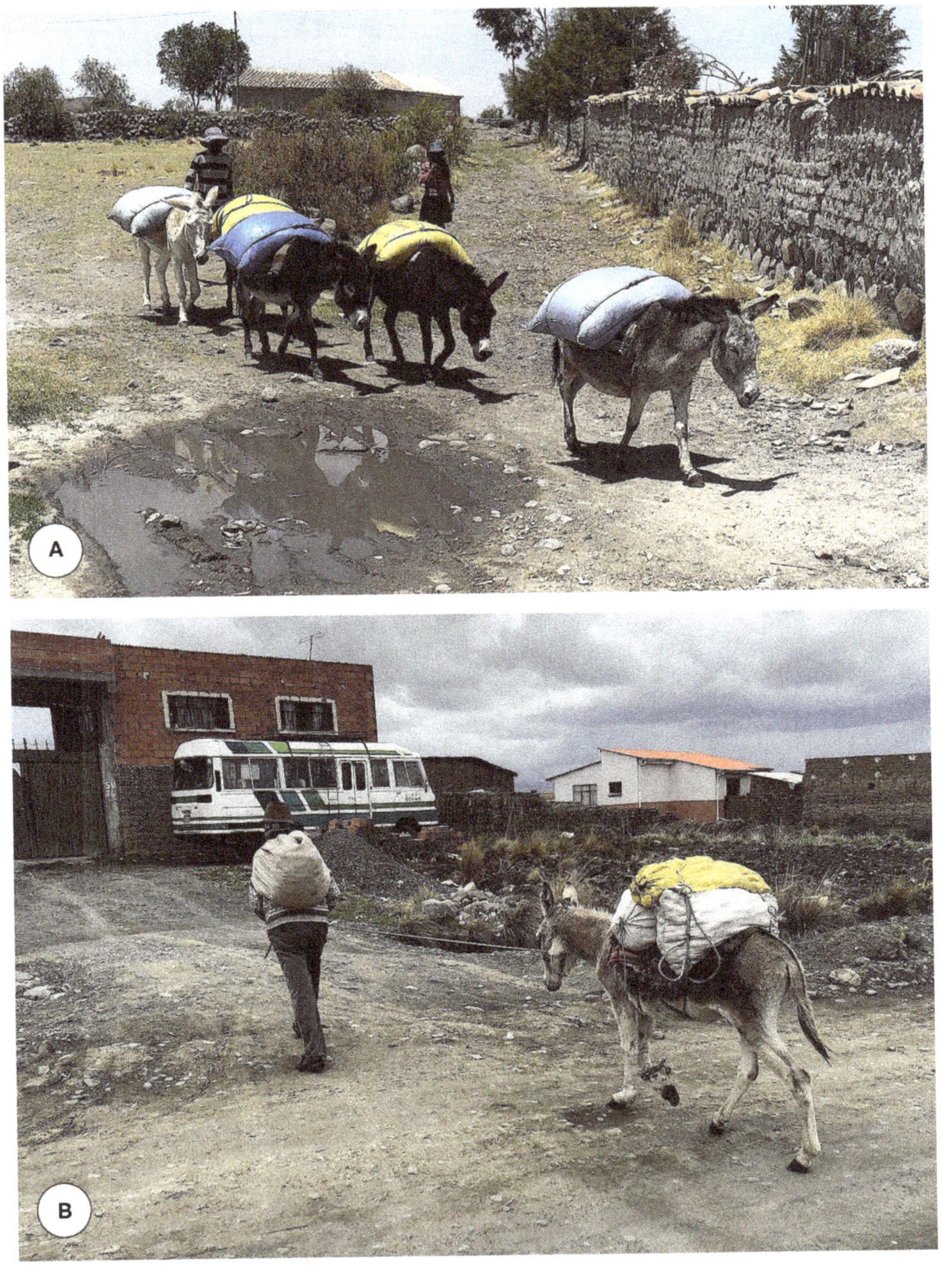

FIGURE 5 | In the Northern Bolivian Altiplano human fascioliasis hyperendemic area, **(A)** donkeys are used for the transport of goods, and **(B)** for movements and travel from one locality/zone to another. Orig. S. Mas-Coma.

species plays an important epidemiological role in the spread of the disease from one zone to another inside the wide endemic area. The participation of the donkey in this disease dissemination takes place in a dual manner. On one side by releasing fasciolid eggs along the routes they follow and on another side by passively transporting the lymnaeid vectors. According to what is known, lymnaeids may remain in dried mud stuck to the feet of animals, then go into hibernation or estivation, and are able to reactivate once in a new location following contact with water or sufficient humidity (5). This becomes even more important in a period as the present one in which the geographical distribution of the disease is spreading throughout the Northern Altiplano due to climate change (47).

Additionally, this fascioliasis spreading capacity of the donkey poses a problem for the implementation of a One Health initiative, because the donkey may give rise to movements of the parasite and the vector from one part to another of the zone selected for control intervention, or the introduction of the parasite and/or the vector from outside into that zone.

This study is an example of the appropriate and complete way to assess the participation of a mammal host species in the transmission and epidemiology of fascioliasis in an endemic area. It illustrates the long-term research complexity and difficulties involved in the needed experimental tasks and field activities in a disease of very high heterogeneity as that caused by liver flukes. To clarify the participation rate of a definitive host species in the case of parasites of low definitive host species specificity as fasciolids by comparing with the participation rates of other definitive host species in the same endemic area becomes crucial to establish correct control measure priorities within a One Health action. All in all, the extreme complexity of a One Health action against fascioliasis becomes evident, further if it is considered that in the Northern Bolivian Altiplano the simplicity is maximum because the disease is only caused by *F. hepatica* and transmitted by only genetically uniform *G. truncatula*, and that the present study only concerns the One Health intervention axis of the mammal reservoirs.

ETHICS STATEMENT

All experimental research was performed with the approval of the Evaluation of Projects concerning Animal Research at University of Valencia (Organo Habilitado para la Evaluación de Proyectos de Experimentación Animal de la Universidad de Valencia) (A1263 915389140), strictly following the institution's guidelines based on Directive 2010/63/EU. Permission for animal research was additionally obtained from the Servicio de Sanidad y Bienestar Animal, Dirección General de Producción Agraria y Ganadería, Consellería de Presidencia y Agricultura, Pesca, Alimentación y Agua, Generalitat Valenciana, Valencia, Spain (No. 2015/VSC/PEA/00001 tipo 2). Animal ethics guidelines regarding animal care were strictly adhered. The study was approved by the Comisión de Etica de la Investigación of the Comité Nacional de Bioética, La Paz (Certificate dated 10 September 2007), Comité de Etica y Bioética de la Facultad de Medicina de la Universidad Mayor de San Andres, UMSA, La Paz - COMETICA (Resolución COMETICA No. 03/2019, dated 23 July 2019), and Comité de Revisión Etica (PAHOERC) of the Pan American Health Organization, PAHO, Washington DC (Dictamen Ref. No. 2018-02-0007, dated 10 September 2019). Written informed consent for participation was not obtained from the owners because all investigations were made after permission was obtained from local Aymara community chiefs (jilakatas and malkus), and with the consent of animal owners.

AUTHOR CONTRIBUTIONS

SM-C performed One Health studies, designed the protocols, wrote the manuscript, and obtained project funding. PB performed the surveys and diagnosis of animals. IRF performed the snail cultures, experimental snail infections, and chronobiological assessments. RA coordinated local research and logistics and participated in surveys. CM-B reviewed donkey physiology and metabolism and analyzed parasite-induced pathological repercussions. PA participated in surveys and diagnosis of animals. MAV performed the experimental mammal infections, statistical analyses, and obtained project funding. MDB performed the egg development studies, designed and participated in the experimental snail infections, participated in surveys, and obtained project funding. All authors contributed to the article and approved the submitted version.

FUNDING

Studies funded by Project No. 2017/ACDE/001583 de Innovación para el Desarrollo of the Agencia Española de Cooperación Internacional para el Desarrollo (AECID), Ministry of Foreign Affairs and Cooperation, Madrid, Spain; by Project No. RLA5049 of the International Atomic Energy Agency (Animal Production and Health section, Joint FAO/IAEA Division of Nuclear Techniques in Food and Agriculture, Department of Nuclear Sciences and Applications, IAEA Headquarters Vienna, Austria); by Health Research Project No. PI16/00520, Subprograma Estatal de Generación de Conocimiento de la Acción Estratégica en Salud (AES) y Fondos FEDER, Plan Estatal de Investigación Científica y Técnica y de Innovación, ISCIII-MINECO, Madrid, Spain; by the Red de Investigación de Centros de Enfermedades Tropicales – RICET (Project No. RD16/0027/0023 of the PN de I+D+I, ISCIII-Subdirección General de Redes y Centros de Investigación Cooperativa RETICS), Ministry of Health and Consumption, Madrid; by Project No. 2016/099 of the PROMETEO Program, Programa of Ayudas para Grupos de Investigación de Excelencia, Generalitat Valenciana, Valencia, Spain; and by Project No. 2017/01 of the V Convocatoria de Proyectos de Cooperación al Desarrollo de la Universidad de Valencia de 2016, Valencia, Spain.

ACKNOWLEDGMENTS

Studies of this article have been performed within the framework of the Worldwide Initiative of WHO against Human Fascioliasis (WHO Headquarters, Geneva, Switzerland). One Health initiative designed within the official meeting Reunión de Análisis con Expertos sobre la Situación Actual y Próximos Pasos para el Control de la Fascioliasis en Bolivia, organized by PAHO/WHO in Hotel Camino Real, Calacoto, La Paz, on 10-12 November 2014, with the participation of (i) Ministerio de Salud de Bolivia, (ii) Ministerio de Desarrollo Rural y Tierras de Bolivia, (iii) Servicio Departamental de Salud de La Paz (SEDES La Paz), (iv) representatives of the Aymara communities from the Northern Altiplano endemic area, (v) delegates from Perú, (vi) experts and advisers of the Programa Regional de Enfermedades Infecciosas Desatendidas of PAHO/WHO, and from the WHO Collaborating Centre on Fascioliasis and its Snail Vectors of Valencia, and (vii) other foreign experts.

The authors acknowledge the facilities provided and the collaboration received from the following Bolivian organisms, institutions and centres, as well as their respective representatives or directors: Servicio Departamental de Salud La Paz (SEDES La Paz); Unidad de Epidemiología of the Bolivian Ministry of Health, La Paz; Office of the Pan American Health Organization in La Paz; Dirección Nacional de Producción Pecuaria and the Instituto Nacional de Biología Animal of Chasquipampa-Calacoto both of the Ministerio de Asuntos Campesinos y Agropecuarios (M.A.C.A.) in La Paz; and Granja de Mejoramiento Ganadero de Kallutaca related to the Programa de Fomento Lechero of the Corporación Regional de Desarrollo de La Paz (CORDEPAZ, El Alto).

REFERENCES

1. Chen MG, Mott KE. Progress in assessment of morbidity due to *Fasciola hepatica* infection: a review of recent literature. *Trop Dis Bull.* (1990) 87:R1–38.
2. Mas-Coma S, Bargues MD, Valero MA. Diagnosis of human fascioliasis by stool and blood techniques: update for the present global scenario. *Parasitology.* (2014) 141:1918–46. doi: 10.1017/S0031182014000869
3. Mas-Coma S. Human fascioliasis emergence risks in developed countries: from individual patients and small epidemics to climate and global change impacts. *Enf Emerg Microbio Clín.* (2020) 38:253–6. doi: 10.1016/j.eimc.2020.01.014
4. World Health Organization. *Sustaining the Drive to Overcome the Global Impact of Neglected Tropical Diseases.* Geneva: Department of Control of Neglected Tropical Diseases, World Health Organization, WHO Headquarters (2013). 128. p
5. Mas-Coma S, Valero MA, Bargues MD. *Fasciola*, lymnaeids and human fascioliasis, with a global overview on disease transmission, epidemiology, evolutionary genetics, molecular epidemiology and control. *Adv Parasitol.* (2009) 69:141–6. doi: 10.1016/S0065-308X(09)69002-3
6. Valero MA, Girones N, Garcia-Bodelon MA, Periago MV, Chico-Calero I, Khoubbane M, et al. Anaemia in advanced chronic fasciolosis. *Acta Trop.* (2008) 108:35–43. doi: 10.1016/j.actatropica.2008.08.007
7. Valero MA, Bargues MD, Khoubbane M, Artigas P, Quesada C, Berinde L, et al. Higher physiopathogenicity by *Fasciola gigantica* than by the genetically close *F. hepatica*: experimental long-term follow-up of biochemical markers. *Trans Roy Soc Trop Med Hyg.* (2016) 110:55–66. doi: 10.1093/trstmh/trv110
8. Mas-Coma S, Agramunt VH, Valero MA. Neurological and ocular fascioliasis in humans. *Adv Parasitol.* (2014) 84:27–149. doi: 10.1016/B978-0-12-800099-1.00002-8
9. Dalton JP, Robinson MW, Mulcahy G, O'Neill SM, Donnelly S. Immunomodulatory molecules of *Fasciola hepatica*: candidates for both vaccine and immunotherapeutic development. *Vet Parasitol.* (2013) 195:272–85. doi: 10.1016/j.vetpar.2013.04.008
10. Girones N, Valero MA, Garcia-Bodelon MA, Chico-Calero MI, Punzon C, Fresno M, et al. Immune supression in advanced chronic fascioliasis: an experimental study in a rat model. *J Infect Dis.* (2007) 195:1504–12. doi: 10.1086/514822
11. O'Neill SM, Brady MT, Callanan JJ, Mulcahy G, Joyce P, Mills KH, et al. *Fasciola hepatica* infection downregulates Th1 responses in mice. *Parasite Immunol.* (2000) 22:147–55. doi: 10.1046/j.1365-3024.2000.00290.x
12. Valero MA, Navarro M, Garcia-Bodelon MA, Marcilla A, Morales M, Garcia JE, et al. High risk of bacterobilia in advanced experimental chronic fasciolosis. *Acta Trop.* (2006) 100:17–23. doi: 10.1016/j.actatropica.2006.09.002
13. Esteban JG, Flores A, Angles R, Strauss W, Aguirre C, Mas-Coma S. A population-based coprological study of human fascioliasis in a hyperendemic area of the bolivian altiplano. *Trop Med Int Health.* (1997) 2:695–99. doi: 10.1046/j.1365-3156.1997.d01-356.x
14. Gonzalez LC, Esteban JG, Bargues MD, Valero MA, Ortiz P, Naquira C, et al. Hyperendemic human fascioliasis in andean valleys: an altitudinal transect analysis in children of cajamarca province, Peru. *Acta Trop.* (2011) 120:119–29. doi: 10.1016/j.actatropica.2011.07.002
15. Ollerenshaw CB. The ecology of the liver fluke (*Fasciola hepatica*). *Vet Rec.* (1959) 71:957–65.
16. Afshan K, Fortes-Lima CA, Artigas P, Valero MA, Qayyum M, Mas-Coma S. Impact of climate change and man-made irrigation systems on the transmission risk, long-term trend and seasonality of human and animal fascioliasis in Pakistan. *Geospat Health.* (2014) 8:317–34. doi: 10.4081/gh.2014.22
17. Valero MA, Perez-Crespo I, Chillon-Marinas C, Khoubbane M, Quesada C, Reguera-Gomez M, et al. *Fasciola hepatica* reinfection potentiates a mixed Th1/Th2/Th17/Treg response and correlates with the clinical phenotypes of anemia. *PLoS ONE.* (2017) 12:e0173456. doi: 10.1371/journal.pone.0173456
18. Valero MA, Girones N, Reguera-Gomez M, Perez-Crespo I, Lopez-Garcia MP, Quesada C, et al. Impact of fascioliasis reinfection on *Fasciola hepatica* egg shedding: relationship with the immune-regulatory response. *Acta Trop.* (2020) 209:105518. doi: 10.1016/j.actatropica.2020.105518
19. Gonzalez-Miguel J, Valero MA, Reguera-Gomez M, Mas-Bargues C, Bargues MD, Simon-Martin F, et al. Numerous *Fasciola* plasminogen-binding proteins may underlie blood-brain barrier leakage and explain neurological disorder complexity and heterogeneity in the acute and chronic phases of human fascioliasis. *Parasitology.* (2019) 146:284–98. doi: 10.1017/S0031182018001464
20. Rondelaud D, Dreyfuss G, Vignoles P. Clinical and biological abnormalities in patients after fasciolosis treatment. *Med Mal Infect.* (2006) 36:466–8. doi: 10.1016/j.medmal.2006.07.018
21. Gandhi P, Schmitt EK, Chen CW, Samantray S, Venishetty VK, Hughes D. Triclabendazole in the treatment of human fascioliasis: a review. *Trans Roy Soc Trop Med Hyg.* (2019) 113:797–804. doi: 10.1093/trstmh/trz093
22. World Health Organization. *Ending the Neglect to Attain the Sustainable Development Goals. A Road Map for Neglected Tropical Diseases 2021-2030.* Geneva: World Health Organization, WHO Headquarters (2020) 47 p. Available online at: https://www.who.int/neglected_diseases/Ending-the-neglect-to-attain-the-SDGs--NTD-Roadmap.pdf
23. Esteban JG, Gonzalez C, Bargues MD, Angles R, Sanchez C, Naquira C, et al. High fascioliasis infection in children linked to a man-made irrigation zone in Peru. *Trop Med Int Health.* (2002) 7:339–48. doi: 10.1046/j.1365-3156.2002.00870.x
24. Espinoza JR, Maco V, Marcos L, Saez S, Neyra V, Terashima A, et al. Evaluation of Fas2-ELISA for the serological detection of *Fasciola hepatica* infection in humans. *Am J Trop Med Hyg.* (2007) 76:977–82. doi: 10.4269/ajtmh.2007.76.977
25. Hillyer GV, Soler de Galanes M, Rodriguez-Perez J, Bjorland J, Silva de Lagrava M, Ramirez Guzman S, et al. Use of the Falcon Assay Screening Test - Enzyme-Linked Immunosorbent Assay (FAST-ELISA) and the Enzyme-Linked Immunoelectrotransfer Blot (EITB) to determine the prevalence of human fascioliasis in the bolivian altiplano. *Am J Trop Med Hyg.* (1992) 46:603–9. doi: 10.4269/ajtmh.1992.46.603
26. Bjorland J, Bryan RT, Strauss W, Hillyer GV, McAuley JB. An outbreak of acute fascioliasis among aymara Indians in the bolivian altiplano. *Clin Inf Dis.* (1995) 21:1228–33. doi: 10.1093/clinids/21.5.1228
27. Malandrini JB, Carnevale S, Velazquez J, Soria CC. Diagnóstico de *Fasciola hepatica* con la técnica de ELISA en el departamento de tinogasta. *Ciencia.* (2009) 4:143–51.
28. Mera y Sierra R, Agramunt VH, Cuervo P, Mas-Coma S. Human fascioliasis in Argentina: retrospective overview, critical analysis and baseline for future research. *Parasit Vectors.* (2011) 4:104. doi: 10.1186/1756-3305-4-104
29. Bargues MD, Malandrini JB, Artigas P, Soria CC, Velasquez JN, Carnevale S, et al. Human fascioliasis endemic areas in Argentina: multigene characterisation of the lymnaeid vectors and climatic-environmental assessment of the transmission pattern. *Parasit Vectors.* (2016) 9:306. doi: 10.1186/s13071-016-1589-z
30. Apt W, Aguilera X, Vega F, Zulantay I, Retamal C, Apt P, et al. Fascioliasis en la población rural de las provincias de curico, talca y linares. *Rev Méd Chile.* (1992) 120:621–6.

31. Artigas P, Bargues MD, Mera y Sierra R, Agramunt VH, Mas-Coma S. Characterisation of fascioliasis lymnaeid intermediate hosts from Chile by DNA sequencing, with emphasis on *Lymnaea viator* and *Galba truncatula*. *Acta Trop.* (2011) 120:245–57. doi: 10.1016/j.actatropica.2011.09.002
32. Mas-Coma S, Angles R, Esteban JG, Bargues MD, Buchon P, Franken M, et al. The northern bolivian altiplano: a region highly endemic for human fascioliasis. *Trop Med Int Health.* (1999) 4:45467. doi: 10.1046/j.1365-3156.1999.00418.x
33. De NV, Le TH, Agramunt VH, Mas-Coma S. Early postnatal and preschool age infection by *Fasciola* spp.: report of five cases from Vietnam and worldwide review. *Am J Trop Med Hyg.* (2020) 103:1578–89. doi: 10.4269/ajtmh.20-0139
34. Villegas F, Angles R, Barrientos R, Barrios G, Valero MA, Hamed K, et al. Administration of triclabendazole is safe and effective in controlling fascioliasis in an endemic community of the Bolivian Altiplano. *PLoS Negl Trop Dis.* (2012) 6:e1720. doi: 10.1371/journal.pntd.0001720
35. Valero MA, Periago MV, Perez-Crespo I, Angles R, Villegas F, Aguirre C, et al. Field evaluation of a coproantigen detection test for fascioliasis diagnosis and surveillance in human hyperendemic areas of Andean countries. *PLoS Negl Trop Dis.* (2012) 6:e1812. doi: 10.1371/journal.pntd.0001812
36. Mas-Coma S, Bargues MD, Valero MA. Human fascioliasis infection sources, their diversity, incidence factors, analytical methods and prevention measures. *Parasitology.* (2018) 145:1665–99. doi: 10.1017/S0031182018000914
37. Ueno H, Arandia R, Morales G, Medina G. Fascioliasis of livestock and snail host for *Fasciola* in the altiplano region of Bolivia. *Nat Inst Anim Health Q.* (1975) 15:61–7.
38. Essack SY. Environment: the neglected component of the one health triad. *Lancet.* (2018) 2:e238–39. doi: 10.1016/S2542-5196(18)30124-4
39. Lubroth J. FAO and the one health approach. *Curr Top Microbiol Immunol.* (2013) 366:65–72. doi: 10.1007/978-3-662-45791-7_262
40. World Health Organization, Food and Agriculture Organization of the United Nations, World Organisation for Animal Health. *Taking a Multisectoral, One Health Approach: A Tripartite Guide to Addressing Zoonotic Diseases in Countries.* FAO - OIE - WHO (2019). 151 p. Available online at: https://apps.who.int/iris/handle/10665/325620
41. Rinaldi L, Gonzalez S, Guerrero J, Carol Aguilera L, Musella V, Genchi C, et al. A one-health integrated approach to control fascioliasis in the cajamarca valley of Peru. *Geospat Health.* (2012) 6:S67–73. doi: 10.4081/gh.2012.124
42. Webster JP, Gower CM, Knowles SCL, Molyneux DH, Fenton A. One health – an ecological and evolutionary framework for tackling neglected zoonotic diseases. *Evol Appl.* (2016) 9:313–33. doi: 10.1111/eva.12341
43. Destoumieux-Garzón D, Mavingui P, Boetsch G, Boissier J, Darriet F, Duboz P, et al. The one health concept: 10 years old and a long road ahead. *Front Vet Sci.* (2018) 5:14. doi: 10.3389/fvets.2018.00014
44. Bargues MD, Mas-Coma S. Reviewing lymnaeid vectors of fascioliasis by ribosomal DNA sequence analyses. *J Helminthol.* (2005) 7 9:257–67. doi: 10.1079/JOH2005297
45. Bargues MD, Artigas P, Mera y Sierra R, Pointier JP, Mas-Coma S. Characterisation of *Lymnaea cubensis, L.* viatrix and *L. neotropica n. sp.*, the main vectors of *Fasciola hepatica* in Latin America, by analysis of their ribosomal and mitochondrial DNA. *Ann Trop Med Parasitol.* (2007) 101:621–41. doi: 10.1179/136485907X229077
46. Bargues MD, Artigas P, Khoubbane M, Flores R, Glöer P, Rojas-Garcia R, et al. *Lymnaea schirazensis*, an overlooked snail distorting fascioliasis data: genotype, phenotype, ecology, worldwide spread, susceptibility, applicability. *PLoS ONE.* (2011) 6:e24567. doi: 10.1371/journal.pone.0024567
47. Bargues MD, Artigas P, Angles R, Osca D, Duran P, Buchon P, et al. Genetic uniformity, geographical spread and anthropogenic habitat modifications of lymnaeid vectors found in a one health initiative in the highest human fascioliasis hyperendemic of the Bolivian Altiplano. *Parasit Vectors.* (2020) 13:171. doi: 10.1186/s13071-020-04045-x
48. Fuentes MV, Coello JR, Bargues MD, Valero MA, Esteban JG, Fons R, et al. Small mammals (Lagomorpha and Rodentia) and fascioliasis transmission in the Northern Bolivian Altiplano endemic zone. *Res Rev Parasitol.* (1997) 57:115–21.
49. Mas-Coma S, Rodriguez A, Bargues MD, Valero MA, Coello JR, Angles R. Secondary reservoir role of domestic animals other than sheep and cattle in fascioliasis transmission in the Northern Bolivian Altiplano. *Res Rev Parasitol.* (1997) 57:39–46.
50. Mas-Coma S, Buchon P, Funatsu IK, Angles R, Artigas P, Valero MA, et al. Sheep and cattle reservoirs in the highest human fascioliasis hyperendemic area: experimental transmission capacity, field epidemiology and control within a one health initiative in Bolivia. *Front Vet Sci.* (in press).
51. Boray JC, Enigk K. Laboratory studies on the survival and infectiivity of Fasciola *hepatica* and *F. gigantica* metacercariae. *Z Tropenmed Parasitol.* (1964) 15:324–31.
52. Bargues MD, Gayo V, Sanchis J, Artigas P, Khoubbane M, Birriel S, et al. DNA multigene characterization of *Fasciola hepatica* and *Lymnaea neotropica* and its fascioliasis transmission capacity in Uruguay, with historical correlation, human report review and infection risk analysis. *PLoS Negl Trop Dis.* (2017) 11:e0005352. doi: 10.1371/journal.pntd.0005352
53. Valero MA, Panova M, Comes AM, Fons R, Mas-Coma S. Patterns in size and shedding of *Fasciola hepatica* eggs by naturally and experimentally infected murid rodents. *J Parasitol.* (2002) 88:308–13. doi: 10.1645/0022-3395.2002.088[0308:PISASO]2.0.CO;2
54. Valero MA, Mas-Coma S. Comparative infectivity of *Fasciola hepatica* metacercariae from isolates of the main and secondary reservoir animal host species in the Bolivian Altiplano high human endemic region. *Folia Parasitol.* (2000) 47:17–22. doi: 10.14411/fp.2000.004
55. Valero MA, Santana M, Morales M, Hernandez JL, Mas-Coma S. Risk of gallstone disease in advanced chronic phase of fascioliasis: an experimental study in a rat model. *J Infect Dis.* (2003) 188:787–93. doi 10.1086/377281
56. Buchon P, Cuenca H, Quiton A, Camacho AM, Mas-Coma S. Fascioliasis in cattle in the human high endemic region of the Bolivian Northern Altiplano. *Res Rev Parasitol.* (1997) 57:71–83.
57. Grock R, Morales G, Vaca JL, Mas-Coma S. Fascioliasis in sheep in the human high endemic region of the Northern Bolivian Altiplano. *Res Rev Parasitol.* (1998) 58:95–101.
58. Dennis WR, Stone WM, Swanson LE. A new laboratory and field diagnostic test for fluke ova in feces. *J Amer Vet Med Ass.* (1954) 124:47–50.
59. Valero MA, Panova M, Mas-Coma S. Phenotypic analysis of adults and eggs of *Fasciola hepatica* by computer image analysis system. *J Helminthol.* (2005) 79:217–25. doi: 10.1079/JOH2005301
60. Pitchford RJ. A check list of definitive hosts exhibiting evidence of the genus *Schistosoma* Weinland, 1858 acquired naturally in Africa and the Middle East. *J Helminthol.* (1977) 51:229–51. doi: 10.1017/S0022149X00007574
61. Gear JHS, Davis DHS, Pitchford RJ. The susceptibility of rodents to schistosome infection, with special reference to *Schistosoma haematobium*. *Bull World Health Organ.* (1966) 35:213–21.
62. Diez-Baños MA, Rojo-Vázquez FA. Influencia de la temperatura en el desarrollo de los huevos de *Fasciola hepatica*. *An Fac Vet León.* (1976) 22:65–75.
63. Valenzuela G. Estudio epidemiológico acerca del desarrollo de huevos de *Fasciola hepatica* en el medio ambiente en Valdivia, Chile. *Bol Chil Parasit.* (1979) 34:31–5.
64. Wilson RA, Smith G, Thomas MR. Fascioliasis. In: Anderson RM. Editor. *The Population Dynamics of Infectious Diseases: Theory and Applications.* London; New York, NY: Chapman and Hall (1982). p. 262–319. doi: 10.1007/978-1-4899-2901-3_9
65. Kendall SB. Nutritional factors affecting the rate of development of *Fasciola hepatica* in *Limnaea truncatula. J Helminthol.* (1993) 23:179–90. doi: 10.1017/S0022149X00032491
66. Rondelaud D. Variabilité interpopulationelle de l'infestation fasciolenne chez le mollusque *Lymnaea truncatula* Müller. influence du contact préalable de la population avec le parasite. *Bull Soc Zool France.* (1993) 118:185–93.
67. Vignoles P, Dreyfuss G, Rondelaud D. Larval development of *Fasciola hepatica* in experimental infections: variations with populations of *Lymnaea truncatula. J Helminthol.* (2002) 76:179–83. doi: 10.1079/JOH2002112
68. Roberts WE. Studies on the life-cycle of *Fasciola hepatica* (Linnaeus) and of its snail host *Limnaea* (*Galba*) *truncatula* (Müller) in the field and under controlled conditions in the laboratory. *Ann Trop Med Parasitol.* (1950) 44:187–206. doi: 10.1080/00034983.1950.11685441
69. Rondelaud D, Barthe D. Les générations rédiennes de *Fasciola hepatica L. Premières* observations chez des Limnées tronquées en fin de cycle parasitaire. *Bull Soc Franç Parasitol.* (1986) 4:29–38.

70. Rondelaud D, Dreyfuss G. *Fasciola hepatica*: the influence of the definitive host on the characteristics of the infection in the snail *Lymnaea truncatula*. *Parasite.* (1995) 2:275–80. doi: 10.1051/parasite/1995023275
71. Mas-Coma S, Funatsu IR, Bargues MD. *Fasciola hepatica* and lymnaeid snails occurring at very high altitude in South America. *Parasitology.* (2001) 123:S115–27. doi: 10.1017/S0031182001008034
72. Dreyfuss G, Rondelaud D. *Fasciola hepatica*: a study of the shedding of cercariae from *Lymnaea truncatula* raised under constant conditions of temperature and photoperiod. *Parasite.* (1994) 4:401–4. doi: 10.1051/parasite/1994014401
73. Hodasi JKM. The output of cercariae of *Fasciola hepatica* by *Lymnaea truncatula* and the distribution of metacercariae on grass. *Parasitology.* (1972) 63:431–56.
74. Audousset JC, Rondelaud D, Dreyfuss G, Vareille-Morel C. Les émissions cercariennes de *Fasciola hepatica* L. *chez* le mollusque Lymnaea truncatula Müller. A propos de quelques observations chronobiologiques. *Bull Soc Franç Parasitol.* (1989) 7:217–24.
75. Bargues MD, Oviedo JA, Funatsu IR, Rodriguez A, Mas-Coma S. Survival of lymnaeid snails from the Bolivian Northern Altiplano after the parasitation by different Bolivian isolates of *Fasciola hepatica* (Linnaeus, 1758) (Trematoda: Fasciolidae), In: Guerra A, Rolán E, Rocha F, editors. *Unitas Malacologica.* Vigo: Instituto de Investigaciones Marinas, CSIC, (1995). p. 443–5.
76. Kimura S, Shimizu A. Studies on the survival and infectivity of *Fasciola gigantica* metacercariae. *Sci Rept Fac Agr Kobe Univ.* (1979) 13:347–49.
77. Hosseini SH, Mesghi B, Eslami A, Bokai S, Sobhani M, Samani RE. Prevalence and biodiversity of helminth parasites in donkeys (*Equus asinus*) in Iran. *Int J Vet Res.* (2009) 3:95–9. Available online at: https://ijvm.ut.ac.ir/article_20633_8927af20c4f9b5b2767176762bc5c686.pdf
78. Atia AH. Prevalence of *Fasciola* sp. infection in donkeys in Baghdad, Iraq. *AlTaqani.* (2008) 21:173–8. Available online at: https://www.iasj.net/iasj?func=article&aId=38607
79. Umur S, Acici M. A survey on helminth infections of equines in the central black sea region, Turkey. *Turk J Vet Anim Sci.* (2009) 33:373–8. doi: 10.3906/vet-0712-6
80. Soykan E, Öge H. The prevalence of liver trematodes in equines in different cities of Turkey. *Turkiye Parazitol Derg.* (2012) 36:152–5. doi: 10.5152/tpd.2012.36
81. Askari Z, Mas-Coma S, Bouwman AS, Boenke N, Stöllner T, Aali A, et al. *Fasciola hepatica* eggs in paleofaeces of the persian onager *Equus hemionus onager*, a donkey from chehrabad archaeological site, dating back to the sassanid empire (224-651 AD), in ancient Iran. *Infect Genet Evol.* (2018) 62:233–43. doi: 10.1016/j.meegid.2018.04.028
82. Getachew M, Innocent GT, Trawford AF, Reid SWJ, Love S. Epidemiological features of fasciolosis in working donkeys in Ethiopia. *Vet Parasitol.* (2010) 169:335–9. doi: 10.1016/j.vetpar.2010.01.007
83. Getachew M, Trawford A, Feseha G, Reid SWJ. Gastrointestinal parasites of working donkeys of Ethiopia. *Trop Anim Health Prod.* (2010) 42:27–33. doi: 10.1007/s11250-009-9381-0
84. Ayele G, Feseha G, Bojia E, Joe A. Prevalence of gastro-intestinal parasites of donkeys in Dugda Bora District, Ethiopia. *Livest. Res. Rural. Dev.* (2006) 18:14–21.
85. Mezgebu T, Tafess K, Tamiru F. Prevalence of gastrointestinal parasites of horses and donkeys in and around Gondar Town, Ethiopia. *Open J Vet Med.* (2013) 3:267–72. doi: 10.4236/ojvm.2013.36043
86. Collins DR. Fascioliasis in Mexican burro. *J Am Vet Med Assoc.* (1961) 139:1321–3.
87. Mera y Sierra RL, Artigas P, Cuervo P, Deis E, Sidoti L, Mas-Coma, et al. Fascioliasis transmission by *Lymnaea neotropica* confirmed by nuclear rDNA and mtDNA sequencing in Argentina. *Vet Parasitol.* (2009) 166:73–9. doi: 10.1016/j.vetpar.2009.08.001
88. Mas-Coma S, Angles R, Strauss W, Esteban JG, Oviedo JA, Buchon P. Human fascioliasis in Bolivia: a general analysis and a critical review of existing data. *Res Rev Parasitol.* (1995) 55:73–93,
89. Valero MA, Darce NA, Panova M, Mas-Coma S. Relationships between host species and morphometric patterns in *Fasciola hepatica* adults and eggs from the Northern Bolivian Altiplano hyperendemic region. *Vet Parasitol.* (2001) 102:85–100. doi: 10.1016/S0304-4017(01)00499-X
90. Mera y Sierra R, Neira G, Bargues MD, Cuervo PF, Artigas P, Logarzo L, et al. Equines as reservoirs of human fascioliasis: transmission capacity, epidemiology and pathogenicity in *Fasciola hepatica* infected mules. *J Helminthol.* (2020) 94:e189. doi: 10.1017/S0022149X20000693
91. Fahmy MFM, El-Attar SR. Pathological study on fascioliasis in camel and solipeds. *Egypt J Com Path Clinic Pathol.* (1990) 3:285–91.
92. Mitchell P. *The Donkey in Human History. An Archaelogical Perspective.* Oxford: Oxford University Press. (2018). 306. p
93. Rossel S, Marshall F, Peters J, Pilgram T, Adams MD, O'Connor D. Domestication of the donkey: timing, processes, and indicators. *Proc Natl Acad Sci USA.* (2007) 105:3715–20. doi: 10.1073/pnas.0709692105
94. Smith DG, Pearson RA. A review of the factors affecting the survival of donkeys in semiarid regions of Sub-Saharan Africa. *Trop Anim Health Prod.* (2005) 37:1–19. doi: 10.1007/s11250-005-9002-5
95. Wickler SJ, Greene HM. The horse and high altitude. *Clin Tech Equine Pract.* (2003) 2:231–7. doi: 10.1053/S1534-7516(03)00066-0
96. Burden FA, Hazell-Smith E, Mulugeta G, Patrick V, Trawford R, Brooks Brownlie HW. Reference intervals for biochemical and haematological parameters in mature domestic donkeys (*Equus asinus*) in the UK. *Equine Vet Educ.* (2016) 28:134–9. doi: 10.1111/eve.12512
97. Herrera BY, Rugeles PC, Vergara GO. Perfil hematológico del burro criollo (*Equus asinus*) colombiano. *Rev Colombiana Cienc Anim.* (2017) 9:158–63. doi: 10.24188/recia.v9.n2.2017.553
98. Madany MOK, Adam SEI. Ligation of the bile duct and acute chloroform toxicity in the donkey. *J Comp Pathol.* (1976) 86:539–46. doi: 10.1016/0021-9975(76)90063-3
99. Mendoza FJ, Toribio RE, Perez-Ecija A. Donkey internal medicine - Part I: metabolic, endocrine, and alimentary tract disturbances. *J Equine Vet Sci.* (2018) 65:66–74. doi: 10.1016/j.jevs.2018.02.001

18

Harnessing Clinical Trial Capacity to Mitigate Zoonotic Diseases: The Role of Expert Scientists

Senait Belay [1,2*]***, Mirutse Giday*** [1,3] ***and Tsegahun Manyazewal*** [1]

[1] Center for Innovative Drug Development and Therapeutic Trials for Africa (CDT-Africa), College of Health Sciences, Addis Ababa University, Addis Ababa, Ethiopia, [2] Faculty of Veterinary Medicine, Hawassa University, Hawassa, Ethiopia, [3] Aklilu Lemma Institute of Pathobiology, Addis Ababa University, Addis Ababa, Ethiopia

Correspondence:
Senait Belay
senaitbelay223@gmail.com

Background: The emergence and resurgence of zoonotic diseases have continued to be a major threat to global health and the economy. Developing countries are particularly vulnerable due to agricultural expansions and domestication of animals with humans. Scientifically sound clinical trials are important to find better ways to prevent, diagnose, and treat zoonotic diseases, while there is a lack of evidence to inform the clinical trials' capacity and practice in countries highly affected with the diseases. This study aimed to investigate expert scientists' perceptions and experiences in conducting clinical trials toward zoonotic diseases in Ethiopia.

Methods: This study employed a descriptive, qualitative study design. It included major academic and research institutions in Ethiopia that had active engagements in veterinary and public health researches. It included the National Veterinary Institute, the National Animal Health Diagnostic and Investigation Center, the College of Veterinary Medicine at Addis Ababa University, the Ethiopian Public Health Institute, the Armauer Hansen Research Institute, and the College of Health Sciences at Addis Ababa University. In-depth interviews were conducted with expert scientists. Data were collected from October 2019 to April 2020. Data analysis was undertaken using open code 4.03 for qualitative data analysis.

Results: Five major themes, with 18 sub-themes, emerged from the in-depth interviews. These were: challenges in the prevention, control, and treatment of zoonotic diseases; One Health approach to mitigate zoonotic diseases; personal and institutional experiences in conducting clinical trials on zoonotic diseases; barriers in conducting clinical trials toward zoonotic diseases; and strategies that promote conducting clinical trials on zoonotic diseases. Conducting clinical trials on zoonotic diseases in Ethiopia is hampered by a lack of clearly articulated ethics and regulatory frameworks, trial experts, financial resources, and good governance.

Conclusion: In Ethiopia, conducting clinical trials on zoonotic diseases deserves due attention. Strengthening institutional and human resources capacity is a pre-condition to harness effective implementation of clinical trials on zoonotic diseases in the country. In

Ethiopia where skilled human resource is scarce, One Health approach has the potential to form multidisciplinary teams to systematically improve clinical trials capacity and outcomes in the country.

Keywords: clinical trial, zoonotic disease, Ethiopia, one health, human resources

BACKGROUND

The importance of zoonotic diseases has increased at global and regional levels in recent years in connection with intensive human and wildlife migration, urbanization, human population growth, increased international travel and trade of animals and products of animal origin, and intensification of animal production (1–3). The emergence and resurgence of zoonotic diseases have continued to be a major threat to global health and the economy. Developing countries have a higher incidence and prevalence of zoonoses, and this is attributed to the lack of adequate control mechanisms, inadequate infrastructure, and inadequate information on their significance and distribution (4, 5). Many of the human diseases that are new, emerging, and re-emerging in these settings are caused by pathogens that originate in animals or products of animal.

Ethiopia has the second largest human population and the largest livestock population and is particularly vulnerable to the effects of zoonotic diseases because the economy is largely dependent on agriculture (6–8). Roughly 80% of households have direct contact with domestic animals, that favor an opportunity for infection and spread of disease (9). Ethiopia also ranks very high in the health burden of zoonotic diseases and in having a large population of poor livestock keepers (10). Since a large number of zoonotic diseases endemically arise in Ethiopia, a prioritization process was essential to categorize the most serious zoonotic diseases that should be co-operatively addressed by animal and public health agencies to exploit the impact on the health of people and animals. The zoonotic diseases prioritization workshop that was conducted in Ethiopia from September 25 to 26, 2019 guided a range of government agencies through the process to prioritize zoonotic diseases of greatest concern for Ethiopia and develop next steps and action plans. In the prioritization process, potential zoonotic diseases of concern were identified through a set of criteria. As a result of the prioritization process, human and animal health agencies co-operatively identified five zoonotic diseases they can jointly start to tackle. These are rabies, anthrax, brucellosis, Rift Valley fever, and zoonotic avian influenza (11).

Control of zoonotic diseases constitutes an important health matter. However, many factors are involved in prevention and control and it cannot be addressed by public health sectors only. Success in reducing the public health significance greatly depends on the level of cooperation between public and veterinary health sectors using one health approach in all aspects of the diagnosis, exchange of information, organization of shared surveillance systems, common training of staff and creation of community awareness. High-level commitment and the ability of national programmers to mobilize the necessary resources and to collaborate closely with other relevant sectors are needed to cope with the common challenges.

Conducting clinical trials toward zoonotic diseases is paramount to reduce the impact of zoonotic diseases on human and human health (12). It finds better ways to prevent, screen, diagnose, and treat the zoonotic diseases. In Ethiopia, the number of clinical trials that have been done keeps growing throughout the years. However, compared to other countries, it is still much lower. Africa, in general, shares only 2.4% of clinical trials generated globally and Ethiopia shares only 2.3% of clinical trials generated out of Africa and the trials are limited in number and variety (13–15). This is due to the existence of many challenges for the conduct of clinical trials that would determine the safety and efficacy of new products and interventions in the country. The tendencies to conduct clinical trials toward zoonotic disease in Ethiopia has not been studies. Thus, this study intended to investigate researchers' and experts' perceptions and experiences of conducting clinical trials toward zoonotic diseases in Ethiopia.

METHODS

Study Setting and Design

This study employed a descriptive, qualitative study design. It included major academic and research institutions in Ethiopia that had active engagements in veterinary and public health researches. It included the National Veterinary Institute (NVI), the National Animal Health Diagnostic and Investigation Center (NAHDIC), the College of Veterinary Medicine at Addis Ababa University (CVM AAU), the Ethiopian Public Health Institute (EPHI), the Armauer Hansen Research Institute (AHRI), and the College of Health Sciences at Addis Ababa University (CHS AAU). The six institutions are all government-owned and have a long history providing research, academic, and disease prevention and treatment services in Ethiopia. NVI was established in 1964 and is currently certified by ISO/QMS to develop, manufacture, sell, and distribute veterinary vaccines as its primary mandate, and it is certified by ISO/IEC to function as a research and development laboratory for some specific laboratory tests (16). NAHDIC, established in 1995, is a national and East African reference laboratory for animal diseases and related public health problems. It has an ISO 17025 certified laboratory for molecular testing, including real-time PCR (17). EPHI works to improve the health of the general public of

Abbreviations: AHARI, Armauer Hansen Research Institute; AI, Avian Influenza; CDC, US Centers for Disease Control and Prevention; CDT-Africa, Center for Innovative Drug Development and Therapeutic Trial for Africa; EPHI, Ethiopian Public Health Institute; EWA, Ethiopian Wildlife Authority; FDA, Food and Drug Administration; GCP, Good Clinical Practice; NAHDIC, National Animal Health Diagnostic and Investigation Center; NVI, National Veterinary Institute; RVF, Rift Valley Fever; WHO, World Health Organization.

Ethiopia through undertaking research on priority health and nutrition issues for evidence-based information and technology transfer, effective public health emergency management, quality laboratory system, and training public health researchers and practitioners for pre-eminent public health interventions (18). CVM AAU, established in 1963, provides teaching, problem-solving research, and community services including treating all species of animals (over 20,000–25,000 patients every year), vaccination, consultancy, ambulatory clinic, artificial insemination, veterinary drug sale, harness making, and animal welfare education of school children among others (19). AHRI, founded in 1970, works to improve medical care, health, and well-being of the public by generating and delivering scientific evidence, developing new tools and methods through biomedical, clinical, and translational research, and to serve as a hub for technology transfer and capacity building in medical research and training (20). CHS AAU provides high quality and regionally relevant health sciences training, research and community services at both undergraduate and post-graduate levels. It is the only institution where some specialized tertiary healthcare services are given (21).

Participants

We followed a purposive sampling method to recruit the participants from the selected study areas. The total number of participants in the study was 14 using data saturation procedures. The Inclusion criteria were holding a proven exhibit primarily leading research activities or research units within the institutions, having a minimum of three publications as the first author, and/or a minimum of 5-year work experience in the research or management of zoonotic research. According to the legal procedure in the institutions, institutional directors, or college deans at each institution should first give verbal approval for a researcher to proceed to contact a participant. Therefore, after getting an approval letter for the study from the Addis Ababa University College of Health Science, CDT-Africa, we contacted institutional directors or college deans at each institution to select the participants. All of the institutional directors or college deans received the letters and gave their verbal approval. Some recruited the participants themselves based on the information they read in the letter, whereas, others allowed us to select by ourselves. Finally, the selected participants agreed and participated in the study.

Data Collection

We conducted a face-to-face, open-ended in-depth interviews to allow participants to discuss their opinions, views, and experiences fully in detail. We prepared a list of questions to be responded to by each participant. All the interviews were m by the primary investigator during work hours in private rooms and the discussions were open for any questions or clarification. The participants themselves scheduled when and where they were to be interviewed, and reported that they were comfortable about their decisions. The language of communication with the participants during the in-depth interviews was English. We conducted an in-depth interview with two researchers to test the validity of the interview questions and gain the necessary experience. When the primary investigator conducted in-depth interviews, she audio-recorded the interviews for later transcription, and she took additional notes. The use of audio records determined by the participants' consent and each of them was asked to and agreed to be recorded, except two who allowed taking notes only. The interviews had nine open-ended questions, uniquely developed for the sole purpose of this study.

Data Analysis and Interpretation

We started analyzing the material during the fieldwork to identify gaps early and produce a good description of topics. The audio files from the in-depth interviews were transcribed and data analysis was undertaken using open code 4.03 for qualitative data analysis (22). To improve the rigor of the study, two investigators were involved in the data analysis. Braun and Clark's reflexive thematic analysis framework (23) was used and the analysis process followed the six phases: familiarization, initial coding, theme construction, reviewing themes, defining themes, and producing the report.

Ethical Clearance and Consideration

Ethical clearance was obtained from the Scientific and Ethics Review Committee of the Centre for Innovative Drug Development and Therapeutic Trials for Africa (CDT-Africa), College of Health Sciences, Addis Ababa University. Letters of ethical clearance as well as a letter of support were submitted to the selected academic and research institutions and researchers, and their consent was obtained. Interviewees were briefed on the purpose of the study without any form of deception before securing informed consent from them and confidentiality maintained entirely.

RESULTS

Demography of the Participants

In total, 14 participants were involved, including two from NVI, two from CVM AAU, two from NAHDIC, four from AHARI, three from CHS AAU, and one from EPHI. **Table 1** summarizes the participants' demographic characteristics.

Study Themes

During the interview sessions, participants reflected upon several concepts around zoonotic diseases, clinical trials, one health approach, and integrative practices of the public and animal health system. Participants were also able to ground these discussions by drawing connections to their experiences in clinical research on zoonotic diseases and how these ideas may have influenced the research world. Many participants in this study reported their appreciation for the opportunity to participate in the interview as the topic is new with an appreciable idea. Some mentioned that the researchers allowed them to talk about issues that are always in their minds and planned to do more in the future. As such, five themes were identified from the data, each containing several sub-themes (**Table 2**). These themes are:-

1. Challenges in the prevention, control, and treatment of zoonotic diseases

TABLE 1 | Participants demographic information.

Participant ID	Name of the institution	Highest level of education	Academic rank/Position in the institution	Service year	Publication as the first Author
CDP001	AHRI	PhD	Research directorate	15 year	18
CDP002	CVM AAU	PhD	Professor	25 year	50
CDP003	EPHI	MSc	Research directorate	10 year	16
CDP004	NVI	PhD	Drug formulation director directorate	18 years	8
CDP005	NAHDIC	MSc	Senior researcher	13 years	6
CDP006	CHS AAU	PhD	Professor	30 years	60
CDP007	AHRI	MSc	Physician	8 years	4
CDP008	AHRI	MSc	Principal Investigator	18 years	15
CDP009	AHRI	PhD	Head of the one health	15 years	20
CDP010	NVI	PhD	Senior researcher	13 years	7
CDP011	CVM AAU	PhD	Associate Professor	18 years	20
CDP012	CHS AAU	PhD	Associate Professor /east Africa one health initiative director	21 year	56
CDP013	CHS AAU	PhD	Associate Professor	10 year	39
CDP014	NAHDIC	MSc	Senior researcher	9 years	4

2. One health approach to mitigate zoonotic diseases
3. Personal and institutional experiences in conducting clinical trials on zoonotic diseases.
4. Barriers in conducting clinical trials toward zoonotic diseases.
5. Strategies that promote conducting clinical trials toward zoonotic diseases.

Theme 1: Challenges in the Prevention, Control, and Treatment of Zoonotic Diseases

The challenges in the prevention, control, and treatment of zoonotic diseases are mentioned in many of the interviews. This theme and its five subthemes and some codes captured participants' perceptions and experiences on the challenges in the prevention, control, and treatment of zoonotic diseases. The codes (subthemes) supported by descriptions and quotes are as follows:

Lack of Integration Between Human and Animal Health Professionals and Sectors

All participants perceived a lack of integration between human and animal health professionals as the main challenge. They mentioned that people who were engaged in the public health profession did not emphasize zoonotic diseases; they did not have the interest to get involved in research concerning zoonotic diseases. They considered dealing with the zoonotic related issue was the responsibility of animal health professionals. Moreover, participants stated that researchers who were professionals in veterinary health and those experts in public health were not collaborating to do research together. Even geographically public health institutes and veterinary health institutes were not in the same area.

> "*Researchers who are working in the field of veterinary health and those who are working in human health are not working collaboratively. That is the most difficult challenge...for example, if you take Addis Ababa University, College of Veterinary Medicine, it is in Bishoftu but the College of Health Sciences in Tikur Anbesa....even geography can be also a problem to work together*"*(CDP013)*. "*...I mean ... people who are engaged in public health, they don't have Knowledge of zoonotic diseases... You know they consider this responsibility is for veterinarians.... They don't give much attention to zoonotic diseases ..... That is a major challenge*" *(CDP010).*

Lack of Trained Manpower and Inadequate Finance

On the other hand, lack of human capacity, limited resources, and other related tools were reported by the majority of participants as challenges in the prevention, control, and treatment of zoonotic diseases. They mentioned that lack of skilled manpower who specialized in the area of zoonotic diseases with knowledge of different aspects of those diseases required to propose, initiate, and conduct of any research intended for zoonotic diseases. Financial scarcity also another challenge in Ethiopia as it is also in most low-income countries; research is considered to be a luxury because of economic constraints. Participants indicated that as long as we do not have experts in the area who can deal with zoonotic diseases and well-organized financial systems, it could be difficult to prevent and control zoonotic diseases.

> "*....I think yes... there are several challenges, in terms of human capacity who are specialized in the field and in terms of resource both financial and another resource...*"*(CDP012)* "*...Because we don't have tools to deal with the infection, to produce drugs such as vaccines, and so on...Even the diagnosis is very difficult for most of these diseases...they need a special laboratory for example diseases that needs complicated diagnostic techniques like brucellosis, anthrax... They need level 3 laboratories, but we do not have these ...*" *(CDP007).*

TABLE 2 | List of the themes and sub-themes (codes) that resulted from the data analysis.

Themes	Sub-themes/Categories/codes
Theme 1: Challenges in the prevention, control, and treatment of zoonotic diseases	1.1 lack of integration between public and veterinary health professionals and sectors, 1.2 Human capacity (lack of skilled personnel, lack of awareness and motivation) 1.3 Inadequate financial and other resources support (lack of funding, inadequate laboratory equipment, lack of infrastructure) 1.4 Limited research, experience (Lack of research materials/facilities, lack of conducive research atmosphere) 1.5 Problems related to awareness and attitude.
Theme 2: One Health approach to mitigate zoonotic diseases	2.1 Implementation of one health 2.2 Silo effect 2.3 Importance of clinical trial and other basic or applied researches intended for zoonotic diseases
Theme 3: Individual and institutional experiences in conducting clinical trials on zoonotic diseases	3.1 Personal experiences 3.2 Institutional experiences
Theme 4: Barriers in conducting clinical trials toward zoonotic diseases	4.1 Ethical and regulatory systems (delay of approval decision, complex and strict ethical and regulatory system) 4.2 Human resources (lack of skilled personnel, lack of awareness and motivation) 4.3 Administrative support, (unsupportive administrative system) 4.4 Budget and infrastructure (lack of funding, inadequate laboratory equipment, lack of infrastructure) 4.5 lack of time
Theme 5: Strategies that promote conducting clinical trials on zoonotic diseases	5.1 Capacity building 5.2 Developing clinical trial industries 5.3 Promoting other applied researches

Limited Research

Others described that there is a lack of baseline data due to limited research in the area and could lead to the irrational use of drugs and the scarcity of vaccines to prevent those diseases. Several neglected zoonotic diseases are not yet researched in Ethiopia.

> *"...... The major challenges are related to issues of limited research in the area of zoonotic diseases and the knowledge and awareness of the community ... " (CDP004).*

Lack of Awareness and Attitude

Besides, lack of knowledge, attitude, and awareness in the society aggravate disease transmission between animals and humans as Ethiopia, a country that has the biggest herd of livestock in Africa where its economy largely depended on agriculture and most of the society lives closer to its animals. People don't know about those diseases and are not aware of how they get diseases from animals.

> *"....We have the biggest herd of livestock in Africa and people are living very close to livestock especially in the rural areas; in the whole pastoral area, there is a close link between animals and people and increased human and animal contact leads to a risk of a high prevalence of zoonotic diseases in the area ... I think this happens due to lack of awareness and scarcity of information in Ethiopia on this topic....."(CDP011).*

Theme 2: One Health and Research Approach Intended for Zoonotic Diseases

This theme reflects the researchers' perceptions and experiences in connection with one health approach and different issues related to clinical trials and other basic or applied researches toward zoonotic diseases. It is divided into three further subthemes: implementation of one health, silo effect and importance of clinical trial and other applied researches intended for zoonotic diseases.

Implementation of One Health

All fourteen participants considered that the implementation of one health in Ethiopia would be a beneficial approach in reducing the burden of zoonotic diseases. They considered that one health would enable earlier detection of zoonotic diseases, and therefore earlier reporting and opportunities for prevention or management of zoonotic transmission from animals to humans. They were asked about their perceptions concerning one health approach and whether they had participated in any project, workshop, conference, and other duties associated with one health initiative. Data suggest that some of them were involved in one health initiative activities and observed challenges and opportunities to implement it. As it is a new concept in Ethiopia, the progress of implementation so far is somehow appreciable, as different ministries are preparing a platform that helps them work together. Other participants also discussed that although some institutions started participating in one health initiative; still there is no proper health implementation in Ethiopia. The participants' further stated that where we have several emerging and re-emerging pathogens, working in isolation on the veterinary pathogen or human pathogens will not lead us any further in the control of zoonotic diseases.

> *"... To my knowledge, there is no proper health implementation in Ethiopia. We have a project in the Somali region. We are starting*

to implement one health initiative, but there is no result to show yet..... In my experience I am seeing that we still are not considering the whole ecosystem and the wildlife as part of the one health approach We started implementing one health but we have not yet exploited the full potential ....The research institute at which I am working, i.e. AHRI, is also involved in one health initiative and it has one health unit that focuses on addressing zoonotic diseases particularly related to bovine tuberculosis and other diseases of interest like Pasteurella, brucellosis and other bacterial diseases" (CDP003). ".....in the case of one health approach,... it is a good idea to improve the diagnosis as well as the controlling and preventing method of transmission from animal to human and vice versa and there is a start of one health approach in Ethiopia in which we are just participating with other institutes working on this..... Our institution (NAHDIC) as one member is participating in prioritizing zoonotic diseases using one health approach...." (CDP002).

Silo Effect

Participants discussed the issue that there were challenges in implementing one health approach. The majority of them mentioned the existence of the silo effect in the implementation of one health and have similar challenges to collaboratively prevent and control zoonotic diseases. Silo Effect in one health refers to lack of information flowing between institutions or parts of an organization and limits the interactions between members of different sectors, thus leading to reduced productivity and capacity of collaborative working.

"....the Silo effect is the first and the most important challenge in the implementation of one health....you know there is no ministry or no office that works on one health ....Since it doesn't belong to one ministry people have their circle and work on that circle and there is a very bad history of working together....as I said the challenges that are faced on issues around working on zoonotic disease are also faced encountered in one health program. ......" (CDP012).

Importance of Clinical Trial and Other Basic or Applied Researches Intended for Zoonotic Diseases

The significance of conducting clinical trials over other basic or applied researches was reported by most of the participants. In this regard, they mentioned that clinical trials had a broad concept. They stated that it was not only developing a new treatment but rather it included so many aspects it *is beyond that; a clinical trial is about vaccine, clinical trial is about diagnostics, a clinical trial is about lifestyle.* They further mentioned that as there was evidence of a gap in the control and prevention of zoonotic diseases in Ethiopia and thus a need for a new intervention in terms of developing new diagnostic tools, vaccines, or treatment.

"....Yes,... because the evidence is always good...I mean my work was involving both clinical trial and leadership of one health partnership. First, we should start by defining and understanding what a clinical trial is. In this perspective, someone is considering clinical trial in the context of developing a new drug but a clinical trial is beyond that; a clinical trial is about. vaccine, clinical trial is about diagnostics, a clinical trial is about any intervention.if we think of for example a trial on vaccine efficacy and safety in this country for several diseases like rabies, do we work on and invest in zoonotic diseases vaccine development, diagnostic development...yes... Clearly... yes... As I said earlier, these are diseases that are highly affecting developing countries Like Ethiopia. The problem is ours and the solution should come from us. ...For example, brucellosis is one of the vaccine-preventable diseases. Anthrax is one that is vaccine-preventable. Rabies is one of the vaccine-preventable diseases. So to answer your question, do we need a clinical trial for those diseases in Ethiopia...." (CDP012). "....Yes, a clinical trial is more important than other basic or applied researches because you do have better, tangible information because a clinical trial is you know it is a method to evaluate the certain drug, or biological things, any kind of intervention have to first evaluate Before putting the ground..... (CDP005).

In contrast, some participants reported that as the magnitude of most of the zoonotic diseases was not well-researched in Ethiopia, where there are inadequate epidemiological and other types of data, conducting clinical trial was not applicable. They thus further suggested that emphasis first be given to other basic or applied studies rather than to clinical trials.

".....For some diseases that we just, don't know enough, basic epidemiological studies would be more important to get a proper idea of what is going on. it may not be the right time to do clinical trials for these diseases because to me we are very far away from knowing the magnitude of these diseases like the rift valley or rabies. but I don't think we know what the magnitude of those diseases is. The first thing is we need to do more work in integration beyond just simply talking about one health. We need to go the grass-root level and get more involved in basic researches..." (CDP009). "... Conducting clinical trials is good. I am not against that but I don't give priority to a clinical trial on the zoonotic disease rather the basic researches. If you do basic researches on zoonotic diseases we can generate evidence. We can do awareness creation works on zoonotic diseases and...I prefer the basic and epidemiological researches on zoonotic diseases than clinical ....Probably it might be because I don't know the magnitude of the problem but before doing a clinical trial, it is good to have adequate information on the burden of the diseases... For instance, understanding the basic characteristics of a pathogen at ultrastructure"(CDP008).

Theme 3: Personal and Individual Experiences in Conducting Clinical Trials on Zoonotic Diseases

Under this theme, participants discussed different issues related to their experiences in connection with clinical trials toward zoonotic diseases as well as institutional level perceptions and experiences.

Concerning personal and institutional experiences, participants claimed that there was a limited experience in conducting clinical trials in Ethiopia in general. The majority of the participants stated that they had never participated in any clinical trial toward zoonotic diseases due to some country-level challenges, such as institutional administrative problems and lack of funding opportunities.

"...I have no experience in conducting clinical trials for zoonotic diseases.... probably one reason is as I said we still do not have much knowledge on the epidemiology of those diseases. The second

thing is a matter of prioritization of government and international bodies... As an institution, yes; I would say it is very low, to be frank. AHRI is more, I can say, working on clinical trial but when you come to specifically zoonotic diseases, it is very low. Like I said, usually, sponsors are interested in other diseases like HIV, TB, and Malaria than zoonotic diseases ... " (CDP010).

On the other hand, few participants reported that they had the experience of conducting clinical trial toward zoonotic diseases involving tuberculosis, leishmaniasis which included vaccine trial, diagnostic trial, and an on-going treatment trial.

"...... ya so, this is the issue so, for example, I did with leishmaniasis And you know that leishmaniasis is a zoonotic disease and therefore we have been conducting a clinical trial. I was involved in at least 7 or 8 clinical trials. Some are completed and some on-going.....so we have new formulation and resumption to the existing treatment are to evaluated we had to come up with the short duration of treatment this has been done and even the guideline. The treatment guideline has been changed as a result of that and there has been also a negative result. Because I said close to 8 clinical trials I was engaged at least one study which was interrupted because the result was discouraging ... not always to be successful and but most of the time we were successful the same thing. It was a treatment trial and evaluation of diagnostic tests ... a couple of diagnostic tests evaluated now the tests are in use in the health system. The result was published and has been translated and public health use in diagnostic and treatment now. in the movement, we have one clinical trial which is vaccines for leishmaniasis, but that is on-going... " (CDP006).

Theme 4: Barriers in Conducting Clinical Trials Toward Zoonotic Diseases

Participants outlined the different barriers they faced or perceived during their research life. Most of the barriers they mentioned were similar to the challenges faced in the prevention and control of zoonotic diseases except for a few of them. The identified ones were barriers related to the handling of ethical and regulatory systems, lack of human capacity, administrative problems, financial scarcity, and other resources for conducting clinical trials. Barriers may differ generally depending on the setting in which the clinical trials are conducted.

Barriers Related to Ethical and Regulatory Systems

The majority of participants indicated difficulties with ethical and regulatory requirements, either at a national or institutional level as the main barrier. Respondents claimed that approval of proposals takes a long time to get approval and that discouraged most researchers to think of and conducting clinical trials on zoonotic diseases.

"... Ya... the main challenges for conducting a clinical trial is ethical clearance and regulatory approval especially in our country Regulators and the ethical clearance are most of the time delay and make the research lose interest... " (CDP005).

Financial Constraints and Other Resources

Most respondents report that clinical trial by itself is complicated. It is costly; it needs a long duration of time and organized documentation. They indicated that in the context of our country, as a developing country, most of the research institutions focus on basic or applied researches which is not financially expensive. Participants highlighted barriers related to infrastructure like lack of standard laboratory to conduct clinical trials was the most frequently cited resource limitation. They indicated that zoonotic diseases posed risk to people and the environment and thus a need for good laboratory facilities, which is not available in the country. The quote from one participant could be taken as evidence that a good laboratory facility is very crucial to conduct the different phases of a clinical trial for zoonotic diseases. Lack of skilled manpower was also the most frequently cited barrier to conduct clinical trials toward zoonotic diseases.

"... it is costly, it takes time, it's complicated ..... and it needs a lot of good practice and good laboratory practice and documentation and ethical clearance also the problem .... you don't get timely feedback, or approvals from ethics committees and that takes time so the protocol would take up to 2 years to get it approval" (CDP006). ".....the human and financial capacities are the main challenges, for example, 5 years ago I was engaging in a project with the main target of building capacity in all East Africa to conduct clinical trial so. Ethiopia was a member and the other country, Kenya, Tanzania, and Uganda. the idea was to build capacity then AHARI was identified as sister institutions that probably to upgrade to be a site where we conduct a clinical trial. So we bought very few basic equipments like freezers, incubators, so on but after a couple of years everything was stopped because of a lack of capacity to run the project... so at this time, we can't even host phase two and other phases of clinical trial... probably we can do just phase one small clinical trial because of lack of capacity to do further phases of a clinical trial" (CDP008).

Barrier Related to Administrative Issue

Participants stated that a lack of support and encouragement from an institution is also another barrier. They reported failure to acquire grants as most of the grants for clinical trials were too competitive. Institutional grants were always keen to basic or applied researches and that resulted in a lack of motivation from research coordinators and administrative bodies. Certain quotations below show these and related opinions:

"...support and encouragement from an institution is the main challenge because institutions give apriority for other epidemiological research rather than clinical trial ... For example. I have submitted a protocol for the university thematic research grant in the genetics and behavior related topic... which was... the effect of genetics on behavior so, we want to do a clinical trial on twins, but finally it got rejected because it's a kind of a clinical trial, basic research people assume that it is a kind of luxury so, getting institutional support was a big challenge" (CDP013). The other problem is administrative support especially from the institutions is limited ....in clinical trial organizational support is crucial... there is reporting for example within 24 hours you know taking immediate action it might have emergencies ... It needs support from the administrative but that is not available and also There is the issue of import of goods and supplies, medication and so on" (CDP006).

Theme 5: Strategies that Promote Conducting Clinical Trials Toward Zoonotic Diseases

Different suggestions were made by respondents on how to improve the conduct of clinical trials toward zoonotic diseases. Most of the suggestions were related to the challenges that have been identified above. Below are some of the common responses:

Capacity Building

The most common promoting factors identified by the study participants included capacity building including change of education system since Ethiopian scientists are not that much aware of and want to do clinical trials. There must be some reform in the educational system to address the need for clinical trials. Higher learning institutions could incorporate modules on clinical trials within their teaching programs for health professionals. The other factor mentioned by participants was related to capacity building of researchers by creating a platform to bring all different researchers together to conduct a clinical trial, which according to them, needs a lot of support to move forward, including from that of funding organizations, and policy and decision-makers. Participants from CVM AAU and CHS AAU mentioned that the following:

> *"...ya.... So what could be done and I think, to begin with, education Not many scientists in Ethiopia are aware and wanting to do clinical trials, there must be some platform whereby ...you know to address the need of clinical trial not only zoonotic diseases but also other diseases. I know there is some initiative in CDT Africa....to promote there is an approach to doing it as educational system.the higher learning institutions could incorporate modules about clinical trial within their teaching program and as far as I know, there is none as the movement so, you know health professionals in general before they graduated they should get a module of a clinical trial in the final year then they will get something about clinical research ... they will get something about ethics and other related issues of clinical trial.....so that is a missing link and the ministry of education and higher education if they can address it which means we will have everyone comes out of school will have an idea of what clinical trial and some might decide to do clinical trials and so have it as a career and I think with that you know the scenario might change for the future,* for example, *EPHI they have a unit for zoonotic disease and also ... Aklilulema institute of pathobiology ....those institutions should be leading this exercise otherwise it becomes an issue for just an interested individual, but there must be an institutional commitment they have to incorporate clinical trials in their programs and this message has to be conveyed to those institute" (CDP006). "ya... one thing we have to improve the capacity of researchers and funding organization they have to make open their doors for such kind of and also policymakers, Decision makers they have to be open to using outputs of clinical trials that conducted. There should be a kind of change of perception about what clinical trial is. the other one, there should be a kind of platform to bring all different professionals to work together in conducting clinical trials for these diseases unless We work together. Clinical trial for zoonotic diseases may not be successful as need." (CDP011).*

Developing Clinical Trial Industries

Other respondents talked about promoting factors in terms of infrastructure and locally developed clinical trial industry to motivate researchers to do clinical trials. The respondents reported that external partners only supported the conduct of a trial that focused on diseases of their interest but not zoonotic diseases that were relevant to the country. The respondents further stressed on the importance of locally developed tools to be self-sufficient in everything.

> *".. I think the first thing is they have to need to do more on capacity building in human and also the infrastructure that is initial thing otherwise I believe Ethiopia is a good site for clinical trial what we are lacking is the human capacity on the other hand. I don't see the particular challenge and particular Solution for zoonotic diseases. it's the same as any other diseases so generally in the clinical trial industry because of we don't have locally Developed tools eternal partners are influenced us ....so we have to be self-sufficient by everything, the local scientific Community development should be We should have new tools and idea we going to do clinical trial" (CDP007).*

Promoting Other Applied Researches

On the other hand, some respondents indicated that to promote conducting clinical trials toward zoonotic diseases, there was a need to first promote epidemiological researches before thinking of conducting clinical trials because of the need to understand the magnitude and the importance of diseases in our country. So we need to have the basic information of the diseases regarding magnitude and epidemiology.

> *"To promote clinical trial.i don't think. It is you know we are on the time to implement clinical trial.it should be established that we have to have to the ground otherwise it should. The country should have some industry working on pharma industry as well as biological things b/c we have to have our capacity rather than importing as a product so that if we are plan to produce or develop drugs, vaccines even we have to change our traditional medicines to market to make the marketable we have to conduct a clinical trial, so it's the time also force us to establish this think we are on the right direction, the government Addis Ababa university. Open this clinical trial-related discipline so it is nice one awarded people to participate in clinical trial". (CDP004).*

DISCUSSION

In this study, in-depth interviews with 14 participants provided information on researchers' perceptions and experiences in conducting clinical trials toward zoonotic diseases, and several issues around zoonotic diseases were mentioned. Participants reported so many challenges in the prevention and control of these diseases in Ethiopia. The main challenge for the effective implementation of zoonoses control reported was the lack of integration between human and animal health professionals. Sectors working on public health, veterinary health, agriculture, and the environment must be aware of the importance to get involved in cooperative efforts in the control of zoonotic diseases. This finding is supported by many studies around the globe, which state the challenges of preventing and control of zoonotic diseases greatly due to lack of cooperation between medical and veterinary sectors in the diagnosis of zoonoses, exchange of information, organization of shared surveillance systems, common training of staff and creation of community awareness (24–27).

An additional challenge mentioned by the respondents was a lack of infrastructure and other resources, such as good laboratory facilities. Participants stated that zoonotic diseases needed at most care while researching because they pose a high risky for humans as well as the environment. The respondents stressed that there was a lack of good laboratory facilities, such as level three and above. Participants believed that funding could become a sensitive issue to conduct clinical trials on zoonotic diseases as such, mostly a problem of developing countries, like Ethiopia. Funding for clinical trials in a developing country comes mostly from Western countries in which pharmaceutical companies are based. In most low-income countries, research is a luxury because of economic constraints. This result was in line with studies reported elsewhere in different African countries (27, 28).

Participant emphasized the significance of one health approach, an interdisciplinary approach to zoonotic diseases, which encourages structured collaboration and coordination between human and animal health sectors, which have also been supported and highlighted in many other studies (29–31). The existence of the "silo effect" between professional sectors was also evident from the findings in this study. Participants perceived that the "silo effect" can inhibit cross-sectional collaboration and communication. This phenomenon has also been reported by several other studies (32, 33). The COVID-19 outbreak is evidence of how emerging animal-source of diseases cause a human health hazard globally (34, 35) and disrupt the healthcare system (36).

Participants stated that highly qualified personnel are required to propose, initiate, and conduct clinical trials. Such human resource development requires relatively stable, well-resourced research and higher education institutes, and well-established science governance systems, which is not the case in Ethiopia because higher learning institutions and teaching hospitals in Ethiopia have poorly prepared their graduates to conduct scientific trials and clinical research. A recent systematic review reports that there are substantial barriers at the system, organization, and individual level that hamper the conduct of clinical trials in developing countries, and that instituting a system for wider implementation of local investigator-initiated trials would address this problem (37).

Ethical and regulatory system obstacles emerged as the second most important barrier. Prolonged ethical and regulatory review time lead to delays in implementing grants and sometimes led grants to expire before recruitment taking place. They also reported lengthy or ill-defined approval processes, significant bureaucracy, and lack of regulatory staff with expertise in reviewing. Similar findings have been reported in several studies around the globe especially in developing countries reporting (37, 38). Complex and unreasonably strict government regulatory systems could worsen the negative feedback loop between limited research capacity and small numbers of trials conducted. Limited researches in the area were also identified as likely barriers to the conduct of clinical trial for zoonotic diseases in Ethiopia.

Strategies for strengthening the conduct of clinical trials toward zoonotic diseases in Ethiopia need to focus on identifying country-specific problems. The study identified some promoting requirements necessary for successfully conducting a clinical trial for zoonotic diseases that are relevant in the future planning of such a strategy. Most of the promoting strategies reported by participants included the establishment of a well-organized educational system and capacity building. The result of this study reinforces the need for an educational system that integrates portions of clinical trial toward zoonotic diseases to provide students and professionals with a holistic understanding of clinical trial and zoonotic diseases as well as to improve intersectoral collaboration. As most of the Ethiopian scientists are interested to involve in clinical trial studies, there must be some mechanism to address such needs. The higher learning institutions may incorporate modules about clinical trials within their teaching programs. A standard guideline and platform should be established that address conducting clinical trials toward zoonotic diseases, especially on neglected zoonotic diseases by bringing together experts from different disciplines. This finding is supported by a study (39) which stated that capacity building is a basic strategy needed to build good clinical industries. Additionally, policymakers should be involved to support clinical trial studies on zoonotic diseases in this country. Successful promotion of conducting clinical trials toward zoonotic diseases requires government and ministerial office involvement. Raising awareness among decision-makers and policy-makers on the burden of zoonoses in humans and animals may assist in securing political commitment and financial support for conducting clinical trials toward zoonotic diseases. Moreover, participants stressed the importance of sharing experiences from other countries that have a success story in conducting clinical trials toward zoonotic diseases as that could encourage them to get involved in such research. In other countries, there are so many clinical trials conducted on zoonotic diseases, including vaccine trials for anthrax, rabies, and other zoonotic diseases (40–43).

This study has limitations in that it focuses on the perspective of participants included and is not necessarily representative of that of their peers as such these views can not be generalized. In the contrary, its unique approach, with a country-level focus and input from prominent experts around Ethiopia who are influential in their corresponding fields including in the areas of public health, veterinary health, and one health, give the study strength. Further large scale studies involving interviews and surveys of stakeholders including representatives from a range of institutions would be beneficial.

CONCLUSION

In Ethiopia, conducting clinical trials on zoonotic diseases deserves due attention. Several challenges hinder conducting clinical trials toward zoonotic diseases. These challenges include ethical and regulatory system barriers, lack of collaboration across different sectors, financial scarcity, lack of human capacity, and administrative related issues. The study illustrates the importance of interdisciplinary collaboration and communication in the field of zoonotic disease control. Strengthening institutional and human resources capacity is a pre-condition to harness effective implementation of clinical trials on zoonotic diseases in the country. In Ethiopia where skilled human resource is scarce, One Health approach has the potential to form multidisciplinary teams to systematically improve clinical trials capacity and outcomes in the country.

ETHICS STATEMENT

The studies involving human participants were reviewed and approved by Scientific and Ethics Review Committee of the Center for Innovative Drug Development and Therapeutic Trials for Africa (CDT-Africa), College of Health Sciences, Addis Ababa University, Addis Ababa, Ethiopia. The patients/participants provided their written informed consent to participate in this study.

AUTHOR CONTRIBUTIONS

SB conceived the study, collected the primary data, analyzed, and wrote the first draft. SB, TM, and MG designed the study. TM and MG supervised the data collection and revised the manuscript. All authors approved the final version for publication.

ACKNOWLEDGMENTS

The authors acknowledge the input of the study participants and the heads of the study sites who enabled the data collection.

REFERENCES

1. Gibb R, Redding DW, Chin KQ, Donnelly CA, Blakburn TM, Newbold T, et al. Zoonotic host diversity increases in human-dominated ecosystems. *Nature.* (2020) 584:398–402. doi: 10.1038/s41586-020-2562-8
2. Ehrenberg JP, Zhou X-N, Fontes G, Rocha EMM, Tanner M, et al. Strategies supporting the prevention and control of neglected tropical diseases during and beyond the COVID-19 pandemic. *Infect Dis Poverty.* (2020) 9:86. doi: 10.1186/s40249-020-00701-7
3. Paul P, Kangalawe RYM, Mboera LEG. Land-use patterns and their implication on malaria transmission in Kilosa District, Tanzania. *Trop Dis Travel Med Vaccines.* (2018) 4:6. doi: 10.1186/s40794-018-0066-4
4. Singh G, Angwafor SA, Njamnshi AK, Fraimow K, Sander JW. Zoonotic and vector-borne parasites and epilepsy in low-income and middle-income countries. *Nat Rev Neurol.* (2020) 16:333–45. doi: 10.1038/s41582-020-0361-3
5. Human zoonotic tuberculosis and livestock exposure in low- and middle-income countries: a systematic review identifying challenges in laboratory diagnosis. *Zoonoses Public Health.* (2020) 67:97–111. doi: 10.1111/zph.12684
6. Gizaw S, Desta H, Alemu B, Tgegne A, Wieland B,. A Tegegne Importance of livestock diseases identified using participatory epidemiology in the highlands of Ethiopia. *Trop Anim Health Prod.* (2020) 52:1745–57. doi: 10.1007/s11250-019-02187-4
7. Abebe E, Gugsa G, Ahmed M. Review on major food-borne zoonotic bacterial pathogens. *J Trop Med.* (2020) 2020:4674235. doi: 10.1155/2020/4674235
8. Alemayehu B, Ayele BT, Kloos H, Ambelu A. Individual and community-level risk factors in under-five children diarrhea among agro-ecological zones in southwestern Ethiopia. *Int J Hyg Environ Health.* (2020) 224:113447. doi: 10.1016/j.ijheh.2019.113447
9. Pieracci EG, Hall AJ, Gharpure R. Prioritizing zoonotic diseases in Ethiopia using a one health approach. One *Health.* (2016) 2:131–5. doi: 10.1016/j.onehlt.2016.09.001
10. Leta S, Mesele F. Spatial analysis of cattle and shoat population in Ethiopia: growth trend, distribution and market access. *Springerplus.* (2014) 3:310. doi: 10.1186/2193-1801-3-310
11. *US Centers for Disease Control and Prevention (US CDC): One Health. Zoonotic Disease Prioritization: Completed OHZDP Workshops.* Available online at: https://www.cdc.gov/onehealth/what-we-do/zoonotic-disease-prioritization/completed-workshops.html#ethiopia (accessed May 26, 2020).
12. Gourlaouen M, Angot A, Mancin M. An inter-laboratory trial as a tool to increase rabies diagnostic capabilities of Sub-Saharan African Veterinary laboratories. *PLoS Negl Trop Dis.* (2020) 14:e0008010. doi: 10.1371/journal.pntd.0008010
13. Deressa BT, Rauch D, Badra EV. Current status of clinical trials in Ethiopia: how much is done? *Ethiop Med J.* (2018) 56:167–74.
14. Fekadu A, Hailu A, Makonnen E. Short-term impact of celebrating the international clinical trial day: experience from Ethiopia. *Trials.* (2017) 18:332. doi: 10.1186/s13063-017-2081-6
15. Manyazewal T, Woldeamanuel Y, Holland DP, Fekadu A, Blumberg HM, Marconi C. Electronic pillbox-enabled self-administered therapy versus standard directly observed therapy for tuberculosis medication adherence and treatment outcomes in Ethiopia (SELFTB): protocol for a multicenter randomized controlled trial. *Trials.* (2020) 21:383. doi: 10.1186/s13063-020-04324-z
16. *National Veterinary Institute (NVI). Ethiopia.* Available online at *https://www.nvi.com.et/* (accessed May 26, 2020).
17. *National Animal Health Diagnostic and Investigation Center (NAHDIC). Ethiopia.* Available online at: *https://nahdic.gov.et/* (accessed May 26, 2020).
18. *Ethiopian Public Health Institute (EPHI). Ethiopia.* Available online at: *https://www.ephi.gov.et/* (accessed May 26, 2020).
19. *College of Veterinary Medicine and Agriculture. Ethiopia.* Available online at: *http://www.aau.edu.et/cvma/* (accessed May 26, 2020).
20. *Armauer Hansen Research Institute (AHRI). Ethiopia.* Available online at: *https://ahri.gov.et/* (accessed May 26, 2020).
21. *College of Health Sciences, Addis Ababa University. Ethiopia.* Available online at: *http://www.aau.edu.et/chs/* (accessed May 26, 2020).
22. Saldana J. *The Coding Manual for Qualitative Researchers.* 2nd ed. London, SAGE Publication Ltd (2013).
23. Willig C, Stainton-Rogers W. *The SAGE Handbook of Qualitative Research in Psychology.* 2nd ed. London: SAGE (2017). doi: 10.4135/9781526405555
24. Seimenis A, Battelli G. Main challenges in the control of zoonoses and related foodborne diseases in the South Mediterranean and Middle East region. *Vet Ital.* (2018) 54:97–106. doi: 10.12834/VetIt.1340.7765.1
25. Stärk KDC, Morgan D. Emerging zoonoses: Tackling the challenges. *Epidemiol Infect.* (2015) 143:2015–7. doi: 10.1017/S0950268815000680
26. Foof and Agriculture Organization of the United Nations (FAO). *Protecting People and Animals from Disease Threats. USAID; USA.* (2019). Available online at: *http://www.fao.org/3/i8747en/I8747EN.pdf* (accessed May 26, 2020).
27. Elelu N, Aiyedun JO, Mohammed IG. Neglected zoonotic diseases in Nigeria: Role of the public health veterinarian. *Pan Afr Med J.* (2019) 32:36. doi: 10.11604/pamj.2019.32.36.15659
28. Kemunto N, Mogoa E, Osoro E, Bitek A, Njenga MK, Thumbi SM. Zoonotic disease research in East Africa. *BMC Infect Dis.* (2018) 18:545. doi: 10.1186/s12879-018-3443-8

29. Wernli D, Jørgensen PS, Parmley EJ, Troell M, Majowicz S, Harbarth S. Evidence for action: a One Health learning platform on interventions to tackle antimicrobial resistance. *Lancet Infect Dis.* (2020) 20:e307–e311. doi: 10.1016/S1473-3099(20)30392-3
30. Natterson-Horowitz B. A physician's view of One Health: challenges and opportunities. *Vet Sci.* (2015) 2:23–5. doi: 10.3390/vetsci2010023
31. Osterhaus A, Vanlangendonck C, Barbeschi M. Make science evolve into a One Health approach to improve health and security: a white paper. One *Health Outlook.* (2020) 2:6. doi: 10.1186/s42522-019-0009-7
32. Implementing One Health as an integrated approach to health in Rwanda. *BMJ Glob Health.* (2017) 2:e000121. doi: 10.1136/bmjgh-2016-000121
33. Harrison S, Baker MG, Benschop J, Death RG, French NP, Harmsworth G, et al. One Health Aotearoa: a transdisciplinary initiative to improve human, animal and environmental health in New Zealand. One *Health Outlook.* (2020) 2:4. doi: 10.1186/s42522-020-0011-0
34. Gautam A, Kaphle K, Shrestha B, Phuyal S. Susceptibility to SARS, MERS, and COVID-19 from animal health perspective. *Open Vet J.* (2020) 10:164–77. doi: 10.4314/ovj.v10i2.6
35. Mushi V. The holistic way of tackling the COVID-19 pandemic: the one health approach. *Trop Med Health.* (2020) 48:69. doi: 10.1186/s41182-020-00257-0
36. Manyazewal T, Woldeamanuel Y, Blumberg HM, Fekadu A, Marconi VC. The fight to end tuberculosis must not be forgotten in the COVID-19 outbreak. *Nat Med.* (2020) 26:811–2. doi: 10.1038/s41591-020-0917-1
37. Alemayehu C, Mitchell G, Nikles J. Barriers for conducting clinical trials in developing countries- a systematic review. *Int J Equity Health.* (2018) 17:37. doi: 10.1186/s12939-018-0748-6
38. Aguilera B, DeGrazia D, Rid A. Regulating international clinical research: an ethical framework for policy-makers. *BMJ Glob Health.* (2020) 5:e002287. doi: 10.1136/bmjgh-2020-002287
39. Levine AC, Barry MA, Agrawal P, Duber HC, Chang MP, Mackey JM, et al. Global health and emergency care: overcoming clinical research barriers. *Acad Emerg Med.* (2017) 24:484–93. doi: 10.1111/acem.13142
40. Giesen A, Gniel D, Malerczyk C. 30 Years of rabies vaccination with Rabipur: a summary of clinical data and global experience. *Expert Rev Vaccines.* (2015) 14:351–61. doi: 10.1586/14760584.2015.1011134
41. A bivalent anthrax-plague vaccine that can protect against two tier-1 bioterror pathogens, *Bacillus anthracis* and *Yersinia pestis. Front Immunol.* (2017) 8:687. doi: 10.3389/fimmu.2017.00687
42. Dodds WJ, Larson LJ, Christine KL, Schultz RD. Duration of immunity after rabies vaccination in dogs: the rabies challenge fund research study. *Can J Vet Res.* (2020) 84:153–8.
43. Nuismer SL, Bull JJ. Self-disseminating vaccines to suppress zoonoses. *Nat Ecol Evol.* (2020) 4:1168–73. doi: 10.1038/s41559-020-1254-y

19

Trichuris trichiura (Linnaeus, 1771) from Human and Non-Human Primates: Morphology, Biometry, Host Specificity, Molecular Characterization and Phylogeny

Julia Rivero, Cristina Cutillas and Rocío Callejón*

Department of Microbiology and Parasitology, Faculty of Pharmacy, University of Seville, Seville, Spain

***Correspondence:**
Cristina Cutillas
cutillas@us.es

Human trichuriasis is a Neglected Tropical Disease, which affects hundreds of millions of persons worldwide. Several studies have reported that non-human primates (NHP) represent important reservoirs for several known zoonotic infectious diseases. In this context, *Trichuris* infections have been found in a range of NHP species living in natural habitats, including colobus monkeys, macaques, baboons, and chimpanzees. To date, the systematics of the genus *Trichuris* parasitizing humans and NHP is unclear. During many years, *Trichuris trichiura* was considered as the whipworm present in humans and primates. Subsequently, molecular studies suggested that *Trichuris* spp. in humans and NHP represent several species that differ in host specificity. This work examines the current knowledge of *T. trichiura* and its relationship to whipworm parasites in other primate host species. A phylogenetic hypothesis, based on three mitochondrial genes (*cytochrome c oxidase* subunit 1, *cytochrome* b, and large subunit rRNA-encoding gene) and two fragments of ribosomal DNA (Internal Transcribed Spacer 1 and 2), allowed us to define a complex of populations of *T. trichiura* hosting in a large variety of NHP species, in addition to humans. These populations were divided into four phylogenetic groups with a different degree of host specificity. From these data, we carry out a new morphological and biometrical description of the populations of *Trichuris* based on data cited by other authors as well as those provided in this study. The presence of *T. trichiura* is analyzed in several NHP species in captivity from different garden zoos as possible reservoir of trichuriasis for humans. This study contributes to clarify questions that lead to identification of new taxa and will determine parasite transmission routes between these primates, allowing the implementation of appropriate control and prevention measures.

Keywords: *Trichuris trichiura*, non-human primates, ribosomal DNA, mitochondrial DNA, zoonoses

INTRODUCTION

Worldwide, ~1.5 billion people, nearly 24% of the world's population, are infected with soil-borne helminths. Soil-borne helminthiasis is widely distributed in tropical and subtropical areas, especially in sub-Saharan Africa, The Americas, China, and East Asia. More than 267 million preschoolers and more than 568 million school-age children live in areas with severe transmission of these parasites and need treatment and preventive interventions. The main species of soil-borne helminths that infect humans are *Ascaris lumbricoides* (roundworm), *Trichuris trichiura* (whipworm), and *Necator americanus* and *Ancylostoma duodenale* (hookworms) (1).

T. trichiura, is the etiological agent of the parasitic disease known as "trichuriasis," which is considered as a Neglected Tropical Disease. *T. trichiura* is the second most common helminth in humans, and Trichuriasis has a worldwide geographical distribution. The prevalence is higher in places with warm and humid weather, where there is a lack of basic sanitation services. Between 30 and 80% of cases are recorded in children, who suffer the greatest parasitic burden and those with the most significant symptoms (2). Transmission of this parasite occurs after ingestion of embryonated eggs. These eggs can enter new hosts through contaminated hands, food, soil, and water. Then these hatch in the intestine, where L1 larvae are released. Larvae penetrate the epithelial layer of the large intestine and grow to adult stage. After mating, the non-embryonated eggs are released from the females and again reach the environment through the host's feces.

Up to date, whipworms isolated from humans and other primates have traditionally been regarded as *T. trichiura* (3–5), while those recovered from pigs and wild boars are known as *Trichuris suis* (6, 7). It is well-known that differentiation between closely related species of *Trichuris* is very difficult due to the phenotypic plasticity of the organisms themselves; host-induced variation, paucity of morphological features, and overlapping morphological characteristics that occur among species (8–11). Thus, many studies on *Trichuris* have focused on the morphological and molecular differentiation of *T. trichiura* and *T. suis*, which are molecularly different but morphologically similar (7, 12–14).

On the other hand, the relationship between *Trichuris* from humans and non-human primates (NHP) in terms of genetic and evolutionary aspects is poorly understood. In recent years, some publications addressed the question of whether *Trichuris* species are shared between humans and NHP or whether there are different species. The genus *Trichuris* is likely a candidate to harbor cryptic species as it has a wide geographical distribution and infects several host species (15). As revealed by recent studies, there is more than one taxon capable of infecting humans and other primates, including individuals in captivity, suggesting that *T. trichiura* should be considered a complex species that includes different cryptic units (16, 17). In addition, based on morpho-biometric and molecular parameters, new species of *Trichuris* have been described in primates, such as *Trichuris rhinopiptheroxella* (18) that was found in the golden snub-nosed monkey (*Rhinopithecus roxellana*), *Trichuris colobae* from *Colobus guereza kikuyuensis* (19), and *Trichuris ursinus* from *Papio ursinus* (20). Therefore, these studies confirmed that *T. trichiura* is not the only whipworm found in primates.

Currently, the systematics of the genus *Trichuris* shows significant gaps. This is due to two main reasons: (i) the lack of comparative morpho-biometric data through the use of multiple parameters and statistical tests applied to the taxonomic study of these species and (ii) the paucity of published research on the genetics of the different *Trichuris* species in humans, NHP, and pigs. Nowadays, researchers have not yet managed to finally establish the degree of divergence between the different genetic lineages that appear to exist in *Trichuris* species parasitizing these hosts.

In this paper, we carried out an update of the morphological and biometric characteristics of *T. trichiura* isolated from human and NHP. Besides, the molecular phylogenetic relationships between these populations are analyzed based on molecular data (mitochondrial and nuclear markers). Furthermore, some phylogenetic hypotheses were inferred for *Trichuris* spp. to shed light on the degree of divergence between different genetic lineages. In addition, the presence of *T. trichiura* was analyzed in several NHP species in captivity from different garden zoos as possible reservoir of trichuriasis for humans.

MATERIALS AND METHODS

Ethics Statement

This study does not require approval by an ethics committee. *Macaca sylvanus* and *C. g. kikuyensis*, from which *Trichuris* specimens were collected from their caeca *postmortem*, died of natural death. The specimens were handled and housed in a zoo in strict accordance with good animal practices. The other specimens and eggs of *Trichuris* sp. were recovered from the feces after routine anthelmintic treatment.

Isolation of Material

In this study, we sampled *Trichuris*'s adults and eggs of a total of five NHP host species, including the Barbary macaque (*M. sylvanus*), vervet monkey (*Chlorocebus aethiops*), patas monkey (*Erythrocebus patas*), Guinea baboon (*Papio papio*), and black and white colobus (*C. g. kikuyuensis*) from the Zoo Castellar (Cádiz, Spain), Selwo Aventura (Málaga, Spain), Zoo Barcelona (Barcelona, Spain), Parque de la Naturaleza de Cabárceno (Cantabria, Spain), and Bioparc Fuengirola (Málaga, Spain), respectively (**Table 1**).

Only three adult whipworm specimens (two females and one male) were collected from Guinea baboon, sixty-five adults (32 females and 33 males) from a male Barbary macaque (17, 21) and five adults from a *C. g. kikuyuensis*. Adult's worms were washed separately in saline solution (0.9% w/v), then frozen at −20°C until posterior studies. Whipworm's eggs were isolated from feces of all NHP species. The sequences successfully obtained of different molecular markers are summarized in the **Table 1**.

The fecal eggs were concentrated using a Sheather's sugar solution (22) and then embryonated at 32°C for 3–4 weeks added with potassium dichromate 0.2% w/v solution to give humidity to the medium and prevent fungal and bacterial growth (23). Subsequently, the worms were measured and genomic DNA, from both worms and eggs, was extracted.

Morphological Study

Three adult whipworms from Guinea baboon were identified according to previous studies (7, 19, 20). We carried out morphological studies as described Oliveros et al. (24) and Skrjabin et al. (25). *Trichuris* specimens were measured according

TABLE 1 | DNA obtained from the samples.

Zoo gardens	Hosts species		N° adults/eggs analyzed	*Trichuris* species	Haplotypes obtained					Number of base pairs/G+C				
	Scientific name	Common name			*cox*1	*cob*	*rrn*L	ITS1	ITS2	*cox*1	*cob*	*rrn*L	ITS1	ITS2
Zoo Castellar	*Macaca sylvanus*	Barbary macaque	43 adults	*T. trichiura*	4 H (*)	5 H (*)	5 H	6 H	8 H (*)	370/38–39.2	520/30.2–31	386–387/29.7–31.3	586–597/63.1–64.3	514–587/63.7–65.2
Selwo Aventura	*Chlorocebus aethiops*	Vervet monkey	5 sample batches of eggs (40–65 eggs/batch)		1 H	1 H	-	2 H	5 H	370/38.6	522/30.1	–	594–601/61.4–62.3	556–580/62.1–64.1
Zoo Barcelona	*Erythrocebus patas*	Patas monkey	1 sample batch of eggs		1 H	1 H	-	1 H	1 H	332/38	520/29.6	–	593/64.1	436/65.6
Parque de la Naturaleza de Cabarceno	*Papio papio*	Guinea baboon	3 adults and 9 sample batches of eggs (40–200 eggs/batch)		1 H	4 H	1 H	2 H	5 H	370/38.6	520/29.6–30.8	387/30	588–607/61.4–64.3	602–611/62.8–63.2
Bioparc Fuengirola	*Colobus guereza kikuyuensis*	Black and white colobus	5 adults	*T. colobae*	-	-	5 H	-	-	-	-	395/30.1–30.9	-	-

H, haplotype; (*) analyzed by Rivero et al. (17).

to parameters reported by Spakulová and Lýsek (26), Suriano and Navone (27), and Robles et al. (28), and a comparative study was carried out with *T. trichiura*'s specimens previously analyzed biometrically and molecularly (7, 14, 17, 21).

Molecular Study

PCR and Sequencing of Specimens

Genomic DNA from adult worms and a pack of 45–200 isolated eggs were extracted using DNeasy Blood and Tissue Kit (Qiagen) according to the manufacturer's protocol. Quality of extractions was assessed using 0.8% agarose gel electrophoresis infused with SYBR® Safe DNA gel stain.

All molecular markers sequenced in the present study [*cox*1, *cob* and *rrn*L mitochondrial DNA (mtDNA) and ITS1 and ITS2 ribosomal DNA (rDNA)] were amplified using the polymerase chain reaction (PCR) by a thermal cycler (Eppendorf AG; Hamburg, Germany). PCR mix, PCR conditions, and PCR primers are summarized in the **Supplementary Table 1**.

The PCR products were checked on SYBR® Safe stained with 2% w/v Tris-borate–EDTA (TBE) agarose gels. Bands were eluted and purified from the agarose gel using the QWizard SV Gel and PCR Clean-Up System Kit (Promega, Madison, WI, U.S.A.). Once purified and concentrated, the products were sequenced by Stab Vida (Lisbon, Portugal).

Phylogenetic Analysis

To assess the similarity among all marker sequences of *Trichuris* sp. obtained in the present study and other *Trichuris* species, the number of nucleotide differences per sequence was analyzed using Compute Pairwise Distances based on the number of differences method of MEGA v7.0 (29).

To obtain a nucleotide sequence alignment file, the MUSCLE alignment method was used in MEGA v7.0 (29). Additional sequences from the National Center for Biotechnology Information (NCBI) GenBank® database were incorporated into the alignments (**Supplementary Table 2**).

Assessment of nucleotide substitution saturation, an indicator of whether the genetic marker is useful, was performed using DAMBE v5.3.32 (30, 31). Saturation was based on the values of Iss (index of substitution saturation) and Iss.c (critical Iss value), where Iss < Iss.c indicated that the genetic marker was not saturated and vice versa. Haplotype diversity (h) and nucleotide diversity (π) were calculated using DnaSP v6.12.03 (32).

All phylogenetic trees were inferred based on nucleotide data and obtained by two methods: Maximum Likelihood (ML) and Bayesian Inference (BI). PHYML package was used to generate ML trees (33), and MrBayes v3.2.6 to generate BI (34). jModelTest was employed to resolve the best-fit substitution model for the parasite data (35). Models of evolution were selected for subsequent analysis according to the Akaike Information Criterion (36). To examine the dataset containing the concatenation of four markers used (ITS1, ITS2, *cox*1, and *cob*), analyses based on BI were partitioned by gene and models for individual genes within partitions were those selected by jModelTest. For ML inference, best-fit nucleotide substitution models included the general time-reversible (GTR) model with gamma-distributed rate variation (G) and a proportion of invariable sites (I), GTR + G (ITS1 and ITS2), GTR + I + G (*cox1*), GTR + I + G (*cob*), and GTR + G (*rrnL*). Support for the topology was examined using bootstrapping (heuristic option) (37) over 1,000 replications to assess the relative reliability of clades. The commands used in MrBayes for BI were *nst* = 6 with gamma rates (ITS1, ITS2, and *rrnL*), *nst* = 6 with invgamma rates (*cox1* and *cob*), and *nst* = mixed (concatenated phylogenetic trees). The standard deviation of split frequencies was used to determine whether the number of generations completed was sufficient; the chain was sampled every 500 generations, and each dataset was run for 10 million generations. Trees from the first million generations were discarded based on an assessment of convergence. Burn-in was determined empirically by examination of the log likelihood values of the chains. The Bayesian Posterior Probabilities (BPP) comprise the percentage converted.

RESULTS

Molecular Analysis

Annotation and Features of Ribosomal and Mitochondrial Genomes

The successfully sequenced specimens, the length of the different sequences, the content of G + C%, and haplotypes of ribosomal and mitochondrial markers analyzed at the present study are shown in **Table 1**. Different repetitive nucleotide sequences, termed ≪ microsatellites ≫, were found in the ITS2 sequences of *Trichuris* sp. from human and different NHP. Thus, Poly (GCA), Poly (CGA), and Poly (GCG) were observed in positions 280, 302, and 344, respectively. Furthermore, Poly (GCA) and Poly (GGC) were found in the ITS1 sequences in positions 77 and 203, respectively. Also, a common area to all species of *Trichuris* was observed in positions 280 (GATCTGGGTGT) and 286 (GCCGCCGGTT) in this ITS1 sequence.

Nucleotide sequence data reported in this study were deposited at the GenBank™, EMBL, and DDBJ databases, and the accession numbers are available in **Supplementary Table 2**.

Phylogenetic Analysis

All phylogenetic trees based on ribosomal and mitochondrial markers (partitioned and concatenated) confirmed the existence of two main clades: clade 1: "*Trichuris suis*" and clade 2: "*Trichuris trichiura*" (**Figures 1–3** and **Supplementary Figures 1–3**).

The alignment of 46 ITS1 and 79 ITS2 rDNA sequences of *Trichuris* species yielded a dataset of 876 and 863 characters, respectively. Based on ITS1 and ITS2 sequences, the concatenated phylogenetic tree revealed the existence of two highly supported phylogenetic groups within clade 2 "*T. trichiura*": One group corresponded to *T. trichiura* lineage (100% ML and 100% BPP) (**Supplementary Table 3**) clustering *Trichuris* sp. from different hosts and geographical regions in six subclades (100% ML and 100% BPP) that included *Trichuris* sp. from *Trachypithecus francoisi* (**Figure 1**). The other 5 subclades (except *Trichuris* sp. from *T. francoisi*) showed a high homology each other, ranging 94.65–99.65% (**Supplementary Table 4**).

The phylogeny inferred on mitochondrial datasets (partitioned and concatenated) revealed similar topologies (**Figure 2** and **Supplementary Figures 1–3**). Thus, four main clades were observed in "*T. trichiura* lineage" where *Trichuris* sp. from *P. papio*, *C. aethiops*, and *E. patas* clustered together in the subclade named 2c with *T. trichiura* from *Homo sapiens* from Uganda and *Trichuris* sp. from other hosts from Africa and Europe (**Figure 2** and **Supplementary Figures 1, 2**).

The multiple alignments of 48 *cox1* nucleotide sequences (including outgroups) yielded a dataset of 296 characters. The phylogenetic tree based on *cox1* showed *Trichuris* from *E. patas*, *C. aethiops*, and *P. papio* clustering in subclade 2c (European and African origin) and related with *Macaca fuscata* (subclade 2d). This marker did not resolve subclade 2a (Asian and USA origin) appearing in polytomy (**Supplementary Figure 1** and **Supplementary Table 3**).

The multiple alignments of 47 *cob* nucleotide sequences (including outgroups) yielded a dataset of 444 characters. The phylogenetic tree based on *cob* was in congruence with *rrnL* phylogenetic inferences of *T. trichiura* lineage. Nevertheless, the sister relationship between subclades 2a, 2b, and 2d was not supported (**Supplementary Figure 2** and **Supplementary Table 3**).

The *rrnL* dataset included 358 aligned positions and 76 taxa, including outgroups. ML and BI methods showed congruence between each other revealing two main clades ("*T. suis* lineage" and "*T. trichiura* lineage") and respect to the sister-group relationships between *Trichuris* spp. from NHP, humans and pigs (**Supplementary Figure 3** and **Supplementary Table 3**). Within clade 2 "*T. trichiura* lineage," phylogenetic trees confirmed the existence of four different subclades highly supported clustering subclade 2b: *T. trichiura* from *H. sapiens* from China and *Papio anubis* from the USA and subclade 2a including the minority haplotype of *T. trichiura* from *M. sylvanus* from Spain; subclade 2c: *T. trichiura* from *P. papio*, *Chlorocebus sabaeus* and *M. sylvanus* from Spain, *H. sapiens* from Uganda, *Papio hamadryas* from Europe, and two haplotypes of *Trichuris* sp. from *M. fuscata* from Europe; and subclade 2d: *T. trichiura* from *M. fuscata* from Europe (**Supplementary Figure 3**). Curiously, the minority haplotype of *M. sylvanus* (subclade 2a) and *M. fuscata* (subclade 2d) (European origin) appeared related with those from Asia and USA (subclade 2b) (**Supplementary Figure 3** and **Supplementary Table 3**). In addition, a sister relationship between *T. trichiura* and *Trichuris* sp. from *T. francoisi* was observed, both species within "*T. trichiura* lineage" (clade 2).

The concatenated dataset of mitochondrial gene (*cox1* and *cob*) sequences (**Figure 2**) revealed the subclade 2c as the main one clustering the majority of *T. trichiura* parasitizing African humans and different NHP from Africa and Europe, showing a sister relationship between 2c and 2d and besides between 2a and 2b (Asian and USA origins) (**Figure 2**).

The concatenated dataset of ribosomal (ITS1 and ITS2) and mitochondrial (*cox1* and *cob*) gene sequences included 2,479 aligned sites and only 13 taxa, since only we could concatenate sequences of the same individual. Phylogenetic analyses of this dataset yielded a tree with branches strongly supported. Thus, the *T. trichiura* population was separated in only three different

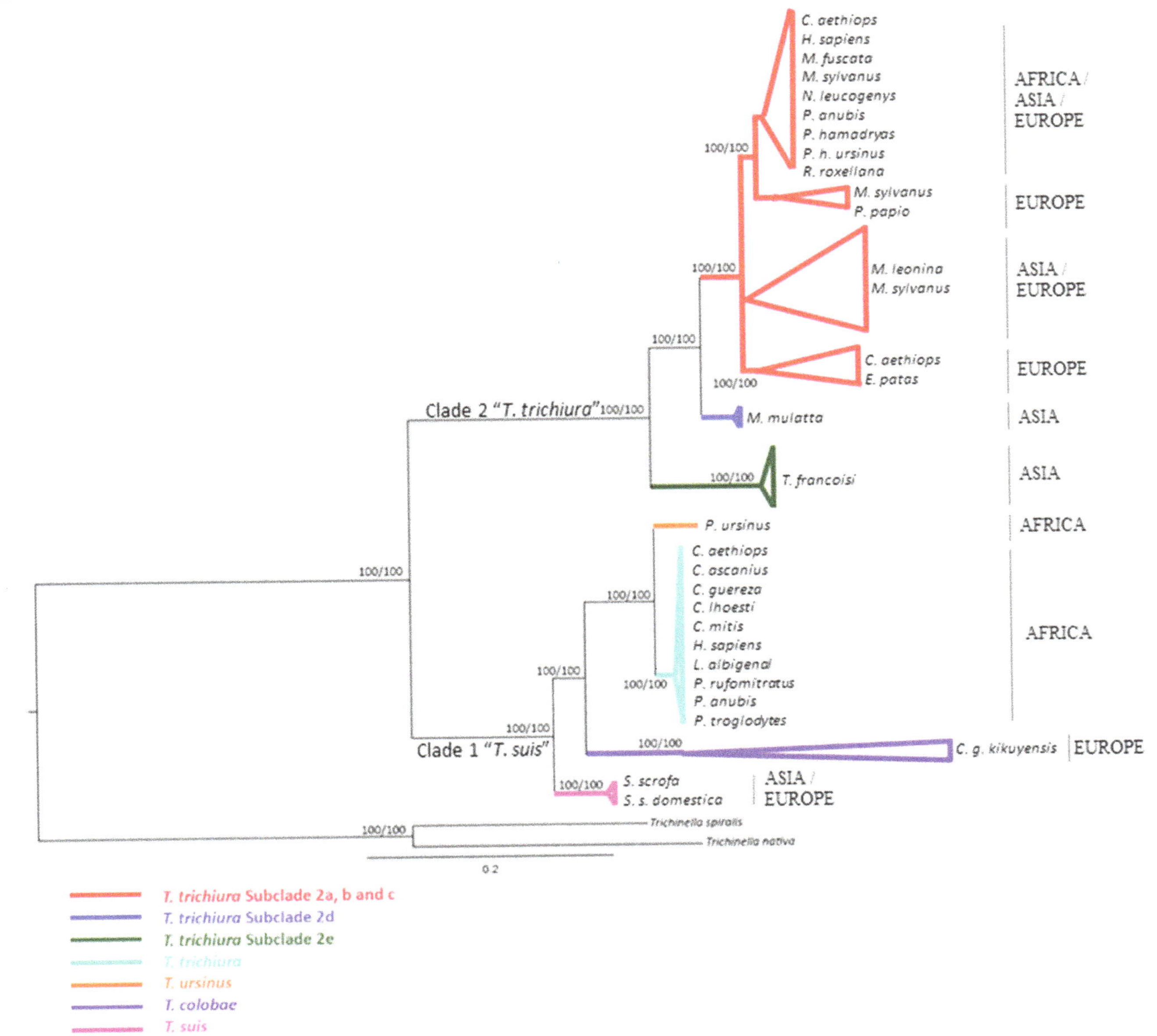

FIGURE 1 | Phylogenetic tree of *Trichuris* species based on combined analysis of ribosomal DNA (ITS1 and ITS2) inferred using Bayesian Inference. Maximum Likelihood bootstrap values of clades are listed first, followed by Bayesian Posterior Probabilities, respectively, for clade frequencies exceeding 60%.

subclades, the subclade 2d not being represented due to the absence of sequences in all the markers. Subclade 2c was the most representative subclade including populations from a high variety of host species (**Figure 3** and **Supplementary Table 3**).

The phylogenetic inferences revealed that the populations of *Trichuris* from *P. papio*, *C. aethiops*, and *E. patas* analyzed in the present study clustered mainly in the subclade of *T. trichiura* (subclade 2c).

Comparative Sequence Analysis

In order to analyze the intraspecific and interspecific similarity in *T. trichiura* and between *T. trichiura* and *Trichuris* spp. parasitizing NHP as well as *T. suis*, we carried out a comparative study considering the different clades and subclades previously described for *Trichuris* spp. hosting humans, NHP, and swine (**Supplementary Tables 4–7**).

Thus, by examining ITS1 and ITS2 sequences, specimens obtained from *P. papio*, *C. aethiops*, and *E. patas* from Spain revealed a high similarity with populations of *T. trichiura* corresponding to subclades 2a, 2b, and 2c and subclade *Macaca mulatta* from different geographical origins (94.65 to 100%) (**Supplementary Table 4**). Further, the similarity was lower when clade 2 (*T. trichiura* lineage) and clade 1 (*T. suis*) were compared (90.62–92.23%).

Mitochondrial sequences (*cox*1 and *cob*) from *T. trichiura* from *P. papio*, *C. aethiops*, and *E. patas* from Spain showed the

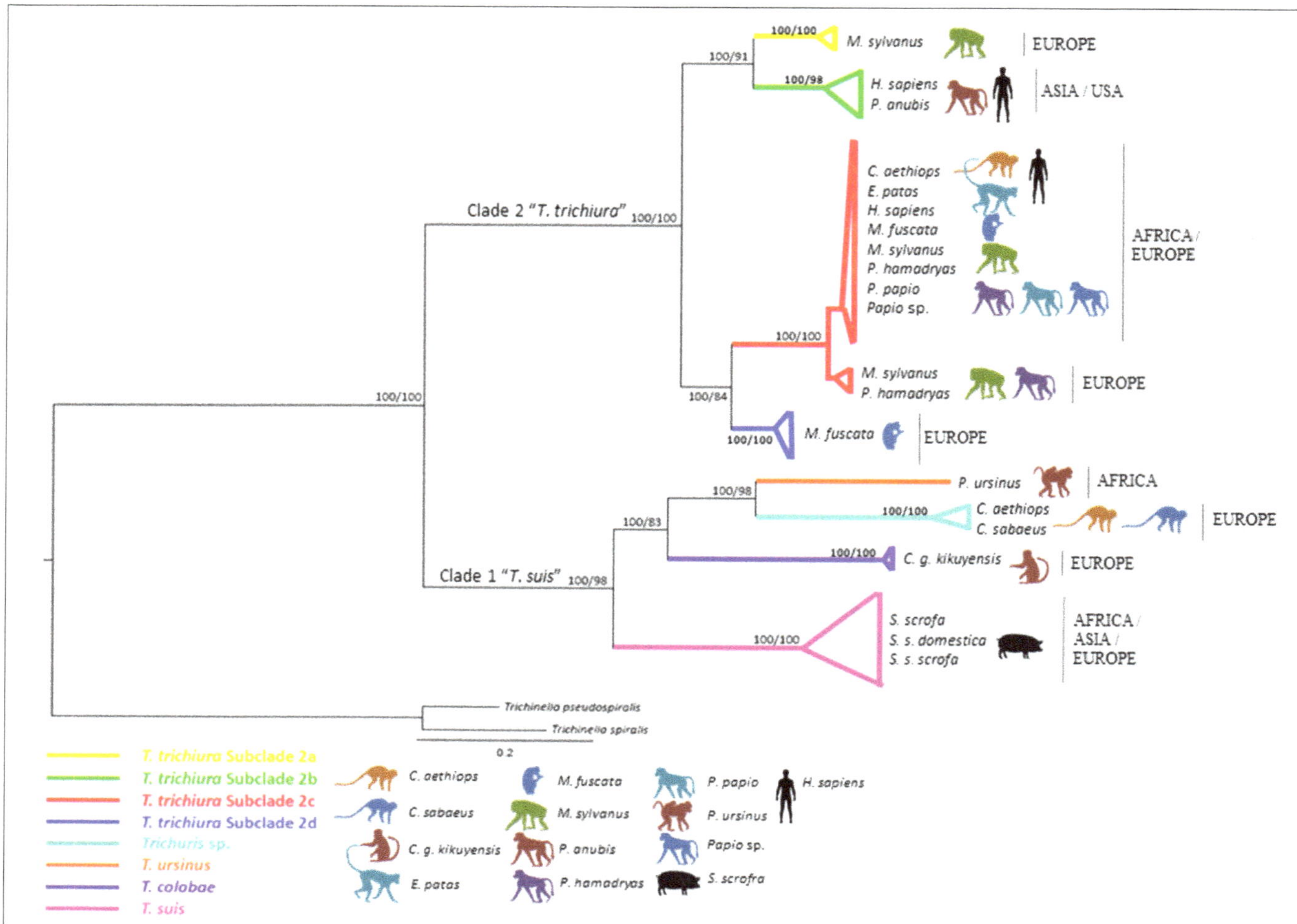

FIGURE 2 | Phylogenetic tree of *Trichuris* species based on combined analysis of mitochondrial DNA (*cox*1 and *cob*) inferred using Bayesian Inference. Maximum Likelihood bootstrap values of clades are listed first, followed by Bayesian Posterior Probabilities, respectively, for clade frequencies exceeding 60%.

highest intraspecific similarity within subclade 2c (97.3 to 100% and 92.12 to 100%, respectively) (**Supplementary Tables 5, 6**). For *rrn*L sequences, similar results were observed for *T. trichiura* from *M. sylvanus* and *P. papio* (97.77–100%). However, based on three mitochondrial markers, *T. trichiura* from *M. sylvanus* showed two different lineages corresponding to subclades 2a and 2c (**Supplementary Table 7**). Based on three mitochondrial markers, the similarity between clade 2 and *T. suis* ranged from 68.47 to 82.68%, values lower than those shown within clade 2.

Analysis of genetic diversity for clade 2 based on ITS and mitochondrial sequences revealed a haplotype diversity of 1.0 and 0.95–0.93, respectively (**Table 2**). In addition, nucleotide diversity based on ITS and *rrn*L sequences was 0.05; nevertheless, mitochondrial genes (*cox*1 and *cob* genes) revealed a higher nucleotide diversity (0.09–0.11) with the maximum values for *cox*1 (0.11) (**Table 2**). Within clade 2 (subclades 2a, 2b, 2c, and 2d), haplotype diversity of mitochondrial genes ranged 0.71–1.0 for *cox*1, 0.67–1.0 for *cob*, and 0.88–1.0 for *rrn*L with the maximum values for subclade 2a. Nucleotide diversity of mitochondrial genes ranged 0.01–0.04 for *cox*1 and *cob* with the maximum values for subclade 2b, and the value for *rrn*L was 0.01 (**Table 2**).

The analysis of nucleotide substitution saturation based on nuclear markers showed Iss > Iss.c ($P < 0.005$), indicating that ITS regions were saturated. Nevertheless, mitochondrial genes (*cox*1, *cob*, and *rrn*L) were not saturated (Iss < Iss.c, $P < 0.005$). Genetic diversity measures for all markers are summarized in **Table 2**.

Update Morphological Description of *T. trichiura* (Linnaeus, 1771)

Taxonomic summary

- Class Enoplea (Order Trichocephalida) (12, 38).
- Host: *H. sapiens* (14), *Pan troglodytes* (7), *M. sylvanus* (17, 21), *P. papio* (present study).

General: This is a parasite with a filiform anterior part and a broad and handle-like posterior part. The thin anterior portion of the parasite displays 2 types of cuticle patterns. One side is distinctly striated with transverse grooves and the other side

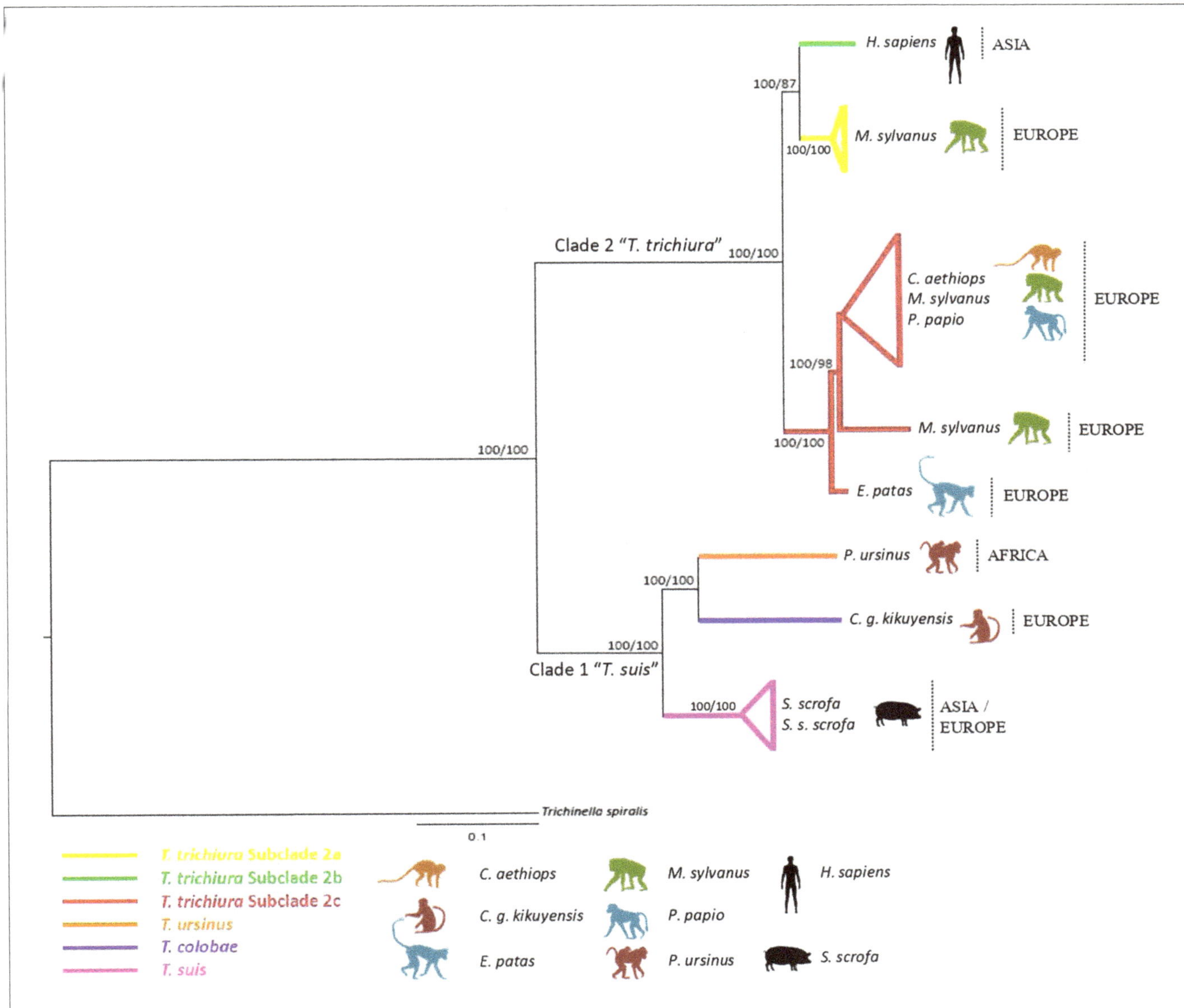

FIGURE 3 | Phylogenetic tree of *Trichuris* species based on combined analysis of mitochondrial DNA (*cox*1, *cob*) and nuclear ribosomal DNA (ITS1 and ITS2) inferred using Bayesian Inference. Maximum Likelihood bootstrap values of clades are listed first, followed by Bayesian Posterior Probabilities, respectively, for clade frequencies exceeding 60%.

in a finely tuberculate band under higher magnification reveals small circular elevated bodies, which are evenly distributed (**Figure 4A**). The ventral side of the anterior part of the body is slightly tapered toward the cephalic end which presents a broad longitudinal elongated "bacillary band" showing typical cuticle inflations (**Figure 4B**). The mouth is surrounded by a group of cephalic papillae arranged in two circles (an inner circle and a lateral circle) with a conspicuous organ, the stylet (**Figure 4C**), protruding from the middle portion of the mouth cavity. Adults present a moniliform esophagus constituted with a short muscular zone and a long stichosome with 1 row of stichocytes (**Figure 4D**), and 1 pair of conspicuous cells at esophagus-intestinal junction level (**Figures 4D, 5A,B**). The site where the esophagus transforms into the intestine corresponds to the place of transition of the thin anterior part into the thick posterior and shows typical glandular cells at this point (**Figures 4D, 5A,B**).

Male: The body is 25–49.3 mm long. The ratio between anterior and posterior body length is 2.6–4:1. The thin anterior part is 1:1.4–1.7 of the entire length of the body. The length of the esophagus is 18–28.9 mm. The width of the body in the esophageal end is 0.15–0.49 mm, and the maximum width (in the posterior part of the body) is 0.39–0.74 mm (**Table 3**). Posterior end of the body ventrally incurved (**Figures 4E–G**).

The genital apparatus of the male is a long tube whose sections differ from each other in structure bearing different functions (**Figure 5A**). The first section of the genital apparatus is the testis, which is very long and strongly convoluted, beginning

TABLE 2 | Summary of genetic measures for *cox*1, *cob*, *rrn*L genes, and ITS region sequences.

	Subclade 2a			**Subclade 2b**			**Subclade 2c**			**Subclade 2d**			***Trichuris trichiura* complex (Clade 2)**			
	***cox*1**	***cob***	***rrn*L**	***cox*1**	***cob***	***rrn*L**	***cox*1**	***cob***	***rrn*L**	***cox*1**	***cob***	***rrn*L**	***cox*1**	***cob***	***rrn*L**	**ITS**
Number of haplotypes/number of sequences	3/3	3/3	2/2	3/4	2/3	10/13	5/13	14/18	15/29	6/6	4/5	5/6	17/26	23/29	31/50	21/22
Haplotype diversity	1.0	1.0	1.0	0.83	0.67	0.95	0.71	0.95	0.88	1.0	0.90	0.93	0.93	0.98	0.95	1.0
Nucleotide diversity	0.02	0.02	0.01	0.04	0.04	0.01	0.01	0.02	0.01	0.02	0.01	0.01	0.11	0.09	0.05	0.05
Nucleotide saturation*	-	-	-	-	-	-	-	-	-	-	-	-	No	No	No	Yes

**Substitution saturation test for partial cox1, cob, rrnL genes, and ITS sequences of Trichuris trichiura (Clade 2). "Yes" indicates that most of this sites have already been changed before (Iss>Iss.c), indicating nucleotide saturation.*

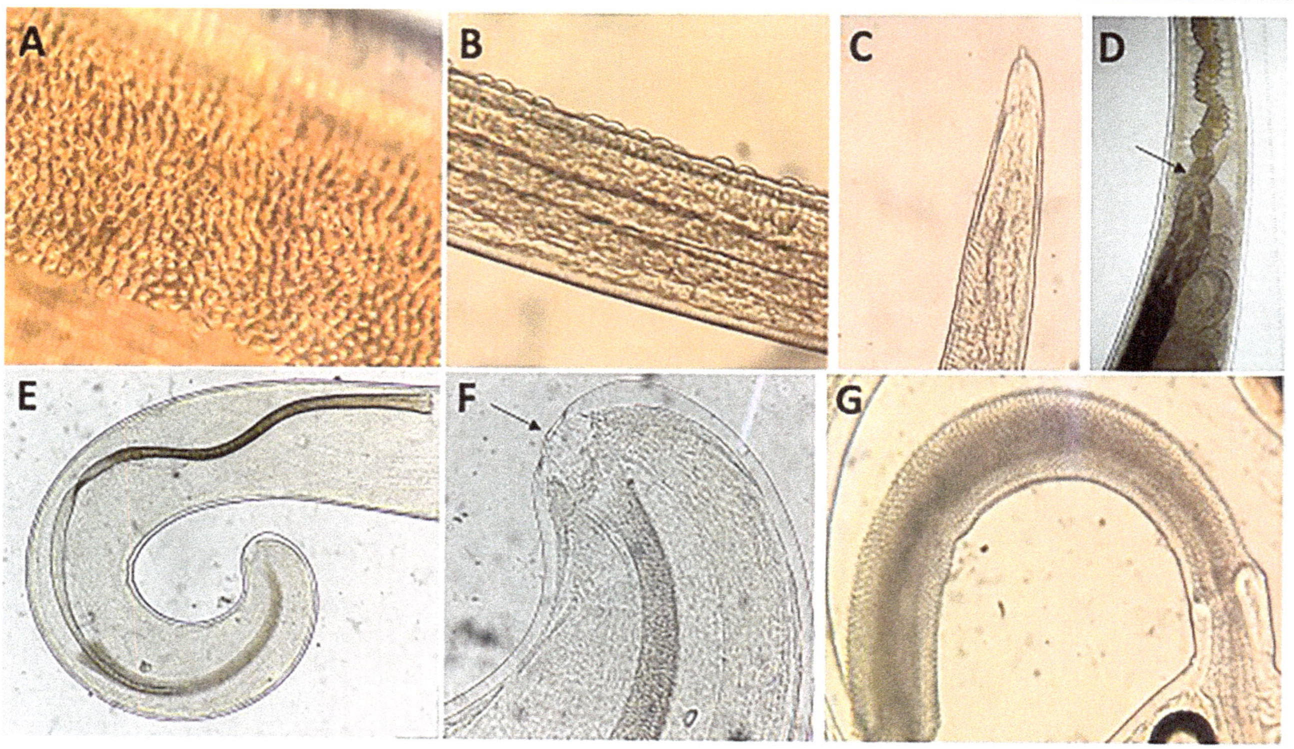

FIGURE 4 | Morphology of males of *T. trichiura*. **(A)** Tuberculate band. **(B)** Bacillary band showing typical cuticular inflations. **(C)** The mouth with the stylet. **(D)** Stichosome with 1 row of stichocytes and 1 pair of conspicuous cells at esophagus–intestinal junction level (arrowed). **(E)** Spicule. **(F)** Papillae pericloacal. **(G)** Spicule sheath.

in the posterior part of the male body, directed anteriorly, and lying along the long axis of the body terminating at a short distance from the transition of the esophagus into the intestine (**Figure 5A**). The testis ends near the union of the ejaculator conduct and intestine. The testis is followed by the vas deferens which at first runs somewhat anteriorly along the intestine, and then, at the level of the esophageal end and somewhat short of it, describes a convolution, turns backward, and terminates in a small constriction, connecting it with the following section of the genital apparatus, the seminal vesicle. The seminal vesicle runs parallel to the intestine but does not describe sharp convolutions and via a narrow tube with thick muscular walls joins the ejaculatory duct, which is 1.07–2.34 mm long (**Figure 5A**). The ejaculatory duct joins the intestine to form the cloaca, which opens at the posterior end of the male body. The cloaca with anus subterminal and one pair of paracloacal papilla not ornamented (**Figure 4F**) was observed when the spicule sheath was invaginated. No cluster of papillae was observed. The proximal cloacal tube is wide and continued with the distal cloacal tube (1.10–2.75 mm) that contains the spicule which projects into the anterior portion of the body in a spicule tube (**Figure 5A**). There is only one spicule, which is elongated with a pointed tip. This spicule presents two chitinized extreme zones and a light central part and is 1.61–3.81 mm long

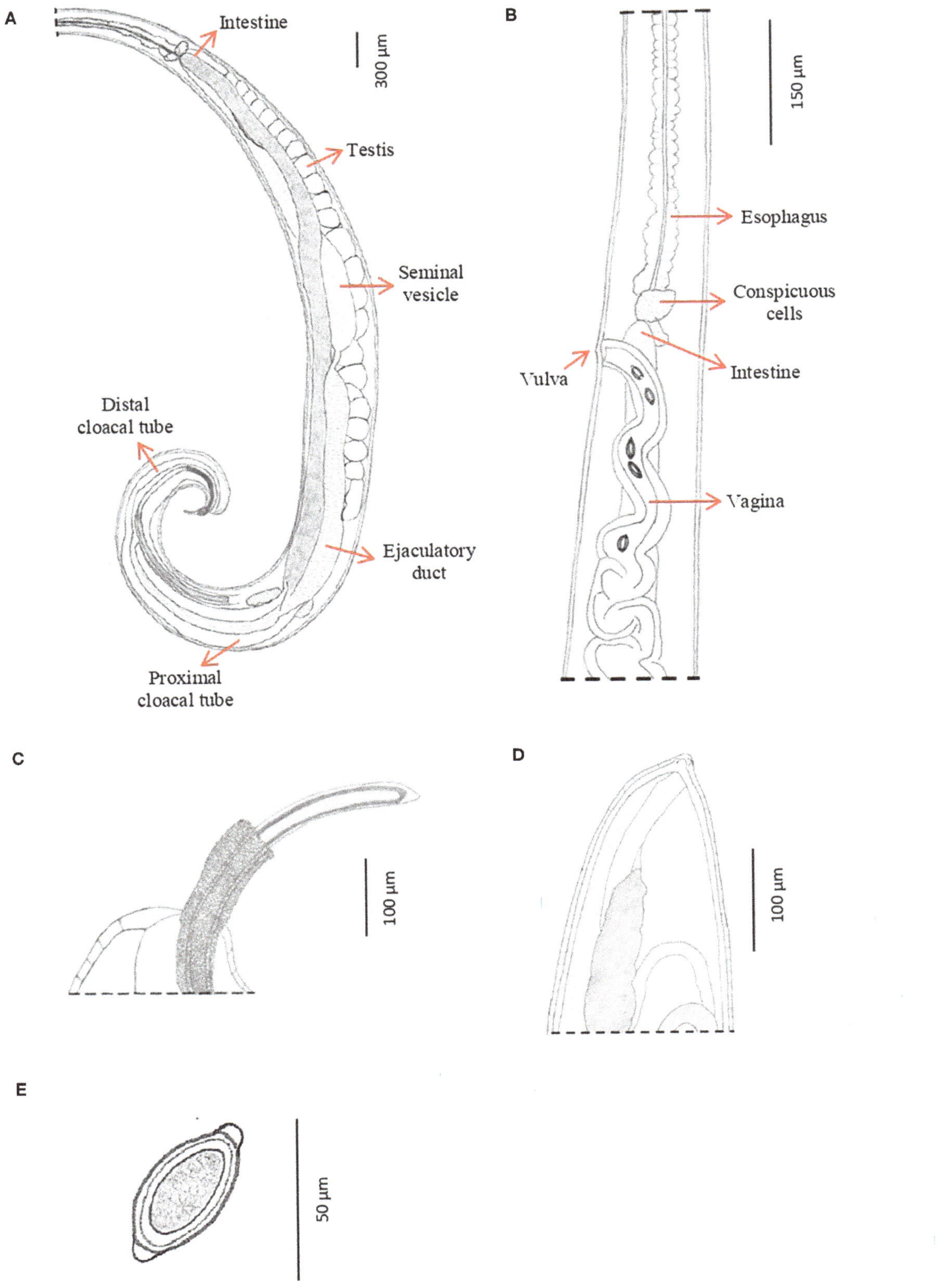

FIGURE 5 | Drawings of *T. trichiura* from *P. papio*. **(A)** Male, posterior end, spiny spicule sheath, spicule, spicule tube and proximal and distal cloacal tube, lateral view. **(B)** Female, esophagus–intestine junction, vulva and vagina, lateral view. **(C)** Male, detail of the posterior end, lateral view. **(D)** Female, posterior end, lateral view. **(E)** Eggs.

TABLE 3 | Biometrical data of males of *T. trichiura*.

	T. trichiura **(Present study, updated)**	***T. trichiura*** **from** ***P. troglodytes*** **[Cutillas et al., (7)]**				***T. trichiura*** **from** ***Homo sapiens*** **[Nissen et al. (14)]**			***T. trichiura*** **from** ***M. sylvanus*** **[García-Sánchez et al. (21)]**				***T. trichiura*** **from** ***P. papio*** **(Present study)**		
	MIN-MAX	**MIN**	**MAX**	**X**	**δ**	**MIN**	**MAX**	**X**	**MIN**	**MAX**	**X**	**δ**	**MIN-MAX**	**X**	**δ**
M1	25.0–49.3	32.0	36.0	33.5	0.19	37.2	49.3	43.9	30.0	39.0	34.5	0.25	25.0	25.0	-
M2	18.0–28.9	18.0	23.0	20.5	0.21	20.9	28.9	25.6	19.0	28.0	21.9	0.27	18.0	18.0	-
LP	7.0–20.4	12.0	14.0	13.0	0.05	14.9	20.4	18.4	8.0	17.0	1.25	0.22	7.0	7.0	-
M3	0.09–0.31	0.09	0.31	0.15	0.02	0.10	0.20	0.15	0.12	0.18	0.14	0.02	0.12	0.12	-
M4	0.39–0.74	0.39	0.60	0.50	0.08	0.50	0.70	0.63	0.49	0.74	0.61	0.07	0.56	0.56	-
M5	0.15–0.49	0.15	0.24	0.2	0.04				0.25	0.49	0.37	0.06	0.35	0.35	-
M6	0.33–0.64	-	-	-	-				0.33	0.64	0.49	0.09	0.50	0.50	-
M7	1.10–1.62	-	-	-	-				1.10	1.57	1.33	0.14	1.62	1.62	-
M8	1.61–3.81	1.61	2.22	1.90	0.23	2.88	3.81	3.19	2.23	3.23	2.65	0.23	2.86	2.86	-
M9	0.22–1.23	0.22	0.22	0.22	-				0.53	1.23	0.93	0.20	0.63	0.63	-
M10	0.01–0.08	0.01	0.06	0.02	0.02				0.04	0.08	0.06	0.01	0.07	0.07	-
M11	0.04–0.09	0.05	0.09	0.07	0.02				0.04	0.08	0.06	0.01	0.05	0.05	-
M12	0.06–0.11	0.09	0.11	0.09	0.01				0.06	0.09	0.07	0.01	0.07	0.07	-
M13	1.79–5.19	1.79	1.95	1.88	0.07				2.90	5.19	4.06	0.58	3.31	3.31	-
M14	1.07–2.34	1.07	1.07	-	-				1.32	2.34	1.97	0.29	1.74	1.74	-
M15	1.10–2.75	1.10	1.10	-	-				1.55	2.75	2.20	0.36	1.35	1.35	-

M1, total body length of adult worm; M2, length of the esophageal region of the body; LP, length of the posterior region of the body; M3, width of the esophageal region of the body; M4, maximum width of the posterior region of the body (thickness); M5, body width in the place of the junction of the esophagus and the intestine; M6, Distance from the head end to beginning of bacillary stripes; M7, length of bacillary stripes; M8, length of spicule; M9, maximum length of spicule sheath; M10, width of the proximal end of the spicule; M11, width of the spicule sheath at the tail end of the body; M12, maximum width of the spicule sheath; M13, distance between the posterior part of the testis and tail end of body; M14, length of ejaculatory duct; M15, length of distal cloacal tube. Б, arithmetic mean. σ, standard deviation.

(**Figures 4E, 5A**). The spicule is surrounded by a peculiar spicule sheath (0.22–1.23 mm long), which may protrude externally together with the spicule (**Figure 4G**). The maximum width of the spicule sheath is 0.06–0.11 mm and is covered throughout its length by densely located chitinous spines from the proximal to distal portion and is cylindrical without a distal bulb (**Figures 4G, 5C** and **Table 3**).

Female: The body is 20–48.6 mm long. The ratio between anterior and posterior body length is 2.1–2.2:1. The thin anterior part is 1: 0.65–0.67 of the entire length of the body. The length of the esophagus is 13–33 mm. The width of the body around the esophageal end is 0.13–0.48 mm, and the maximum width (in the posterior part of the body) is 0.38–0.90 mm (**Table 4**). The uterus is unpaired. The vulva is located at esophagus-intestine junction level (**Figures 5B, 6A,B**). This part of body thereafter changes into a transversely striated body cuticle. The vulva is non-protrusive and has no ornamentation (**Figures 6A,B**). The vagina has strong walls and, when everted, shows small papillae (**Figure 6B**). This vagina is long and presents one zone straight near the vulva while presenting circumvolutions nearly the uterus (**Figures 5B, 6A**). The ovary is long and continues with the oviduct in the back of the body (**Figure 6C**). The anus lies, subterminal, at the tip of the tail (**Figures 5D, 6D**). The eggs are barrel-shaped with clear, mucoid-appeared polar plugs, in addition to a vitelline membrane, and have a triple shell, the outermost layer of which is brown (**Figure 5E**).

DISCUSSION

In the present paper, we address an updated morphological and biometric description of *T. trichiura*, based on the results provided in the present study as well as on previous studies by different authors who characterized this species combining the analysis of morphological, biometric, and molecular characteristics. Thus, for the emendation of the description of *T. trichiura*, we have considered the populations of *P. troglodytes* (7), *H. sapiens* (14), *M. sylvanus* (17, 21), and *P. papio* (present study). For many years, different authors have based on the description of *T. trichiura* isolated from humans and NHP, on morphological and biometric characteristics exclusively (6, 25, 39–43), which was not molecularly confirmed to have corresponded to *T. trichiura*.

Thus, we found that females of *T. trichiura* are characterized by a non-protrusive vulva without ornamentation. However, some authors have described the vulva with a surface covered with spines like those of the male's spicule sheath (6, 25). Likewise, based on the morphological characteristics of males, *T. trichiura* is characterized by the presence of a lanceolate spicule that tapers at the end (41). However, Tenora et al. (42) observed a spicule with a cylindrical end in isolated samples of *H. sapiens*. Furthermore, males of *T. trichiura* isolated from *P. papio* and *M. sylvanus* presented a spicule with two chitinized extreme zones and a lighter central part (17). This feature was not observed in

TABLE 4 | Biometrical data of females of *T. trichiura*.

	***T. trichiura* (Present study, updated)**	***T. trichiura* from *P. troglodytes* [Cutillas et al. (7)]**				***T. trichiura* from *H. sapiens* [Nissen et al. (14)]**			***T. trichiura* from *M. sylvanus* [García-Sánchez et al. (21)]**				***T. trichiura* from *P. papio* (Present study)**			
	MIN-MAX	**MIN**	**MAX**	**X**	**δ**	**MIN**	**MAX**	**X**	**MIN**	**MAX**	**X**	**δ**	**MIN**	**MAX**	**X**	**δ**
F1	20–48.6	20.0	42.0	33.4	0.78	29.1	48.6	38.4	30.0	38.0	34.1	0.25	24.0	28.0	26	0.28
F2	13–33	13.0	33.0	25.3	0.68	16.2	32.1	25.6	18.0	26.0	21.9	0.23	17.0	20.0	18.5	0.21
LP	6–15.60	6.0	10.0	8.1	0.14	10.5	15.60	13.7	09.0	14.0	12.1	0.16	7	8	7.5	0.07
F3	0.09–0.20	0.09	0.19	0.14	0.04	0.11	0.20	0.17	0.13	0.18	0.15	0.01	0.14	0.15	0.14	0.00
F4	0.38–0.90	0.38	0.64	0.45	0.08	0.52	0.90	0.73	0.64	0.81	0.72	0.05	0.60	0.63	0.62	0.02
F5	0.13–0.48	0.13	0.23	0.17	0.03				0.36	0.48	0.42	0.03	0.31	0.41	0.36	0.07
F6	0.38–0.76	0.48	0.64	0.56	0.11				0.42	0.76	0.50	0.09	0.38	0.42	0.40	0.03
F7	0.36–1.71	0.36	0.63	0.50	0.19				0.90	1.71	1.44	0.21	1.08	1.35	1.22	0.19
F8	0.68–1.99	0.68	1.29	0.96	0.20				0.73	1.99	1.12	0.35	0.87	0.91	0.89	0.03
F9	0.02–0.09	0.03	0.05	0.04	0.01				0.02	0.09	0.05	0.02	0.05	0.05	0.05	0.00
F10	0.33–0.11	0.11	0.24	0.15	0.05				0.15	0.33	0.25	0.05	0.18	0.19	0.18	0.01
F11	0.13–0.84	0.13	0.24	0.21	0.04				0.40	0.84	0.61	0.14	0.35	0.37	0.36	0.01
F12	0.19–0.62	0.32	0.53	0.44	0.11				0.19	0.48	0.30	0.09	0.56	0.62	0.59	0.04
F13	0.05–0.81	0.66	0.67	0.67	0.01				0.05	0.14	0.11	0.04	0.73	0.81	0.77	0.06

F1, total body length of adult worm; F2, length of the esophageal region of the body; LP, length of the posterior region of body; F3, width of the esophageal region of the body; F4, maximum width of the posterior region of the body (thickness); F5, body width in the place of the junction of the esophagus and the intestine; F6, distance from the head end to beginning of bacillary stripes; F7, length of bacillary stripes; F8, length of vagina; F9, diameter of vulva turned over the surface of the body; F10, distance of vulva from the place of junction of the esophagus and the intestine; F11, distance of the posterior loop of the uterus from the tail end of the body; F12, distance of the tail end of the body and posterior fold of the seminal receptacle; F13, length of the muscular zone of the esophagus. X̄, arithmetic mean. σ, standard deviation.

males of *T. trichiura* described by several authors who exclusively carried out morphological and biometric studies (6, 7, 25, 39–42).

On the other hand, the spicule sheath is cylindrical without a distal bulb with triangular spines; however, other authors described these spines with different shapes and sizes, some of them with blunt points in *T. trichiura* from humans and NHP (25, 42). Besides, we found that the males of *T. trichiura* are characterized by the presence of a pair of paracloacal papillae which are observed when the sheath is invaginated (17); however, a proximal group of small papillae is not observed, as described by Ooi et al. (6) in a morpho-biometric study carried out on samples of monkeys, baboons, and humans. These papillae cluster was described in *T. colobae* by Cutillas et al. (19) who characterized a new species of *Trichuris* present in *C. g. kikuyuensis* based on morphological, biometric, and molecular data. This fact could suggest that the descriptions carried out by Ooi et al. (6) of *Trichuris* populations from humans and NHP based exclusively on morphological and biometric characters could correspond to different species closed to *T. trichiura*.

Biometrically, there is a concordance between the measures of *T. trichiura* obtained by different authors and those provided in the present paper, since all the values overlapped within the range of defined measures. However, regarding males, Dinnik et al. (40) reported that the maximum total body length and the maximum length of the anterior part [total body length of adult worm (M1) and length of esophageal region of body (M2)] were slightly larger (52 and 34 mm, respectively). Furthermore, the maximum width of the posterior region of body (thickness) (M4), length of spicule (M8), and length of ejaculatory duct (M14) has also been reported as slightly higher by Skrjabin et al. (25) (M4 = 0.76 mm, M8 = 3.9 mm, and M14 = 3.9 mm). Regarding females, the maximum total body length of adult worm (M1) showed slightly higher values in the studies of Dinnik et al. (40), Skrjabin et al. (25), and Vigot-Fréres (39) (50, 52.7, and 50 mm, respectively). In addition, the maximum length of the esophageal region of body (M2) and the maximum body width in the place of junction of esophagus and the intestine (F5) were slightly higher (35.6 and 0.50 mm, respectively) in the data provided by Skrjabin et al. (25).

In addition, there are differences in the population of *Trichuris* sp. from chimpanzees showing a shorter size of the males and females collected from chimpanzees with respect to *T. trichiura* from *H. sapiens*, *M. sylvanus*, and *P. papio*. García-Sánchez et al. (21) who reported the differentiation of *Trichuris* species using a morphometric approach cited these results previously. The occurrence of different biometrical measurements in the same species may be explained by the phenotypic plasticity of these organisms themselves (8–11).

Morphological and biometric data for *T. trichiura* provided in the present study allow the differentiation of this species with respect to other species of *Trichuris* parasitizing NHP such as *T. colobae* (19) and *T. ursinus* (20). The typical *T. trichiura* spicule has a clear central part, which is not present in that of *T. colobae* and *T. ursinus*. Furthermore, the typical papilla group is only present in *T. colobae* (19). Females of *T. trichiura* and *T. ursinus* appear to have a non-protrusive vulva (20); nevertheless, females of *T. colobae* present a vulva like a crater with papillae (19). The vagina is very long and straight in *T. ursinus* (20) but appear with circumvolutions in *T. trichiura*.

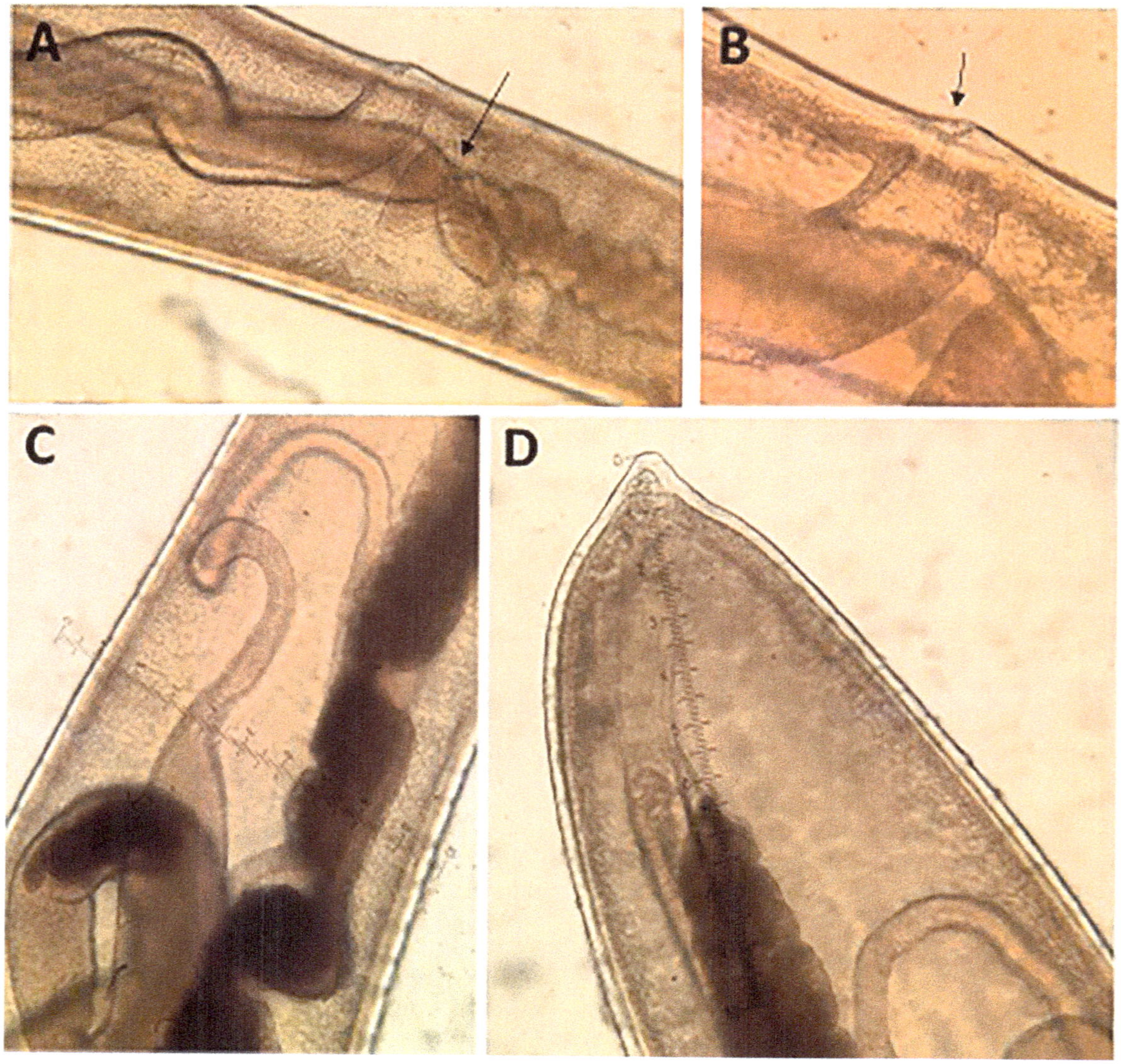

FIGURE 6 | Morphology of females of *T. trichiura*. **(A)** Esophagus–intestinal junction level (arrowed), vulva and vagina. **(B)** Vulva (arrowed). **(C)** Oviduct. **(D)** Posterior end.

With respect to the biometric characteristics, most of the measurements do not allow the specific differentiation between *T. trichiura* and other *Trichuris* spp. of NHP since these values overlapped for most of the measurements. However, males of *T. trichiura* have a smaller range of values in terms of distance from the end of the head to beginning of bacillary stripes and length of bacillary stripes (M6 and M7) compared to *T. colobae*, and values of length of minor bacillary stripes regarding *T. ursinus*. Regarding the specific differentiation of females based on biometric measurements, *T. trichiura* presents a lower range of values of length of bacillary stripes and distance of the tail end of the body and posterior fold of the seminal receptacle (F7 and F12) respect to *T. colobae*. In addition, the maximum and minimum values of distance of the vulva from the place of junction of the esophagus and the intestine were below than those observed in *T. ursinus* (19, 20).

From a molecular point of view, molecular markers which have been used by different authors to resolve species-level questions in *Trichuris* include the ITS1 and ITS2 nuclear regions (7, 44–53), 18S nuclear rRNA gene (38, 53, 54), mtDNA 16S rRNA gene (*rrn*L) (17, 50, 55), and protein-coding mitochondrial genes, including the 13 common genes obtained from the mitochondrial complete genome (12, 16, 56), *cox*1 mtDNA partial gene (17, 20, 38, 53, 55, 57), and *cob* mtDNA partial gene (17, 20, 55, 57, 58).

Different ITS rDNA types have been cited by different authors in some species of *Trichuris* (45–47). These sequence differences among ITS repeats in the rDNA array appeared to be a consequence of (intrachromosomal) mutational exchange during DNA replication (59). Thus, different reports suggest that different sequence types are most likely to be a result of base changes at certain positions in the sequence of a proportion of rDNA repeats because of mutational exchange during DNA replication, the extent of which appears to differ depending on the taxonomic group (60–63).

The results observed in ITS sequences revealed a percentage of similarity between 2a, 2b, 2c, and 2d subclades higher than those previously observed by other authors for species of the genus *Trichuris* (50, 57). Genetic analysis revealed that ITS regions were saturated and showed poor nucleotide diversity for clade 2 (*T. trichiura*). Thus, ITS sequences were not useful to infer the phylogenetic relationships between the different populations of *T. trichiura* (clade 2). On the other hand, some sequences from *T. trichiura* from Uganda and Cameroon (4) appeared within clade 1, suggesting that this population could be included on *T. ursinus* due to the high interpopulation similarity observed between both populations (**Supplementary Table 4** and **Figure 1**). Therefore, the different genetic lineages within *T. trichiura* were delimited exclusively based on analysis of the mitochondrial genes in agreement with Chan et al. (64), who evaluated the utility of mitochondrial and ribosomal genes for molecular systematics of parasitic nematodes. ITS regions accumulated substitutions substantially more slowly than mtDNA and showed nucleotide saturation.

Studies of interpopulation similarity between the different 2a, 2b, 2c, and 2d subclades, based on the mitochondrial markers (*cox*1 and *cob*), revealed a range of similarity lower than those observed by ITS sequences, and similar to those observed among other clearly defined species such as for example *T. suis* and *T. colobae*, *T. colobae*, and *T. ursinus* [cited by present authors, **Supplementary Tables 5, 6** and previously by Callejón et al. (20) and Rivero et al. (17)]. However, this similarity range showed higher values between *rrn*L sequences presenting a strong resolution of the different *T. trichiura* lineages (**Supplementary Table 7**). These results agree with those of Chan et al. (64), who evaluated the utility of mitochondrial ribosomal genes for molecular systematics of parasitic nematodes. These authors cited that 18S and 28S rRNA genes as well as 12S (*rrn*S) and 16S (*rrn*L) rRNA and *cox*1 genes showed a higher resolution for phylogenetic studies indicating that these five genes have potentially to be used as markers. Furthermore, they demonstrated that mitochondrial 12S and 16S genes present a resolution power at both lower and higher taxonomic levels for species and clade discrimination (64). For this reason and considering the similarity values observed in the different markers, we suggest that the populations of *T. trichiura* corresponding to the 2a, 2b, 2c, and 2d subclades correspond to different genetic lineages.

On the other hand, within clade 2 "*T. trichiura* lineage," results based on *rrn*L revealed an interpopulation similarity of 83.80–86.31% between *T. trichiura* populations and *Trichuris* sp. from *T. francoisi*. Hence, we suggest that this species has a close relationship with *T. trichiura*. Our results agree with Liu et al. (12) who considered that *Trichuris* populations from *T. francoisi* are a new species of *Trichuris*.

The phylogeny inferred from mitochondrial datasets revealed the same topology of those based on rDNA with respect to the two main clades (clade 1 and clade 2). We were able to identify several genetically distinct subgroups (subclades) of whipworms, which were present in the sampled primates. The subclades 2b and 2c showed a broad host range and were not restricted to NHP species. However, the subclades 2a and 2d showed a higher host specificity corresponding with the *T. trichiura* population from *M. sylvanus* and *H. sapiens* (subclade 2a) and *M. fuscata* (subclade 2d) exclusively. In agreement to this study, similar results were observed on *Trichuris* sp. from *M. fuscata* (44, 55). This population also showed two potentially distinct entities of *Trichuris* present in two different subclades: subclade 2d [analogous to subclade MF reported by Cavallero et al. (44, 55)] and subclade 2c. These authors suggested the possibility of two different sources of infection for Japanese macaques corresponding with two *Trichuris* taxa, one potentially able to also infect humans.

In our study, all phylogenetic trees (partitioned and concatenated) reported the existence of two main clades, which has been previously reported (3, 7, 12, 17, 20, 33, 44, 55, 58). A clear differentiation between *T. suis* (clade 1) and *T. trichiura* (clade 2) can be confirmed according to our results. Within clade 2 "*T. trichiura* lineage," *T. trichiura* can be also divided into 4 subclades, suggesting a complex of different genetic lineages. The analysis of the intraspecific similarity between the populations of *T. trichiura* from *P. papio*, *C. aethiops*, and *E. patas* from Spain revealed their highest value when compared with the populations of *T. trichiura* belonging to subclade 2c [previously described by Rivero et al. (17)] in all analyzed markers.

In addition to *T. trichiura*, a complex of *Trichuris* species showed infecting primates (*Trichuris* sp. from *T. francoisi* within clade 2 "*T. trichiura* lineage" and from *C. aethiops* from Italy and *C. sabaeus* from Czech Republic within clade 1 "*T. suis* lineage"). Different authors (17, 65) have previously reported the presence of several groups of *T. trichiura*. These results emphasize that the taxonomy and genetic variations of *Trichuris* are more complicated than previously acknowledged (65). Ravasi et al. (3) identified two distinct *Trichuris* genotypes that infect both humans and NHP. These authors identified "heterozygotes" confirming the identification of two distinct *Trichuris* genotypes in primates. On the other hand, Nissen et al. (14) identified "heterozygote" worms isolated from humans suggesting that *T. trichiura* might consist of several subspecies, some being found mainly in NHP. Ghai et al. (66) suggested that the *Trichuris* taxon should be considered a multi-host pathogen that is capable of infecting wild primates and humans. Finally, Betson et al. (5) reported that *Trichuris* infecting primates represents a complex of cryptic species with some species being able to infect both humans and NHP.

On the other hand, the existence of populations of *Trichuris* sp. associated with clade 1 "*T. suis* lineage" (based on all partitioned and concatenated markers) could indicate the possible origin of the change of host from NHP to pigs and, therefore, the origin of a new species, *T. suis*. This fact has been suggested by Hawash et al. (16) who found evidence of an African origin of *T. trichiura* that was later transmitted with human ancestors to Asia and then to South America. These authors suggested the possibility of a change of host to pigs in Asia where *T. suis* appears to have been transmitted globally by a combination of natural host dispersion and anthropogenic factors.

The present work examines the taxonomy, genetics, and phylogeny of *T. trichiura* parasitizing human and NHP and its relationship to *Trichuris* spp. from other NHP host species. A similar analysis was carried out on whipworms from humans (5). These authors suggested the existence of zoonotic transmission, especially regarding *T. trichiura* infections in NHP and, possibly, also for *T. suis* from pigs and *Trichuris vulpis* from dogs. In consequence, *Trichuris* may represent different species with the potential differences in endemicity, which may have important implications for implementing effective control strategies (5).

Several studies have reported that NHP represent an important reservoir for several known zoonotic infectious diseases (67–69). In this context, *Trichuris* infections have been found in a range of NHP species living in natural habitats including colobus monkeys, macaques, baboons, and chimpanzees (70–78). Based on molecular studies described above, some *Trichuris* species seem to be specific to a particular NHP, while others likely have the potential to circulate between humans and NHP, as they are genetically identical. This is particularly important when humans and NHP live in close proximity, as it is becoming increasingly common with human encroachment on pristine habitats and NHP accessing gardens and farms in search of food, and it has significant implications for human health and wildlife conservation (5).

The taxonomic, genetic, and phylogenetic results obtained in the present study confirm that *T. trichiura* exists as a complex (four subclades) with different host affinities and cross-infection capabilities corresponding with four different genetic lineages. Specifically, two of the four subclades show little host specificity and can develop trichuriasis in a wider variety of NHP species (*C. sabaeus*, *C. aethiops*, *M. fuscata*, *M. sylvanus*, *E. patas*, *P. papio*, *P. hamadryas*, *Papio* sp., and *P. anubis*) shared with humans. For this reason, we suggest the existence of a possible reservoir in the previously mentioned NHP species for human trichuriasis, which constitutes a serious public health risk (17). However, previous studies showed that the majority of the population of *M. fuscata* was included in a specific subclade [2d, subclade MF cited by Cavallero et al. (44, 55)] including only specimens from macaques.

Therefore, considering the following arguments for the taxonomic and phylogenetic study of populations of *T. trichiura*: (i) ITS regions were saturated and accumulated substitutions substantially slowly than mtDNA; therefore, they are not good genetic markers to delimit different genetic lineages. This is in agreement with previous studies where intraspecific variation was not observed when using nuclear DNA (64) suggesting that is not a useful genetic marker for intraspecies discrimination. (ii) The mitochondrial genes *cox*1, *cob*, and *rrn*L were not saturated, indicating that these three genes could have potential to be used as markers. Nevertheless, although *cox*1 presents the advantage for the extensive availability of database sequences, allowing for thorough comparisons of unknown sequences, *cox*1 sequences showed a high intraspecific variability which hinders resolution between closely related species. (iii) Nucleotide diversity showed that the *rrn*L gene present a lower intraspecific variability than *cox*1 and *cob* genes. However, *rrn*L interspecific genetic distance values allowed the phylogenetic resolution of the different *T. trichiura* subclades. Whence, *rrn*L was used successfully for inter-lineage discrimination of closely related populations within the *T. trichiura* lineage.

We suggest the utility of *rrn*L rRNA gene as a useful genetic marker for *Trichuris* species discrimination. Different authors who evaluated the utility of different mitochondrial genes for phylogenetic analyses (64, 79–81) have cited similar results. Future studies should focus on developing sequence databases for rRNA genes, which can serve as alternative genetic.

In conclusion, the present work provides an extensive study of biometric, morphological and molecular data for the unification of criteria that allows an update description of *T. trichiura* as well as a complex taxonomic, genetic, and phylogenetic study of the cited species applying multiple genetic markers to whipworm populations collected from humans and NHP from sympatric areas and worldwide locations. This study provides useful results for future studies aimed at the identification of new subspecies and hybridization events between existing species and enables a much clearer and more detailed understanding of dispersal patterns. This will reveal parasite transmission routes between these primates and will allow the implementation of appropriate control and prevention measures.

AUTHOR CONTRIBUTIONS

JR, RC, and CC contribute conception, design of the study, and wrote the manuscript. All the authors contributed to the manuscript revision and read and approved the submitted version.

FUNDING

This work was financially supported by FEDER/Ministry of Science and Innovation, State Research Agency (CGL2017-83057). The Junta de Andalucía (BIO-338), and a grant from the V and VI Plan Propio de Investigación of the University of Seville, Spain.

ACKNOWLEDGMENTS

The authors thank Zoo Castellar (Cádiz, Spain) for providing samples of *Trichuris* sp. from *M. sylvanus* which naturally died. Further, we thank to Zoo Barcelona, Selwo Aventura (Málaga), Parque de la Naturaleza de Cabárceno (Cantabria) and Bioparc Fuengirola (Málaga) from Spain.

REFERENCES

1. World Health Organization. Soil-transmitted helminth infections (2020). Available online at: https://www.who.int/es/news-room/fact-sheets/detail/soil-transmitted-helminth-infections (accessed March 2, 2020).
2. Mcdowell MA, Rafati S, editors. *Neglected Tropical Diseases – Middle East and North Africa*. Wien: Springer-Verlag Wien (2014). p. 281.
3. Ravasi DF, O'Riain MJ, Davids F, Illing N. Phylogenetic evidence that two distinct *Trichuris* genotypes infect both humans and non-human primates. *PLoS ONE*. (2012) 7:e44187. doi: 10.1371/journal.pone.0044187
4. Ghai RR, Chapman CA, Omeja PA, Davies TJ, Goldberg TL. Nodule worm infection in humans and wild primates in Uganda: cryptic species in a newly identified region of human transmission. PLoS Negl Trop Dis. (2014) 8:e2641. doi: 10.1371/journal.pntd.0002641
5. Betson M, Søe M, Nejsum P. Human trichuriasis: whipworm genetics, phylogeny, transmission and future research directions. *Curr Trop Med Rep*. (2015) 2:209–17. doi: 10.1007/s40475-015-0062-y
6. Ooi HK, Tenora F, Itoh K, Kamiya M. Comparative study of *Trichuris trichiura* from nonhuman primates and from man, and their differences with *Trichuris suis*. *J Vet Med Sci*. (1993) 55:363–6. doi: 10.1292/jvms.55.363
7. Cutillas C, Callejón R, De Rojas M, Tewes B, Úbeda JM, Ariza C, et al. *Trichuris suis* and *Trichuris trichiura* are different nematode species. *Acta Trop*. (2009) 111:299–307. doi: 10.1016/j.actatropica.2009.05.011
8. Knight RA. Morphological differences in *Trichuris ovis* associated with different host species. *J Parasitol*. (1984) 70:842–3.
9. Spakulová M. Discriminant analysis as a method for the numerical evaluation of taxonomic characters in male trichurid nematodes. *Syst Parasitol*. (1994) 29:113–9. doi: 10.1007/BF00009807
10. Robles MdR, Navone GT. Redescription of *Trichuris laevitestis* (Nematoda: trichuridae) from *Akodon azarae* and *Scapteromys aquaticus* (Sigmodontinae: Cricetidae) in Buenos Aires province, Argentina. *J Parasitol*. (2006) 92:1053–7. doi: 10.1645/GE-827R.1
11. Robles MdR. New species of *Trichuris* (Nematoda: Trichuridae) from *Akodon montensis* Thomas, 1913, of the Paranaense Forest in Argentina. *J Parasitol*. (2011) 97:319–27. doi: 10.1645/GE-2434.1
12. Liu GH, Gasser RB, Su A, Nejsum P, Peng L, Lin RQ, et al. Clear genetic distinctiveness between human-and pig-derived *Trichuris* based on analysis of mitochondrial datasets. *PLoS Negl Trop Dis*. (2012) 6:e1539. doi: 10.1371/journal.pntd.0001539
13. Liu GH, Zhou W, Nisbet AJ, Xu MJ, Zhou DH, Zhao GH, et al. Characterization of *Trichuris trichiura* from humans and *T. suis* from pigs in China using internal transcribed spacers of nuclear ribosomal DNA. *J Helminthol*. (2014) 88:64–8. doi: 10.1017/S0022149X12000740
14. Nissen S, Aljubury A, Hansen TV, Olsen A, Christensen H, Thamsborg SM, et al. Genetic analysis of *Trichuris suis* and *Trichuris trichiura* recovered from humans and pigs in a sympatric setting in Uganda. *Vet Parasitol*. (2012) 188:68–77. doi: 10.1016/j.vetpar.2012.03.004
15. Nadler S, De Leon G. Integrating molecular and morphological approaches for characterizing parasite cryptic species: implications for parasitology. *Parasitology*. (2011) 138:1688–709. doi: 10.1017/S003118201000168X
16. Hawash MB, Andersen LO, Gasser RB, Stensvold C, Nejsum P. Mitochondrial genome analyses suggest multiple *Trichuris* species in humans, baboons, and pigs from different geographical regions. *PLoS Negl Trop Dis*. (2015) 9:e0004059. doi: 10.1371/journal.pntd.0004059
17. Rivero J, García-Sánchez A, Zurita A, Cutillas C, Callejón R. *Trichuris trichiura* isolated from *Macaca sylvanus*: morphological, biometrical, and molecular study. *BMC Vet Res*. (2020) 16:445. doi: 10.1186/s12917-020-02661-4
18. Wang H, Zhang H, Song L, Zhu L, Chen M, Ren G, et al. Morphological and molecular confirmation of the validity of *Trichuris rhinopiptheroxella* in the endangered golden snub-nosed monkey (*Rhinopithecus roxellana*). *J Helminthol*. (2019) 93:601–7. doi: 10.1017/S0022149X18000500
19. Cutillas C, De Rojas M, Zurita A, Oliveros R, Callejón R. *Trichuris colobae* n. sp. (Nematoda: Trichuridae), a new species of *Trichuris* from *Colobus guereza kikuyensis*. *Parasitol Res*. (2014) 113:2725–32. doi: 10.1007/s00436-014-3933-6
20. Callejón R, Halajian A, Cutillas C. Description of a new species, *Trichuris ursinus* n. sp. (Nematoda: Trichuridae) from *Papio ursinus* Keer, 1792 from South Africa. *Infect Genet Evol*. (2017) 51:182–93. doi: 10.1016/j.meegid.2017.04.002
21. García-Sánchez ÁM, Rivero J, Zurita A, Callejón R, Cutillas C. Differentiation of *Trichuris* species using a morphometric approach. *Int J Parasitol Parasites Wildl*. (2019) 9:218–23. doi: 10.1016/j.ijppaw.2019.05.012
22. Gupta SK, Singla LD. Veterinary diagnostics. In: Gupta RP, Garg SR, Nehra V, Lather D, editors. Chapter 6: *Diagnostic Trends in Parasitic Diseases of Animals*. Delhi: Statish Serial Publishing House (2013). p. 81–112.
23. Horii Y, Usui M. Experimental transmission of *Trichuris ova* from monkeys to man. *Trans R Soc Trop Med Hyg*. (1985) 79:423. doi: 10.1016/0035-9203(85)90403-1
24. Oliveros R, Cutillas C, Aris P, Guevara D. Morphologic, biometric and isoenzyme characterization of *Trichuris suis*. *Parasitol Res*. (1998) 84:513–5. doi: 10.1007/s004360050438
25. Skrjabin KI, Shikhobalova NP, Orlow IV. Essentials of Nematodology, vol. VI. In: Greenberg D, editors. Translated by Birron A. *Trichocephalidae* and *Capillariidae* of animals and the man and the diseases caused by them. Jerusalem: Keter Press Wiener Binder Ltd. (1957).
26. Spakulová M, Lýsek H. A biometric study of two populations of *Trichocephalus suis* Schrank, 1788 from swine and wild boars. *Helminthologia*. (1981) 18:91–8.
27. Suriano DM, Navone GT. Three new species of the genus *Trichuris* Roederer, 1761 (Nematoda: Trichuridae) from Cricetidae and Octodontidae rodents in Argentina. *Res Re Parasitol*. (1994) 54:39–46.
28. Robles MdR, Navone GT, Notarnicola J. A new species of *Trichuris* (Nematoda: Trichuridae) from *Phyllotini rodents* in Argentina. *J Parasitol*. (2006) 92:100–4. doi: 10.1645/GE-GE-552R.1
29. Kumar S, Stecher G, Tamura K. MEGA7: molecular evolutionary genetics analysis version 7.0 for bigger datasets. *Mol Biol Evol*. (2016) 33:1870–4. doi: 10.1093/molbev/msw054
30. Xia X, Xie Z, Salemi M, Chen L, Wang Y. An index of substitution saturation and its application. *Mol Phylogenetics Evol*. (2003) 26:1–7. doi: 10.1016/s1055-7903(02)00326-3
31. Xia X, Lemey P. Assessing substitution saturation with DAMBE. 2nd ed. In: Lemey P, Salemi M, Vandamme AM, editors. *The Phylogenetic Handbook: A Practical Approach to DNA and Protein Phylogeny*. Oxford: Cambridge University Press. (2009). p. 615–30.
32. Rozas J, Ferrer-Mata A, Sánchez-DelBarrio JC, Guirao-Rico S, Librado P, Ramos-Onsins SE, et al. DnaSP v6: DNA sequence polymorphism analysis of large datasets. *Mol Biol Evol*. (2017) 34:3299–302. doi: 10.1093/molbev/msx248
33. Guindon S, Gascuel O. A simple, fast, and accurate algorithm to estimate large phylogenies by maximum likelihood. *Syst Biol*. (2003) 52:696–704. doi: 10.1080/10635150390235520
34. Ronquist F, Huelsenbeck JP. MrBAYES 3: Bayesian phylogenetic inference under mixed models. Bioinformatics. (2003) 19:1572–4. doi: 10.1093/bioinformatics/btg180
35. Posada D. jModelTest: phylogenetic model averaging. *Mol Biol Evol*. (2008) 25:1253–6. doi: 10.1093/molbev/msn083
36. Posada D, Buckley TR. Model selection and model averaging in phylogenetics: advantages of akaike information criterion and bayesian approaches over likelihood ratio tests. *Syst Biol*. (2004) 53:793–808. doi: 10.1080/10635150490522304
37. Felsenstein J. Confidence limits on phylogenies: an approach using the bootstrap. *Evolution*. (1985) 39:783–91. doi: 10.1111/j.1558-5646.1985.tb00420.x
38. Callejón R, Nadler S, De Rojas M, Zurita A, Petrášová J, Cutillas C. Molecular characterization and phylogeny of whipworm nematodes inferred from DNA sequences of *cox1* mtDNA and 18S rDNA. *Parasitol Res*. (2013) 112:3933–49. doi: 10.1007/s00436-013-3584-z
39. Frères V, Neveu-Lemaire M. Traité d'helminthologie médicale et vétérinaire. (1936) S1-16:641–2. doi: 10.4269/ajtmh.1936.s1-16.641
40. Dinnik NN. Meditsinskaya Parazitologiya i Parazitarnye Boleznl, 1. (1938). p. 1907.
41. Zaman V. Scanning electron microscopy of *Trichuris trichiura* (Nematoda). *Acta Trop*. (1984) 41:287–92.
42. Tenora F, Hovorka I, Hejlkova D. A supplement to the scanning electron microscopy of some *Trichocephalus* spp. (Nematoda). *Helminthologia*. (1988) 25:227–34.

43. Tenora F, Stanek M, Spakulová M. On the possibility of morphological differentiation of *Trichocephalus trichiurus* (L., 1771) and *T. suis* (Schrank, 1788) species. In: *Conference Aktuálne otázky humánnej parazitológie.* (1992).
44. Cavallero S, De Liberato C, Friedrich KG, Di Cave D, Masella V, D'Amelio S, et al. Genetic heterogeneity and phylogeny of *Trichuris* spp. from captive non-human primates based on ribosomal DNA sequence data. *Infect Genet Evol.* (2015) 34:450–6. doi: 10.1016/j.meegid.2015.06.009
45. Oliveros R, Cutillas C, de Rojas M, Arias P. Characterazition of four species of *Trichuris* (Nematoda: Enoplida) by their second internal transcribed spacer ribosomal DNA sequence. *Parasitol Res.* (2000) 86:1008–13. doi: 10.1007/pl00008519
46. Cutillas C, Oliveros R, De Rojas M, Guevara DC. Determination of *Trichuris muris* from murid hosts and *Trichuris* arvicolae (Nematoda) from arvicolid rodents by amplification and sequentiation of the ITS1-5.8S-ITS2 segment of the ribosomal DNA. *Parasitol Res.* (2002) 88:574–82. doi: 10.1007/s00436-002-0596-5
47. Cutillas C, Oliveros R, De Rojas M, Guevara DC. Determination of *Trichuris skrjabini* by sequencing of the ITS1-5.8S-ITS2 segment of the ribosomal DNA: comparative molecular study of different species of trichurids. *J Parasitol.* (2004) 90:648–52. doi: 10.1645/GE-3295RN
48. Cutillas C, De Rojas M, Ariza C, Úbeda JM, Guevara DC. Molecular identification of *Trichuris vulpis* and *Trichuris suis* isolated from different hosts. *Parasitol Res.* (2007) 100:383–9. doi: 10.1007/s00436-006-0275-z
49. Callejón R, Gutiérrez-Avilés L, Halajian A, Zurita A, de Rojas M, Cutillas C. Taxonomy and phylogeny of *Trichuris globulosa* Von Linstow, 1901 from camels. A review of *Trichuris* species parasitizing herbivorous. *Infect Genet Evol.* (2015) 34:61–74. doi: 10.1016/j.meegid.2015.06.011
50. Callejón R, Halajian A, De Rojas M, Marrugal A, Guevara DC, Cutillas C. 16S partial gene DNA and internal transcribed spacers ribosomal DNA as differential markers of *Trichuris discolor* populations. *Vet Parasitol.* (2012) 186:350–63. doi: 10.1016/j.vetpar.2011.11.033
51. Salaba O, Rylková K, Vadlejch J, Petrtýl M, Schánková Š, Brožová A, et al. The first determination of *Trichuris* sp. from roe deer by amplification and sequentiation of the ITS1-5.8S-ITS2 segment of ribosomal DNA. *Parasitol Res.* (2013) 112:955–60. doi: 10.1007/s00436-012-3215-0
52. Robles MdR, Cutillas C, Panei CJ, Callejón R. Morphological and molecular characterization of a new *Trichuris* species (Nematoda-Trichuridae), and phylogenetic relationships of *Trichuris* species of cricetid rodents from Argentina. *PLoS ONE.* (2014) 9:e112069. doi: 10.1371/journal.pone.0112069
53. DoleŽalová J, Oborník M, Hajdušková E, Jirku M, PetrŽelková KJ, Bolechová P, et al. How many species of whipworms do we share? Whipworms from man and other primates form two phylogenetic lineages. *Folia Parasitol (Praha).* (2015) 62:1–12. doi: 10.14411/fp.2015.063
54. Guardone L, Deplazes P, Macchioni F, Magi M, Mathis A. Ribosomal and mitochondrial DNA analysis of Trichuridae nematodes of carnivores and small mammals. *Vet Parasitol.* (2013) 197:364–9. doi: 10.1016/j.vetpar.2013.06.022
55. Cavallero S, Nejsum P, Cutillas C, Callejón R, DoleŽalová J, Modrý D, et al. Insights into the molecular systematics of *Trichuris* infecting captive primates based on mitochondrial DNA analysis. *Vet Parasitol.* (2019) 272:23–30. doi: 10.1016/j.vetpar.2019.06.019
56. Liu GH, Gasser RB, Nejsum P, Wang Y, Chen Q, Song HQ, et al. Mitochondrial and nuclear ribosomal DNA evidence supports the existence of a new *Trichuris* species in the endangered françois' leaf-monkey. *PLoS ONE.* (2013) 8:e66249. doi: 10.1371/journal.pone.0066249
57. Callejón R, Robles MdR, Panei CJ, Cutillas C. Molecular diversification of *Trichuris* spp. from Sigmodontinae (Cricetidae) rodents from Argentina based on mitochondrial DNA sequences. *Parasitol Res.* (2016) 115:2933–45. doi: 10.1007/s00436-016-5045-y
58. Callejón R, Cutillas C, Nadler SA. Nuclear and mitochondrial genes for inferring *Trichuris* phylogeny. *Parasitol Res.* (2015) 114:4591–9. doi: 10.1007/s00436-015-4705-7
59. Schlötterer C, Tautz D. Chromosomal homogeneity of *Drosophila* ribosomal DNA arrays suggests intrachromosomal exchanges drive concerted evolution. *Curr Biol.* (1994) 4:777–83. doi: 10.1016/s0960-9822(00)00175-5
60. Wesson DM, Porter CH, Collins FH. Sequence and secondary structure comparisons of ITS rDNA in mosquitoes (Diptera: Culicidae). *Mol Phylogenet Evol.* (1992) 1:253–69. doi: 10.1016/1055-7903(92)90001-w
61. Campbell AJ, Gasser RB, Chilton NB. Differences in a ribosomal DNA sequence of *Strongylus* species allows identification of single eggs. *Int J Parasitol.* (1995) 25:359–65. doi: 10.1016/0020-7519(94)00116-6
62. Hoste H, Chilton NB, Gasser RB, Beveridge I. Differences in the second internal transcribed spacer (ribosomal DNA) between five species of *Trichostrongylus* (Nematoda: Trichostrongylidae). *Int J Parasitol.* (1995) 25:75–80. doi: 10.1016/0020-7519(94)00085-3
63. Gasser RB, Stewart LE, Speare R. Genetic markers in ribosomal DNA for hookworm identification. *Acta Trop.* (1996) 62:15–21. doi: 10.1016/s0001-706x(96)00015-0
64. Chan AHE, Chaisiri K, Morand S, Saralamba N, Thaenkham U. Evaluation and utility of mitochondrial ribosomal genes for molecular systematics of parasitic nematodes. *Parasit Vectors.* (2020) 13:364. doi: 10.1186/s13071-020-04242-8
65. Xie Y, Zhao B, Hoberg EP, Li M, Zhou X, Gu X, et al. Genetic characterisation and phylogenetic status of whipworms (*Trichuris* spp.) from captive non-human primates in China, determined by nuclear and mitochondrial sequencing. *Parasit Vectors.* (2018) 11:516. doi: 10.1186/s13071-018-3100-5
66. Ghai RR, Simons ND, Chapman CA, Omeja PA, Davies TJ, Ting N, et al. Hidden population structure and cross-species transmission of whipworms (*Trichuris* sp.) in humans and non-human primates in Uganda. *PLoS Negl Trop Dis.* (2014) 8:e3256. doi: 10.1371/journal.pntd.0003256
67. Geerts S, Gryseels B. Anthelmintic resistance in human helminths: a review. *Tropical Med Int Health.* (2001) 6:915–21. doi: 10.1046/j.1365-3156.2001.00774.x
68. World Health Organization. Helminth control in school-age children. A guide for managers of control programmes. Available online at: https://apps.who.int/iris/bitstream/handle/10665/44671/9789241548267_eng.pdf?sequence=1 (2011) (accessed September, 2011).
69. Global Burden of Disease Study 2013 Collaborators. *Global, regional, and national incidence, prevalence, and years lived with disability for 301 acute and chronic diseases and injuries in 188 countries, 1990–2013: a systematic analysis for the Global Burden of Disease Study. Lancet.* (2015) 386:743–800. doi: 10.1016/S0140-6736(15)60692-4
70. Arizono N, Yamada M, Tegoshi T, Onishi K. Molecular identification of *Oesophagostomum* and *Trichuris* eggs isolated from wild Japanese macaques. *Korean J Parasitol.* (2012) 50:253–7. doi: 10.3347/kjp.2012.50.3.253
71. Gillespie TR, Lonsdorf EV, Canfield EP, Meyer DJ, Nadler Y, Raphael J, et al. Demographic and ecological effects on patterns of parasitism in eastern chimpanzees (*Pan troglodytes* schweinfurthii) in Gombe National Park, Tanzania. *Am J Phys Anthropol.* (2010) 143:534–44. doi: 10.1002/ajpa.21348
72. Kooriyama T, Hasegawa H, Shimozuru M, Tsubota T, Nishida T, Iwaki T. Parasitology of five primates in Mahale Mountains National Park Tanzania. *Primates.* (2012) 53:365–75. doi: 10 1007/s10329-012-0311-9
73. Levecke B, Dorny P, Vercammen F, Visser LG, Van EM, Vercruysse J, et al. Transmission of *Entamoeba nuttalli* and *Trichuris trichiura* from non-human primates to humans. *Emerg Infect Dis.* (2015) 21:1871–2. doi: 10.3201/eid2110.141456
74. Li M, Zhao B, Li B, Wang Q, Niu L, Deng J, et al. Prevalence of gastrointestinal parasites in captive non-human primates of twenty-four zoological gardens in China. *J Med Primatol.* (2015) 44:168–73. doi: 10.1111/jmp.12170
75. Muriuki SMK, Murugu RK, Munene E, Karere GM, Chai DC. Some gastro-intestinal parasites of zoonotic (public health) importance commonly observed in old world non-human primates in Kenya. *Acta Trop.* (1998) 71:73–82. doi: 10.1016/s0001-706x(98)00040-0
76. Pourrut X, Diffo JLD, Somo RM, Bilong Bilong CF, Delaporte E, LeBreton M, et al. Prevalence of gastrointestinal parasites in primate bushmeat and pets in Cameroon. *Vet Parasitol.* (2011) 175:187–91. doi: 10.1016/j.vetpar.2010.09.023
77. Yao C, Walkush J, Shim D, Cruz K, Ketzis J. Molecular species identification of *Trichuris trichiura* in African green monkey on St. Kitts, West Indies. *Vet Parasitol Reg Stud Reports.* (2018) 11:22–6. doi: 10.1016/j.vprsr.2017.11.004

78. Zanzani SA, Gazzonis AL, Epis S, Manfredi MT. Study of the gastrointestinal parasitic fauna of captive non-human primates (Macaca fascicularis). *Parasitol Res.* (2016) 115:307–12. doi: 10.1007/s00436-015-4748-9
79. Medina M, Walsh PJ. Molecular systematics of the order Anaspidea based on mitochondrial DNA sequence (12S, 16S, and COI). *Mol Phylogenet Evol.* (2000) 15:41–58. doi: 10.1006/mpev.1999.0736
80. Paternina LE, Verbel Vergara D, Bejarano EE. Comparación y utilidad de las regiones mitocondriales de los genes 16S y *COX1* para los análisis genéticos en garrapatas (Acari: Ixodidae). *Biomedica.* (2016) 36:295–302. doi: 10.7705/biomedica.v36i2.3116
81. Chan AHE, Chaisiri K, Dusitsittipon S, Jakkul W, Charoennitiwat V, Komalamisra C, et al. Mitochondrial ribosomal genes as novel genetic markers for discrimination of closely related species in the *Angiostrongylus cantonensis* lineage. *Acta Trop.* (2020) 211:105645. doi: 10.1016/j.actatropica.2020.105645

The Constant Threat of Zoonotic and Vector-Borne Emerging Tropical Diseases: Living on the Edge

Alfonso J. Rodriguez-Morales[1,2,3,4], Alberto E. Paniz-Mondolfi[5,6], Álvaro A. Faccini-Martínez[7], Andrés F. Henao-Martínez[8], Julian Ruiz-Saenz[9], Marlen Martinez-Gutierrez[9,10], Lucia E. Alvarado-Arnez[3], Jorge E. Gomez-Marin[11], Ruben Bueno-Marí[12,13], Yenddy Carrero[14], Wilmer E. Villamil-Gomez[15,16], D. Katterine Bonilla-Aldana[17], Ubydul Haque[18], Juan D. Ramirez[19], Juan-Carlos Navarro[20], Susana Lloveras[21], Kovy Arteaga-Livias[4,22], Cristina Casalone[23], Jorge L. Maguiña[4], Angel A. Escobedo[24], Marylin Hidalgo[25], Antonio C. Bandeira[26], Salim Mattar[27], Jaime A. Cardona-Ospina[1,2] and Jose A. Suárez[28]*

[1] Grupo de Investigación Biomedicina, Faculty of Medicine, Fundacion Universitaria Autonoma de las Americas, Pereira, Colombia, [2] Emerging Infectious Diseases and Tropical Medicine Research Group, Instituto para la Investigación en Ciencias Biomédicas - Sci-Help, Pereira, Colombia, [3] Coordinación Nacional de Investigación, Universidad Privada Franz Tamayo (UNIFRANZ), Cochabamba, Bolivia, [4] Master Program on Clinical Epidemiology and Biostatistics, Universidad Científica del Sur, Lima, Peru, [5] Department of Pathology, Molecular and Cell-Based Medicine, Laboratory of Microbiology, Icahn School of Medicine at Mount Sinai, New York, NY, United States, [6] Instituto de Investigaciones Biomédicas IDB/Incubadora Venezolana de la Ciencia, Barquisimeto, Venezuela, [7] Department of Pathology, University of Texas Medical Branch, Galveston, TX, United States, [8] Department of Medicine, Division of Infectious Diseases, School of Medicine, University of Colorado Denver, Aurora, CO, United States, [9] Grupo de Investigación en Ciencias Animales - GRICA, Facultad de Medicina Veterinaria y Zootecnia, Universidad Cooperativa de Colombia, Bucaramanga, Colombia, [10] Infettare, Facultad de Medicina, Universidad Cooperativa de Colombia, Medellín, Colombia, [11] Grupo de Estudio en Parasitologia Molecular (GEPAMOL) Group, Facultad de Ciencias de la Salud, Universidad del Quindío, Armenia, Colombia, [12] Departamento de Investigación y Desarrollo (I+D), Laboratorios Lokímica, Paterna, Spain, [13] Área de Parasitología, Departamento de Farmacia y Tecnología Farmaceútica y Parasitología, Universidad de Valencia, Burjasot, Spain, [14] Facultad de Ciencias de la Salud, Carrera de Medicina, Universidad Técnica de Ambato, Ambato, Ecuador, [15] Infectious Diseases and Infection Control Research Group, Hospital Universitario de Sincelejo, Sincelejo, Colombia, [16] Programa Del Doctorado de Medicina Tropical, SUE Caribe, Universidad Del Atlántico, Barranquilla, Colombia, [17] Semillero de Investigación en Zoonosis (SIZOO), Grupo de Investigación BIOECOS, Fundacion Universitaria Autonoma de las Americas, Pereira, Colombia, [18] Department of Biostatistics and Epidemiology, University of North Texas Health Science Center, Fort Worth, TX, United States, [19] Centro de Investigaciones en Microbiología y Biotecnología-UR (CIMBIUR), Facultad de Ciencias Naturales, Universidad del Rosario, Bogotá, Colombia, [20] Research Group of Emerging Diseases, Ecoepidemiology and Biodiversity, Health Sciences Faculty, Universidad Internacional SEK, Quito, Ecuador, [21] Sección Zoopatología Médica, Hospital de Infecciosas FJ Muñiz, Buenos Aires, Argentina, [22] Faculty of Medicine, Universidad Nacional Hermilio Valdizán, Huánuco, Peru, [23] Istituto Zooprofilattico del Piemonte, Torino, Italy, [24] Department of Epidemiology, Institute of Gastroenterology, Havana, Cuba, [25] Infectious Diseases Group, Facultad de Ciencias, Pontificia Universidad Javeriana, Bogotá, Colombia, [26] Faculdade de Medicina, UniFTC, Salvador, Brazil, [27] Instituto de Investigaciones Biologicas del Tropico, Universidad de Cordoba, Monteria, Colombia, [28] Investigador SNI Senacyt Panamá, Instituto Conmemorativo Gorgas de Estudios de la Salud (ICGES), Panama, Panama

***Correspondence:**
Alfonso J. Rodriguez-Morales
alfonso.rodriguez@uam.edu.co

Keywords: vector-borne diseases, zoonotic diseases, emerging, SARS-CoV-2/COVID-2, tropical diseases, challenges

Emerging diseases have significantly impacted the last few decades (1–10). The emergence and re-emergence of vector-borne and zoonotic diseases in Africa, Asia, and Latin America have reshaped the epidemiological landscape of these continents. The impact of these diseases and the establishment of local transmission in traditionally non-endemic areas, due to migration and travel, have been revealed over the last years. Diseases such as Chikungunya (11–16), Zika (17–24), Yellow Fever (25–28), Dengue (29–33), Oropouche, Madre de Dios virus, Iquitos virus (34, 35), Mayaro Fever (36, 37), Ebola (38–42), Nipah virus, arenaviruses such as Lassa (43), Machupo (44,

45), Chapare (45, 46), Junin (47), zoonotic Malaria (48), Severe Fever with Thrombocytopenia Syndrome (49), Plague (50), Crimean-Congo Hemorrhagic Fever, Acute Orally Transmitted Chagas Disease (51–54), Visceral and Diffuse Cutaneous Leishmaniasis (55, 56), Toxoplasmosis (57–59), Tick-Borne Diseases (60, 61), Rift Valley Fever, Tuberculosis (62), Leprosy (63–67), Avian Influenza (68–70), Orthohantavirus (71–75), and Toxocariasis (76, 77) have posed a significant impact to human health. Furthermore, zoonotic epidemics and pandemic coronaviruses, such as the Severe Acute Respiratory Syndrome (SARS), the Middle East Respiratory Syndrome (MERS) (78–82), and the ongoing SARS-CoV-2/COVID-19 (83, 84) pandemic, have caused a profound economical and social disruption threatening to overwhelm public health systems globally (85) (**Table 1**). Most of these pathogens can even cocirculate and coinfect a significant proportion of inhabitants within the same territories (11, 87–94). For example, in arboviral diseases, the occurrence of coinfections has been widely reported -such as Dengue with Chikungunya and/or with Zika virus- and affects diverse populations, including pregnant women and immunocompromised patients (94–97). This may obscure clinical suspicion, as signs and symptoms for many of these pathogens may overlap. In endemic areas, this becomes a particularly pressing issue that must be taken into account in order to ensure accurate diagnosis and provide appropriate management. The ChikDenMaZika syndrome has been previously adopted as a mnemonic device to include Chikungunya, Dengue, Mayaro, and Zika in the broad differential of acute febrile illnesses due to arboviral agents (95). More recently, emerging coinfections, including bacterial and parasitic diseases, such as tuberculosis and Chagas disease, have also been reported (98).

Current times call for more comprehensive ecoepidemiological and bioecosocial approaches (20, 99). Scarce funding and the lack of research (39, 43, 61, 81) in tropical medicine are entirely unacceptable. Human immunodeficiency virus (HIV)/acquired immune deficiency syndrome (AIDS), tuberculosis (TB), and malaria combined receive approximately 70% of neglected diseases funding. As mentioned here, emerging tropical diseases, such as those mentioned here, are worldwide in scope, and many have significant regional implications. Therefore, a different funding paradigm that improves their situation is needed (100). The world is no longer a place with distant countries and shielded territories. Instead, ever increasing interconnectivity has turned it into a "small" global village, where the health status of underprivileged areas may undermine not only their lives and development but extend to the wealthiest. The Ebola crisis in 2014 highlighted how high-consequence emerging diseases could spill over to Europe and North America (38, 40). The ongoing 2020-2021 pandemic of COVID-19, which has reached as far as Antarctica, affecting almost all countries worldwide, is another clear example (8, 29, 84, 101–112). As was expected, coinfections between tropical pathogens and COVID-19 are also now increasingly being reported, especially with dengue (30). Dengue affects over 100 countries worldwide and puts about 2.5-3.9 billion people at risk of infection (113, 114). Within the next century, nearly a billion people are at risk of exposure to virus transmission by both main *Aedes* spp., *Ae. aegypti*, and *Ae. albopictus* (also Chikungunya and Zika) in the worst-case scenario (115). The recent first detection of *Ae. vittatus* in the Dominican Republic and the Americas generated concern in the region, requiring enhanced surveillance to understand the range and public health risks of this potential invasive mosquito species, deserving more studies (116). Most of these emerging tropical diseases are vector-borne, zoonotically transmitted, or environmentally spread through direct contact, food or water ingestion, as well as a consequence of environmental alterations (including the effects of climate change) (117–125), becoming significant sources of mortality and morbidity worldwide (2).

TABLE 1 | Lessons learned from the COVID-19 pandemic in Latin America.

- Avoid fragmentation and segmentation of the health system
- Enhance data integration between sectors
- Improve transfer of inputs and deployment of personnel
- Better linking of health and safety authorities
- Build up a strong capacity for molecular (RT-PCR) testing
- Validate rapid tests for complementary diagnosis
- Improve primary care interventions before admission to ICU
- Improve ICU capacities including facilities, equipment, and personnel
- Better management and monitoring of non-COVID patients
- Promote education of human resources, including health professionals
- Improve health personnel's working conditions (salaries, PPE, among others)
- Enhance medical training during the pandemic
- Warrant medicinal oxygen supplement
- Monitor transparency in health authorities' decision-making documents
- Use of medications with evidence and develop evidence-based guidelines
- Provide appropiate information about public health policy and decision-making processes
- Develop more capacities in biotechnology (for development of tests, treatments, and vaccines)

Modified from Herrera-Añazco et al. (86).

The impact of these diseases extends well beyond the acute constellation of symptoms, leading in a considerable proportion of patients to chronic sequelae and complications, which can be long lasting and severely incapacitating, as is the case with Chikungunya (15, 126–132), Zika (17, 133–135), Ebola, Chagas disease (52), and even for COVID-19 (136–139).

Many tools have been deployed to counteract emerging infectious diseases. Amongst these are active surveillance (some supported by artificial intelligence) (140–142), leading to the rapid identification of novel pathogens by genome sequencing and phylogenetic tracing studies (36, 105, 107, 143–146) based on computing methods to predict possible interspecies barriers spillover between humans and animals (147). Coupling biotechnological approaches with social sciences—the holistic understanding of humans and their interactions in the disease ecosystems—is also a critical element needed when studying emerging infectious diseases (148, 149).

One of the most significant challenges when studying tropical infectious diseases relies on their complexity and heterogeneity, which usually requires a deep understanding not only of the disease itself but its overall context. In order to better approach these diseases one must keep a broader vision of designing proposed interventions, including multilevel ecoepidemiological studies ranging from molecular and omics to satellite epidemiology (use of data and images derived from geospatial technologies, e.g., satellites, for the study of the occurrence and distribution of health-related events in specified populations, and the application of this knowledge to control the health problems) of pathogens, vectors, hosts, abiotic variables, and other socio-environmental factors (125, 150, 151). While more research is required to fill in the numerous gaps in knowledge for many of these diseases, particular attention should be placed in designing strategies to develop methods to forecast these diseases not only in vulnerable and underserved populations from low-income countries but also in those poverty pockets located in high-income countries. A whole chapter to be considered in emerging tropical diseases is vaccines development. Innovative global partnership between public, private, philanthropic, and civil society organisations, such as the Coalition for Epidemic Preparedness Innovations (CEPI), launched in 2017, are important to develop vaccines to stop future epidemics. To accelerate the development of vaccines against emerging infectious diseases and enable equitable access to these vaccines for people during outbreaks is crucial. Nevertheless, more funding to understand biology, pathogenesis, epidemiology, prevention, and treatment of emerging tropical diseases are urgently needed and expected (152–154).

Tropical Medicine is no more a clinical specialty of "exotic diseases," as it was conceived at its beginnings, and is no more about "diseases for those entering the jungle." One dramatic change is the urban installation of diseases that before were observed only after sylvatic or primary forest exposure. The increase of urban outbreaks of Chagas disease in South America is now a horrific reality in Brazil (155–157), Venezuela (158), and Colombia (159, 160), and it is also a new reality for visceral leishmaniasis (161–164). The integrated work of public health experts, veterinarians, entomologists, and parasitologists is an urgent need to face these new challenges and transformations of tropical diseases. Tropical diseases also include non-infectious diseases, such as animal bites and stings (e.g. myiasis and tungiasis) (165, 166). Snake bites, scorpion stings, and spider bites, account for a significant amount of the morbidity and mortality in tropical countries in these changing scenarios, including ecotourism, rural migration, and other related factors (167–170).

There is no doubt that "many things are wrong in the world today", as the legendary American rock n'roll band Aerosmith has been singing since the 90s. We are "living on the edge", the edge of neglect and of a surge of many emerging infectious diseases with no hope for resolution in the foreseeable future. Furthermore, "it sure ain't no surprise" that poverty, inequality, climate change, deforestation, migration, urbanization, wildlife trade, among many other factors, have all contributed to the emergence of novel tropical diseases and the resurgence of other endemic diseases (171). There is no spare place for the arrival of emerging pathogens, and over time pathogens tend to adapt to new environments leading to unforeseen consequences. The next epidemic, the next pandemic, is just around the corner (68). In response to this latent threat, we need to gather real-time information and build collaborative networks aimed to enhance surveillance activities in order to develop high-priority medical countermeasures to prevent and control emerging tropical diseases. Research in Zoonotic and Vector-Borne Emerging Tropical Diseases remains the most critical aspect and the foundation to determine the drivers of emerging and re-emerging infectious diseases.

With that vision, our new Section *Emerging Tropical Diseases* in the journal Frontiers in Tropical Diseases offers to contribute to the scientific advancement and fill in the many knowledge gaps based on a multi and transdisciplinary approach. Our team of Associate Editors is comprised of a diverse group of experts from different countries, diverse backgrounds, and varied interrelated expertises in a wide range of conditions within the tropical diseases spectrum of diseases, following the One Health approach vision (8, 172).

Grand challenges exist in the fight against the threat of emerging tropical diseases. In the laboratory, our daily work, in the hospitals, in the field, in the community, and in many other places, our shared goal is to understand the drivers of emergence and address their root-causes. We are working collaboratively in social networks to reduce the impact of emerging tropical diseases. Let's work on this together! We value your work and welcome your submissions to this new section of *Frontiers in Tropical Diseases*.

AUTHOR CONTRIBUTIONS

All authors contributed to manuscript conception and design, literature review, manuscript preparation, and critical review. All authors contributed to the article and approved the submitted version.

ACKNOWLEDGMENTS

AR-M is the Specialty Chief Editor in Emerging Tropical Diseases of Frontiers in Tropical Diseases. The remaining authors of this article are their Associate Editors. This is a collaborative article of the Network NHEPACHA.

REFERENCES

1. Alfaro-Toloza P, Clouet-Huerta DE, Rodriguez-Morales AJ. Chikungunya, the Emerging Migratory Rheumatism. *Lancet Infect Dis* (2015) 15(5):510–2. doi: 10.1016/S1473-3099(15)70160-X
2. McArthur DB. Emerging Infectious Diseases. *Nurs Clin North Am* (2019) 54 (2):297–311. doi: 10.1016/j.cnur.2019.02.006
3. Shi Z. Emerging Infectious Diseases Associated With Bat Viruses. *Sci China Life Sci* (2013) 56(8):678–82. doi: 10.1007/s11427-013-4517-x
4. Liu SL, Saif L. Emerging Viruses Without Borders: The Wuhan Coronavirus. *Viruses* (2020) 12(2):130. doi: 10.3390/v12020130
5. Gill CM, Beckham JD, Piquet AL, Tyler KL, Pastula DM. Five Emerging Neuroinvasive Arboviral Diseases: Cache Valley, Eastern Equine

Encephalitis, Jamestown Canyon, Powassan, and Usutu. *Semin Neurol* (2019) 39(4):419–27. doi: 10.1055/s-0039-1687839

6. Millan-Oñate J, Rodríguez-Morales AJ, Camacho-Moreno G, Mendoza-Ramírez H, Rodríguez-Sabogal IA, Álvarez-Moreno C. A New Emerging Zoonotic Virus of Concern: The 2019 Novel Coronavirus (Covid-19). *Infectio* (2020) 24(3):187–92. doi: 10.22354/in.v24i3.848
7. Carrion M, Madoff LC. ProMED-mail: 22 Years of Digital Surveillance of Emerging Infectious Diseases. *Int Health* (2017) 9(3):177–83. doi: 10.1093/inthealth/ihx014
8. Bonilla-Aldana DK, Dhama K, Rodriguez-Morales AJ. Revisiting the One Health Approach in the Context of COVID-19: A Look Into the Ecology of This Emerging Disease. *Adv Anim Vet Sci* (2020) 8(3):234–7. doi: 10.17582/journal.aavs/2020/8.3.234.237
9. de Wit E, van Doremalen N, Falzarano D, Munster VJ. SARS and MERS: Recent Insights Into Emerging Coronaviruses. *Nat Rev Microbiol* (2016) 14 (8):523–34. doi: 10.1038/nrmicro.2016.81
10. Rodriguez-Morales AJ. Zika and Microcephaly in Latin America: An Emerging Threat for Pregnant Travelers? *Travel Med Infect Dis* (2016) 14 (1):5–6. doi: 10.1016/j.tmaid.2016.01.011
11. Rodriguez-Morales AJ, Villamil-Gomez WE, Franco-Paredes C. The Arboviral Burden of Disease Caused by Co-Circulation and Co-Infection of Dengue, Chikungunya and Zika in the Americas. *Travel Med Infect Dis* (2016) 14(3):177–9. doi: 10.1016/j.tmaid.2016.05.004
12. Escalera-Antezana JP, Murillo-Garcia DR, Rodriguez-Morales AJ. Chikungunya in Bolivia: Still a Neglected Disease? *Arch Med Res* (2018) 49(4):288. doi: 10.1016/j.arcmed.2018.09.002
13. Zambrano LI, Sierra M, Lara B, Rodriguez-Nunez I, Medina MT, Lozada-Riascos CO, et al. Estimating and Mapping the Incidence of Dengue and Chikungunya in Honduras During 2015 Using Geographic Information Systems (Gis). *J Infect Public Health* (2017) 10(4):446–56. doi: 10.1016/j.jiph.2016.08.003
14. Bonilla-Aldana DK, Bonilla-Aldana JL, Garcia-Bustos JJ, Lozada CO, Rodriguez-Morales AJ. Geographical Trends of Chikungunya and Zika in the Colombian Amazonian Gateway Department, Caqueta, 2015-2018 - Implications for Public Health and Travel Medicine. *Travel Med Infect Dis* (2020) 35:101481. doi: 10.1016/j.tmaid.2019.101481
15. Rodriguez-Morales AJ, Cardona-Ospina JA, Fernanda Urbano-Garzon S, Sebastian Hurtado-Zapata J. Prevalence of Post-Chikungunya Infection Chronic Inflammatory Arthritis: A Systematic Review and Meta-Analysis. *Arthritis Care Res (Hoboken)* (2016) 68(12):1849–58. doi: 10.1002/acr.22900
16. Rodriguez-Morales AJ, Paniz-Mondolfi AE. Venezuela: Far From the Path to Dengue and Chikungunya Control. *J Clin Virol* (2015) 66:60–1. doi: 10.1016/j.jcv.2015.02.020
17. Villamil-Gomez WE, Guijarro E, Castellanos J, Rodriguez-Morales AJ. Congenital Zika Syndrome With Prolonged Detection of Zika Virus RNA. *J Clin Virol* (2017) 95:52–4. doi: 10.1016/j.jcv.2017.08.010
18. Cardona-Ospina JA, Henao-SanMartin V, Acevedo-Mendoza WF, Nasner-Posso KM, Martinez-Pulgarin DF, Restrepo-Lopez A, et al. Fatal Zika Virus Infection in the Americas: A Systematic Review. *Int J Infect Dis* (2019) 88:49–59. doi: 10.1016/j.ijid.2019.08.033
19. Zambrano LI, Fuentes-Barahona IC, Soto-Fernandez RJ, Zuniga C, da Silva JC, Rodriguez-Morales AJ. Guillain-Barre Syndrome Associated With Zika Virus Infection in Honduras, 2016-2017. *Int J Infect Dis* (2019) 84:136–7. doi: 10.1016/j.ijid.2019.05.008
20. Rodriguez-Morales AJ, Ruiz P, Tabares J, Ossa CA, Yepes-Echeverry MC, Ramirez-Jaramillo V, et al. Mapping the Ecoepidemiology of Zika Virus Infection in Urban and Rural Areas of Pereira, Risaralda, Colombia, 2015-2016: Implications for Public Health and Travel Medicine. *Travel Med Infect Dis* (2017) 18:57–66. doi: 10.1016/j.tmaid.2017.05.004
21. Rodriguez-Morales AJ, Galindo-Marquez ML, Garcia-Loaiza CJ, Sabogal-Roman JA, Marin-Loaiza S, Ayala AF, et al. Mapping Zika Virus Disease Incidence in Valle Del Cauca. *Infection* (2017) 45(1):93–102. doi: 10.1007/s15010-016-0948-1
22. Nishiura H, Mizumoto K, Villamil-Gomez WE, Rodriguez-Morales AJ. Preliminary Estimation of the Basic Reproduction Number of Zika Virus Infection During Colombia Epidemic, 2015-2016. *Travel Med Infect Dis* (2016) 14(3):274–6. doi: 10.1016/j.tmaid.2016.03.016
23. Zambrano LI, Vasquez-Bonilla WO, Fuentes-Barahona IC, Claudio da Silva J, Valle-Reconco JA, Medina MT, et al. Spatial Distribution of Zika in Honduras During 2016-2017 Using Geographic Information Systems (GIS) - Implications for Public Health and Travel Medicine. *Travel Med Infect Dis* (2019) 31:101382. doi: 10.1016/j.tmaid.2019.01.017
24. Hamer DH, Barbre KA, Chen LH, Grobusch MP, Schlagenhauf P, Goorhuis A, et al. Travel-Associated Zika Virus Disease Acquired in the Americas Through February 2016: A GeoSentinel Analysis. *Ann Intern Med* (2017) 166(2):99–108. doi: 10.7326/M16-1842
25. Rifakis PM, Benitez JA, De-la-Paz-Pineda J, Rodriguez-Morales AJ. Epizootics of Yellow Fever in Venezuela (2004-2005): An Emerging Zoonotic Disease. *Ann N Y Acad Sci* (2006) 1081:57–60. doi: 10.1196/annals.1373.005
26. Reno E, Quan NG, Franco-Paredes C, Chastain DB, Chauhan L, Rodriguez-Morales AJ, et al. Prevention of Yellow Fever in Travellers: An Update. *Lancet Infect Dis* (2020) 20(6):e129–e37. doi: 10.1016/S1473-3099(20)30170-5
27. Chaves T, Orduna T, Lepetic A, Macchi A, Verbanaz S, Risquez A, et al. Yellow Fever in Brazil: Epidemiological Aspects and Implications for Travelers. *Travel Med Infect Dis* (2018) 23:1–3. doi: 10.1016/j.tmaid.2018.05.001
28. Ortiz-Martinez Y, Patino-Barbosa AM, Rodriguez-Morales AJ. Yellow Fever in the Americas: The Growing Concern About New Epidemics. *F1000Res* (2017) 6:398. doi: 10.12688/f1000research.11280.1
29. Navarro JC, Arrivillaga-Henriquez J, Salazar-Loor J, Rodriguez-Morales AJ. Covid-19 and Dengue, Co-Epidemics in Ecuador and Other Countries in Latin America: Pushing Strained Health Care Systems Over the Edge. *Travel Med Infect Dis* (2020) 37:101656. doi: 10.1016/j.tmaid.2020.101656
30. Cardona-Ospina JA, Arteaga-Livias K, Villamil-Gomez WE, Perez-Diaz CE, Katterine Bonilla-Aldana D, Mondragon-Cardona A, et al. Dengue and COVID-19, Overlapping Epidemics? An Analysis From Colombia. *J Med Virol* (2021) 93(1):522–7. doi: 10.1002/jmv.26194
31. Zambrano LI, Rodriguez E, Espinoza-Salvado IA, Rodriguez-Morales AJ. Dengue in Honduras and the Americas: The Epidemics are Back! *Travel Med Infect Dis* (2019) 31:101456. doi: 10.1016/j.tmaid.2019.07.012
32. Quintero-Herrera LL, Ramirez-Jaramillo V, Bernal-Gutierrez S, Cardenas-Giraldo EV, Guerrero-Matituy EA, Molina-Delgado AH, et al. Potential Impact of Climatic Variability on the Epidemiology of Dengue in Risaralda, Colombia, 2010-2011. *J Infect Public Health* (2015) 8(3):291–7. doi: 10.1016/j.jiph.2014.11.005
33. Zambrano LI, Rodriguez E, Espinoza-Salvado IA, Fuentes-Barahona IC, Lyra de Oliveira T, Luciano da Veiga G, et al. Spatial Distribution of Dengue in Honduras During 2016-2019 Using a Geographic Information Systems (GIS)-Dengue Epidemic Implications for Public Health and Travel Medicine. *Travel Med Infect Dis* (2019) 32:101517. doi: 10.1016/j.tmaid.2019.101517
34. Navarro JC, Giambalvo D, Hernandez R, Auguste AJ, Tesh RB, Weaver SC, et al. Isolation of Madre De Dios Virus (Orthobunyavirus; Bunyaviridae), an Oropouche Virus Species Reassortant, From a Monkey in Venezuela. *Am J Trop Med Hyg* (2016) 95(2):328–38. doi: 10.4269/ajtmh.15-0679
35. Aguilar PV, Barrett AD, Saeed MF, Watts DM, Russell K, Guevara C, et al. Iquitos Virus: A Novel Reassortant Orthobunyavirus Associated With Human Illness in Peru. *PloS Negl Trop Dis* (2011) 5(9):e1315. doi: 10.1371/journal.pntd.0001315
36. Auguste AJ, Liria J, Forrester NL, Giambalvo D, Moncada M, Long KC, et al. Evolutionary and Ecological Characterization of Mayaro Virus Strains Isolated During an Outbreak, Venezuela, 2010. *Emerg Infect Dis* (2015) 21 (10):1742–50. doi: 10.3201/eid2110.141660
37. Aguilar-Luis MA, Del Valle-Mendoza J, Sandoval I, Silva-Caso W, Mazulis F, Carrillo-Ng H, et al. A Silent Public Health Threat: Emergence of Mayaro Virus and Co-Infection With Dengue in Peru. *BMC Res Notes* (2021) 14 (1):29. doi: 10.1186/s13104-021-05444-8
38. Rodriguez-Morales AJ, Marin-Rincon HA, Sepulveda-Arias JC, Paniz-Mondolfi AE. Assessing the Potential Migration of People From Ebola Affected West African Countries to Latin America. *Travel Med Infect Dis* (2015) 13(3):264–6. doi: 10.1016/j.tmaid.2014.12.015
39. Cruz-Calderon S, Nasner-Posso KM, Alfaro-Toloza P, Paniz-Mondolfi AE, Rodriguez-Morales AJ. A Bibliometric Analysis of Global Ebola Research. *Travel Med Infect Dis* (2015) 13(2):202–4. doi: 10.1016/j.tmaid.2015.02.007

40. Cardona-Ospina JA, Giselle-Badillo A, Calvache-Benavides CE, Rodriguez-Morales AJ. Ebola Virus Disease: An Emerging Zoonosis With Importance for Travel Medicine. *Travel Med Infect Dis* (2014) 12(6 Pt A):682–3. doi: 10.1016/j.tmaid.2014.10.014
41. Rodriguez-Morales AJ, Henao DE, Franco TB, Mayta-Tristan P, Alfaro-Toloza P, Paniz-Mondolfi AE. Ebola: A Latent Threat to Latin America. Are We Ready? *Travel Med Infect Dis* (2014) 12(6 Pt A):688–9. doi: 10.1016/j.tmaid.2014.11.002
42. Patino-Barbosa AM, Arroyave-Valencia F, Garcia-Ramirez LM, Vallejo-Atehortua E, Arciniegas-Pantoja M, Rodriguez-Morales AJ, et al. Healthcare Students' and Workers' Knowledge About Epidemiology and Symptoms of Ebola in One City of Colombia. *J Hosp Infect* (2015) 90(4):356–8. doi: 10.1016/j.jhin.2015.05.001
43. Almeida-Guerrero A, Olaya-Gomez JC, Sanchez-Ramirez N, Murillo-Garcia DR, Cardona-Ospina JA, Lagos-Grisales GJ, et al. Mitigation of the Global Impact of Lassa Fever: Have We Investigated Enough About This Arenavirus? - A Bibliometric Analysis of Lassa Fever Research. *Travel Med Infect Dis* (2018) 24:13–4. doi: 10.1016/j.tmaid.2018.06.012
44. Rodriguez-Morales AJ, Castañeda-Hernández DM, Escalera-Antezana JP, Alvarado-Arnez LE. Organisms of Concern But Not Foodborne or Confirmed Foodborne: Bolivian Hemorrhagic Fever Virus (Machupo Virus)☆. *Reference Module Food Sci: Elsevier* (2019). doi: 10.1016/B978-0-08-100596-5.22639-5
45. Silva-Ramos CR, Faccini-Martínez ÁA, Calixto O-J, Hidalgo M. Bolivian Hemorrhagic Fever: A Narrative Review. *Travel Med Infect Dis* (2021) 40:102001. doi: 10.1016/j.tmaid.2021.102001
46. Escalera-Antezana JP, Rodriguez-Villena OJ, Arancibia-Alba AW, Alvarado-Arnez LE, Bonilla-Aldana DK, Rodriguez-Morales AJ. Clinical Features of Fatal Cases of Chapare Virus Hemorrhagic Fever Originating From Rural La Paz, Bolivia, 2019: A Cluster Analysis. *Travel Med Infect Dis* (2020) 36:101589. doi: 10.1016/j.tmaid.2020.101589
47. Vanella JM, Gonzalez LE, Paglini S, Marquez A. [Laboratory Evidence of the Activity of Junin Virus in the Southeast of Cordoba: Hypothesis on Its Epidemiology]. *Dia Med* (1964) 36:290–1.
48. Rodriguez-Morales AJ. Malaria: An Eradicable Threat? *J Infect Dev Ctries* (2008) 2(1):1–2. doi: 10.3855/jidc.316
49. Rodriguez-Morales AJ, Ramirez-Jaramillo V, Patino-Barbosa AM, Bedoya-Arias HA, Henao-SanMartin V, Murillo-Garcia DR, et al. Severe Fever With Thrombocytopenia Syndrome - A Bibliometric Analysis of an Emerging Priority Disease. *Travel Med Infect Dis* (2018) 23:97–8. doi: 10.1016/j.tmaid.2018.04.010
50. Rodriguez-Morales AJ, Escalera-Antezana JP, Alvarado-Arnez LE. Is Plague Globally Reemerging? *Infectio* (2019) 23:7–9. doi: 10.22354/in.v23i1.748
51. Franco-Paredes C, Villamil-Gomez WE, Schultz J, Henao-Martinez AF, Parra-Henao G, Rassi A Jr, et al. A Deadly Feast: Elucidating the Burden of Orally Acquired Acute Chagas Disease in Latin America - Public Health and Travel Medicine Importance. *Travel Med Infect Dis* (2020) 36:101565. doi: 10.1016/j.tmaid.2020.101565
52. Chadalawada S, Sillau S, Archuleta S, Mundo W, Bandali M, Parra-Henao G, et al. Risk of Chronic Cardiomyopathy Among Patients With the Acute Phase or Indeterminate Form of Chagas Disease: A Systematic Review and Meta-Analysis. *JAMA Netw Open* (2020) 3(8):e2015072. doi: 10.1001/jamanetworkopen.2020.15072
53. Madigan R, Majoy S, Ritter K, Luis Concepcion J, Marquez ME, Silva SC, et al. Investigation of a Combination of Amiodarone and Itraconazole for Treatment of American Trypanosomiasis (Chagas Disease) in Dogs. *J Am Vet Med Assoc* (2019) 255(3):317–29. doi: 10.2460/javma.255.3.317
54. Villamil-Gomez WE, Echeverria LE, Ayala MS, Munoz L, Mejia L, Eyes-Escalante M, et al. Orally Transmitted Acute Chagas Disease in Domestic Travelers in Colombia. *J Infect Public Health* (2017) 10(2):244–6. doi: 10.1016/j.jiph.2016.05.002
55. Villamil-Gomez WE, Calderon-Gomezcaseres A, Rodriguez-Morales AJ. Visceral Leishmaniasis in a Patient With Systemic Lupus Erythematosus From Colombia, Latin America. *Infez Med* (2019) 27(1):106–8.
56. Arteaga-Livias K, Santos-Huerta M, Damaso-Mata B, Panduro-Correa V, Gonzales-Zamora JA, Rodriguez-Morales AJ. Disseminated Cutaneous Leishmaniasis in a Pediatric Patient From Peru. *J Trop Pediatr* (2020). doi: 10.1093/tropej/fmaa051
57. Hernandez-de-Los-Rios A, Murillo-Leon M, Mantilla-Muriel LE, Arenas AF, Vargas-Montes M, Cardona N, et al. Influence of Two Major Toxoplasma Gondii Virulence Factors (ROP16 and ROP18) on the Immune Response of Peripheral Blood Mononuclear Cells to Human Toxoplasmosis Infection. *Front Cell Infect Microbiol* (2019) 9:413. doi: 10.3389/fcimb.2019.00413
58. Pfaff AW, de-la-Torre A, Rochet E, Brunet J, Sabou M, Sauer A, et al. New Clinical and Experimental Insights Into Old World and Neotropical Ocular Toxoplasmosis. *Int J Parasitol* (2014) 44(2):99–107. doi: 10.1016/j.ijpara.2013.09.007
59. El Bissati K, Levigne P, Lykins J, Adlaoui EB, Barkat A, Berraho A, et al. Global Initiative for Congenital Toxoplasmosis: An Observational and International Comparative Clinical Analysis. *Emerg Microbes Infect* (2018) 7(1):1–14. doi: 10.1038/s41426-018-0164-4
60. Rodriguez-Morales AJ, Bonilla-Aldana DK, Idarraga-Bedoya SE, Garcia-Bustos JJ, Cardona-Ospina JA, Faccini-Martinez AA. Epidemiology of Zoonotic Tick-Borne Diseases in Latin America: Are We Just Seeing the Tip of the Iceberg? *F1000Res* (2018) 7:1988. doi: 10.12688/f1000research.17649.1
61. Rodriguez-Morales AJ, Bonilla-Aldana DK, Escalera-Antezana JP, Alvarado-Arnez LE. Research on Babesia: A Bibliometric Assessment of a Neglected Tick-Borne Parasite. *F1000Res* (2018) 7:1987. doi: 10.12688/f1000research.17581.1
62. Cubillos-Angulo JM, Arriaga MB, Melo MGM, Silva EC, Alvarado-Arnez LE, de Almeida AS, et al. Polymorphisms in Interferon Pathway Genes and Risk of Mycobacterium Tuberculosis Infection in Contacts of Tuberculosis Cases in Brazil. *Int J Infect Dis* (2020) 92:21–8. doi: 10.1016/j.ijid.2019.12.013
63. Alvarado-Arnez LE, Amaral EP, Sales-Marques C, Duraes SM, Cardoso CC, Nunes Sarno E, et al. Association of IL10 Polymorphisms and Leprosy: A Meta-Analysis. *PloS One* (2015) 10(9):e0136282. doi: 10.1371/journal.pone.0136282
64. Franco-Paredes C, Marcos LA, Henao-Martinez AF, Rodriguez-Morales AJ, Villamil-Gomez WE, Gotuzzo E, et al. Cutaneous Mycobacterial Infections. *Clin Microbiol Rev* (2018) 32(1):e00069–18. doi: 10.1128/CMR.00069-18
65. Sales-Marques C, Cardoso CC, Alvarado-Arnez LE, Illaramendi X, Sales AM, Hacker MA, et al. Genetic Polymorphisms of the IL6 and NOD2 Genes are Risk Factors for Inflammatory Reactions in Leprosy. *PloS Negl Trop Dis* (2017) 11(7):e0005754. doi: 10.1371/journal.pntd.0005754
66. de Toledo-Pinto TG, Ferreira AB, Ribeiro-Alves M, Rodrigues LS, Batista-Silva LR, Silva BJ, et al. Sting-Dependent 2'-5' Oligoadenylate Synthetase-Like Production is Required for Intracellular Mycobacterium Leprae Survival. *J Infect Dis* (2016) 214(2):311–20. doi: 10.1093/infdis/jiw144
67. Franco-Paredes C, Rodriguez-Morales AJ. Unsolved Matters in Leprosy: A Descriptive Review and Call for Further Research. *Ann Clin Microbiol Antimicrob* (2016) 15(1):33. doi: 10.1186/s12941-016-0149-x
68. Bonilla-Aldana DK, Aguirre-Florez M, Villamizar-Pena R, Gutierrez-Ocampo E, Henao-Martinez JF, Cvetkovic-Vega A, et al. After SARS-CoV-2, Will H5N6 and Other Influenza Viruses Follow the Pandemic Path? *Infez Med* (2020) 28(4):475–85.
69. Philippon DAM, Wu P, Cowling BJ, Lau EHY. Avian Influenza Human Infections At the Human-Animal Interface. *J Infect Dis* (2020) 222(4):528–37. doi: 10.1093/infdis/jiaa105
70. Dhama K, Chauhan R, Kataria J, Mahesh M, Simmi T. Avian Influenza: The Current Perspectives. *J Immunol Immunopathol* (2005) 7(2):1–33.
71. Chandy S, Mathai D. Globally Emerging Hantaviruses: An Overview. *Indian J Med Microbiol* (2017) 35(2):165–75. doi: 10.4103/ijmm.IJMM_16_429
72. Kruger DH, Figueiredo LTM, Song J-W, Klempa B. Hantaviruses—Globally Emerging Pathogens. *J Clin Virol* (2015) 64:128–36. doi: 10.1016/j.jcv.2014.08.033
73. Enria DA, Pinheiro F. Rodent-Borne Emerging Viral Zoonosis: Hemorrhagic Fevers and Hantavirus Infections in South America. *Infect Dis Clinics North America* (2000) 14(1):167–84. doi: 10.1016/S0891-5520(05)70223-3
74. Chand S, Thapa S, Kon S, Johnson SC, Poeschla EM, Franco-Paredes C, et al. Hantavirus Infection With Renal Failure and Proteinuria, Colorado, USA, 2019. *Emerg Infect Dis* (2020) 26(2):383–5. doi: 10.3201/eid2602.191349
75. Escalera-Antezana JP, Torrez-Fernandez R, Montalvan-Plata D, Montenegro-Narvaez CM, Aviles-Sarmiento JL, Alvarado-Arnez LE, et al.

Orthohantavirus Pulmonary Syndrome in Santa Cruz and Tarija, Bolivia, 2018. *Int J Infect Dis* (2020) 90:145–50. doi: 10.1016/j.ijid.2019.10.021
76. Gomez-Marin JE, Londono AL, Cabeza-Acevedo N, Torres E, Navarrete-Moncada L, Bueno O, et al. Ocular Toxocariasis in Parasitology Consultation in Quindio, Colombia: Description of Cases and Contact Studies. *J Trop Pediatr* (2021) 67(1):fmaa096. doi: 10.1093/tropej/fmaa096
77. Rodriguez-Morales AJ, Bonilla-Aldana DK, Gallego-Valencia V, Gómez-DeLaRosa SH, López-Echeverri C, Peña-Verjan NM, et al. Toxocariasis in Colombia: More Than Neglected. *Curr Trop Med Rep* (2020) 7(1):17–24. doi: 10.1007/s40475-020-00199-x
78. Bonilla-Aldana DK, Cardona-Trujillo MC, Garcia-Barco A, Holguin-Rivera Y, Cortes-Bonilla I, Bedoya-Arias HA, et al. Mers-CoV and SARS-CoV Infections in Animals: A Systematic Review and Meta-Analysis of Prevalence Studies. *Infez Med* (2020) 28(suppl 1):71–83. doi: 10.20944/preprints202003.0103.v1
79. Dhama K, Patel SK, Sharun K, Pathak M, Tiwari R, Yatoo MI, et al. Sars-CoV-2 Jumping the Species Barrier: Zoonotic Lessons From SARS, MERS and Recent Advances to Combat This Pandemic Virus. *Travel Med Infect Dis* (2020) 37:101830. doi: 10.1016/j.tmaid.2020.101830
80. Rabaan AA, Al-Ahmed SH, Haque S, Sah R, Tiwari R, Malik YS, et al. SARS-Cov-2, SARS-CoV, and MERS-COV: A Comparative Overview. *Infez Med* (2020) 28(2):174–84.
81. Bonilla-Aldana DK, Quintero-Rada K, Montoya-Posada JP, Ramirez-Ocampo S, Paniz-Mondolfi A, Rabaan AA, et al. SARS-Cov, MERS-CoV and Now the 2019-Novel CoV: Have We Investigated Enough About Coronaviruses? - *A Bibliometric Analysis Travel Med Infect Dis* (2020) 33:101566. doi: 10.1016/j.tmaid.2020.101566
82. Al-Tawfiq JA, Rodriguez-Morales AJ. Super-Spreading Events and Contribution to Transmission of MERS, SARS, and SARS-CoV-2 (Covid-19). *J Hosp Infect* (2020) 105(2):111–2. doi: 10.1016/j.jhin.2020.04.002
83. Sanchez-Duque JA, Arce-Villalobos LR, Rodriguez-Morales AJ. [Coronavirus Disease 2019 (COVID-19) in Latin America: Role of Primary Care in Preparedness and Response]. *Aten Primaria* (2020) 52 (6):369–72. doi: 10.1016/j.aprim.2020.04.001
84. Dhama K, Khan S, Tiwari R, Sircar S, Bhat S, Malik YS, et al. Coronavirus Disease 2019-COVID-19. *Clin Microbiol Rev* (2020) 33(4):e00028–20. doi: 10.1128/CMR.00028-20
85. Hashem NM, Gonzalez-Bulnes A, Rodriguez-Morales AJ. Animal Welfare and Livestock Supply Chain Sustainability Under the COVID-19 Outbreak: An Overview. *Front Vet Sci* (2020) 7:582528. doi: 10.3389/fvets.2020.582528
86. Herrera-Anazco P, Uyen-Cateriano A, Mezones-Holguin E, Taype-Rondan A, Mayta-Tristan P, Malaga G, et al. Some Lessons That Peru did Not Learn Before the Second Wave of COVID-19. *Int J Health Plann Manage* (2021). doi: 10.1002/hpm.3135
87. Carrillo-Hernandez MY, Ruiz-Saenz J, Villamizar LJ, Gomez-Rangel SY, Martinez-Gutierrez M. Co-Circulation and Simultaneous Co-Infection of Dengue, Chikungunya, and Zika Viruses in Patients With Febrile Syndrome At the Colombian-Venezuelan Border. *BMC Infect Dis* (2018) 18(1):61. doi: 10.1186/s12879-018-2976-1
88. Haqqi A, Awan UA, Ali M, Saqib MAN, Ahmed H, Afzal MS. Covid-19 and Dengue Virus Coepidemics in Pakistan: A Dangerous Combination for an Overburdened Healthcare System. *J Med Virol* (2021) 93(1):80–2. doi: 10.1002/jmv.26144
89. Sanchez-Duque JA, Orozco-Hernandez JP, Marin-Medina DS, Cvetkovic-Vega A, Aveiro-Robalo TR, Mondragon-Cardona A, et al. Are We Now Observing an Increasing Number of Coinfections Between SARS-CoV-2 and Other Respiratory Pathogens? *J Med Virol* (2020) 92(11):2398–400. doi: 10.1002/jmv.26089
90. Alberca RW, Yendo TM, Leuzzi Ramos YA, Fernandes IG, Oliveira LM, Teixeira FME, et al. Case Report: Covid-19 and Chagas Disease in Two Coinfected Patients. *Am J Trop Med Hyg* (2020) 103(6):2353–6. doi: 10.4269/ajtmh.20-1185
91. Touzard-Romo F, Tape C, Lonks JR. Co-Infection With SARS-CoV-2 and Human Metapneumovirus. *R I Med J (2013)* (2020) 103(2):75–6.
92. Rodriguez JA, Rubio-Gomez H, Roa AA, Miller N, Eckardt PA. Co-Infection With SARS-COV-2 and Parainfluenza in a Young Adult Patient With Pneumonia: Case Report. *IDCases* (2020) 20:e00762. doi: 10.1016/j.idcr.2020.e00762
93. Rodriguez-Morales AJ, Suarez JA, Risquez A, Delgado-Noguera L, Paniz-Mondolfi A. The Current Syndemic in Venezuela: Measles, Malaria and More Co-Infections Coupled With a Breakdown of Social and Healthcare Infrastructure. Quo Vadis? *Travel Med Infect Dis* (2019) 27:5–8. doi: 10.1016/j.tmaid.2018.10.010
94. Villamil-Gomez WE, Gonzalez-Camargo O, Rodriguez-Ayubi J, Zapata-Serpa D, Rodriguez-Morales AJ. Dengue, Chikungunya and Zika Co-Infection in a Patient From Colombia. *J Infect Public Health* (2016) 9 (5):684–6. doi: 10.1016/j.jiph.2015.12.002
95. Paniz-Mondolfi AE, Rodriguez-Morales AJ, Blohm G, Marquez M, Villamil-Gomez WE. Chikdenmazika Syndrome: The Challenge of Diagnosing Arboviral Infections in the Midst of Concurrent Epidemics. *Ann Clin Microbiol Antimicrob* (2016) 15(1):42. doi: 10.1186/s12941-016-0157-x
96. Villamil-Gomez WE, Rodriguez-Morales AJ, Uribe-Garcia AM, Gonzalez-Arismendy E, Castellanos JE, Calvo EP, et al. Zika, Dengue, and Chikungunya Co-Infection in a Pregnant Woman From Colombia. *Int J Infect Dis* (2016) 51:135–8. doi: 10.1016/j.ijid.2016.07.017
97. Villamil-Gomez WE, Rodriguez-Morales AJ. Reply: Dengue RT-PCR-Positive, Chikungunya IgM-positive and Zika Rt-PCR-positive Co-Infection in a Patient From Colombia. *J Infect Public Health* (2017) 10 (1):133–4. doi: 10.1016/j.jiph.2016.02.003
98. Villamil-Gomez WE, Silvera LA, Henao-Palencia S, Contreras-Arrieta J, Caceres JF, Ortiz-Martinez Y, et al. Coinfection of Trypanosoma Cruzi and Mycobacterium Tuberculosis in a Patient From Colombia. *J Infect Public Health* (2016) 9(1):113–5. doi: 10.1016/j.jiph.2015.09.004
99. Rifakis PM, Benitez JA, Rodriguez-Morales AJ, Dickson SM, De-La-Paz-Pineda J. Ecoepidemiological and Social Factors Related to Rabies Incidence in Venezuela During 2002-2004. *Int J BioMed Sci* (2006) 2(1):1–6.
100. Macleod CK, Bright P, Steer AC, Kim J, Mabey D, Parks T. Neglecting the Neglected: The Objective Evidence of Underfunding in Rheumatic Heart Disease. *Trans R Soc Trop Med Hyg* (2019) 113(5):287–90. doi: 10.1093/trstmh/trz014
101. Rodriguez-Morales AJ, Sánchez-Duque JA, Hernández-Botero S, Pérez-Díaz CE, Villamil-Gómez WE, Méndez CA, et al. Preparación Y Control De La Enfermedad Por Coronavirus 2019 (COVID-19) En América Latina. *Acta Med Peruana* (2020) 37(1):3–7. doi: 10.35663/amp.2020.371.909
102. Pathak M, Patel SK, Jigyasa R, Tiwari R, Dhama K, Sah R, et al. Global Threat of SARS-CoV-2/COVID-19 and the Need for More and Better Diagnostic Tools. *Arch Med Res* (2020) 51(5):450–2. doi: 10.1016/j.arcmed.2020.04.003
103. Mousavi SH, Zahid SU, Wardak K, Azimi KA, Reza Hosseini SM, Wafaee M, et al. Mapping the Changes on Incidence, Case Fatality Rates and Recovery Proportion of COVID-19 in Afghanistan Using Geographical Information Systems. *Arch Med Res* (2020) 51(6):600–2. doi: 10.1016/j.arcmed.2020.06.010
104. Cimerman S, Chebabo A, Cunha CAD, Rodriguez-Morales AJ. Deep Impact of COVID-19 in the Healthcare of Latin America: The Case of Brazil. *Braz J Infect Dis* (2020) 24(2):93–5. doi: 10.1016/j.bjid.2020.04.005
105. Rodriguez-Morales AJ, Rodriguez-Morales AG, Mendez CA, Hernandez-Botero S. Tracing New Clinical Manifestations in Patients With COVID-19 in Chile and Its Potential Relationship With the SARS-CoV-2 Divergence. *Curr Trop Med Rep* (2020) 7:75–8. doi: 10.1007/s40475-020-00205-2
106. Bonilla-Aldana DK, Villamil-Gómez WE, Rabaan AA, Rodriguez-Morales AJ. Una Nueva Zoonosis Viral De Preocupación Global: COVID-19, Enfermedad Por Coronavirus 2019. *Iatreia* (2020) 33(2):107–10. doi: 10.17533/udea.iatreia.85
107. Rodriguez-Morales AJ, Balbin-Ramon GJ, Rabaan AA, Sah R, Dhama K, Paniz-Mondolfi A, et al. Genomic Epidemiology and its Importance in the Study of the COVID-19 Pandemic. *Infez Med* (2020) 28(2):139–42.
108. Ahmad T, Khan M, Haroon, Musa TH, Nasir S, Hui J, et al. Covid-19: Zoonotic Aspects. *Travel Med Infect Dis* (2020) 36:101607. doi: 10.1016/j.tmaid.2020.101607
109. Escalera-Antezana JP, Lizon-Ferrufino NF, Maldonado-Alanoca A, Alarcon-De-la-Vega G, Alvarado-Arnez LE, Balderrama-Saavedra MA, et al. Clinical Features of the First Cases and a Cluster of Coronavirus Disease 2019 (Covid-19) in Bolivia Imported From Italy and Spain. *Travel Med Infect Dis* (2020) 35:101653. doi: 10.1016/j.tmaid.2020.101653
110. Rodriguez-Morales AJ, Cardona-Ospina JA, Gutierrez-Ocampo E, Villamizar-Pena R, Holguin-Rivera Y, Escalera-Antezana JP, et al.

Clinical, Laboratory and Imaging Features of COVID-19: A Systematic Review and Meta-Analysis. *Travel Med Infect Dis* (2020) 34:101623. doi: 10.1016/j.tmaid.2020.101623

111. Rodriguez-Morales AJ, Gallego V, Escalera-Antezana JP, Mendez CA, Zambrano LI, Franco-Paredes C, et al. Covid-19 in Latin America: The Implications of the First Confirmed Case in Brazil. *Travel Med Infect Dis* (2020) 35:101613. doi: 10.1016/j.tmaid.2020.101613
112. Ahmad T, Haroon , Dhama K, Sharun K, FM K, Ahmed I, et al. Biosafety and Biosecurity Approaches to Restrain/Contain and Counter SARS-CoV-2/ Covid-19 Pandemic: A Rapid-Review. *Turk J Biol* (2020) 44(Special issue 1):132–45. doi: 10.3906/biy-2005-63
113. Nuraini N, Fauzi IS, Fakhruddin M, Sopaheluwakan A, Soewono E. Climate-Based Dengue Model in Semarang, Indonesia: Predictions and Descriptive Analysis. *Infect Dis Model* (2021) 6:598–611. doi: 10.1016/j.idm.2021.03.005
114. Hussen MO, Sayed ASM, Abushahba MFN. Sero-Epidemiological Study on Dengue Fever Virus in Humans and Camels At Upper Egypt. *Vet World* (2020) 13(12):2618–24. doi: 10.14202/vetworld.2020.2618-2624
115. Ryan SJ, Carlson CJ, Mordecai EA, Johnson LR. Global Expansion and Redistribution of Aedes-borne Virus Transmission Risk With Climate Change. *PloS Negl Trop Dis* (2019) 13(3):e0007213. doi: 10.1371/ journal.pntd.0007213
116. Alarcon-Elbal PM, Rodriguez-Sosa MA, Newman BC, Sutton WB. The First Record of Aedes Vittatus (Diptera: Culicidae) in the Dominican Republic: Public Health Implications of a Potential Invasive Mosquito Species in the Americas. *J Med Entomol* (2020) 57(6):2016–21. doi: 10.1093/jme/tjaa128
117. Chowdhury FR, Ibrahim QSU, Bari MS, Alam MMJ, Dunachie SJ, Rodriguez-Morales AJ, et al. The Association Between Temperature, Rainfall and Humidity With Common Climate-Sensitive Infectious Diseases in Bangladesh. *PloS One* (2018) 13(6):e0199579. doi: 10.1371/journal.pone.0199579
118. Rodriguez-Morales AJ. Climate Change, Climate Variability and Brucellosis. *Recent Pat Antiinfect Drug Discovery* (2013) 8(1):4–12. doi: 10.2174/ 1574891X11308010003
119. Rodriguez-Morales AJ. [Climate Change, Rainfall, Society and Disasters in Latin America: Relations and Needs]. *Rev Peru Med Exp Salud Publica* (2011) 28(1):165–6. doi: 10.1590/S1726-46342011000100032
120. Chowdhury FR, Ibrahim QSU, Bari MS, Alam MMJ, Dunachie SJ, Rodriguez-Morales AJ, et al. Correction: The Association Between Temperature, Rainfall and Humidity With Common Climate-Sensitive Infectious Diseases in Bangladesh. *PloS One* (2020) 15(4):e0232285. doi: 10.1371/journal.pone.0232285
121. Mattar S, Morales V, Cassab A, Rodriguez-Morales AJ. Effect of Climate Variables on Dengue Incidence in a Tropical Caribbean Municipality of Colombia, Cerete, 2003-2008. *Int J Infect Dis* (2013) 17(5):e358–9. doi: 10.1016/j.ijid.2012.11.021
122. Cardenas R, Sandoval CM, Rodriguez-Morales AJ, Franco-Paredes C. Impact of Climate Variability in the Occurrence of Leishmaniasis in Northeastern Colombia. *Am J Trop Med Hyg* (2006) 75(2):273–7. doi: 10.4269/ ajtmh.2006.75.273
123. Zambrano LI, Sevilla C, Reyes-Garcia SZ, Sierra M, Kafati R, Rodriguez-Morales AJ, et al. Potential Impacts of Climate Variability on Dengue Hemorrhagic Fever in Honduras, 2010. *Trop BioMed* (2012) 29(4):499–507.
124. Herrera-Martinez AD, Rodriguez-Morales AJ. Potential Influence of Climate Variability on Dengue Incidence Registered in a Western Pediatric Hospital of Venezuela. *Trop BioMed* (2010) 27(2):280–6.
125. Cardenas R, Sandoval CM, Rodriguez-Morales AJ, Vivas P. Zoonoses and Climate Variability. *Ann N Y Acad Sci* (2008) 1149:326–30. doi: 10.1196/ annals.1428.094
126. Rodriguez-Morales AJ, Simon F. Chronic Chikungunya, Still to be Fully Understood. *Int J Infect Dis* (2019) 86:133–4. doi: 10.1016/j.ijid.2019.07.024
127. Rodriguez-Morales AJ, Cardona-Ospina JA, Villamil-Gomez W, Paniz-Mondolfi AE. How Many Patients With Post-Chikungunya Chronic Inflammatory Rheumatism can We Expect in the New Endemic Areas of Latin America? *Rheumatol Int* (2015) 35(12):2091–4. doi: 10.1007/s00296-015-3302-5
128. Rodriguez-Morales AJ, Restrepo-Posada VM, Acevedo-Escalante N, Rodriguez-Munoz ED, Valencia-Marin M, Castrillon-Spitia JD, et al. Impaired Quality of Life After Chikungunya Virus Infection: A 12-Month Follow-Up Study of its Chronic Inflammatory Rheumatism in La Virginia, Risaralda, Colombia. *Rheumatol Int* (2017) 37(10):1757–8. doi: 10.1007/ s00296-017-3795-1
129. Rodriguez-Morales AJ. Letter to the Editor: Chikungunya Virus Infection-an Update on Chronic Rheumatism in Latin America. *Rambam Maimonides Med J* (2017) 8(1):e0013. doi: 10.5041/RMMJ.10288
130. Rodriguez-Morales AJ, Villamil-Gomez W, Merlano-Espinosa M, Simone-Kleber L. Post-Chikungunya Chronic Arthralgia: A First Retrospective Follow-Up Study of 39 Cases in Colombia. *Clin Rheumatol* (2016) 35 (3):831–2. doi: 10.1007/s10067-015-3041-8
131. Rodriguez-Morales AJ, Calvache-Benavides CE, Giraldo-Gomez J, Hurtado-Hurtado N, Yepes-Echeverri MC, Garcia-Loaiza CJ, et al. Post-Chikungunya Chronic Arthralgia: Results From a Retrospective Follow-Up Study of 131 Cases in Tolima, Colombia. *Travel Med Infect Dis* (2016) 14(1):58–9. doi: 10.1016/j.tmaid.2015.09.001
132. Rodriguez-Morales AJ, Gil-Restrepo AF, Ramirez-Jaramillo V, Montoya-Arias CP, Acevedo-Mendoza WF, Bedoya-Arias JE, et al. Post-Chikungunya Chronic Inflammatory Rheumatism: Results From a Retrospective Follow-Up Study of 283 Adult and Child Cases in La Virginia, Risaralda, Colombia. *F1000Res* (2016) 5:360. doi: 10.12688/ f1000research.8235.2
133. Alvarado-Socarras JL, Idrovo AJ, Contreras-Garcia GA, Rodriguez-Morales AJ, Audcent TA, Mogollon-Mendoza AC, et al. Congenital Microcephaly: A Diagnostic Challenge During Zika Epidemics. *Travel Med Infect Dis* (2018) 23:14–20. doi: 10.1016/j.tmaid.2018.02.002
134. Rodriguez-Morales AJ, Cardona-Ospina JA, Ramirez-Jaramillo V, Gaviria JA, Gonzalez-Moreno GM, Castrillon-Spitia JD, et al. Diagnosis and Outcomes of Pregnant Women With Zika Virus Infection in Two Municipalities of Risaralda, Colombia: Second Report of the ZIKERNCOL Study. *Travel Med Infect Dis* (2018) 25:20–5. doi: 10.1016/j.tmaid.2018.06.006
135. Alvarado-Socarras JL, Aux-Cadena CP, Murillo-Garcia DR, Rodriguez-Morales AJ. Ophthalmologic Evaluation in Infants of Mothers With Zika: A Report From Colombia. *Travel Med Infect Dis* (2019) 32:101449. doi: 10.1016/j.tmaid.2019.07.005
136. Wijeratne T, Crewther S. Covid-19 and Long-Term Neurological Problems: Challenges Ahead With Post-COVID-19 Neurological Syndrome. *Aust J Gen Pract* (2021) 50. doi: 10.31128/AJGP-COVID-43
137. Chun HJ, Coutavas E, Pine A, Lee AI, Yu V, Shallow M, et al. Immuno-Fibrotic Drivers of Impaired Lung Function in post-COVID-19 Syndrome. *medRxiv* (2021). doi: 10.1101/2021.01.31.21250870
138. Soriano JB, Waterer G, Penalvo JL, Rello J. Nefer, Sinuhe and Clinical Research Assessing post-COVID-19 Syndrome. *Eur Respir J* (2021). doi: 10.1183/13993003.04423-2020
139. Borg K, Stam HJ. Rehabilitation of post-Covid - 19 Syndrome - Once Again a Call for Action! *J Rehabil Med* (2021) 53(1):jrm00132. doi: 10.2340/ 16501977-2783
140. Walsh DP, Ma TF, Ip HS, Zhu J. Artificial Intelligence and Avian Influenza: Using Machine Learning to Enhance Active Surveillance for Avian Influenza Viruses. *Transbound Emerg Dis* (2019) 66(6):2537–45. doi: 10.1111/ tbed.13318
141. Thiebaut R, Cossin S. Section Editors for the IYSoPH, Epidemiology I. Artificial Intelligence for Surveillance in Public Health. *Yearb Med Inform* (2019) 28(1):232–4. doi: 10.1055/s-0039-1677939
142. Chiappelli F, Balenton N, Khakshooy A. Future Innovations in Viral Immune Surveillance: A Novel Place for Bioinformation and Artificial Intelligence in the Administration of Health Care. *Bioinformation* (2018) 14(5):201–5. doi: 10.6026/97320630014201
143. Cardona-Ospina JA, Rojas-Gallardo DM, Garzon-Castano SC, Jimenez-Posada EV, Rodriguez-Morales AJ. Phylodynamic Analysis in the Understanding of the Current COVID-19 Pandemic and its Utility in Vaccine and Antiviral Design and Assessment. *Hum Vaccin Immunother* (2021), 1–8. doi: 10.1080/21645515.2021.1880254
144. Rabaan AA, Al-Ahmed SH, Sah R, Al-Tawfiq JA, Haque S, Harapan H, et al. Genomic Epidemiology and Recent Update on Nucleic Acid-Based Diagnostics for COVID-19. *Curr Trop Med Rep* (2020) 7:113–9. doi: 10.1007/s40475-020-00212-3
145. Auguste AJ, Lemey P, Bergren NA, Giambalvo D, Moncada M, Moron D, et al. Enzootic Transmission of Yellow Fever Virus, Venezuela. *Emerg Infect Dis* (2015) 21(1):99–102. doi: 10.3201/eid2101.140814

146. Solano D, Navarro JC, Leon-Reyes A, Benitez-Ortiz W, Rodriguez-Hidalgo R. Molecular Analyses Reveal Two Geographic and Genetic Lineages for Tapeworms, Taenia Solium and Taenia Saginata, From Ecuador Using Mitochondrial DNA. *Exp Parasitol* (2016) 171:49–56. doi: 10.1016/j.exppara.2016.10.015
147. Rendon-Marin S, Martinez-Gutierrez M, Whittaker GR, Jaimes JA, Ruiz-Saenz J. Sars CoV-2 Spike Protein in Silico Interaction With ACE2 Receptors From Wild and Domestic Species. *Front Genet* (2021) 12(27):571707. doi: 10.3389/fgene.2021.571707
148. Elsinga J, Grobusch MP, Tami A, Gerstenbluth I, Bailey A. Health-Related Impact on Quality of Life and Coping Strategies for Chikungunya: A Qualitative Study in Curacao. *PloS Negl Trop Dis* (2017) 11(10):e0005987. doi: 10.1371/journal.pntd.0005987
149. Proos R, Matheron H, Vas Nunes J, Falama A, Sery Kamal P, Grobusch MP, et al. Perspectives of Health Workers on the Referral of Women With Obstetric Complications: A Qualitative Study in Rural Sierra Leone. *BMJ Open* (2020) 10(12):e041746. doi: 10.1136/bmjopen-2020-041746
150. Porta M. *A Dictionary of Epidemiology: Books.Google.Com.* International Association of Epidemiology and Oxford Press (2014). doi: 10.1093/acref/9780199976720.001.0001
151. Rodríguez-Morales AJ. Ecoepidemiología Y Epidemiología Satelital: Nuevas Herramientas En El Manejo De Problemas En Salud Pública. *Rev Peruana Medicina Exp y Salud Publica* (2005) 22:54–63.
152. Brende B, Farrar J, Gashumba D, Moedas C, Mundel T, Shiozaki Y, et al. CEPI-a New Global R&D Organisation for Epidemic Preparedness and Response. *Lancet* (2017) 389(10066):233–5. doi: 10.1016/S0140-6736(17)30131-9
153. Gouglas D, Christodoulou M, Plotkin SA, Hatchett R. Cepi: Driving Progress Toward Epidemic Preparedness and Response. *Epidemiol Rev* (2019) 41 (1):28–33. doi: 10.1093/epirev/mxz012
154. Plotkin SA. Vaccines for Epidemic Infections and the Role of CEPI. *Hum Vaccin Immunother* (2017) 13(12):2755–62. doi: 10.1080/21645515.2017.1306615
155. de Sousa Pereira H, Scofield A, Junior PSB, Lira Dos Santos D, de Sousa Siqueira J, Chaves JF, et al. Chagas Disease in Urban and Periurban Environment in the Amazon: Sentinel Hosts, Vectors, and the Environment. *Acta Trop* (2021) 217:105858. doi: 10.1016/j.actatropica.2021.105858
156. Bastos CJ, Aras R, Mota G, Reis F, Dias JP, de Jesus RS, et al. Clinical Outcomes of Thirteen Patients With Acute Chagas Disease Acquired Through Oral Transmission From Two Urban Outbreaks in Northeastern Brazil. *PloS Negl Trop Dis* (2010) 4(6):e711. doi: 10.1371/journal.pntd.0000711
157. Shikanai-Yasuda MA, Carvalho NB. Oral Transmission of Chagas Disease. *Clin Infect Dis* (2012) 54(6):845–52. doi: 10.1093/cid/cir956
158. Noya BA, Perez-Chacon G, Diaz-Bello Z, Dickson S, Munoz-Calderon A, Hernandez C, et al. Description of an Oral Chagas Disease Outbreak in Venezuela, Including a Vertically Transmitted Case. *Mem Inst Oswaldo Cruz* (2017) 112(8):569–71. doi: 10.1590/0074-02760170009
159. Diaz ML, Leal S, Mantilla JC, Molina-Berrios A, Lopez-Munoz R, Solari A, et al. Acute Chagas Outbreaks: Molecular and Biological Features of Trypanosoma Cruzi Isolates, and Clinical Aspects of Acute Cases in Santander, Colombia. *Parasit Vectors* (2015) 8:608. doi: 10.1186/s13071-015-1218-2
160. Rueda K, Trujillo JE, Carranza JC, Vallejo GA. [Oral Transmission of Trypanosoma Cruzi : A New Epidemiological Scenario for Chagas' Disease in Colombia and Other South American Countries]. *Biomedica* (2014) 34 (4):631–41. doi: 10.7705/biomedica.v34i4.2204
161. Lacerda AFA, Oliveria DS, Salomao JVF, Oliveira LGR, Monte-Alegre A, Santos J, et al. Clinical, Epidemiological and Transmission Cycle Aspects of Leishmaniasis Urbanization in Barreiras, Bahia, Brazil. *Spat Spatiotemporal Epidemiol* (2021) 36:100395. doi: 10.1016/j.sste.2020.100395
162. da Silva Santana Cruz C, Soeiro Barbosa D, Oliveira VC, Cardoso DT, Guimaraes NS, Carneiro M. Factors Associated With Human Visceral Leishmaniasis Cases During Urban Epidemics in Brazil: A Systematic Review. *Parasitology* (2021) 148 (6):639–47. doi: 10.1017/S0031182021000019
163. Ribeiro CJN, Dos Santos AD, Lima S, da Silva ER, Ribeiro BVS, Duque AM, et al. Space-Time Risk Cluster of Visceral Leishmaniasis in Brazilian Endemic Region With High Social Vulnerability: An Ecological Time Series Study. *PloS Negl Trop Dis* (2021) 15(1):e0009006. doi: 10.1371/journal.pntd.0009006
164. Zambrano-Hernandez P, Ayala-Sotelo MS, Fuya-Oviedo P, Montenegro-Puentes CA, Aya-Vanegas NM, Aguilera-Jaramillo G, et al. [Urban Outbreak of Visceral Leishmaniasis in Neiva (Colombia)]. *Rev Salud Publica (Bogota)* (2015) 17(4):514–27. doi: 10.15446/rsap.v17n4.44663
165. Osorio-Pinzon J, Palencia A, Cruz-Calderon S, Rodriguez-Morales AJ. Myiasis and Tungiasis. *Curr Trop Med Rep* (2021). doi: 10.1007/s40475-021-00233-6
166. Shepard Z, Rios M, Solis J, Wand T, Henao-Martínez AF, Franco-Paredes C, et al. Common Dermatologic Conditions in Returning Travelers. *Curr Trop Med Rep* (2021). doi: 10.1007/s40475-021-00231-8
167. Pecchio M, Suarez JA, Hesse S, Hersh AM, Gundacker ND. Descriptive Epidemiology of Snakebites in the Veraguas Province of Panama, 2007-2008. *Trans R Soc Trop Med Hyg* (2018) 112(10):463–6. doi: 10.1093/trstmh/try076
168. Reyes-Lugo M, Sanchez T, Finol HJ, Sanchez EE, Suarez JA, Guerreiro B, et al. Neurotoxic Activity and Ultrastructural Changes in Muscles Caused by the Brown Widow Spider Latrodectus Geometricus Venom. *Rev Inst Med Trop Sao Paulo* (2009) 51(2):95–101. doi: 10.1590/S0036-46652009000200007
169. Benitez JA, Rifakis PM, Vargas JA, Cabaniel G, Rodriguez-Morales AJ. Trends in Fatal Snakebites in Venezuela, 1995-2002. *Wilderness Environ Med* (2007) 18(3):209–13. doi: 10.1580/06-WEME-BR-076R.1
170. De Roodt AR, Salomon OD, Lloveras SC, Orduna TA. [Poisoning by Spiders of Loxosceles Genus]. *Medicina (B Aires)* (2002) 62(1):83–94.
171. Bonilla-Aldana DK, Suarez JA, Franco-Paredes C, Vilcarromero S, Mattar S, Gomez-Marin JE, et al. Brazil Burning! What is the Potential Impact of the Amazon Wildfires on Vector-Borne and Zoonotic Emerging Diseases? - A Statement From an International Experts Meeting. *Travel Med Infect Dis* (2019) 31:101474. doi: 10.1016/j.tmaid.2019.101474
172. Bonilla-Aldana DK, Holguin-Rivera Y, Perez-Vargas S, Trejos-Mendoza AE, Balbin-Ramon GJ, Dhama K, et al. Importance of the One Health Approach to Study the SARS-CoV-2 in Latin America. *One Health* (2020) 10:100147. doi: 10.1016/j.onehlt.2020.100147

Dogs as New Hosts for the Emerging Zoonotic Pathogen *Anaplasma capra*

Ke Shi[1,2†], *Junqiang Li*[1,3†], *Yaqun Yan*[1,2], *Qian Chen*[1], *Kunlun Wang*[1], *Yongchun Zhou*[1], *Dongfang Li*[1], *Yuancai Chen*[1], *Fuchang Yu*[1,2], *Yongshuai Peng*[1], *Longxian Zhang*[1,2] and *Changshen Ning*[1,2*]

[1] College of Animal Science and Veterinary Medicine, Henan Agricultural University, Zhengzhou, China, [2] International Joint Research Laboratory for Zoonotic Diseases of Henan, Zhengzhou, China, [3] Scientific Research Experiment Center & Laboratory Animal Center, Henan University of Chinese Medicine, Zhengzhou, China

***Correspondence:**
Changshen Ning
nnl1986@163.com

† These authors have contributed equally to this work

Anaplasma capra is an emerging zoonotic tick-borne pathogen with a broad host range, including many mammals. Dogs have close physical interactions with humans and regular contact with the external environment. Moreover, they have been previously reported to be hosts of *Anaplasma phagocytophilum*, *A. platys*, *A. ovis*, and *A. bovis*. To confirm whether dogs are also hosts of *A. capra*, pathogen DNA was extracted from blood samples of 521 dogs, followed by PCR amplification of the citrate synthase (*gltA*) gene, heat shock protein (*groEL*) gene, and major surface protein 4 (*msp4*) gene of the *A. capra*. A total of 12.1% (63/521) of blood samples were shown to be *A. capra*-positive by PCR screening. No significant differences were observed between genders ($P = 0.578$) or types ($P = 0.154$) of dogs with *A. capra* infections. However, significantly higher *A. capra* infections occurred in dogs with regular contact with vegetation ($P = 0.002$), those aged over 10 years ($P = 0.040$), and during the summer season ($P = 0.006$). Phylogenetic analysis based on *gltA*, *groEL*, and *msp4* sequences demonstrated that the isolates obtained in this study were clustered within the *A. capra* clade, and were distinct from other *Anaplasma* species. In conclusion, dogs were shown to be a host of the human pathogenic *A. capra*. Considering the affinity between dogs and humans and the zoonotic tick-borne nature of *A. capra*, dogs should be carefully monitored for the presence of *A. capra*.

Keywords: *Anaplasma capra*, dogs, hosts, tick-borne, zoonotic

INTRODUCTION

Vector-borne diseases are major causes of morbidity and mortality in dogs and are potentially of great public health importance because of their zoonotic nature and the role of pets as reservoirs (Xu et al., 2015; Cui et al., 2017; Maggi and Krämer, 2019). In the last few years, the number and range of species kept as companion animals have risen, and they are maintaining increasingly close interactions with humans in industrialized societies (Cito et al., 2016). Although the phenomenon of all companion animals, especially dogs and cats, sharing the same environment as humans is long-standing (Fang et al., 2015; Cui et al., 2017), urbanization has affected the emergence and increasing incidence of tick-borne diseases (TBD) (Fang et al., 2015). Together, these changes in human activity and the increased contact between humans, their pets, and nature have contributed to the rising abundance of tick exposure (Uspensky, 2014; Fang et al., 2015). Dogs are particularly unusual companion animals because of their outdoor nature and close relationship with humans. They can therefore act as good sentinels for human tick-borne infections, suggesting that their role as hosts of ticks and tick-borne pathogens should be monitored (Hornok et al., 2013; Vlahakis et al., 2018).

Anaplasma species are zoonotic pathogens with tick vectors and mammalian reservoir hosts (Li et al., 2015). To date, three *Anaplasma* species have been identified as human pathogens: *A. phagocytophilum*, *A. ovis*, and *A. capra* (Chen et al., 1994; Chochlakis et al., 2010; Li et al., 2015). *A. phagocytophilum* was first confirmed as the causative agent of human granulocytic anaplasmosis (HGA) in the USA in 1994 (Chen et al., 1994). In China, the first suspected human case was described in Anhui in 2006 (Zhang et al., 2008). The severity of HGA ranges from an asymptomatic infection to a mild or severe febrile illness with multiple organ failure or even death (Li et al., 2015). Besides humans, hosts of *A. phagocytophilum* include domestic and wild animals such as cattle, sheep, goats, horses, dogs, hares, yaks, and rodents (Fang et al., 2015). An *A. ovis* variant was first identified in a patient with fever, hepatosplenomegaly, and lymphadenopathy in Cyprus in 2007 (Chochlakis et al., 2010). Hosts of this pathogen include domestic goats, sheep, deer, wild boar, and domestic dogs (Yabsley et al., 2005; Aktas et al., 2010; Pereira et al., 2016; Cui et al., 2017; Wei et al., 2017). *A. capra* is a novel *Anaplasma* species so-called because it was originally found in asymptomatic goats; soon after, it was identified in 28 patients in Heilongjiang, China (Beyer and Carlyon, 2015; Li et al., 2015; Yang et al., 2018). Clinical features of *A. capra* infection in humans include the acute onset of fever, headache, and malaise, but it is very difficult to distinguish from other acute febrile illnesses, thus leading to misdiagnosis (Li et al., 2015). Subsequent reports have shown that *A. capra* is widely distributed throughout China (Yang et al., 2018). It appears to have a broad host range and genetic diversity, with other mammalian hosts including goats, sheep, cattle, deer, serows, takins, and Reeves' muntjacs worldwide (Sato et al., 2009; Sun et al., 2015; Yang et al., 2017, 2018; Peng et al., 2018; Seo et al., 2018).

As one of the main mammalian hosts of *Anaplasma* species, dogs have been shown to carry *A. phagocytophilum*, *A. platys*, *A. ovis*, and *A. bovis* pathogens in recent years in China (Zhang et al., 2012; Li et al., 2014; Cui et al., 2017). However, there are no reports about dogs as hosts of *A. capra* worldwide. To provide further information about the host range, clinical symptoms, and risk factors of *A. capra* infections, the detection of this pathogen was carried out in dogs in Henan Province, China.

MATERIALS AND METHODS

Sample Collection

During 2013–2018, blood sample collection from dogs was carried out at six sampling sites in Zhengzhou city, Henan Province, central China. These included three pet hospitals (Pet clinic 1, Pet clinic 2, and Pet clinic 3) and three rescue centers for stray dogs (Stray dog rescue center 1, Stray dog rescue center 2, and Stray dog rescue center 3). Blood samples from pet clinics were obtained during outpatient testing, and detailed medical records were also collected. Blood samples from stray dog rescue centers were collected from a random proportion (5–10%) of dogs with the assistance of an experienced veterinarian. All blood samples were collected from the anterior tibial vein of the dogs with the help of a pet doctor or local veterinarian.

A total of 521 EDTA-K2 whole blood samples from different types of dogs were collected. Information about pet dogs, including age, gender, and clinical features, was obtained from sampling records, descriptions of chief complaints, and veterinarian diagnoses. However, few documents about stray dogs were available, and a review of their clinical symptoms suggested that they were healthy.

DNA Extraction

Pathogen genomic DNA was extracted from 200 μL blood samples using a Blood DNA Kit (Omega Biotek Inc., Norcross, GA, USA) according to the manufacturer's protocol. The quantity and quality of the extracted DNA were evaluated using a NanoDrop^{TM} 2000 spectrophotometer (Thermo Fisher Scientific, Waltham, MA), and it was stored at −20°C before use.

PCR Amplification

DNA samples were screened for the presence of *A. capra* by PCR amplification of the citrate synthase gene (*gltA*), heat shock protein gene (*groEL*), and major surface protein 4 gene (*msp4*) using previously described primers and PCR conditions (**Table 1**). Each DNA sample was screened for all three *A. capra* genes, and the successful amplification of any one of the three genes was taken to indicate positive infection. Each PCR reaction was conducted at least twice using nuclease-free water as a negative control, and DNA extracted from sheep infected with *A. capra* (GenBank accession nos. MG879297, MH174929, and MH174932) was used as a positive control. PCR reactions were performed in an ABI 2720 thermal cycler (Life Technologies Holdings Pte Ltd., Singapore). The products were examined by agarose gel electrophoresis and visualized after staining with GelRed (Biotium Inc., Hayward, CA).

Sequencing and Phylogenetic Analysis

Positive PCR products were purified using Montage PCR filters (Millipore, Bedford, MA) and sequenced using a BigDye Terminator v 3.1 cycle sequencing kit (Applied Biosystems, Foster City, CA) on an ABI 3730 DNA analyzer (Applied Biosystems). Nucleotide sequences were confirmed by bidirectional sequencing and by sequencing a new PCR product if necessary. They were then compared with reference sequences downloaded from the National Center for Biotechnology Information (https://www.ncbi.nlm.nih.gov/) using ClustalX 2.1 (http://www.clustal.org/) to determine new variant strains of *A. capra*.

Phylogenetic trees were conducted by Bayesian inference (BI) and Monte Carlo Markov Chain methods in MrBayes v 3.2.6 (http://mrbayes.sourceforge.net/). FigTree v 1.4.4 (http://tree.bio.ed.ac.uk/software/figtree/) was used to visualize and edit the maximum clade credibility tree generated by these analyses. Posterior probability values were estimated based on

TABLE 1 | Primers and PCR amplification conditions of *A. capra*.

Target gene	Primer name	Primer sequence (5′–3′)	Annealing temperature	Amplicon size	References
glt A	Outer-f	GCGATTTTAGAGTGYGGAGATTG	55°C	1031 bp	Li et al., 2015
	Outer-r	TACAATACCGGAGTAAAAGTCAA			
	Inner-f	TCATCTCCTGTTGCACGGTGCCC	60°C	594 bp	Yang et al., 2017
	Inner-r	CTCTGAATGAACATGCCCACCCT			
groEL	Forward	TGAAGAGCATCAAACCCGAAG	55°C	874 bp	Yang et al., 2017
	Reverse	CTGCTCGTGATGCTATCGG			
msp4	Forward	GGGTTCTGATATGGCATCTTC	53°C	656 bp	
	Reverse	GGGAAATGTCCTTATAGGATTCG			

1,000,000 generations with four simultaneous tree building chains, with trees being saved every 100th generation. A 50% majority rule consensus tree for each analysis was constructed based on the final 75% of trees generated by BI.

Sequences similarity were further analyzed by DNAStar Laser-gene program (DNAStar Inc., Madison, WI, USA) to evaluated the homology of the sequences obtained in the present with the sequences downloaded from the National Center for Biotechnology Information (https://www.ncbi.nlm.nih.gov/) (**Figure S2**).

Statistical Analysis

Variations in *A. capra* infection of dogs at different locations, seasons, age groups, genders, clinical signs, and use of vermifuge were analyzed by Fisher's exact test with SPSS (version 22.0) software. Differences were considered statistically significant if $P < 0.05$. Odds ratios (ORs) and their 95% confidence intervals (95% CIs) were estimated to explore the strength of the association between *A. capra*-positivity and the conditions tested. Then, the significant different correlation factors were used to process the canonical correspondence analysis by canoco5 (http://www.canoco5.com) (**Figure S1**).

Nucleotide Sequence Accession Numbers

The representative sequences obtained in this study have been submitted and deposited in the GenBank database with the following accession numbers: *gltA* (MK838608 and MK838609), *groEL* (MK862099), and *msp4* (MK838605- MK838607).

Ethics Statement

This study was carried out in accordance with the Chinese Laboratory Animal Administration Act (1988) after it was reviewed and its protocol was approved by the Research Ethics Committee of Henan Agricultural University. Appropriate permission was gained from the dog owners before the collection of blood specimens.

RESULTS

Infection of Dogs With *A. capra*

A total of 63 of the 521 dog blood samples were *A. capra*-positive by PCR screening (12.1%, 95% CI: 9.3–14.9). The infection rates of *A. capra* in pet dogs and stray dogs were 12.9% (59/458, 95% CI: 9.8–16.0) and 6.3% (4/63, 95% CI: 0.2–12.5), respectively. There were no significant differences in the infection ratio of *A. capra* in pet dogs and stray dogs ($P = 0.154$) (**Table 2**).

Distribution of *A. capra* Infections

A. capra infections in dogs with different types of samples were analyzed (**Table 2**). *A. capra* infections were found in five of the six sampling sites, at rates ranging from 0–18.5%, with significant differences among sites ($P = 0.002$). Additionally, higher infection rates were observed in dogs older than 10 years (33.3%, 95% CI: 6.3–60.4), and lower rates were seen in dogs aged 3–6 months compared with other age groups (6.5%, 95% CI: 1.4–11.5) ($P = 0.040$). As expected, the highest infections were documented in the summer months (20.4%, 95% CI: 13.7–27.1) ($P = 0.006$), and in dogs with anemic symptoms such as pale mucous membranes ($P = 0.019$). However, there were no differences in infection rates between dogs of different genders ($P = 0.578$), nor in those with influenza-like illness symptoms including fever, cough, malaise, and depression ($P = 0.370$), nor in those administered vermifuge in the last month ($P = 0.651$).

Sequences and Phylogenetic Analysis

Of the 63 *A. capra*-positive specimens, 26 were PCR-positive based on *gltA*, 17 based on *groEL*, and 61 based on *msp4*. Sequence analysis showed that *gltA* sequences were divided into two distinct sequence types: one (including 20 isolate sequences, MK838608) shared 100% identity with *A. capra* isolates from China, with previous hosts including humans (KM206274), goats (KM869310), sheep (KM869280), and ticks (MG940871 and MH029895). The others (including six isolates sequences, MK838609) showed 99.7% identity with *A. capra* isolates from humans (KM206274) (**Figure S2A**). Phylogenetic analysis based on *gltA* sequences revealed that the two types were in the same *Anaplasma* species clade (**Figure 1**). These isolates were closely related to *A. capra*, but distinct from other known *Anaplasma* species (**Figure 1**).

Sequence analysis revealed that *groEL* gene sequences obtained in this study (MK862099) were 100% identical to each other. Findings showed that the sequence had two single nucleotide polymorphisms (SNPs; G→A and T→A substitutions at positions 445 and 827, respectively) compared with the human isolate sequence (KM206275), and shared 99.9% identity with sequences isolated from sheep (KX417341), goats (KJ700629), and ticks (KX987393) (**Figure S2B**). Phylogenetic analysis based on *groEL* gene sequences

TABLE 2 | Univariable and multivariable analyses of risk factors associated with *A. capra* in dogs.

Variables	No. tested	No. positive	Infection rate (%) 95% CI	OR 95% CI	*P*
Sampling sites[a]					
Pet clinic 1	233	43	18.5 (13.4–23.5)	1	0.002
Pet clinic 2	77	3	3.9 (0.0–8.3)	0.179 (0.054–0.595)	0.001
Pet clinic 3	148	13	8.8 (4.2–13.4)	0.425 (0.220–0.822)	0.006
Stray dog rescue center1	20	3	15.0 (0.0–32.1)	0.780 (0.219–2.780)	1.000
Stray dog rescue center2	24	1	4.2 (0.0–12.8)	0.192 (0.025–1.462)	0.090
Stray dog rescue center3	19	0	0.0		
Kinds of dogs[a]					
Pet dogs	458	59	12.9 (9.8–16.0)	1	
Dogs in Stray dog rescue center	63	4	6.3 (0.2–12.5)	0.458 (0.161–1.309)	0.154
Seasons[a]					
Spring (Mar.-May)	354	33	9.3 (6.3–12.4)	0.401 (0.233–0.689)	0.001
Summer (Jun. –Aug.)	142	29	20.4 (13.7–27.1)	1	0.006
Autumn (Sep. –Nov.)	10	0	0.0		
Winter (Dec. –Feb.)	15	1	6.7(0–21.0)	0.278 (0.035–2.204)	0.306
Age groups[b]					
>10 year	15	5	33.3 (6.3–60.4)	1	0.040
5–10 year	40	7	17.5 (5.2–29.8)	0.424 (0.110–1.634)	0.274
1–5 year	147	20	13.6 (8.0–19.2)	0.315 (0.098–1.017)	0.059
6–12 month	92	9	9.8 (3.6–16.0)	0.217 (0.061–0.776)	0.026
3–6 month	93	6	6.5 (1.4–11.5)	0.138 (0.036–0.535)	0.007
<3 month	71	12	16.9 (8.0–25.8)	0.407 (0.118–1.406)	0.164
Unknown	63	4	6.3 (0.2–12.5)		
Gender[b]					
Female	202	28	13.9 (9.1–18.7)	1	
Male	256	31	12.1 (8.1–16.1)	0.856 (0.495–1.481)	0.578
Unknown	63	4	6.3 (0.2–12.5)		
Influenza-like illness symptoms[c]					
Yes	312	37	11.9(8.3–15.5)	1	
No	146	22	15.1(9.2–20.9)	1.319 (0.747–2.329)	0.370
Unknown	63	4	6.3 (0.2–12.5)		
Anemia symptoms or not[c]					
Yes	18	6	33.3(9.2–57.5)	1	
No	440	53	12.0(9.0–15.1)	0.274 (0.099–0.760)	0.019
Unknown	63	4	6.3 (0.2–12.5)		
Vermifuge used or not[b]					
Yes	136	20	14.7 (8.7–20.7)	1	
No	322	39	12.1 (8.5–15.7)	0.854 (0.479–1.524)	0.651
Unknown	63	4	6.3 (0.2–12.5)		
Total	521	63	12.1 (9.3–14.9)		

[a] *Sampling record.*
[b] *Chief complaint.*
[c] *Veterinarian diagnosis.*

demonstrated that the isolates were clustered within the *A. capra* clade, but distinct from other well-defined *Anaplasma* species (**Figure 1**).

For *msp4* gene sequences, we acquired three different sequences (MK838605–MK838607) from dogs in the present study. One (KM838607) shared 100% identity with those of *A. capra* isolates from humans (KM206277), and the others had one (T→C at position 320) or two (C→T and T→C substitutions at positions 246 and 320, respectively) SNPs compared with the human sequence (KM206277), and shared 99.7–99.8% similarity with sequences of *Anaplasma* spp. from humans (KM206277), goats (KJ700631), sheep (KX417357), and ticks (KR261641) (**Figure S2C**). Phylogenetic analysis based on *msp4* sequences demonstrated that the isolates were clustered within the *A. capra* clade, but distinct from other well-defined *Anaplasma* species (**Figure 1**).

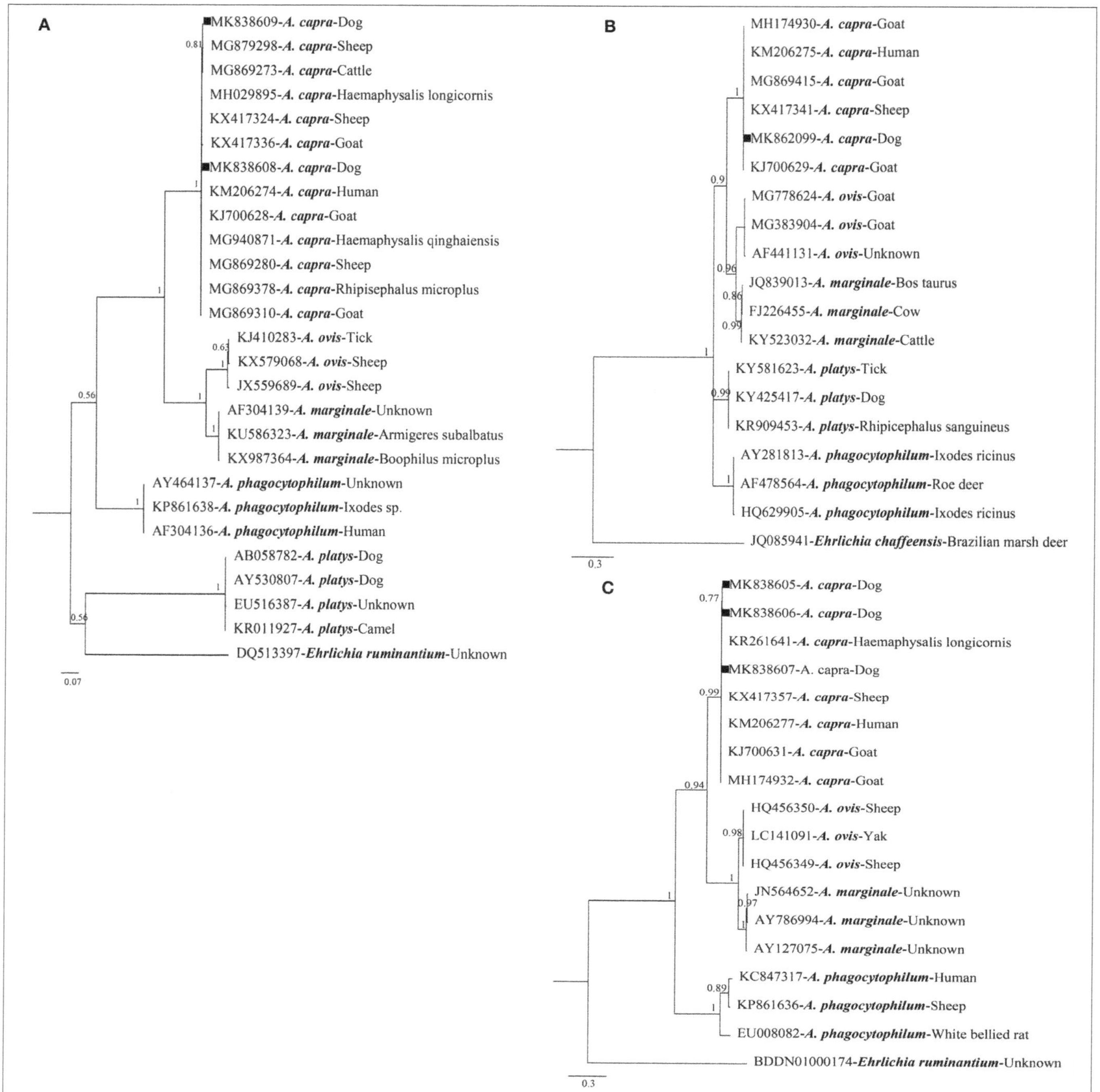

FIGURE 1 | Bayesian phylogenetic analysis of *A. capra* based on *gltA* **(A)**, *groEL* **(B)**, and *msp4* **(C)** sequences. Significant posterior probabilities are indicated at branches. Sample names include GenBank accession numbers followed by *Anaplasma* spp. *Ehrlichia ruminantium* and *Ehrlichia chaffeensis* were used as outgroups. The sequences identified in this study are marked by squares.

DISCUSSION

The natural infection cycle of *Anaplasma* species is dependent upon the presence of tick vectors and infected vertebrate reservoir hosts (de la Fuente et al., 2016). *Anaplasma* species are transmitted by ixodid ticks transstadially rather than transovarially, so reservoir hosts play a crucial role in the maintenance and spread of these pathogens (Yang et al., 2018). Currently, a number of vertebrate animals are considered competent hosts for *Anaplasma*, including humans, cattle, sheep, goats, dogs, horses, and deer (Stuen et al., 2013). Moreover, dogs have been reported as hosts of *A. phagocytophilum*, *A. platys*, *A. ovis*, and *A. bovis* (Zhang et al., 2012; Li et al., 2014; Cui et al., 2017).

Host and environmental factors are thought to play an important role in the epidemiology of TBD in dogs (Abd Rani et al., 2011). Furthermore, high-quality vegetative cover may have increased the abundance and diversity of ticks (Fang et al., 2015). A previous study showed that TBD were less likely to infect dogs from refuges and animals fed nutritious diets, even after adjusting for the presence of ticks, than free-roaming strays (Abd Rani et al., 2011). However, we found no difference in the natural infection rate of *A. capra* between pet and stray dogs ($P = 0.154$).

The novel tick-transmitted zoonotic *A. capra* was identified in dogs from five of six sampling sites in the present study, with a total infection rate of 12.1% (63/521). Likewise, *A. ovis*, *A. bovis*, and *A. phagocytophilum* have been identified in dogs in Henan with prevalences of 6.2%, 4.1%, and 0.4%, respectively (Cui et al., 2017), suggesting that *Anaplasma* species are common pathogens of dogs in Henan. We detected the highest infection rate in Pet clinic 1 ($P = 0.002$), which is located in a suburban area of the city surrounded by rich vegetation. Similar findings were previously observed for the tick-borne fever with thrombocytopenia syndrome which was also significantly associated with vegetation-rich regions (Liu et al., 2014; Fang et al., 2015).

We observed the highest *A. capra* infection rate in dogs older than 10 years of age. Similarly, other canine vector-borne disease pathogens such as *A. phagocytophilum* and *B. burgdorferi* were detected at higher infection rates in Korean dogs aged over 2 years (Lim et al., 2010), while no significant difference in *A. platys* infection was observed among various groups of dogs (Kamani et al., 2013). Dogs aged over 10 years, so-called elderly dogs, may have a poor physical condition and be more easily infected by pathogens. Furthermore, *A. capra* infection may be chronic and persistent infection, so the potential role of elderly dogs as carriers of *A. capra* should be noted. We observed no difference in infection rate between dogs of different genders, which is consistent with previous reports about tick-borne pathogens (Lim et al., 2010; Hornok et al., 2013; Peng et al., 2018).

Our study also revealed a high prevalence of *A. capra* infection during the summer season. Similar results were reported for *Anaplasma* species such as *A. bovis*, *A. ovis*, and *A. capra* in sheep, goats, and cattle (Belkahia et al., 2017; Seo et al., 2018). All *Anaplasma* species are transmitted to their natural hosts by ticks, and the warm summer season offers favorable conditions for tick distribution (Belkahia et al., 2017). Thus far, *A. capra* has also been detected in ticks such as *Ixodes persulcatus*, *Haemaphysalis longicornis*, and *Haemaphysalis qinghaiensis* in many places in China (Peng et al., 2018). From spring to autumn, ticks are found throughout China and demonstrate extended periods of activity; therefore with rising tick numbers, the risks of host infection with tick-borne pathogens also increase (Chvostáč et al., 2018; Jaimes-Dueñez et al., 2018).

Clinical features of human infection by *A. capra* include an influenza-like illness such as fever, headache, malaise, and chills (Li et al., 2015). In the present study, we found no difference in *A. capra* infections between dogs with and without influenza-like illness symptoms. However, a significant difference was detected between dogs with and without symptoms of anemia such as pale mucous membranes. However, Li and colleagues (Li et al., 2015) did not describe morulae or other forms of *A. capra* in peripheral blood smears, but instead found that *A capra* was more closely related to species that infect mammalian erythrocytes; thus, they anticipated intracellular *A capra* infection in mammalian erythrocytes. The correlation of anemia with *A. capra* infection should nonetheless be verified in a future study, while the present study describes the clinical features of *A. capra* infection in dogs for the first time.

Phylogenetic analysis of *A. capra* based on *gltA*, *groEL*, and *msp4* showed that the isolate sequences obtained in the present study, as well as those previously isolated from sheep, ticks, goats, and humans, formed an independent clade clearly distinct from other members of *Anaplasma* species (Li et al., 2015; Yang et al., 2017; Guo et al., 2018; Peng et al., 2018; **Figure 1**). For *gltA*, one sequence (MK838608) obtained in this study shared 100% identity with an *A. capra* isolate (KM206274) from humans, while the other sequence (MK838609) shared 99.7% identity with the same isolates from humans (Li et al., 2015). For *groEL*, the sequence acquired from dogs (MK862099) shared 99.9% identity with the sequence from humans (KM206275), and three different *msp4* sequences obtained in the present study shared 99.7–100% similarity with sequences of *Anaplasma* species from humans (KM206277) (Li et al., 2015). Phylogenetic analysis indicated that *A. capra* identified in this study was highly similar to sequences obtained from humans (KM206274, KM206275, and KM206277), in view of the affinity between dogs and humans, indicating that a high level of attention should be paid to *A. capra* infection in dogs for public health reasons.

A large proportion of *A. capra* sequences (20/26) obtained from dogs in this study showed 100% identity with isolates from ticks, sheep, goats, and humans (Li et al., 2015; Yang et al., 2017; Guo et al., 2018; Peng et al., 2018). Furthermore, many domestic animals like dogs may serve as a suitable reservoir or a dead end host of *Anaplasma* species in urban areas (Schorn et al., 2011). Companion animals are becoming increasingly popular in China, and the transport of dogs to other areas adds to the spread of pathogens (Stuen et al., 2013). Considering dogs as hosts both of *Anaplasma* species and ticks, together with the growing affinity between humans and dogs, we should not ignore their important role in spreading *A. capra* infection in areas where tick vectors are abundant.

CONCLUSION

The present study documents dogs as a new host for *A. capra* for the first time. It is noteworthy that older dogs are more readily infected by *A. capra*. The risk factor for infection is predicted to increase with rising numbers of ticks in hot seasons and with increasing contact between dogs and ticks. Hence, we advise that dog owners prevent their pets from entering woods, copses, mountainsides, and grass close to rivers during peak tick seasons to limit vector contact. Further research should also evaluate whether dogs are competent reservoirs of *A. capra*.

ETHICS STATEMENT

The animal study was reviewed and approved by Chinese Laboratory Animal Administration Act (1988); Research Ethics Committee of Henan Agricultural University. Written informed consent was obtained from the owners for the participation of their animals in this study.

AUTHOR CONTRIBUTIONS

CN conceived the study. CN and LZ designed the experiments. KS, YY, QC, KW, YZ, and YP performed the experiments. KS, DL, YC, and FY performed data analysis. KS, JL, and CN wrote the manuscript. All authors approved the final version of the manuscript.

ACKNOWLEDGMENTS

We thank Sarah Williams, Ph.D., from Liwen Bianji, Edanz Group China (www.liwenbianji.cn), for editing the English text of a draft of this manuscript.

SUPPLEMENTARY MATERIAL

Figure S1 | Results of Canonical correspondence Analysis (CCA) between the prevalence of *A. capra* and several variables.

Figure S2 | The homology analysis of *A. capra* based on *gltA* **(A)**, *groEL* **(B)**, and *msp4* **(C)** sequences.

REFERENCES

1. Abd Rani, P. A., Irwin, P. J., Coleman, G. T., Gatne, M., and Traub, R. J. (2011). A survey of canine tick-borne diseases in India. *Parasit. Vectors*. 4:141. doi: 10.1186/1756-3305-4-141
2. Aktas, M., Altay, K., and Dumanli, N. (2010). Molecular detection and identification of *Anaplasma* and *Ehrlichia* species in cattle from Turkey. *Ticks Tick Borne Dis.* 2, 62–65. doi: 10.1016/j.ttbdis.2010.11.002
3. Belkahia, H., Ben Said, M., El Mabrouk, N., Saidani, M., Cherni, C., Ben Hassen, M., et al. (2017). Seasonal dynamics, spatial distribution and genetic analysis of *Anaplasma* species infecting small ruminants from Northern Tunisia. *Infect. Genet. Evol.* 54, 66–73. doi: 10.1016/j.meegid.2017.06.016
4. Beyer, A. R., and Carlyon, J. A. (2015). Of goats and men: rethinking anaplasmoses as zoonotic infections. *Lancet Infect. Dis.* 15, 619–620. doi: 10.1016/S1473-3099(15)70097-6
5. Chen, S. M., Dumler, J. S., Bakken, J. S., and Walker, D. H. (1994). Identification of a granulocytotropic *Ehrlichia* species as the etiologic agent of human disease. *J. Clin. Microbiol.* 32, 589–595.
6. Chochlakis, D., Ioannou, I., Tselentis, Y., and Psaroulaki, A. (2010). Human anaplasmosis and *Anaplasma ovis* variant. *Emerging Infect. Dis.* 16, 1031–1032. doi: 10.3201/eid1606.090175
7. Chvostác˘, M., Špitalská, E., Václav, R., Vaculová, T., Minichová, L., and Derdáková, M. (2018). Patterns in the prevalence and diversity of tick-borne *Borrelia burgdorferi Sensu Lato, Anaplasma phagocytophilum* and *Rickettsia* spp. in an Urban Temperate Forest in South Western Slovakia. *Int. J. Environ. Res. Public Health.* 15:E994. doi: 10.3390/ijerph15050994
8. Cito, F., Rijks, J., Rantsios, A. T., Cunningham, A. A., Baneth, G., Guardabassi, L., et al. (2016). Prioritization of companion animal transmissible diseases for policy intervention in Europe. *J. Comp. Pathol.* 155, S18–26. doi: 10.1016/j.jcpa.2015.01.007
9. Cui, Y., Yan, Y., Wang, X., Cao, S., Zhang, Y., Jian, F., et al. (2017). First molecular evidence of mixed infections of *Anaplasma* species in dogs in Henan, China. *Ticks Tick Borne Dis.* 8, 283–289. doi: 10.1016/j.ttbdis.2016.12.001
10. de la Fuente, J., Estrada-Peña, A., Cabezas-Cruz, A., and Kocan, K. M. (2016). *Anaplasma phagocytophilum* uses common strategies for infection of ticks and vertebrate hosts. *Trends Microbiol.* 24, 173–180. doi: 10.1016/j.tim.2015.12.001
11. Fang, L. Q., Liu, K., Li, X. L., Liang, S., Yang, Y., Yao, H. W., et al. (2015). Emerging tick-borne infections in mainland China: an increasing public health threat. *Lancet Infect. Dis.* 15, 1467–1479. doi: 10.1016/S1473-3099(15)00177-2
12. Guo, W. P., Huang, B., Zhao, Q., Xu, G., Liu, B., Wang, Y. H., et al. (2018). Human- pathogenic *Anaplasma* spp., and *Rickettsia* spp. in animals in Xi'an, China. *PLoS Negl. Trop. Dis.* 12:e0006916. doi: 10.1371/journal.pntd.0006916
13. Hornok, S., Dénes, B., Meli, M. L., Tánczos, B., Fekete, L., Gyuranecz, M., et al. (2013). Non-pet dogs as sentinels and potential synanthropic reservoirs of tick-borne and zoonotic bacteria. *Vet Microbiol.* 167, 700–703. doi: 10.1016/j.vetmic.2013.08.011
14. Jaimes-Dueñez, J., Triana-Chávez, O., and Mejía-Jaramillo, A. M. (2018). Genetic, host and environmental factors associated with a high prevalence of *Anaplasma marginale. Ticks Tick Borne Dis.* 9, 1286–1295. doi: 10.1016/j.ttbdis.2018.05.009 Kamani, J., Baneth, G., Mumcuoglu, K. Y., Waziri, N. E., Eyal, O., Guthmann, Y., et al. (2013). Molecular detection and characterization of tick-borne pathogens in dogs and ticks from Nigeria. *PLoS Negl. Trop. Dis.* 7:e2108. doi: 10.1371/journal.pntd.0002108
15. Li, H., Zheng, Y. C., Ma, L., Jia, N., Jiang, B. G., Jiang, R. R., et al. (2015). Human infection with a novel tick-borne *Anaplasma* species in China: a surveillance study. *Lancet Infect. Dis.* 15, 663–670. doi: 10.1016/S1473-3099(15)70051-4
16. Li, H. T., Sun, L. S., Chen, Z. M., Hu, J. S., Ye, C. D., Jia, K., et al. (2014). Detection of *Anaplasma platys* in dogs using real-time loop-mediated isothermal amplification. *Vet J.* 199, 468–470. doi: 10.1016/j.tvjl.2013.11.012
17. Lim, S., Irwin, P. J., Lee, S., Oh, M., Ahn, K., Myung, B., et al. (2010). Comparison of selected canine vector-borne diseases between urban animal shelter and rural hunting dogs in Korea. *Parasit. Vectors.* 3:32. doi: 10.1186/1756-3305-3-32
18. Liu, K., Cui, N., Fang, L. Q., Wang, B. J., Lu, Q. B., Peng, W., et al. (2014). Epidemiologic features and environmental risk factors of severe fever with thrombocytopenia syndrome, Xinyang, China. *PLoS Negl. Trop. Dis.* 8:e2820. doi: 10.1371/journal.pntd.0002820
19. Maggi, R. G., and Krämer, F. (2019). A review on the occurrence of companion vector-borne diseases in pet animals in Latin America. *Parasit. Vectors.* 12, 145. doi: 10.1186/s13071-019-3407-x
20. Peng, Y., Wang, K., Zhao, S., Yan, Y., Wang, H., Jing, J., et al. (2018). Detection and phylogenetic characterization of *Anaplasma capra*: an emerging pathogen in sheep and goats in China. *Front. Cell. Infect. Microbiol.* 8:283. doi: 10.3389/fcimb.2018.00283
21. Pereira, A., Parreira, R., Nunes, M., Casadinho, A., Vieira, M. L., Campino, L., et al. (2016). Molecular detection of tick-borne bacteria and protozoa in cervids and wild boars from Portugal. *Parasit. Vectors.* 9:251. doi: 10.1186/s13071-016-1535-0
22. Sato, M., Nishizawa, I., Fujihara, M., Nishimura, T., Matsubara, K., and Harasawa, R. (2009). Phylogenetic analysis of the 16S rRNA gene of *Anaplasma* species detected from Japanese serows (*Capricornis crispus*). *J. Vet. Med. Sci.* 71, 1677–1679. doi: 10.1292/jvms.001677
23. Schorn, S., Pfister, K., Reulen, H., Mahling, M., Manitz, J., Thiel, C., et al. (2011). Prevalence of Anaplasma phagocytophilum in Ixodes ricinus in Bavarian public parks, Germany. *Ticks Tick Borne Dis.* 2, 196–203. doi: 10.1016/j.ttbdis.2011.09.009
24. Seo, M. G., Ouh, I. O., Lee, H., Geraldino, P. J. L., Rhee, M. H., Kwon, O. D., et al. (2018). Differential identification of *Anaplasma* in cattle and potential of cattle to serve as reservoirs of *Anaplasma capra*, an emerging tick-borne zoonotic pathogen. *Vet. Microbiol.* 226, 15–22. doi: 10.1016/j.vetmic.2018.10.008
25. Stuen, S., Granquist, E. G., and Silaghi, C. (2013). *Anaplasma phagocytophilum*— a widespread multi-host pathogen with highly adaptive strategies. *Front. Cell. Infect. Microbiol.* 3:31. doi: 10.3389/fcimb.2013.00031

26. Sun, X. F., Zhao, L., Wen, H. L., Luo, L. M., and Yu, X. J. (2015). *Anaplasma* species in China. *Lancet Infect. Dis.* 15, 1263–1264. doi: 10.1016/S1473-3099(15)00377-1
27. Uspensky, I. (2014). Tick pests and vectors (Acari: Ixodoidea) in European towns: introduction, persistence and management. *Ticks Tick Borne Dis.* 5, 41–47. doi: 10.1016/j.ttbdis.2013.07.011
28. Vlahakis, P. A., Chitanga, S., Simuunza, M. C., Simulundu, E., Qiu, Y., Changula, K., et al. (2018). Molecular detection and characterization of zoonotic *Anaplasma* species in domestic dogs in Lusaka, Zambia. *Ticks Tick Borne Dis.* 9, 39–43. doi: 10.1016/j.ttbdis.2017.10.010
29. Wei, R., Liu, H. B., Jongejan, F., Jiang, B. G., Chang, Q. C., Fu, X., et al. (2017). Cultivation of *Anaplasma ovis* in the HL-60 human promyelocytic leukemia cell line. *Emerg. Microbes Infect.* 6:e83. doi: 10.1038/emi.2017.70
30. Xu, D., Zhang, J., Shi, Z., Song, C., Zheng, X., Zhang, Y., et al. (2015). Molecular detection of vector-borne agents in dogs from ten provinces of China. *Parasit. Vectors.* 8:501. doi: 10.1186/s13071-015-1120-y
31. Yabsley, M. J., Davidson, W. R., Stallknecht, D. E., Varela, A. S., Swift, P. K., Devos, J. C. Jr., et al. (2005). Evidence of tick-borne organisms in mule deer (*Odocoileus hemionus*) from the western United States. *Vector Borne Zoonotic Dis.* 5, 351–362. doi: 10.1089/vbz.2005.5.351
32. Yang, J., Liu, Z., Niu, Q., Liu, J., Han, R., Guan, G., et al. (2017). A novel zoonotic *Anaplasma* species is prevalent in small ruminants: potential public health implications. *Parasit. Vectors.* 10:264. doi: 10.1186/s13071-017-2182-9
33. Yang, J., Liu, Z., Niu, Q., Mukhtar, M. U., Guan, G., Liu, G., et al. (2018). A novel genotype of "*Anaplasma capra*" in wildlife and its phylogenetic relationship with the human genotypes. *Emerg. Microbes Infect.* 7:210. doi: 10.1038/s41426-018-0212-0
34. Zhang, L., Liu, H., Xu, B., Lu, Q., Li, L., Chang, L., et al. (2012). *Anaplasma phagocytophilum* infection in domestic animals in ten provinces/cities of China. *Am. J. Trop. Med. Hyg.* 87, 185–189. doi: 10.4269/ajtmh.2012.12-0005
35. Zhang, L., Liu, Y., Ni, D., Li, Q., Yu, Y., Yu, X. J., et al. (2008). Nosocomial transmission of human granulocytic anaplasmosis in China. *JAMA* 300, 2263–2270. doi: 10.1001/jama.2008.626

22

Nipah Virus–Another Threat from the World of Zoonotic Viruses

Krzysztof Skowron[1], Justyna Bauza-Kaszewska[2], Katarzyna Grudlewska-Buda[1], Natalia Wiktorczyk-Kapischke[1], Maciej Zacharski[3], Zuzanna Bernaciak[1] and Eugenia Gospodarek-Komkowska[1]*

[1] *Department of Microbiology, Ludwik Rydygier Collegium Medicum in Bydgoszcz, Nicolaus Copernicus University in Toruń, Bydgoszcz, Poland,* [2] *Department of Microbiology and Food Technology, Jan and Jędrzej Śniadecki University of Technology in Bydgoszcz, Bydgoszcz, Poland,* [3] *Department of Biochemistry and Molecular Biology, Wrocław University of Environmental and Life Sciences, Wrocław, Poland*

***Correspondence:**
Maciej Zacharski
maciej.zacharski@upwr.edu.pl

Among the diseases that pose a serious threat to public health, those caused by viruses are of great importance. The Nipah virus (NiV) belonging to the *Paramyxoviridae* family was reported in Malaysia in 1998/1999. Due to its high mortality in humans, its zoonotic nature, the possibility of human-to-human transmission, and the lack of an available vaccine, the World Health Organization (WHO) has recognized it as a global health problem. Depending on strain specificity, neurological symptoms and severe respiratory disorders are observed in NiV infection. In most confirmed cases of NiV epidemics, the appearance of the virus in humans was associated with the presence of various animal species, but generally, bats of *Pteropus* species are considered the most important natural animal NiV reservoir and vector. Consumption of contaminated food, contact with animals, and "human-to-human" direct contact were identified as NiV transmission routes. Due to the lack of vaccines and drugs with proven effectiveness against NiV, treatment of patients is limited to supportive and prophylactic.

Keywords: Nipah, transmission routes, epidemics, diagnosis, health treat, vaccine, pandemic potential

INTRODUCTION

One of the consequences of the ongoing Severe Acute Respiratory Syndrome Coronavirus 2 (SARS-CoV-2) pandemic is the increased interest in various aspects related to its origin, virulence mechanisms, potential sources of infection, and modes of transmission. Increasing research to develop an effective epidemic reduction strategy leads to a deeper understanding of the factors that shape its dynamics and the means of controlling it. Paradoxically, the outbreak of a global epidemic may therefore bring beneficial effects in the context of the prevention and monitoring of other infectious agents with epidemiological potential.

Viruses are the cause of diseases that pose a serious threat to public health. Marburg, coronaviruses: Middle East Respiratory Syndrome (MERS) and Severe Acute Respiratory Syndrome Coronavirus 1 (SARS-CoV-1), Human Immunodeficiency Virus (HIV), Hendra, Nipah virus (NiV) and those responsible for Crimean-Congo hemorrhagic fever, Lassa fever, Ebola, Influenza A virus subtype H1N1, Asian highly pathogenic avian influenza (HPAI) A(H5N1) virus or Rift Valley Fever (RVF) caused numerous epidemics in recent years. These epidemics were characterized by high morbidity and mortality, mainly in developing countries in Asia, Africa, and South America (Jones et al., 2008; Aiyar and Pingali, 2020).

The NiV virus, due to its high mortality in humans, its zoonotic nature, the possibility of human-to-human transmission, and the lack of an available vaccine, has been recognized by the World Health Organization (WHO) as a global health problem and included in the list of epidemic threats treated as a priority in research and development activities (R&D Blueprint) (Anderson et al., 2019; World Health Organization [WHO], 2021c). In turn, the Centers for Disease Control and Prevention (CDC) and the National Institute of Allergy and Infectious Diseases (NIAID) classified NiV as category C in the classification of pathogens that pose a terrorist threat (Ochani et al., 2019). The latest information confirms the emergence of the NiV virus in India in September 2021 (World Health Organization [WHO], 2021b).

The study aimed to characterize the NiV virus in the context of its epidemiological potential and to evaluate the effectiveness of previous preventive and intervention measures. Conclusions and observations resulting from such an analysis may constitute suggestions for the development of a scheme of action in the event of an outbreak of an epidemic on a larger than just a local scale.

NIPAH VIRUS–GENERAL CHARACTERISTICS

The name of the NiV derives from the name of the village of Sungai Nipah (Nipah River Village) in Negeri Sembilan state, Malaysia, where the presence of NiV [IgM antibodies in cerebrospinal fluid (CSF) against Hendra viral antigens] was first confirmed in patient serum samples with symptoms of encephalitis in 1999 (Chua et al., 1999; Parashar et al., 2000). NiV first appeared in Malaysia and Singapore in 1998/1999 (Centers for Disease Control and Prevention [CDC], 1999). The detailed molecular, antigenic and serological analysis made it eligible for the *Paramyxoviridae* family and the genus *Henipavirus*. Paramyxoviruses include many known types of pathogenic viruses, such as the measles virus (MV, genus *Morbillivirus*) or mumps virus (MuV, genera *Rubulavirus*). In turn, the Henipavirus genus, in addition to NiV, also includes three species that are harmless to humans: Cedar virus, Ghanaian bat virus and Mojiang virus, and the highly pathogenic Hendra virus (HeV) (Shoemaker and Choi, 2020). The pathogenic potential of Ghanaian bat virus (Drexler et al., 2012) and Mojiang virus (Wu et al., 2014) are unknown as these have not been isolated, but identified through sequencing data. Sequencing showed a high 80% similarity of NiV and HeV viruses in terms of nucleotide homology (Sharma et al., 2019; Thakur and Bailey, 2019).

Morphologically, NiV resembles other paramyxoviruses: it is a pleomorphic, spherical, or thread-like enveloped virus with a size of 40–1900 nm, containing a single layer of surface protrusions with an average length of approximately 17 nm (Ang et al., 2018; Sharma et al., 2019).

Nipah virus has single-stranded RNA of negative polarity. RNA viruses, due to their extremely short generation time and faster evolution, show an increased probability of infection of new host species, although they are already considered the main etiological factors responsible for 25–44% of recently emerging infectious diseases (Harcourt et al., 2001; Carrasco-Hernandez et al., 2017; Devnath and Al Masud, 2021). NiV has six genes, with a genome size ranging from 18,246 to 18,252, depending on the strain (Harcourt et al., 2001; Chakraborty et al., 2019). The NiV genome contains six transcription units that encode the main structural proteins of the virus: nucleocapsid (N), phosphoprotein (P), matrix protein (M), fusion protein (F), attachment glycoprotein (G), and the large protein or RNA polymerase protein (L) (**Figure 1**). The P gene, in addition to the phosphoprotein, also encodes the NiV proteins C, V, and W, which are responsible for pathogenicity (Wang et al., 2001; Martinez-Gil et al., 2017; Sun et al., 2018; Hauser et al., 2021). Physically related G and F proteins play a key role in binding and fusion to the host cell during the first stage of the viral life cycle. After attaching to the EphrinB2/B3 receptor and entering the cell, the NiV genome is released and replicated. After the transcription catalyzed by the L and P proteins, the viral messenger RNA is translated into the main structural proteins (Hauser et al., 2021). The N protein is responsible, among others, for the proper course of viral replication and transcription. The M protein plays an important role in the final stage of assembling the virion from the genome and proteins, encapsulating and releasing the virus from the host cell (Sun et al., 2018).

Nipah virus mainly enters cells through the fusion of the virus with the cell membrane on the plasma membrane. Cellular expression of NiV glycoproteins can induce cell-membrane fusion (syncytium formation) through the interaction of G and F glycoproteins. The fusion of the virus and host cell membranes (which is pH independent) begins with the binding of G to its host receptor (ephrinB2 or ephrinB3) (Negrete et al., 2005). This is followed by protein conformational changes. F moves from its pre-fusion (PF) conformation to its intermediate hairpin conformation (PHI), causing the fusion peptide to be inserted into the host cell membrane (Aguilar et al., 2010). F then enters the thermodynamically stable six-helical beam (6HB) conformation. The intermediate steps include: the fusion of external flakes (hemifusion), the formation of fusion pores and the widening of the fusion pores (Aguilar et al., 2016). These critical steps in the membrane fusion cascade are necessary for the initiation of infection. Wong et al. (2021) showed that G and ephrinB2 form clusters and that ephrinB2 oligomerization is necessary for F activation. Researchers found no evidence of stable F-G protein complexes before or after activation.

NIPAH VIRUS EPIDEMICS

Malaysia

The first human cases of NiV were reported among pig farmers in September 1998 during an epidemic in Malaysia. Initially, they were mistaken for cases of Japanese encephalitis (JE), but both transmission through direct contact with pigs and its occurrence in adults were not typical of infections caused by this infectious agent (Centers for Disease Control and Prevention [CDC], 1999). In May 1999, after the new virus was isolated from the CSF of a patient with Sungai Nipah, NiV was officially recognized as

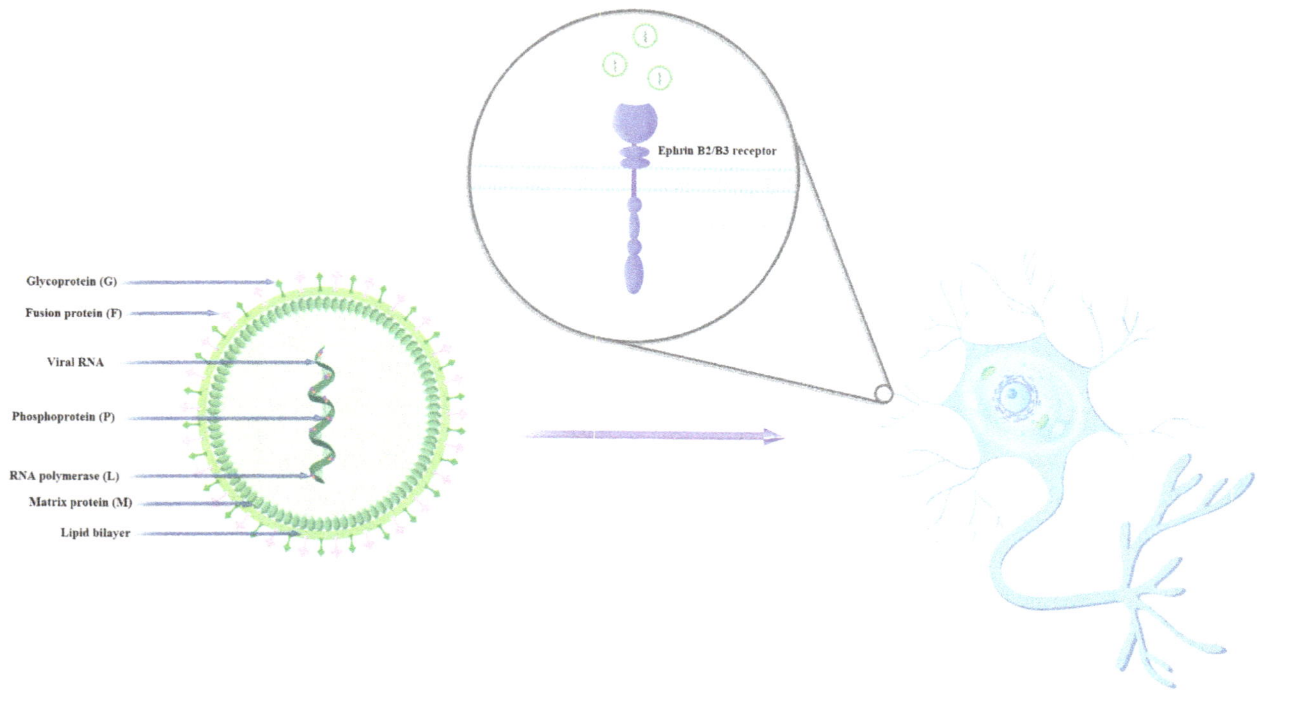

FIGURE 1 | Structure and mechanism of NiV infection of human nerve cells.

the cause of reported infections (Chua, 2003). Most of the cases were in men who worked with pigs and very few of the patients were young children (Lam and Chua, 2002). Typical symptoms reported by the patients included fever, headache, and decreased consciousness. Depending on the source, the number of cases during the epidemic in Malaysia ranged from 238 to 265 and the number of deaths from 105 to 109, which suggested very high mortality, confirmed during subsequent epidemics (**Table 1**; Looi and Chua, 2007; Aditi and Shariff, 2019; Ambat et al., 2019).

Singapore

Detected in Singapore in March 1999, NiV infections involving the respiratory system and the brain affected slaughterhouse workers who received pigs from Malaysia. Of the 11 cases, 1 was fatal. The median age was 44 years (range 24-66). All patients were men; ten were Chinese, and one Indian (Paton et al., 1999). The epidemic ended with the introduction of a ban on the import of pigs from Malaysia (Chua, 2003; Aditi and Shariff, 2019).

Bangladesh

In Bangladesh, NiV outbreaks occurred almost annually from 2001 to 2013, mainly in the winter months. They were detected in many parts of the country, some of which appeared several times. Mortality during the first epidemic in 2001 was 69%, and in 2013 it increased to 83%. In total, from April 2001 to March 31, 2012, the number of NiV cases was 209, of which 161 (77%) were fatal (Ambat et al., 2019; Anderson et al., 2019). Gurley et al. (2007) showed that NiV was an ethological factor in the outbreak in the Faridpur district of Bangladesh in April–May 2004. Bangladesh epidemic NiV genomic sequences are presented by Lo et al. (2012). Researchers showed that NiV genomic sequences from patients (two diagnosed in 2008 and three in 2010) constituted a separate genetic group (Lo et al., 2012). Additionally, Lo et al. (2012) proposed the determination of the previously identified NiV strains. Their division assumes that NiV genomic sequences from Malaysia and Cambodia are defined as the M genotype, while the B genotype are sequences obtained from Bangladesh and India. Scientists and doctors were particularly interested in the Bangladesh-specific way of transmitting the virus through the consumption of date palm juice and the transmission between people as a result of direct contact with their secretions of various origins, including the respiratory tract (Aditi and Shariff, 2019).

India

As in Bangladesh, India's NiV outbreaks have occurred several times, though not as frequently. The first outbreak of NiV cases was recorded in 2001 in West Bengal, a region across the border from the NiV belt in Bangladesh (Aditi and Shariff, 2019). Confirmed infections and deaths were the highest at the time, at 66 and 45, respectively. The second NiV outbreak occurred in the same region in 2007, with five cases and five deaths (Arankalle et al., 2011). In May 2018, 18 NiV infections were reported in the state of Kerala, mainly characterized by acute respiratory syndrome and encephalitis. At least 17 infected people died then, which means that this NiV outbreak is characterized by the highest mortality, exceeding 90% (Ambat et al., 2019; Plowright et al., 2019). Phylogenetic analysis by Arunkumar et al. (2019) showed that the percent identity of gene fragments of the NiV outbreak that occurred in Kerala, India (May–June 2018) with genotype B NiV (AY988601–Bangladesh 2004)

TABLE 1 | Morbidity, transmission route, and fatality rate of NiV infections in different NiV epidemic (Ang et al., 2018; Ambat et al., 2019; Sharma et al., 2019; Hauser et al., 2021).

Country	Year/regions	Primary route of transmission	Cases	Death	Fatality rate [%]
Malaysia	1998–1999	Contact with pigs	265	105	39.6
Singapore	1999	Contact with pigs	11	1	9
India	2001 Siliguri	Human-to-human–close direct contact Contact with bats from the *Pteropus* spp.	66	45	68.2
	2007 Nadia		5	5	100
	2018 Kerala		18	17	94.4
	2021 Kerala		1	1	100.0
Bangladesh	2001 Meherpur	Consumption of contaminated fruits and palm sap Person-to-person–close direct contact	13	9	69.2
	2003–2007 Naogaon, Rajbari, Tangail, Kushtia, Natore, Pabna, Thakurgaon		99	78	78.8
	2008–2015 Manikganj, Rajbari, Gaibandha, Nilphamari, Rangpur, Faridpur, Gopalganj, Kurigram, Comilla, Dinajpur, Lalmonirhat, Joypurhat, Naogaon, Natore, Pabna, Magura, Ponchoghor		139	106	76.3
Philippines	2014	Contact with horses Consumption of horse meat	17	9	52.9

was 97.37–98.64%. The Kerala NiVs were shown to clustered with genotype B viruses but created variations within the clade (Arunkumar et al., 2019). In turn, the phylogenetic analysis by Yadav et al. (2019) based on four human and three fruit bats (*Pteropus medius*) samples from the 2018 outbreak in Kerala, India, found that human NiV was 96.15% similar to the Bangladeshi strain, but 99.7–100% similar to bat virus, meaning bats were the source of the epidemic. Recent reports of NiV cases date from 2019, when a single NiV case was confirmed in the Ernakulam district, culminating in a full recovery of the patient (Sahay et al., 2020).

In 2021, a 12-year-old boy died from the NiV infection on the 5th of September in Kerala's Kozhikode district. Samples taken after contact-tracing from friends, family members, and health workers were negative (World Health Organization [WHO], 2021b).

Philippines

The epidemic in the southern part of the Philippines occurred in 2014 and included 17 cases. It was characterized by high mortality, exceeding 80%. The infections were mainly associated with exposure to or consumption of horse meat, and the responsible strain was closely related to the Malaysian strain (Ching et al., 2015; Aditi and Shariff, 2019; Ambat et al., 2019). Fruit bats were the most likely source of horse infection (Ching et al., 2015).

SYMPTOMS OF NIPAH VIRUS INFECTION

The incubation period for the NiV virus ranges from 4 to 45 days (World Health Organization [WHO], 2021a), with typical symptoms not appearing until after a clinically quiescent period of 4 days to 2 weeks (Ochani et al., 2019; Thakur and Bailey, 2019). Disease caused by NiV infection can be overt or asymptomatic in nature. Cases of such subclinical infections were reported during the NiV epidemics in Malaysia and Singapore, although the percentages for all confirmed cases varied. In Malaysia, it ranged from 8 to 17%, while in Singapore it was even more than 45% (Tan et al., 1999; Parashar et al., 2000; Chan et al., 2002; Chua, 2003; Sharma et al., 2019). In turn, during the epidemic in Bangladesh, asymptomatic infections did not occur or were sporadic (Hsu et al., 2004). They were also rare in India. It confirmed a lower risk of subclinical infections in people who had physical contact with those infected with NiV, but without exposure to their body fluids (Kumar et al., 2019). Recurrence of latent infection has been observed up to months or years after acute infection (Thakur and Bailey, 2019).

Nipah virus infection can affect many major organs, including the brain, lungs, heart, kidneys, and spleen (Thakur and Bailey, 2019). Initial symptoms of NiV resemble flu-like infections, with fever, headache, dizziness, and vomiting (Thakur and Bailey, 2019). However, these symptoms can very quickly turn into an encephalitic syndrome that, in addition to headache and fever, is characterized by serious neurological symptoms. A decrease in consciousness was observed in patients, accompanied by convulsions and visible cerebellar symptoms along with tachycardia (Sharma et al., 2019). In studies conducted in Malaysia, more than 50% of the patients had a low level of consciousness and pronounced brain stem dysfunction (Chua, 2003). However, during the Bangladesh epidemic, the number of infected patients with similar symptoms was much higher, exceeding 90% (Sharma et al., 2019). The result of deep mental disorientation may be a coma appearing after 1–2 days (Singh et al., 2019).

In addition to neurological symptoms, severe respiratory disorders are also observed in NiV infection. Coughs, colds, and shortness of breath, and in extreme cases, acute respiratory distress syndrome, were especially frequently diagnosed during epidemics in Bangladesh and India. These problems are estimated to account for half to two-thirds of the cases. The lower number of patients who declared these symptoms during the epidemics in Malaysia and Singapore was due to differences between the NiV strains responsible for the disease in these regions and the higher frequency of human-to-human transmission confirmed in Bangladesh and India (Goh et al., 2000; Chua, 2003; Sharma et al., 2019; Thomas et al., 2019). Information about the symptoms of NiV infection is summarized in **Table 2**.

The effects of the virus on the host's organism depend on the type of strain responsible for the outbreak of a specific infection outbreak. Out of the NiV strains responsible for causing disease in humans tested so far, there are two main strains characterized–the Malaysian strain (NiV-MY) and the NiV Bangladesh (NiV-BD) (Ang et al., 2018; Devnath and Al Masud, 2021). The analyses showed that the NiV genome in Bangladesh and India is 18,252 nucleotides long and is six nucleotides longer than the Malaysian one (Ang et al., 2018; Aditi and Shariff, 2019). In turn, the nucleotide sequences of NiV strains from the Indian regions of Siliguri and Kerala showed 99 and 97% similarity to the strain from Bangladesh, respectively (Pallivalappil et al., 2020). Genetic differences between strains translate into epidemiological effects caused by them. NiV infections in Malaysia have been less severe, with lower mortality and more subclinical cases (Kumar et al., 2019). In Bangladesh and India, genetically similar strains caused a significantly higher number of deaths, although this was also partly related to the low quality of healthcare in these countries and the incidence of new virus outbreaks (Ochani et al., 2019; Sharma et al., 2019; Thakur and Bailey, 2019). The higher infection rate confirmed for the NiV strain from Bangladesh, related to the mode of human-to-human transmission, suggests the possibility of rapid mutation formation (Devnath and Al Masud, 2021). During the epidemic in India in 2001, the clinical symptoms observed in the Siliguri were similar to those of NiV cases diagnosed in neighboring Bangladesh (Chadha et al., 2006).

TABLE 2 | Clinical manifestations of NiV infection.

NiV MY	NiV BD
Primary influenza-like symptoms:	
fever 95%	*fever 100%*
headache 75%	*headache 73%*
vomiting 32%	*vomiting 58%*
Characteristic severe symptoms:	
• Reduced level of consciousness 72%	• Altered mental status or unconsciousness 90%
• Hyporeflexia 60%	• Areflexia/hyporeflexia 65%
• Encephalitis–segmental myoclonus 32–54%	• Segmental myoclonus–not reported
• Brain stem dysfunction: o abnormal pupils 52% o hypertension 43% o tachycardia 42%	• Respiratory symptoms: o *atypical pneumonia* o *cough 62%* o *respiratory difficulty 69%* o *acute respiratory distress syndrome 63%*
	• Severe weakness 72%

However, the 2018 NiV outbreak in Kerala was characterized by significantly higher mortality than in Siliguri and the occurrence of heart muscle dysfunction in patients–a symptom that had not been reported in previous epidemics (Pallivalappil et al., 2020). The mean disease duration from symptom onset to death was 16 days in Malaysia and only 4–6 days in Bangladesh and India (Ang et al., 2018; Pallivalappil et al., 2020).

NIPAH VIRUS TRANSMISSION

Animals as a Source of Nipah Virus

Nipah Virus belongs to the group of zoonotic viruses whose source and vector enabling transmission and multiplication are wild and domesticated animals. In some cases of NiV epidemics, depending on the location of the outbreak, the appearance of the virus in humans was associated with the presence of various animal species. Initially, the search for a natural animal NiV reservoir focused on bats in which the HeV, closely related to NiV, was previously detected (Chua, 2003). In Malaysia, the presence of NiV has been confirmed in species *Pteropus hypomelanus*, *Pteropus lylei*, and *Pteropus vampyrus* (Sharma et al., 2019). In India, early research to identify the NiV vector was carried out in insectivorous bats (*Megaderma spasma*), however, its presence was finally confirmed in fruit bats also of the genus *Pteropus*, e.g., *Pteropus giganteus* (Plowright et al., 2019; Thakur and Bailey, 2019). Following the detection of the NiV case in India in 2019, the presence of virus and IgG antibodies was confirmed in bats of the species *P. medius* (Sudeep et al., 2021). The highest degree of sequence similarity of NiV genes from infected bats and Indian patients compared to Malaysia, Cambodia, and Bangladesh clearly suggests that bats were the most likely source of human infection during this epidemic. It could have occurred by eating fruit contaminated with bat saliva or by inhaling an aerosol containing droplets of contaminated urine or saliva (Yadav et al., 2019). Raw date palm juice may also be an important source of the virus, which confirms that the dates of the NiV epidemics in Bangladesh coincide with the palm fruit harvesting and juice production periods (December–May) (Aditi and Shariff, 2019).

The presence of NiV was detected in 9–25% of serologically tested bat samples (antibodies against NiV detected by enzyme—linked immunosorbent assay) from Malaysia, Cambodia, Thailand, and Bangladesh (Sharma et al., 2019). The lack of characteristic clinical symptoms both in wild NiV-positive bats and in individuals intentionally vaccinated with the virus suggests that NiV may have been present in the organisms of these animals for a long time and cause sporadic infections in humans and animals. Only the development of appropriate diagnostic methods, including real-time RT-PCR (TaqMan) tests based on the identification of the specific sequence of the N gene, allowed its identification and monitoring (Thakur and Bailey, 2019). Currently, when looking for evidence of the presence of NiV in bats, but also in other animals, their secretions like saliva, urine, or feces are examined (Looi and Chua, 2007; Sharma et al., 2019; Sudeep et al., 2021).

Although bats are the primary natural reservoir for the NiV virus, pigs were the source of human infection during the Malaysian epidemic (Looi and Chua, 2007). They act as an intermediate host and become infected by eating fruit contaminated by bats (**Figure 2**; Thakur and Bailey, 2019). In pigs, NiV causes the syndrome of airway inflammation and encephalitis. The acute form of the disease with fever and cough occurs mainly in animals under 6 months of age. Neurological symptoms include muscle twitching, weakness of the hind legs, and paresis of varying severity (Singh et al., 2019). Despite the incidence of up to 100%, pig mortality from NiV infection is relatively low (Mohd Nor et al., 2000).

In Malaysia, NiV transmission to humans has occurred through close contact with infected pigs (**Figure 2**). Pig virus isolates in the southern regions of the country had identical gene sequences to those of humans (Abu Bakar et al., 2004). A clear link has been established between infection and the performance of activities related to pig breeding, e.g., drug application, insemination, or disposal of dead animals (Parashar et al., 2000; Thakur and Bailey, 2019). As in Malaysia, cases of NiV infection in Singapore resulted from direct contact with pigs or their feces and involved slaughterhouse workers (Paton et al., 1999; Chan et al., 2002; Aditi and Shariff, 2019).

In Bangladesh and India, the involvement of pigs as the virus vectors and the impact of these animals on the scale of infection have not been observed (Centers for Disease Control and Prevention [CDC], 1999; Thakur and Bailey, 2019). On the other hand, the presence of NiV in people who did not declare contact with pigs was an incentive to search for other potential virus hosts that could pose a threat to humans. Among the various animal species (birds, bats, pigs, and dogs) tested after the epidemic in Bangladesh, no virus was detected in them, and antibodies were found only in bats, which confirms that they could be a source of accidental infection (Hsu et al., 2004). Although NiV has been shown to infect dogs and cats by contact with infected pigs and their secretions, there is no definitive confirmation of their relevance to human infection. The end of the epidemic in Malaysia as a result of the massive destruction of pig herds proves the negligible role of other animals in the spread of NiV (Parashar et al., 2000; Chua, 2003; Mills et al., 2009).

Nipah Virus infection has also been found among hospital workers. NiV nosocomial transmission was reported during the outbreak in Siliguri, India (Chadha et al., 2006). Detection of NiV RNA on a hospital surface indicates that infected patients are transmitting the virus into an environment that could provide an opportunity for NiV transmission to hospital staff. Gurley et al. (2007) showed that environmental samples collected from

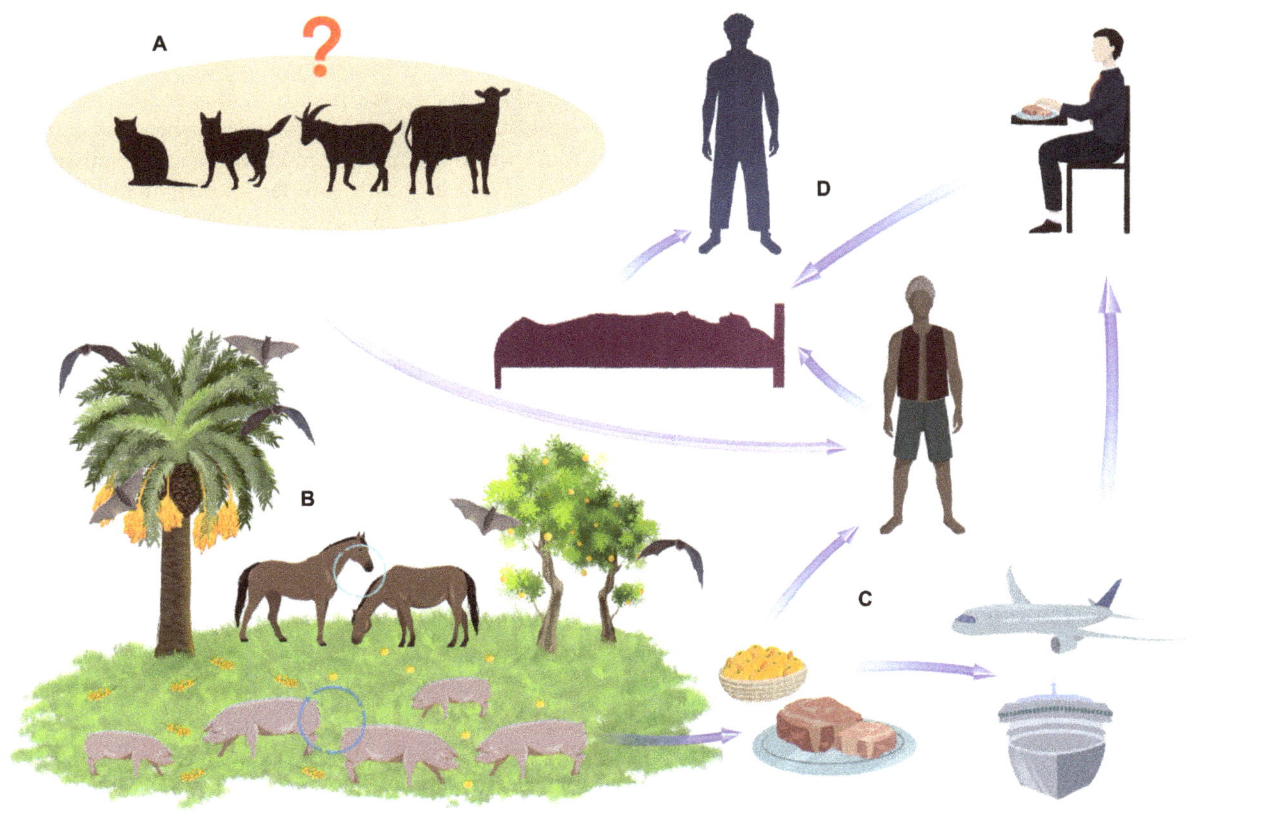

FIGURE 2 | Potential transmission routes of NiV. Pets and some farm animals, such as cows and sheep, are unconfirmed routes of transmission NiV **(A)**. Bats are the natural reservoir of the NiV. When they eat date fruit, the NiV can infect other animals such as pigs and horses, which eat the remains of falling fruit **(B)**. Virus can transmitted to humans through the consumption of the date palm sap or by meat exported all over the world **(C)**. Close contact wit NiV affected human in different situations e.g., in hospital can lead to spread of the virus to other person **(D)**.

hospital areas were contaminated with NiV (RT-PCR). The lifetime of NiV on the surface is not known exactly.

Human-to-Human Transmission

Studies on the spread of NiV during the Bangladesh epidemic led to the conclusion that it was primarily the result of human-to-human transmission of the virus through direct contact with patients and their natural secretions. The primary infection came from a source that is difficult to establish. Probably these were the secretions of the *Pteropus* genus bats (Montgomery et al., 2008). A 2003 study found the presence of the virus within shared households, which could indicate human-to-human transmission (by the respiratory route), but at the same time did not rule out the possibility of external infection. The reason for these doubts was the lack of infections in hospital staff who came into contact with patients (Hsu et al., 2004). However, another study conducted in Bangladesh in 2001–2014 suggests that, in 82 (33.06%) of 248 patients, NiV infection could have been the result of person-to-person transmission of the disease (Nikolay et al., 2020). In contrast, Gurley et al. (2007) found that 92% of patients had close contact with another affected person before becoming ill, and five cases were likely related to secondary and tertiary NiV transmission from person to person. This mode of transmission of the virus was also confirmed during an epidemic in India, both in 2001 in West Bengal and in 2018 in Kerala. Infections occurred in a hospital setting and repeatedly affected healthcare professionals, as well as people visiting patients in hospitals where cases of NiV had been confirmed (Chadha et al., 2006; Thomas et al., 2019).

RISK FACTORS

The age and sex of infected people are ranked as basic factors that can determine susceptibility to NiV infection. Studies conducted during the Malaysia epidemic indicate that NiV affected mainly male adults, whose average age ranged from 37 to 44 years (75–81.6%) (Goh et al., 2000; Parashar et al., 2000; Chua, 2003). At the time of the Bangladesh outbreak in early 2004, most NiV-infected patients were young boys under the age of 15. However, it is suspected that the low average age of the infected (11.5 years) was related to the frequency of infection-risk-increasing activities i.e., climbing trees with bats carrying NiV. This factor rather than young age was considered relevant in this case (Montgomery et al., 2008). The analysis of Bangladesh NiV cases between 2001 and 2014 showed that the median age of the patients was 24 years and most of them (64%) were men (Nikolay et al., 2020). However, detailed analyses showed significant differences between the regions of the country. The median age of patients with confirmed or probable NiV infection was 12 years in the Naogaon region, and 38 years in the Meherpur region. A shorter time from the first symptoms of the disease to death (4 days vs. 6 days) was also observed in younger Naogaon patients. These results suggest that both children and adults are susceptible to NiV infection (Hsu et al., 2004). Patients infected with NiV in India in Siliguri province were over 15 years old and the female to male ratio was 1.4:1 (Chadha et al., 2006). Also, the subsequent Kerala epidemic affected mainly men, while the mean age of those infected was 41 years (Thomas et al., 2019).

The high percentage of infections in men observed during various epidemics of NiV may be a direct result of their occupations related to close contact with infected animals or their secretions. In Malaysia, where pigs have been confirmed as the intermediate NiV hosts and contact with them has been the predominant mode of virus transmission to humans, the majority (70%) of infections were in pig farmers and piggery workers (Chua, 2003). Subsequent studies confirmed these data, stating that more than 90% of patients lived or worked on a pig farm, performed work involving exposure to pigs, or had contact with these animals or their urine or feces (Parashar et al., 2000). More than 40% of these people reported the deaths of animals with which they had contact (Goh et al., 2000).

When assessing the degree of risk resulting from contact with pigs, one must also take into account the prevailing method of breeding them in a given region. In Malaysia it is practiced to keep them in large pigsties. Whereas in Bangladesh, which is a Muslim country, the scale of their production is limited, and small herds are usually kept by one person. This limits the possibility of virus transmission both between animals and from animals to humans. It is assumed that, *inter alia*, for this reason, pigs were not involved in the outbreaks in Bangladesh (Looi and Chua, 2007; Aditi and Shariff, 2019). Also in India, pig breeding is carried out on a smaller scale than in Malaysia (Ang et al., 2018).

In addition to people working with animals, healthcare workers are a professional group particularly vulnerable to NiV infection. They were frequently diagnosed with an infection, especially during these epidemics, when the human–human route was the dominant mode of NiV transmission. Working and staying in health care facilities significantly increases the risk of exposure to viruses that enter the environment as a result of coughing and sneezing and are transferred to particles suspended in the air, which is especially dangerous in poorly ventilated rooms. In Bangladesh, the presence of virus RNA on hospital surfaces was proven, but these studies did not conclusively determine the possibility of infection by this route (Gurley et al., 2017). Contact with patients' body fluids is also a factor that increases the risk of virus transmission to hospital staff (Sayed et al., 2019). In Malaysia, after examining more than 600 health care workers, both exposed and not exposed to contact with patients, no cases were observed, although some of the respondents confirmed needle-stick injuries and exposure of mucous membranes and skin to body fluids (Mounts et al., 1999). During the epidemics that appeared in Bangladesh in 2001–2014, three infections among medical workers were reported (Nikolay et al., 2020). In India, in 2001, the predominant source of infection in the Siliguri region was contact with infected people in healthcare facilities. The 75% of patients were previously staying in a hospital environment including the employees of such facilities (Chadha et al., 2006). During the last confirmed epidemic in the Kerala region in India (2018), hospital transmission of the virus was observed in three hospitals and two health care workers were infected (Thomas et al., 2019). In the context of the increased risk of NiV infection in hospital conditions, which was observed during the epidemic in

Bangladesh and India, it is worth emphasizing the importance of regularly confirmed negligence in basic hygiene practices, such as washing hands or the use of personal protective equipment (Chadha et al., 2006; Sayed et al., 2019).

The increased risk of the viral infection also applies to family members caring for patients at home. In the case of countries where NiV outbreaks have occurred so far, this model is supported by the cultural norms (Thakur and Bailey, 2019). Family groups in which family members became infected during caregiving were identified as clusters of infections in India (Thomas et al., 2019). It is also suspected that religious practices specific to some of the countries may influence the spread of the NiV virus. The majority of Bangladeshi Muslims do not eat pork and avoid contact with pigs, which may have influenced the way the virus is transmitted in the country bypassing the intermediate host (Montgomery et al., 2008). On the other hand, the practice of washing corpses, including those who died as a result of NiV infection, before the funeral, consistent with the Islamic funeral ritual, could contribute to the transmission of the virus to family members (Ambat et al., 2019).

The factors determining the scale and intensity of individual epidemics were also climatic phenomena independent of humans, such as catastrophes, which, combined with the progressive anthropogenic degradation of the natural environment, may modify the living conditions of the animal hosts of the NiV virus.

There are hypotheses linking the NiV outbreak with the El Niño anomaly in 1997–1998 and the drought it caused, which exacerbated the 1997 anthropogenic fires in Indonesia. The resulting dense fog limited the flowering and fruiting of the forest trees. This resulted in the migration of forest fruit bats from their wild habitats to cultivated orchards located near human inhabited places and their farm animals (Looi and Chua, 2007). In Malaysia, the original transfer of NiV from bats to domestic pigs and eventually to humans and other animals was found to occur at a pig farm near which fruit trees were planted. They were to provide a source of additional income and provide shade, and they turned out to be an excellent habitat for NiV-infected bats, whose secretions contaminated the pig feed and water (Chua, 2003; Daszak et al., 2013).

The reduction of the forest area and the progressive urbanization process also destroy the bats' habitats which, in search of food, move near human settlements. Hunger-induced high stress levels and lowered immunity cause an increase in viremia in their organisms and the virus titer in the urine, semen, and saliva they excrete (Ambat et al., 2019).

NIPAH VIRUS DIAGNOSTICS

Many methods are used in the diagnosis of NiV. Virus isolation in Vero cells, producing cytopathic effects (characterized by syncytia formation and cell death, and an ensuing vasculitis) within 3 days, is used to confirm new NiV foci. Samples from which NiV can be isolated are CSF, respiratory swabs (in viral transport medium), blood, and urine, but all testing procedures must be performed in BSL-4 laboratories (Aditi and Shariff, 2019; Sharma et al., 2019).

Among serological tests based on the detection of IgM and IgG antibodies, ELISA is a simple and inexpensive test (Aditi and Shariff, 2019; Ambat et al., 2019; Sharma et al., 2019). However, it is not 100% specific and may produce false results. Molecular methods provide a higher level of sensitivity and specificity. The polymerase chain reaction (PCR) technique used until recently as a standard has already been replaced by more and more sensitive and specific ones, including conventional reverse transcription PCR (RT-PCR), nested RT-PCR, real-time RT-PCR with the use of intercalating dyes (qPCR), real-time RT-PCR with the use of hydrolysis probes (TaqMan), multiplex bead-based real-time RT-PCR or the RT-LAMP assay. RT-PCR tests for NiV have targeted a highly conserved region of the N, M, or P gene in the viral genome (Guillaume et al., 2004; Ma et al., 2019; Mazzola and Kelly-Cirino, 2019; Ochani et al., 2019; Thakur and Bailey, 2019).

TREATMENT

Due to the lack of an effective drug against NiV, the management of patients is limited to supportive and prophylactic treatment (Chakraborty et al., 2019; Sharma et al., 2019). The basic clinical practices in the case of confirmation of NiV infection are maintenance of airway patency, prophylaxis of venous thrombosis, and maintenance of fluid and electrolyte balance (Aditi and Shariff, 2019; Ambat et al., 2019). Mechanical ventilation is used in severe respiratory symptoms. People infected with NiV are also given broad-spectrum antibiotics (Ambat et al., 2019).

Various active substances have been tested in the search for a drug that inhibits NiV proliferation. However, the effectiveness of ribavirin administered during the epidemic in Malaysia is debatable, as is the effectiveness of acyclovir used in Singapore (Ambat et al., 2019; Sharma et al., 2019; Devnath and Al Masud, 2021). The antimalarial drug chloroquine showed effectiveness in inhibiting NiV in cell cultures, which could not be confirmed in animal models (Aditi and Shariff, 2019; Ambat et al., 2019; Ochani et al., 2019). Promising results were observed after the application of the drug Favipiravir (T-705) and the monoclonal antibodies m102.4 in animals (Sayed et al., 2019; Singh et al., 2019; Devnath and Al Masud, 2021). The monoclonal antibody m102.4 is in phase I human trials (Playford et al., 2020). Eighty-six treatments related adverse events were reported, with similar rates in the placebo and treated groups. No deaths have been recorded (Playford et al., 2020). Lo et al. (2020) evaluated the *in vitro* antiviral activity of GRFT (Griffithsin) and its synthetic trimeric tandemer (3mG) against NiV and other viruses from four virus families. Researchers demonstrated that a preliminary *in vivo* evaluation of oxidation-resistant GRFT (Q-GRFT) showed significant protection against a lethal NiV challenge in golden Syrian hamsters. GRFT is a high mannose oligosaccharide-binding lectin that has shown a broad spectrum *in vivo* activity against viruses (Lo et al., 2020).

VACCINES

Clinical trials with vaccines to protect against NiV are limited due to the lack of new viral outbreaks. The effectiveness of potential preparations is tested in animal models. To date, research has included over 10 vaccines based on viral vectors, mRNA, recombinant protein subunits, or virus-like particles (Broder et al., 2016; Amaya and Broder, 2020). The most studied so far is the subunit vaccine based on soluble recombinant Hendra G-glycoprotein (HeV-sG), also inducing a cross-immune response against NiV. It has been proven to be completely effective in protecting against NiV MY, NiV BD, and HeV in horses, cats, ferrets, and non-human primates, while it did not show effectiveness in pigs (Mungall et al., 2006; McEachern et al., 2008; Bossart et al., 2012; Pallister et al., 2013; Middleton et al., 2014; Mire et al., 2014). The only vaccine officially approved and registered by the Australian Pesticides and Veterinary Medicines Authority (APVMA) vaccine is Equivac produced by Zoetis, Inc. It is used in the prophylactic treatment of horses (Aditi and Shariff, 2019; Ambat et al., 2019; Ochani et al., 2019; Geisbert et al., 2021). Geisbert et al. (2021) conducted two studies on this NiV vaccine. The first one showed that a single dose of vaccination was effective, and the second one showed that the period of 7 days after the first dose was effective in protecting African green monkey (AGM) from the debris form of NiV. Studies conducted in an animal model similar to the human organism–the AGM model confirm the effectiveness of a single dose of this vaccine, which may constitute the basis for its potential use in the event of sudden outbreaks of NiV infection (Geisbert et al., 2021).

Animal studies have also shown the efficacy of recombinant vesicular stomatitis viruses (rVSV recombinant vesicular stomatitis viruses, rMV recombinant measles virus) (Yoneda et al., 2013; Debuysscher et al., 2014; Ang et al., 2018). Yoneda et al. (2013) conducted a study of the effectiveness of recombinant rMV in hamsters and AGM. Researchers demonstrated an increase in anti-NiV antibodies in the serum of hamsters within 3 weeks after inoculation. The hamsters showed no signs of disease and no mortality. Immunization with AGM with two doses of the vaccine protected the monkeys from clinical signs of disease, and levels of antibodies to the NiV G protein were induced. Also, Debuysscher et al. (2014) assessed the recombinant rMV expressing NiV glycoproteins (G or F) or nucleoprotein (N) in a Syrian hamster model. The results were promising as even the first dose of vaccination produced a high humoral immune response (Debuysscher et al., 2014).

The search for new vaccines is constantly ongoing. A vaccine designed by Soltan et al. (2021) is a multi-strain vaccine based on the highest-ranked CTL, HTL, and BCL epitopes from selected NiV proteins. The vaccine design was analyzed for allergenicity and toxicity, physicochemical features, antigenicity, and solubility (computational analysis). The designed vaccine was shown to be non-toxic and non-allergenic (Soltan et al., 2021). However, experimental trials are required to prove the practical effectiveness of this potential vaccine construct. Another attempt to design a vaccine against NiV was made by Loomis et al. (2020). Researchers assessed antigenicity and structural integrity protein subunit vaccines (F and G proteins, stabilized pre-F and G to form a chimeric protein) using kinetic binding assays, electron microscopy and other biophysical properties. Vaccine efficacy was assessed in a mouse model. Mice immunized with all the pre-F designs showed similar levels of pre-F and post-F binding. All mice immunized with multimeric G forms induced only G-specific antibody responses, while mice immunized with pre-F/G or pre-F + G chimeras generated antibody responses directed against both F and monomeric G proteins. Loomis et al. (2020) confirmed that the NiV G glycoprotein is an effective vaccine immunogen and it is feasible to design both pre-F and G as a single vaccine construct which confers greater diversity in responses to antigenic sites (Loomis et al., 2020). Loomis et al. (2020) confirmed that the F NiV protein pre-fusion induces stronger neutralizing activity than post-fusion F, thus confirming the importance of stabilizing the pre-fusion conformation for increasing immunogenicity. In another study by Loomis et al. (2021), an attempt was made to stabilize the fusion protein (F) in its pre-fusion trimeric (pre-F) conformation to increase expression and immunogenicity using design principles based on protein structure. Loomis et al. (2021) have shown that Pre-F and G induce potent neutralizing antibody responses as mRNA vaccines.

Vaccinations are an important part of the fight against the epidemic. Continued work on new vaccines against NiV is necessary, especially in view of clinical trials.

PREVENTION

Due to the limited possibilities of effective treatment and the lack of a vaccine, it seems justified to focus the efforts of scientists and institutions responsible for monitoring epidemiological threats on preventing NiV emergence and their effective supervision.

Preventive strategies to limit the appearance of new and the spread of already initiated epidemic outbreaks relate primarily to avoiding direct contact with the hosts of the virus (fruit bats and pigs) and their secretions and avoiding consumption of contaminated food. On the one hand, it is recommended to carefully check and wash the fruit of the trees where bats live. On the other hand, procedures are implemented to limit their access to places and vessels used to collect date palm juice (bamboo skirt method) (Ambat et al., 2019; Sharma et al., 2019). It is also recommended not to plant fruit trees that attract bats near the piggery (Ang et al., 2018). During work requiring direct contact with farm animals, especially during slaughter and disposal procedures, appropriate protective clothing is required (Aditi and Shariff, 2019).

Implementation of actions raising public awareness of the risks associated with the outbreak of the virus and the importance of preventive measures is another factor that may help to the risk of the new outbreak. Local television, radio channels, and printed media informed local societies, for example, on the dangers of drinking contaminated date palm juice, recommending that its consumption should be limited (Aditi and Shariff, 2019). Similar attempts to eliminate the consumption of fresh juices turned out to be ineffective, as they contradicted the prevailing social and cultural norms (Ang et al., 2018).

An important preventive measure that can effectively reduce the scale of the spread of NiV is to prevent the spread of the virus through direct human-human contact. Washing hands, disinfecting with 70% ethanol, wearing gloves and other protective equipment, and avoiding direct contact with body fluids are standard rules for caring for a person infected or just suspected of having NiV infection (Sharma et al., 2019). In a hospital setting, sharing food and bed between patients is unacceptable.

It is important to evaluate the disinfection efficiency against NiV. Both chemical and physical methods. Like other paramyxoviruses, NiV is easily deactivated by soaps, detergents and many disinfectants. Sodium hypochlorite has been recommended for disinfection of pig farms in Malaysia (Spiclera, 2016). Eickmann et al. (2020) demonstrated an effective reduction of NiV infectivity in platelet and plasma concentrates using UV-C and MB/light (increasing doses of visible light). Treatment with 0.2 J cm^2 UV-C reduced the infectivity of NiV ($\geq$4.3 log) to the limit of detection (LOD) in platelet concentrates, and treatment with MB (120 J/cm^2) reduced NiV ($\geq$2.7 log) to LOD in the plasma.

Transmission of infections to healthcare professionals can be reduced by ensuring access to hand hygiene facilities, regular and appropriate use of personal protective equipment, and isolating patients with meningitis. It is of particular importance to follow appropriate procedures during funeral ceremonies–wearing gloves and masks, washing hands thoroughly with soap and water immediately after contact with the corpse (Ambat et al., 2019).

In the regions along the NiV belt, surveillance is also carried out to enable early detection of virus outbreaks, analysis of its strains, and monitoring of the relationship between environmental factors and the dynamics of epidemic development. For this purpose, specialized research teams are established to identify suspected cases of infection in humans and analyze the possibility of the emergence of new species of potential reservoir hosts of the virus responsible for its transmission to humans (Aditi and Shariff, 2019; Ambat et al., 2019).

NIPAH VIRUS–PANDEMIC POTENTIAL

The situation of the global COVID-19 pandemic, which has resulted in the deaths of nearly 5 million people, encourages scientists to conduct research that will stop the spread of the virus, reduce its effects and help to develop an effective strategy for recognizing, preventing, and managing the emergence of other pathogens with epidemic potential.

One of the features indicating the viral pandemic potential is the rapid and effective transmission of the pathogen from person to person, especially in the absence of immunity in exposed people. This route of NiV transmission was confirmed to be extremely important during the epidemics in Bangladesh and India. Infection may occur as a result of direct contact with an infected person or their secretions, and an additional risk is posed by the possibility of virus transmission with saliva particles in patients with severe respiratory symptoms and accompanying cough (Luby et al., 2009). Many studies indicate that respiratory tract secretion is the main source of infection in accompanying patients and confirm the relationship between virus transmission through this route and the degree of manifestation of symptoms of advanced changes in the respiratory system (Luby, 2013).

The airborne route is also the main mode of transmission of the SARS-CoV-2 virus, which results in the introduction of general orders to apply appropriate protective measures in the pandemic society (Dhand and Li, 2020).

The high mortality characteristic of NiV is a factor that can limit the spread of a virus that does not infect another due to the death of the host. However, it is worth taking into account that the current NiV outbreaks were usually detected in sparsely populated villages (Devnath and Al Masud, 2021). It can be assumed that in the event of an epidemic in a highly populated place, the increase in infections rate could be much higher, especially since, according to WHO, the incubation period for NiV in extreme cases may last 45 days. People-to-people contacts are favored by the growth of the human population globalization, trade, or contemporary travel patterns (Carrasco-Hernandez et al., 2017). Taking into account the risk associated with the appearance of a certain percentage of subclinical cases, the rank of NiV as a potential source of another global epidemic increases.

Amidst the known and tested strains of NiV so far, differences have been observed in transmission methods, the symptoms type and severity, and finally the size of genomes confirmed by molecular analyses. Indirectly, this indicates the need to include the risk of the emergence of mutations, e.g., facilitating the human-to-human viral transmission, in the assessment of the NiV pandemic potential. Such suggestions were made when sequencing of a NiV genome fragment from a Filipino patient (2014) showed a high degree of similarity to the Malaysian strain. However, while in the case of the epidemic in Malaysia no human-to-human transmission was recorded, this possibility has already been confirmed in the Philippines (Ching et al., 2015). RNA viruses, due to their commonly observed high rate of nucleotide substitutions, poor ability to correct mutation errors, and the resulting adaptability to new hosts, are regarded as extremely dangerous and require close supervision (Jones et al., 2008).

In addition to human-human contact, NiV infection can occur through contact with animals. The primary reservoir of NiV is bats, which are likely to have also been a source of COVID-19 infections in humans (Zhou et al., 2020). The detection of henipaviruses in bats in China and West Africa may suggest that the diseases they cause will also appear outside of Asia and Australia (Halpin and Rota, 2014; Kasloff et al., 2019). The range of NiV hosts, unlike other paramyxoviruses, is surprisingly wide, resulting from the virus binding to the ephrin B-2 and B-3 receptors, common in mammalian epithelial cells (Luby, 2014). The possibility of domestic and farm animals infection creates additional opportunity of NiV transmission to humans (Ang et al., 2018). Recent studies show that pigs excluded as a source of the virus during an epidemic in Bangladesh are susceptible to NiV-B infection without evidence of clinical disease. The presence of an infectious virus in the nasal wash may indicate the possibility that asymptomatically infected pigs infect susceptible animals and spread the virus (Kasloff et al., 2019).

CONCLUSION

Drawing conclusions from the COVID-19 pandemic, we must be prepared for the fact that any zoonotic virus, especially one with the ability to human-to-human transmission, can be very dangerous and contribute to a global pandemic. An important argument justifying the concerns about the emergence of NiV in the human population is the lack of vaccines and drugs with proven effectiveness. Attempts to develop them do not bring the expected results, and in combination with the problems in the healthcare efficiency revealed during the ongoing COVID-19 epidemic, both in the poorest and highly developed countries, they can result in serious consequences on a global scale (Ang et al., 2018; Gurley et al., 2020).

AUTHOR CONTRIBUTIONS

KS, JB-K, and KG-B: conceptualization. KG-B and MZ: formal analysis. KS, JB-K, and NW-K: writing—original draft preparation. KS, KG-B, and MZ: writing—review and editing. ZB, KG-B, and NW-K: visualization. KS and EG-K: supervision. KS and JB-K: project administration. All authors have read and agreed to the published version of the manuscript.

FUNDING

The publication was financed under the Leading Research Groups support project from the subsidy increased for the period 2020-2025 in the amount of 2% of the subsidy referred to Art. 387 (3) of the Law of July 20, 2018 on Higher Education and Science, obtained in 2019.

REFERENCES

1. Abu Bakar, S., Chang, L. Y., Ali, A. R., Sharifah, S. H., Yusoff, K., and Zamrod, Z. (2004). Isolation and molecular identification of *Nipah virus* from pigs. *Emerg. Infect. Dis.* 10, 2228–2230. doi: 10.3201/eid1012.040452
2. Aditi, and Shariff, M. (2019). *Nipah virus* infection: a review. *Epidemiol. Infect.* 147:e95. doi: 10.1017/S09502688190000
3. Aguilar, H. C., Aspericueta, V., Robinson, L. R., Aanensen, K. E., and Lee, B. (2010). A quantitative and kinetic fusion protein-triggering assay can discern distinct steps in the *Nipah virus* membrane fusion cascade. *J. Virol.* 84, 8033–8041.
4. Aguilar, H. C., Henderson, B. A., Zamora, J. L., and Johnston, G. P. (2016). Paramyxovirus glycoproteins and the membrane fusion process. *Curr. Clin. Microbiol. Rep.* 3, 142–154.
5. Aiyar, A., and Pingali, P. (2020). Pandemics and food systems - towards a proactive food safety approach to disease prevention & management. *Food Sec.* 12, 749–756. doi: 10.1007/s12571-020-01074-3
6. Amaya, M., and Broder, C. C. (2020). Vaccines to emerging viruses: *Nipah* and *Hendra*. *Annu. Rev. Virol.* 7, 447–473.
7. Ambat, A. S., Zubair, S. M., Prasad, N., Pundir, P., Rajwar, E., Patil, D. S., et al. (2019). *Nipah virus*: a review on epidemiological characteristics and outbreaks to inform public health decision making. *J. Infect. Public Health* 12, 634–639. doi: 10.1016/j.jiph.2019.02.013
8. Anderson, D. E., Islam, A., Crameri, G., Todd, S., Islam, A., Khan, S. U., et al. (2019). Isolation and full-genome characterization of *Nipah viruses* from bats, Bangladesh. *Emerg. Infect. Dis.* 25, 166–170. doi: 10.3201/eid2501.18 0267
9. Ang, B., Lim, T., and Wang, L. (2018). *Nipah virus* infection. *J. Clin. Microbiol.* 56, 1875–1817. doi: 10.1128/JCM.01875-17
10. Arankalle, V. A., Bandyopadhyay, B. T., Ramdasi, A. Y., Jadi, R., Patil, D. R., Rahman, M., et al. (2011). Genomic characterization of *Nipah virus*, West Bengal, India. *Emerg. Infect. Dis.* 17, 907–909. doi: 10.3201/eid1705.100968
11. Arunkumar, G., Chandni, R., Mourya, D. T., Singh, S. K., Sadanandan, R., Sudan, P., et al. (2019). *Nipah* investigators people and health study group. outbreak investigation of *Nipah virus* disease in Kerala, India, 2018. *J. Infect. Dis.* 219, 1867–1878. doi: 10.1093/infdis/jiy612
12. Bossart, K. N., Rockx, B., Feldmann, F., Brining, D., Scott, D., LaCasse, R., et al. (2012). A *Hendra virus* G glycoprotein subunit vaccine protects African green monkeys from *Nipah virus* challenge. *Sci. Transl. Med.* 4:146ra107. doi: 10.1126/ scitranslmed.3004241
13. Broder, C. C., Weir, D. L., and Reid, P. A. (2016). *Hendra virus* and *Nipah virus* animal vaccines. *Vaccine* 34, 3525–3534.
14. Carrasco-Hernandez, R., Jácome, R., López Vidal, Y., and Ponce de León, S. (2017). Are RNA viruses candidate agents for the next global pandemic? A review. *ILAR J.* 58, 343–358. doi: 10.1093/ilar/ilx026
15. Centers for Disease Control and Prevention [CDC] (1999). Update: outbreak of *Nipah virus*–Malaysia, and Singapore, 1999. *MMWR Morb. Mortal Wkly. Rep.* 48, 335–337.
16. Chadha, M. S., Comer, J. A., Lowe, L., Rota, P. A., Rollin, P. E., Bellini, W. J., et al. (2006). *Nipah virus*-associated encephalitis outbreak, Siliguri, India. *Emerg. Infect. Dis.* 12, 235–240. doi: 10.3201/eid1202.051247
17. Chakraborty, S., Deb, B., Barbhuiya, P. A., and Uddin, A. (2019). Analysis of codon usage patterns and influencing factors in *Nipah virus*. *Virus Res.* 263, 129–138. doi: 10.1016/j.virusres.2019.01.011
18. Chan, K. P., Rollin, P. E., Ksiazek, T. G., Leo, Y. S., Goh, K. T., Paton, N. I., et al. (2002). A survey of *Nipah virus* infection among various risk groups in Singapore. *Epidemiol. Infect.* 128, 93–98. doi: 10.1017/s0950268801006422
19. Ching, P. K., de los Reyes, V. C., Sucaldito, M. N., Tayag, E., Columna-Vingno, A. B., Malbas, F. F., et al. (2015). Outbreak of henipavirus infection, Philippines, 2014. *Emerg. Infect. Dis.* 21, 328–331. doi: 10.3201/eid2102.141433
20. Chua, K. B. (2003). *Nipah virus* outbreak in Malaysia. *J. Clin. Virol.* 26, 265–275. doi: 10.1016/s1386-6532(02)00268-8
21. Chua, K. B., Goh, K. J., Wong, K. T., Kamarulzaman, A., Tan, P. S., Ksiazek, T. G., et al. (1999). Fatal encephalitis due to *Nipah virus* among pig-farmers in Malaysia. *Lancet* 354, 1257–1259. doi: 10.1016/S0140-6736(99)04299-3
22. Daszak, P., Zambrana-Torrelio, C., Bogich, T. L., Fernandez, M., Epstein, J. H., Murray, K. A., et al. (2013). Interdisciplinary approaches to understanding disease emergence: the past, present, and future drivers of *Nipah virus* emergence. *Proc. Natl. Acad. Sci. U.S.A.* 110(Suppl. 1), 3681–3688.
23. Debuysscher, B., Scott, D., Marzi, A., Prescott, J., and Feldmann, H. (2014). Single-dose live-attenuated *Nipah virus* vaccines confer complete protection by eliciting antibodies directed against surface glycoproteins. *Vaccine* 32, 2637– 2644. doi: 10.1016/j.vaccine.2014.02.087
24. Devnath, P., and Al Masud, H. M. A. (2021). The *Nipah virus*: a potential pandemic agent in the context of the current severe acute respiratory syndrome coronavirus-2 pandemic. *New Microb. New Infect.* 41, 1–6. doi: 10.1016/j.nmni. 2021.100873
25. Dhand, R., and Li, J. (2020). Coughs and sneezes: their role in transmission of respiratory viral infections, including SARS-CoV-2. *Am. J. Respir. Crit. Care Med.* 202, 651–659. doi: 10.1164/rccm.202004-1263PP
26. Drexler, J., Corman, V., Müller, M., Maganga, G. D., Vallo, P., Binger, T., et al. (2012). Bats host major mammalian paramyxoviruses. *Nat. Commun.* 3:796. doi: 10.1038/ncomms1796
27. Eickmann, M., Gravemann, U., Handke, W., Tolksdorf, F., Reichenberg, S., Müller, T. H., et al. (2020). Inactivation of three emerging viruses - severe acute respiratory syndrome coronavirus, Crimean-Congo haemorrhagic

fever virus and *Nipah virus* - in platelet concentrates by ultraviolet C light and in plasma by methylene blue plus visible light. *Vox Sang.* 115, 146–151. doi: 10.1111/vox. 12888

28. Geisbert, T. W., Bobb, K., Borisevich, V., Geisbert, J. B., Agans, K. N., Cross, R. W., et al. (2021). A single dose investigational subunit vaccine for human use against *Nipah virus* and *Hendra virus*. *NPJ Vaccines* 6:23. doi: 10.1038/ s41541-021- 00284-w
29. Goh, K. J., Tan, C. T., Chew, N. K., Tan, P. S., Kamarulzaman, A., Sarji, S. A., et al. (2000). Clinical features of *Nipah virus* encephalitis among pig farmers in Malaysia. *N. Engl. J. Med.* 342, 1229–1235. doi: 10.1056/ NEJM200004273421701
30. Guillaume, V., Lefeuvre, A., Faure, C., Marianneau, P., Buckland, R., Lam, S. K., et al. (2004). Specific detection of *Nipah virus* using real-time RT-PCR (TaqMan). *J. Virol. Methods* 15, 229–237.
31. Gurley, E. S., Hegde, S. T., Hossain, K., Sazzad, H. M. S., Hossain, M. J., Rahman, M., et al. (2017). Convergence of humans, bats, trees, and culture in *Nipah virus* transmission, Bangladesh. *Emerg. Infect. Dis* 23, 1446–1453. doi: 10.3201/ eid2309.161922
32. Gurley, E. S., Montgomery, J. M., Hossain, M. J., Bell, M., Azad, A. K., Islam, M. R., et al. (2007). Person-to-person transmission of *Nipah virus* in a Bangladeshi community. *Emerg. Infect. Dis.* 13, 1031–1037. doi: 10.3201/ eid1307.061128
33. Gurley, E. S., Spiropoulou, C. F., and de Wit, E. (2020). Twenty years of *Nipah virus* research: where do we go from here? *J. Infect. Dis.* 221, S359–S362. doi: 10.1093/infdis/jiaa078
34. Halpin, K., and Rota, P. A. (2014). Review of *Hendra virus* and *Nipah virus* infections in man and other animals. *Zoonoses Infect. Affect. Hum. Anim.* 22, 997–1012. doi: 10.1007/978-94-017-9457-2_40
35. Harcourt, B. H., Tamin, A., Halpin, K., Ksiazek, T. G., Rollin, P. E., Bellini, W. J., et al. (2001). Molecular characterization of the polymerase gene and genomic termini of *Nipah virus*. *Virology* 287, 192–201. doi: 10.1006/ viro.2001. 1026
36. Hauser, N., Gushiken, A. C., Narayanan, S., Kottilil, S., and Chua, J. V. (2021). Evolution of *Nipah virus* infection: past, present, and future considerations. *Trop. Med. Infect. Dis.* 6:24. doi: 10.3390/tropicalmed6010024
37. Hsu, V. P., Hossain, M. J., Parashar, U. D., Ali, M. M., Ksiazek, T. G., Kuzmin, I., et al. (2004). *Nipah virus* encephalitis reemergence, Bangladesh. *Emerg. Infect. Dis.* 10, 2082–2087. doi: 10.3201/eid1012.040701
38. Jones, K., Patel, N., Levy, M., Storeygard, A., Balk, D., Gittleman, J. L., et al. (2008). Global trends in emerging infectious diseases. *Nature* 451, 990–993. doi: 10.1038/nature06536
39. Kasloff, S. B., Leung, A., Pickering, B. S., Smith, G., Moffat, E., Collignon, B., et al. (2019). Pathogenicity of *Nipah henipavirus* Bangladesh in a swine host. *Sci. Rep.* 9:5230. doi: 10.1038/s41598-019-40476-y
40. Kumar, C. P. G., Sugunan, A. P., Yadav, P., Kurup, K. K., Aarathee, R., Manickam, P., et al. (2019). Infections among contacts of patients with *Nipah virus*, India. *Emerg. Infect. Dis.* 25, 1007–1010. doi: 10.3201/eid2505.181352
41. Lam, S. K., and Chua, K. B. (2002). *Nipah virus* encephalitis outbreak in Malaysia. *Clin. Infect. Dis.* 34, 48–51. doi: 10.1086/338818
42. Lo, M. K., Lowe, L., Hummel, K. B., Sazzad, H. M., Gurley, E. S., Hossain, M. J., et al. (2012). Characterization of *Nipah virus* from outbreaks in Bangladesh, 2008-2010. *Emerg. Infect. Dis.* 18, 248–255. doi: 10.3201/ eid1802.111492
43. Lo, M. K., Spengler, J. R., Krumpe, L. R. H., Welch, S. R., Chattopadhyay, A., Harmon, J. R., et al. (2020). Griffithsin inhibits *Nipah virus* entry and fusion and can protect syrian golden hamsters from lethal *Nipah virus* challenge. *J. Infect. Dis.* 221(Suppl._4), 480–S492. doi: 10.1093/infdis/jiz630
44. Looi, L. M., and Chua, K. B. (2007). Lessons from the *Nipah virus* outbreak in Malaysia. *Malays. J. Pathol.* 29, 63–67.
45. Loomis, R. J., DiPiazza, A. T., Falcone, S., Ruckwardt, T. J., Morabito, K. M., Abiona, O. M., et al. (2021). Chimeric fusion (F) and attachment (G) glycoprotein antigen delivery by mRNA as a candidate *Nipah* vaccine. *Front. Immunol.* 12:772864. doi: 10.3389/fimmu.2021.772864
46. Loomis, R. J., Stewart-Jones, G. B. E., Tsybovsky, Y., Caringal, R. T., Morabito, K. M., McLellan, J. S., et al. (2020). Structure-based design of *Nipah virus* vaccines: a generalizable approach to paramyxovirus immunogen development. *Front. Immunol.* 11:842. doi: 10.3389/fimmu.2020.00842
47. Luby, S. P. (2013). The pandemic potential of *Nipah virus*. *Antiviral Res.* 100, 38–43. doi: 10.1016/j.antiviral.2013.07.011
48. Luby, S. P. (2014). Viruses: *Nipah virus*. *Encyclopaedia Food Saf.* 2, 214–217.
49. Luby, S. P., Gurley, E. S., and Hossain, M. J. (2009). Transmission of human infection with *Nipah virus*. *Clin. Infect. Dis.* 49, 1743–1748. doi: 10.1086/647951
50. Ma, L., Chen, Z., Guan, W., Chen, Q., and Liu, D. (2019). Rapid and specific detection of all known *Nipah virus* strains' sequences with reverse transcription- loop-mediated isothermal amplification. *Front. Microbiol.* 10:418. doi: 10.3389/ fmicb.2019.00418
51. Martinez-Gil, L., Vera-Velasco, N. M., and Mingarro, I. (2017). Exploring the human-*Nipah virus* protein-protein interactome. *J. Virol.* 91:e01461-17. doi: 10.1128/jvi.01461-17
52. Mazzola, L. T., and Kelly-Cirino, C. (2019). Diagnostics for *Nipah virus*: a zoonotic pathogen endemic to Southeast Asia. *BMJ Glob Health* 4:e001118.
53. McEachern, J. A., Bingham, J., Crameri, G., Green, D. J., Hancock, T. J., Middleton, D., et al. (2008). A recombinant subunit vaccine formulation protects against lethal *Nipah virus* challenge in cats. *Vaccine* 26, 3842–3852. doi: 10.1016/j. vaccine.2008.05.016
54. Middleton, D., Pallister, J., Klein, R., Feng, Y. R., Haining, J., Arkinstall, R., et al. (2014). *Hendra virus* vaccine, a one health approach to protecting horse, human, and environmental health. *Emerg. Infect. Dis.* 20, 372–379. doi: 10.3201/ eid2003.131159
55. Mills, J. N., Alim, A. N., Bunning, M. L., Lee, O. B., Wagoner, K. D., Amman, B. R., et al. (2009). *Nipah virus* infection in dogs, Malaysia, 1999. *Emerg. Infect. Dis.* 15, 950–952. doi: 10.3201/eid1506.080453
56. Mire, C. E., Geisbert, J. B., Agans, K. N., Feng, Y. R., Fenton, K. A., Bossart, K. N., et al. (2014). A recombinant *Hendra virus* G glycoprotein subunit vaccine protects nonhuman primates against *Hendra virus* challenge. *J. Virol.* 88, 4624–4631. doi: 10.1128/JVI.00005-14
57. Mohd Nor, M. N., Gan, C. H., and Ong, B. L. (2000). *Nipah virus* infection of pigs in peninsular Malaysia. *Rev. Sci. Tech. Off. Int. Epiz.* 19, 160–165.
58. Montgomery, J. M., Hossain, M. J., Gurley, E., Carroll, G. D., Croisier, A., Bertherat, E., et al. (2008). Risk factors for *Nipah virus* encephalitis in Bangladesh. *Emerg. Infect. Dis* 14, 1526–1532. doi: 10.3201/eid1410.060507
59. Mounts, A. W., Kaur, H., Parashar, U. D., Ksiazek, T. G., Cannon, D., Arokiasamy, T., et al. (1999). A cohort study of health care workers to assess nosocomial transmissibility of *Nipah virus*, Malaysia. *J. Infect. Dis.* 183, 810–813. doi: 10. 1086/318822
60. Mungall, B. A., Middleton, D., Crameri, G., Bingham, J., Halpin, K., Russell, G., et al. (2006). Feline model of acute *Nipah virus* infection and protection with a soluble glycoprotein-based subunit vaccine. *J. Virol.* 80, 12293–12302. doi: 10.1128/JVI.01619-06
61. Negrete, O., Levroney, E., Aguilar, H., Bertolotti-Ciarlet, A., Nazarian, R., Tajyar, S., et al. (2005). EphrinB2 is the entry receptor for *Nipah virus*, an emergent deadly paramyxovirus. *Nature* 436, 401–405. doi: 10.1038/nature03838
62. Nikolay, B., Salje, H., Khan, A. K. M. D., Sazzad, H. M. S., Satter, S. M., Rahman, M., et al. (2020). A framework to monitor changes in transmission and epidemiology of emerging pathogens: lessons from *Nipah virus*. *J. Infect. Dis.* 221, S363–S369.
63. Ochani, R. K., Batra, S., Shaikh, A., and Asad, A. (2019). *Nipah virus* - the rising epidemic: a review. *Infez. Med.* 27, 117–127.
64. Pallister, J. A., Klein, R., Arkinstall, R., Haining, J., Long, F., White, J. R., et al. (2013). Vaccination of ferrets with a recombinant G glycoprotein subunit vaccine provides protection against *Nipah virus* disease for over 12 months. *Virol. J.* 10:237. doi: 10.1186/1743-422X-10-237
65. Pallivalappil, B., Ali, A., Thulaseedharan, N. K., Karadan, U., Chellenton, J., Dipu, P., et al. (2020). Dissecting an outbreak: a clinico-epidemiological study of *Nipah virus* infection in Kerala, India, 2018. *J. Glob. Infect. Dis.* 12, 21–27. doi: 10.4103/jgid.jgid_4_19
66. Parashar, U. D., Sunn, L. M., Ong, F., Mounts, A. W., Arif, M. T., Ksiazek, T. G., et al. (2000). Case-control study of risk factors for human infection with a new zoonotic paramyxovirus, *Nipah virus*, during a 1998-1999 outbreak of severe encephalitis in Malaysia. *J. Infect. Dis.* 181, 1755–1759. doi: 10.1086/315457
67. Paton, N. I., Leo, Y. S., Zaki, S. R., Auchus, A. P., Lee, K. E., Ling, A. E., et al. (1999). Outbreak of *Nipah-virus* infection among abattoir workers in

Singapore. *Lancet* 354, 1253–1256. doi: 10.1016/S0140-6736(99)04379-2
68. Playford, E. G., Munro, T., Mahler, S. M., Elliott, S., Gerometta, M., Hoger, K. L., et al. (2020). Safety, tolerability, pharmacokinetics, and immunogenicity of a human monoclonal antibody targeting the G glycoprotein of henipaviruses in healthy adults: a first-in-human, randomised, controlled, phase 1 study. *Lancet Infect. Dis.* 220, 445–454. doi: 10.1016/S1473-3099(19)30 634-6
69. Plowright, R. K., Becker, D. J., Crowley, D. E., Washburne, A. D., Huang, T., Nameer, P. O., et al. (2019). Prioritizing surveillance of *Nipah virus* in India. *PLoS Negl. Trop. Dis.* 13:e0007393. doi: 10.1371/journal.pntd.0007393
70. Sahay, R. R., Yadav, P. D., Gupta, N., Shete, A. M., Radhakrishnan, C., Mohan, G., et al. (2020). Experiential learnings from the *Nipah virus* outbreaks in Kerala towards containment of infectious public health emergencies in India. *Epidemiol. Infect.* 23:e90. doi: 10.1017/S0950268820000825
71. Sayed, A., Bottu, A., Qaisar, M., Mane, M. P., and Acharya, Y. (2019). *Nipah virus*: a narrative review of viral characteristics and epidemiological determinants. *Public Health* 173, 97–104. doi: 10.1016/j.puhe.2019.05.019
72. Sharma, V., Kaushik, S., Kumar, R., Yadav, J. P., and Kaushik, S. (2019). Emerging trends of *Nipah virus*: a review. *Rev. Med. Virol.* 29:e2010. doi: 10.1002/rmv. 2010
73. Shoemaker, T., and Choi, M. J. (2020). *Henipaviruses. INFECTIOUS AGENT.* Atlanta: CDC Yellow Book.
74. Singh, R. K., Dhama, K., Chakraborty, S., Tiwari, R., Natesan, S., Khandia, R., et al. (2019). *Nipah virus*: epidemiology, pathology, immunobiology and advances in diagnosis, vaccine designing and control strategies - a comprehensive review. *Vet. Q.* 39, 26–55. doi: 10.1080/01652176.2019.1580827
75. Soltan, M. A., Eldeen, M. A., Elbassiouny, N., Mohamed, I., El-damasy, D. A., Fayad, E., et al. (2021). Proteome based approach defines candidates for designing a multitope vaccine against the *Nipah virus*. *Int. J. Mol. Sci.* 22:9330. doi: 10.3390/ijms22179330
76. Spiclera, A. R. (2016). *Nipah Virus Infection*. Available online at: https://www.cfsph. iastate.edu/Factsheets/pdfs/nipah.pdf (accessed December 3, 2021).
77. Sudeep, A. B., Yadav, P. D., Gokhale, M. D., Balasubramanian, R., Gupta, N., Shete, A., et al. (2021). Detection of *Nipah virus* in *Pteropus medius* in 2019 outbreak from Ernakulam district, Kerala, India. *BMC Infect. Dis.* 21:162. doi: 10.1186/s12879-021-05865-7
78. Sun, B., Jia, L., Liang, B., Chen, Q., and Liu, D. (2018). Phylogeography, transmission, and viral proteins of *Nipah virus*. *Virol. Sin.* 33, 385–393. doi: 10.1007/s12250-018-0050-1
79. Tan, K. S., Tan, C. T., and Goh, K. J. (1999). Epidemiological aspects of *Nipah virus* infection. *Neurol. J. Southeast Asia* 4, 77–81.
80. Thakur, N., and Bailey, D. (2019). Advances in diagnostics, vaccines and therapeutics for *Nipah virus*. *Microbes Infect.* 21, 278–286. doi: 10.1016/j.micinf. 2019.02.002
81. Thomas, B., Chandran, P., Lilabi, M. P., George, B., Sivakumar, C. P., Jayadev, V. K., et al. (2019). *Nipah virus* infection in Kozhikode, Kerala, South India, in 2018: epidemiology of an outbreak of an emerging disease. *Indian J. Commun. Med.* 44, 383–387. doi: 10.4103/ijcm.IJCM_198_19
82. Wang, L., Harcourt, B. H., Yu, M., Tamin, A., Rota, P. A., Bellini, W. J., et al. (2001). Molecular biology of *Hendra* and *Nipah viruses*. *Microbes Infect.* 3, 279–287. doi: 10.1016/s1286-4579(01)01381-8
83. Wong, J. J., Chen, Z., Chung, J. K., Groves, J. T., and Jardetzky, T. S. (2021). EphrinB2 clustering by *Nipah virus* G is required to activate and trap F intermediates at supported lipid bilayer-cell interfaces. *Sci. Adv.* 7:eabe1235. doi: 10.1126/sciadv.abe1235
84. World Health Organization [WHO] (2021c). *R&D Blueprint and Nipah Virus*. Available online at: https://www.who.int/teams/blueprint/nipah (accessed September 1, 2021).
85. World Health Organization [WHO] (2021a). *Nipah Virus*. Available online at: https://www.who.int/news-room/fact-sheets/detail/nipah-virus (accessed December 1, 2021).
86. World Health Organization [WHO] (2021b). *Nipah Virus Disease – India*. Available online at: https://www.who.int/emergencies/disease-outbreak-news/ item/nipah-virus-disease---india (accessed September 3, 2021).
87. Wu, Z., Yang, L., Yang, F., Ren, X., Jiang, J., Dong, J., et al. (2014). Novel henipa-like virus, mojiang paramyxovirus, in rats, China, 2012. *Emerg. Infect. Dis.* 20, 1064–1066. doi: 10.3201/eid2006.13 1022
88. Yadav, P. D., Shete, A. M., Kumar, G. A., Sarkale, P., Sahay, R. R., Radhakrishnan, C., et al. (2019). *Nipah virus* sequences from humans and bats during *Nipah* outbreak, Kerala, India, 2018. *Emerg. Infect. Dis.* 25, 1003–1006. doi: 10.3201/eid2505.181076
89. Yoneda, M., Georges-Courbot, M. C., Ikeda, F., Ishii, M., Nagata, N., Jacquot, F., et al. (2013). Recombinant measles virus vaccine expressing the *Nipah virus* glycoprotein protects against lethal *Nipah virus* challenge. *PLoS One* 8:e58414. doi: 10.1371/journal.pone.0058414
90. Zhou, P., Yang, X. L., Wang, X. G., Hu, B., Zhang, L., Zhang, W., et al. (2020). A pneumonia outbreak associated with a new coronavirus of probable bat origin. *Nature* 579, 270–273. doi: 10.1038/s41586-020- 2012-7

23

Zoonotic Tick-Borne Pathogens in Temperate and Cold Regions of Europe—A Review on the Prevalence in Domestic Animals

*Andrea Springer, Antje Glass, Anna-Katharina Topp and Christina Strube**

Institute for Parasitology, Centre for Infection Medicine, University of Veterinary Medicine Hannover, Hanover, Germany

***Correspondence:**
Christina Strube
christina.strube@tiho-hannover.de

Ticks transmit a variety of pathogens affecting both human and animal health. In temperate and cold regions of Europe (Western, Central, Eastern, and Northern Europe), the most relevant zoonotic tick-borne pathogens are tick-borne encephalitis virus (TBEV), *Borrelia* spp. and *Anaplasma phagocytophilum*. More rarely, *Rickettsia* spp., *Neoehrlichia mikurensis,* and zoonotic *Babesia* spp. are identified as a cause of human disease. Domestic animals may also be clinically affected by these pathogens, and, furthermore, can be regarded as sentinel hosts for their occurrence in a certain area, or even play a role as reservoirs or amplifying hosts. For example, viraemic ruminants may transmit TBEV to humans via raw milk products. This review summarizes the role of domestic animals, including ruminants, horses, dogs, and cats, in the ecology of TBEV, *Borrelia* spp., *A. phagocytophilum*, *Rickettsia* spp., *N. mikurensis,* and zoonotic *Babesia* species. It gives an overview on the (sero-)prevalence of these infectious agents in domestic animals in temperate/cold regions of Europe, based on 148 individual prevalence studies. Meta-analyses of seroprevalence in asymptomatic animals estimated an overall seroprevalence of 2.7% for TBEV, 12.9% for *Borrelia burgdorferi* sensu lato (s.l.), 16.2% for *A. phagocytophilum* and 7.4% for *Babesia divergens*, with a high level of heterogeneity. Subgroup analyses with regard to animal species, diagnostic test, geographical region and decade of sampling were mostly non-significant, with the exception of significantly lower *B. burgdorferi* s.l. seroprevalences in dogs than in horses and cattle. More surveillance studies employing highly sensitive and specific test methods and including hitherto non-investigated regions are needed to determine if and how global changes in terms of climate, land use, agricultural practices and human behavior impact the frequency of zoonotic tick-borne pathogens in domestic animals.

Keywords: *Borrelia*, *Rickettsia*, *Anaplasma*, *Babesia*, *Neoehrlichia mikurensis*, tick-borne encephalitis, tick-borne diseases, vector-borne diseases

INTRODUCTION

Many tick-borne diseases (TBDs) are so-called meta-zoonoses, i.e., they may be transmitted to humans as well as animals via their invertebrate tick host (1). In temperate/cold regions of Europe, the hard tick *Ixodes ricinus* is the most important vector of TBDs in terms of both animal and human (public) health, followed by *Dermacentor reticulatus* and *Dermacentor marginatus* (2).

Meta-zoonotic pathogens transmitted by *I. ricinus* include tick-borne encephalitis virus (TBEV), *Borrelia* spp., *Anaplasma phagocytophilum*, *Rickettsia* spp., *Neoehrlichia mikurensis* and zoonotic *Babesia* spp., while ticks of the genus *Dermacentor* may transmit *Rickettsia* spp. to both animals and humans, among others (3). In addition, *D. reticulatus* is now also recognized as a vector for TBEV (4).

Ixodes ricinus has a broad host spectrum, including birds, various wild and domestic animals as well as humans, and occurs in a wide variety of habitats throughout Europe, as far north as 66° N (Norway), close to the Arctic Circle (5). The species' range has continuously expanded northward as well as into higher altitudes during the past decades, probably driven by climatic and environmental changes (6, 7). Similarly, the distribution of *D. reticulatus* is expanding in several European countries (8, 9). A northward spread has been documented in the Baltic countries (10) as well as in Germany (11), but the species has not been documented in Scandinavia to date. In contrast, the distribution of *D. marginatus* seems to be comparatively stable with a northern distribution limit at ~51° N in central Germany (11). In addition to the range expansion of different tick species, changes in human behavior toward more outdoor activities increase the risk of tick bites (2).

In consequence, the incidence and public health burden of TBDs seem to be increasing in Europe. Lyme borreliosis (LB), caused by spirochaetes of the *Borrelia burgdorferi* sensu lato (s.l.) complex and transmitted primarily by *I. ricinus*, is the most common TBD in humans in the Northern Hemisphere. In Europe, annual incidence rates vary between 0.001 and 464 cases/100,000 inhabitants (12). In the Netherlands, a more than 2-fold increase of medical consultations and hospital admissions due to LB was noted from 1994 to 2005 (13). A similar increase in diagnosed LB cases was observed in the United Kingdom from 1998 to 2016 (14). Likewise, the incidence of tick-borne encephalitis, a flavivirus infection transmitted also primarily by *I. ricinus*, has increased significantly since the year 1990 in several European countries (15). The geographic pattern of this disease is also changing, with new transmission foci emerging in previously unaffected regions and countries, e.g., in the Netherlands in 2016 (16) and in the United Kingdom in 2018 (17).

In addition to rising disease incidences, several new tick-borne pathogens have been described in recent decades (18). Although known already since 1995 (19), pathogenicity of *Borrelia miyamotoi*, a tick-transmitted relapsing-fever spirochaete, was first reported in 2011 (20). Similarly, *N. mikurensis* was isolated from ticks and mammals (21) years before being recognized as a human (22) and probably veterinary (23) pathogen. Furthermore, the list of emerging zoonotic tick-borne pathogens relevant in Europe includes several *Rickettsia* spp. (18) and *Babesia* spp. (24). *Borrelia miyamotoi*, *N. mikurensis*, *Rickettsia helvetica* and the relevant zoonotic *Babesia* spp. are all transmitted by *I. ricinus*, which constitutes the main vector of zoonotic TBDs in central and northern Europe. In contrast, *D. marginatus*, the vector of *Rickettsia slovaca*, has a rather limited geographic distribution, and *D. reticulatus*, the vector of *Rickettsia raoultii*, rarely bites humans (11). Therefore, these tick species are of minor importance regarding zoonotic infections.

Domestic animals may also be clinically affected by these pathogens, and, furthermore, can be regarded as sentinel hosts for their occurrence in a certain area, or even play a role as reservoir hosts. Additionally, viraemic ruminants may directly transmit TBEV to humans via raw milk products, causing large outbreaks (25). In this review, we summarize the role of domestic animals, including ruminants, horses, dogs, and cats, in the ecology of TBEV, *Borrelia* spp., *A. phagocytophilum*, *Rickettsia* spp., *N. mikurensis*, and zoonotic *Babesia* species. Unlike for humans, no systematic surveillance of TBDs in domestic animals exists, making it difficult to assess whether the patterns of increasing disease incidence observed in humans can also be found in other species. Therefore (sero-)prevalence data on the mentioned pathogens in domestic animals in temperate and cold regions of Europe are compiled to analyze temporal and regional trends, the influence of the utilized diagnostic test and to identify knowledge gaps requiring further attention.

METHODS

Literature Survey

Systematic literature search on (sero-)prevalence data in temperate and cold regions of Europe [Northern, Western, Central, and Eastern Europe (excluding Russia); see **Figure 1** for included countries] was conducted in the PubMed database in May and July 2020, using combinations of the term "prevalence" with each of "animals," "ruminants," "horses," "dogs," "cats" and each of "TBEV," "*Borrelia*," "*Anaplasma*," "*Rickettsia*," "*Neoehrlichia*," and "*Babesia*."

Further records were obtained by searching the bibliographies of relevant articles and via incidental findings using other databases, e.g., Google Scholar. Original publications in English and different national languages (e.g., German, French, if available) were included. Articles that did not refer to the considered geographical region, did not contain (sero-)prevalence data, e.g., clinical case reports, or that presented data from only one herd/flock, were excluded.

Meta-Analyses

For TBEV, *B. burgdorferi* s.l., *A. phagocytophilum* and *Babesia divergens* seroprevalence, data based on healthy/asymptomatic animals or randomly selected diagnostic samples were subjected to meta-analyses, to gain a comprehensive picture on TBD prevalence in the general domestic animal population. As the number of studies retrieved for the remaining pathogens was low, no meta-analyses were conducted. If studies reported data on healthy and symptomatic groups, only data referring to the healthy group were extracted, because seroprevalences in symptomatic animals may be higher than in the general population.

Random-effects meta-analysis of proportions was conducted with the package "meta" (v. 4.13-0) (26) in R v. 4.0.2 (27), using the inverse variance method with logit transformation and restricted maximum likelihood estimation of the between-study variance (τ^2). To assess heterogeneity between studies, *Q*-tests were performed and the I^2 statistic was assessed, with values ≥50% considered heterogeneous. To evaluate possible sources

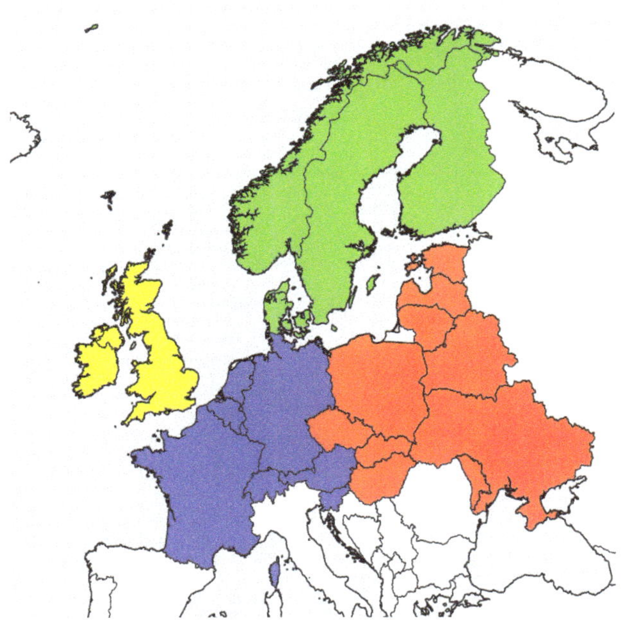

FIGURE 1 | European countries considered in the literature survey on (sero-)prevalence of tick-borne zoonotic diseases in domestic animals. Geographical regions are indicated by different colors: Scandinavia (green), British Isles (yellow), Western continental (blue), and Eastern continental Europe (red).

of heterogeneity, subgroup analyses were performed according to animal species, type of diagnostic test used, geographical region and decade of sampling. For analyses according to geographical region, the considered countries were classified into Eastern or Western continental Europe, Scandinavia or British Isles (**Figure 1**). In cases when studies did not report the period of sampling, it was assumed that the decade of sampling corresponded to the decade of data publication. In subgroup analyses, a common τ^2 was assumed across subgroups.

If studies reported more than one seroprevalence rate, referring to different species, geographic regions, or data acquisition periods, these were considered separately. Since observational prevalence studies are unlikely to suffer from publication bias, i.e., low prevalence rates have a similar probability of being published as higher prevalence rates (28), no assessment of publication bias was performed.

RESULTS

In total, 7,552 publications were assessed for eligibility and 7,404 were excluded because they were not relevant with regard to the considered pathogens or geographical range, consisted of clinical case reports referring to single animals or herds, dealt only with imported animals or did not contain sufficient data. The selection process during the literature survey is depicted in **Figure 2**, with a final dataset containing 148 articles. Of these, 65 reported data on *A. phagocytophilum*, 55 on *B. burgdorferi* s.l., 35 on TBEV, 18 on zoonotic *Babesia* species, 9 on *Rickettsia* spp., and 5 on *N. mikurensis*. Some publications contained data on more than one of these pathogens.

An overview of the roles of domestic animals regarding the considered tick-borne pathogens is given in **Figure 3**. In the following, these roles as well as the (sero-)prevalence rates are discussed in detail for each infectious agent.

Tick-Borne Encephalitis Virus

Tick-borne encephalitis is regarded as the most important arthropod-borne viral disease in Europe (29). It is caused by a flavivirus which is mainly transmitted by *I. ricinus*, but the vector potential of *D. reticulatus* has also been shown (4). Unlike other tick-associated pathogens, it is not consistently distributed throughout the range of its vectors, but occurs in a patchy pattern in delimited geographic areas, termed microfoci or "hotspots." In these foci, it circulates between rodents and ticks and occasionally spills over to domestic animals and humans (29). In recent decades, a geographical spread of the virus has been observed in Europe with new transmission foci having recently emerged in the Netherlands (16) and the United Kingdom (17).

TBEV may cause severe neurologic disease in humans, horses, dogs, and probably also in ruminants (**Figure 3**). Furthermore, most domestic animals are regarded as useful sentinels for human TBE risk (30), with the exception of cats for which no data exist, explaining the comparatively large number of retrieved studies.

In total, 36 studies were retrieved (eight containing data on cattle, seven on sheep, 10 on goats, seven on horses, and 13 on dogs). As cross-reactions with other flaviviruses (e.g., West Nile virus, Louping Ill virus) in serological tests are common, only studies which confirmed positive samples via seroneutralisation test (SNT), considered the gold standard of TBEV serology (31), were included in the meta-analysis of seroprevalence ($N = 20$, with 39 animal cohorts). Therefore, subgroup analysis according to diagnostic test was not performed. The estimated overall prevalence was 2.8%, with a significant level of heterogeneity ($I^2 = 95.8\%$; 95% CI: 95.0–96.5%; $P < 0.001$). No significant differences between animal species ($\chi^2 = 2.6$, df $= 4$, $P = 0.622$; **Figure 4**) nor between decades ($\chi^2 = 4.4$, df $= 2$, $P = 0.110$) or regions ($\chi^2 = 1.9$, df $= 2$, $P = 0.390$) were found.

Ruminants

Domestic ruminants develop viraemia upon TBEV infection, which usually lasts a few days, but remain mostly asymptomatic (32). However, they excrete TBEV in milk during the viraemic phase, potentially leading to human infection via raw milk products like unpasteurized milk or raw milk cheese. In goat milk, infective virus can be detected for up to 19 days post infection (33). Such alimentary transmission often causes clusters of cases [e.g., (34, 35)] and is regarded as the second most important route of human infection (25).

In addition, a few clinical cases of neurologic disease in small ruminants due to TBEV have been described (36, 37). Possibly, clinical cases in these species are often overlooked or misinterpreted, e.g., as *Listeria monocytogenes* infection (36), and may be more common than previously thought. Furthermore, ruminants are regarded as useful sentinel species for TBEV occurrence. They have a comparatively restricted range of

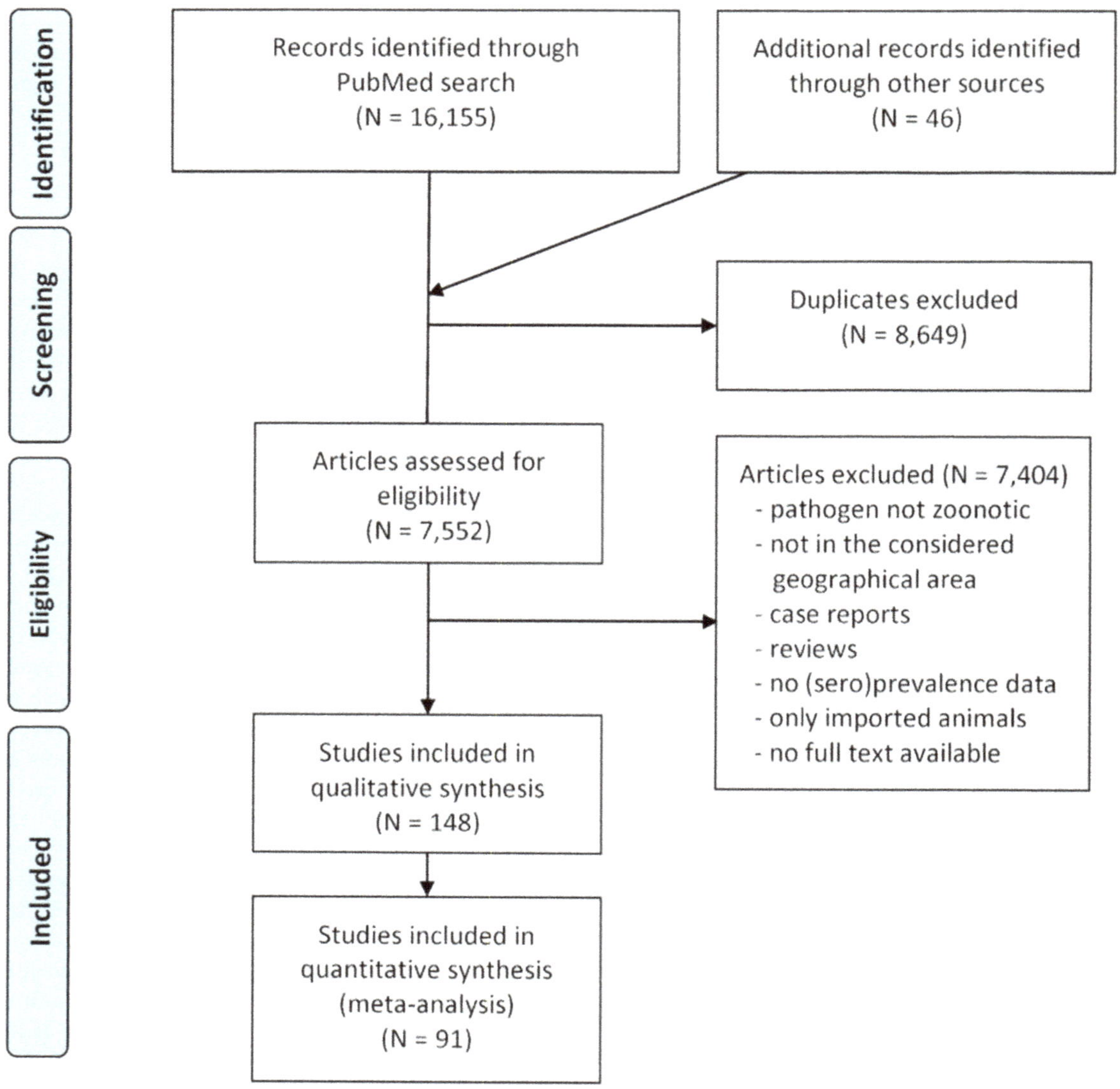

FIGURE 2 | PRISMA flow-chart detailing the selection process applied during the literature survey.

activity, i.e., they travel less than dogs and horses, and show persistence of antibodies for up to 28 months post infection (38). Therefore, several studies have been conducted on TBEV seroprevalence in domestic ruminants, particularly in goats and sheep (**Supplementary Table 1**).

Studies on cattle ($N = 8$, two from Norway, one each from Belgium, Finland, Hungary, Lithuania, the Netherlands, and Poland) reported seroprevalences ranging from 0.0% in the Netherlands (39) to 26.5% in Hungary (40) (**Supplementary Table 1**). One Norwegian study assessed TBEV excretion in milk and found 5.4% PCR-positive samples (41).

Seven studies reported seroprevalence data on sheep (two each from Sweden and Germany, one each from Hungary, Lithuania, and Slovakia), with values ranging from 0.0% in northern Germany (42) to 25.6% in farms with high lamb morbidity and mortality in Sweden (43). However, no confirmation of positive samples by SNT was performed in the latter study, so that cross-reactions with other flavivirus infections, e.g., louping ill, which has previously been detected in Norwegian sheep (44), cannot be ruled out. Seroprevalence in the 10 studies reporting data on goats (four from Germany, one each from Austria, Lithuania, the Netherlands, and Poland) ranged from 0.0% in the northern German federal state of Mecklenburg-Western Pomerania, which is not regarded as a TBEV risk area (45), to 14.6% in the Swiss canton of Ticino (46). Direct pathogen detection in sheep and goats, e.g., by PCR, was not reported in the considered studies.

Horses

As in ruminants, TBEV infections in horses are mostly asymptomatic (47). However, cases of encephalomyelitis with symptoms such as anorexia, ataxia, spasms, and epileptic seizures

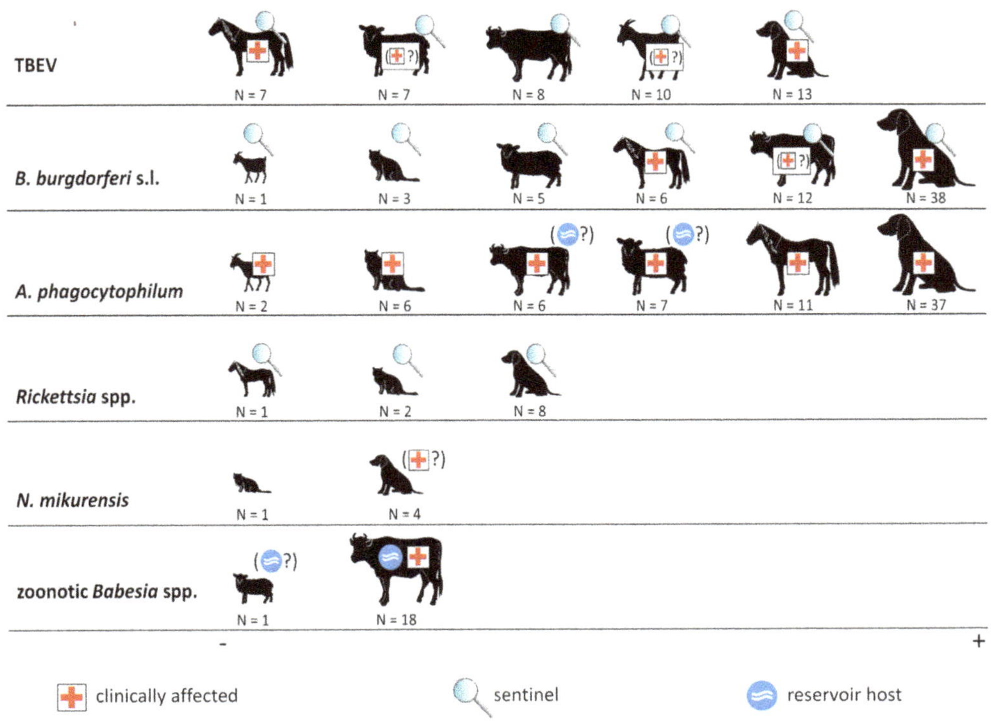

FIGURE 3 | Animal species and tick-borne pathogens. The size of animal icons corresponds to the number of studies. Symbols indicate the role of each animal species in the ecology of the respective pathogen. Symbols in brackets indicate that this role is uncertain. *Borrelia miyamotoi* is not shown as no (sero-)prevalence studies regarding this pathogen in domestic animals were retrieved.

have been described (48, 49). Mild neurologic deficits may persist after recovery (49).

The literature survey resulted in the identification of seven studies on TBEV seroprevalence in horses (three from Germany, two from Austria, one each from Hungary and Slovakia; **Supplementary Table 1**), with values ranging from 0.0% in Hungary (40) to 33.0% in a TBEV risk area in Bavaria, Germany (49). All of these studies confirmed positive samples by SNT (**Supplementary Table 1**).

Dogs and Cats

In dogs, a similar TBE disease course as in humans with severe, often fatal neurological manifestations due to encephalitis has been described (50). However, high seroprevalence rates in some areas indicate that only a small proportion of infected dogs develops disease, whereas most infections remain asymptomatic (47). Because dogs usually accompany their owners, they are regarded as valuable sentinels for human TBEV risk. However, as companions of man, they often have a travel history, which makes assessment of TBE risk in a certain area based on dog sera less reliable compared to other sentinel animals (30).

In the present survey, 13 studies presenting data on TBEV (sero-)prevalence in dogs were identified (three from Germany, two from the Czech Republic, one each from Austria, Belgium, Denmark, Finland, the Netherlands, Norway, and Poland, and one study reporting data on dogs from different European countries; **Supplementary Table 1**). Seroprevalence ranged from 0.0% in the Netherlands (39) to 53.6% in dogs with neurological signs in Germany (51). However, positive results were not confirmed by SNT in the latter study, so that the possibility of cross-reactions with other flaviviruses needs to be considered. Cross-reactions also appear probable in light of the high seroprevalence detected in healthy dogs (30.4%) in the same study, compared with an estimated overall seroprevalence of 1.4% based on asymptomatic dogs when positive samples were confirmed by SNT (**Figure 4**). Nevertheless, another study including dogs with neurological illness determined a TBEV infection rate of 12.6% by real-time PCR (52), indicating that TBEV prevalence among dogs with neurologic disease may be substantial.

No cases of TBEV infections in cats have been published to date. Preliminary data of a study including more than 200 cats from a TBE-endemic area in Germany showed no seropositive individuals (personal communication with Martin Pfeffer, Institute of Animal Hygiene and Veterinary Public Health, University of Leipzig, and Gerhard Dobler, Bundeswehr Institute of Microbiology, Munich).

Borrelia burgdorferi s.l.

The *B. burgdorferi* s.l. complex currently comprises 22 recognized species of spirochaetal bacteria (53), at least nine of which occur in European tick populations (54). Of those, *Borrelia afzelii* and *Borrelia garinii* are the most prevalent and constitute the most important agents of human LB throughout Europe (54, 55).

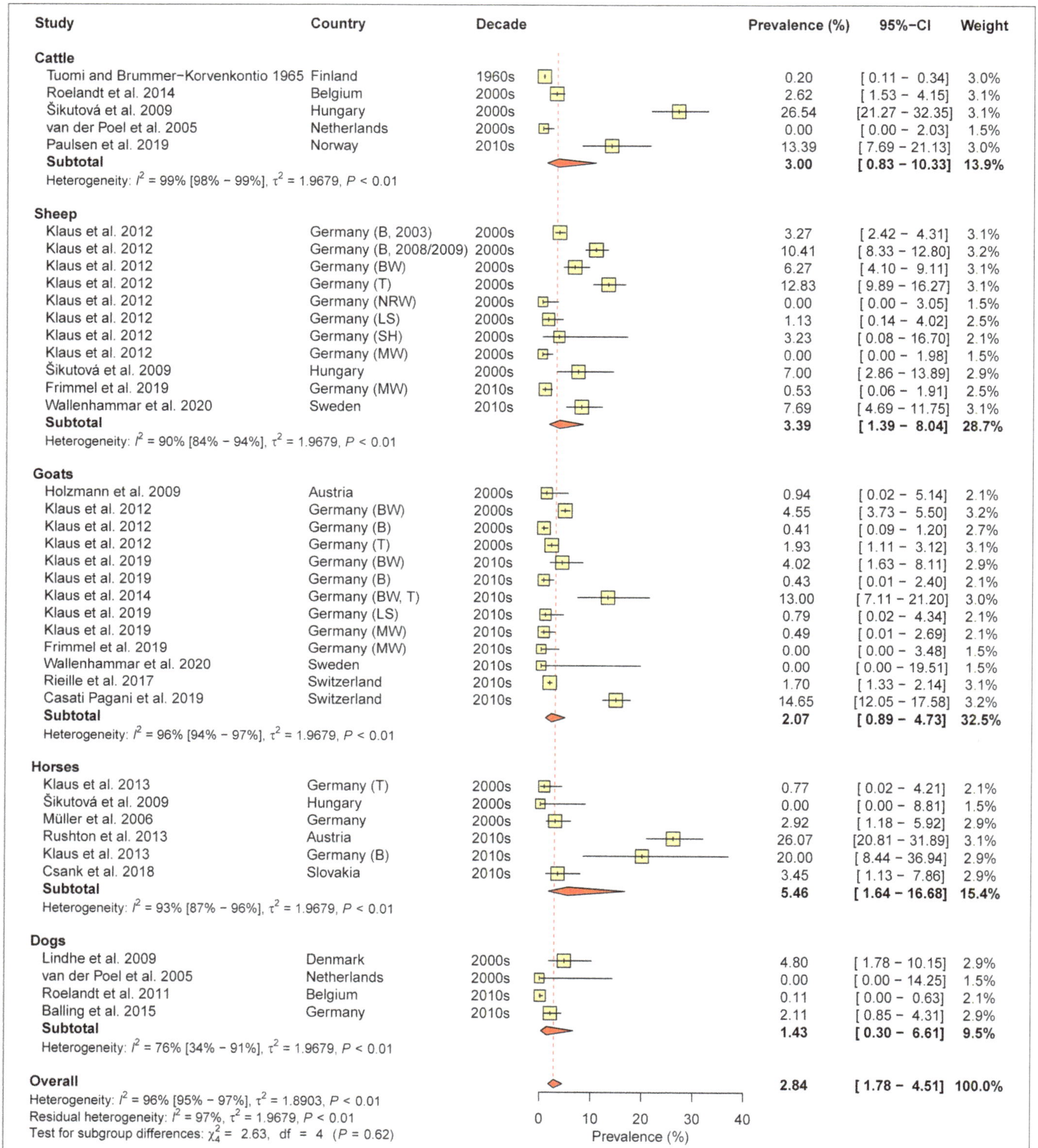

FIGURE 4 | Forest plot displaying the results of random-effects meta-analysis of tick-borne encephalitis virus seroprevalence in domestic animals, with subgroup analysis according to animal species. Individual study results are shown as yellow squares, corresponding in size to the weight of the study on the overall prevalence estimate. Error bars indicate 95% confidence intervals (CI). Pooled prevalences are shown as red diamonds and the red dotted vertical line indicates the estimated overall prevalence.

Borrelia burgdorferi s.l. predominantly circulates between *Ixodes* ticks (in Europe *I. ricinus*) and wild mammals (e.g., *B. afzelii*, *B. bavariensis*), birds (e.g., *B. garinii*, *B. valaisiana*), or reptiles (*B. lusitaniae*) as reservoir hosts (56).

In total, 53 studies reporting *B. burgdorferi* s.l. (sero-)prevalence rates in domestic animals were retrieved (**Supplementary Table 2**). Since a vaccine against borreliosis in dogs was introduced to the European market at the end of the 1990s, it is important to distinguish between vaccinated and naturally exposed dogs when evaluating seroprevalence (57). Antibodies against the variable major protein-like sequence expressed (VlsE) and one of its invariable regions, the C6 peptide, as well as the outer surface protein OspF indicate natural exposure, because these antigens are not present in the available vaccines (58). Therefore, dog seroprevalence studies conducted after 1995 were only considered in the meta-analysis if they were based on a C6 or OspF assay.

Meta-analysis of seroprevalence, including 48 animal cohorts (13 cattle, 3 sheep, 9 horse, 21 dog, and 2 cat cohorts) from 30 publications, estimated an overall seroprevalence of 12.4% (95% CI: 0.1–17.2%) with a significant level of heterogeneity (I^2 = 98.0%; 95% CI: 97.8–98.3%; $P < 0.001$). Subgroup analysis indicated a significant effect of animal species ($\chi^2 = 24.4$, df = 4, $P < 0.001$), with a lower seroprevalence in dogs (5.8%, 95% CI: 3.7–8.9%) than in cattle (23.6%, 95% CI: 14.8–35.4%) and horses (22.5%, 95% CI: 12.6–36.9%; **Figure 5**). In contrast, there were no significant differences according to decade ($\chi^2 = 4.7$, df = 3, $P = 0.193$), diagnostic test used ($\chi^2 = 3.3$, df = 2, $P = 0.193$), and geographical region ($\chi^2 = 2.9$, df = 2, $P = 0.230$) when analyzing all 48 cohorts.

Due to the significant effect of animal species, further analyses were conducted on the data subset for dogs, as this species had the largest sample size (21 cohorts from 16 studies). In the data subset on dogs, a significant effect of diagnostic test was found ($\chi^2 = 7.5$, df = 2, $P = 0.023$), with a lower seroprevalence determined by a C6-based rapid ELISA (3.1%, 95% CI: 1.5–6.0%) than by conventional ELISA (11.2%, 95% CI: 6.0–20.0%; **Supplementary Figure 1**). In contrast, no significant effect of geographical region ($\chi^2 = 2.4$, df = 2, $P = 0.302$) nor decade of sampling ($\chi^2 = 3.5$, df = 3, $P = 0.324$) was found in dogs.

Ruminants

Species-specific *Borrelia*-host associations are thought to be primarily driven by variation in resistance toward host defense mechanisms, particularly complement (59). Different species of the *B. burgdorferi* s.l. complex differ in their level of susceptibility toward inactivation of sera from certain animals *in vitro* [e.g., (60, 61)]. Notably, all tested members of the *B. burgdorferi* s.l. complex display high sensitivity toward serum complement from several ruminant species, including deer, bison, and cattle (59). Thus, these species seem to be irrelevant as *B. burgdorferi* s.l. reservoirs. In contrast, ticks feeding on these species may even lose their *Borrelia* infection, as suggested by prevalence patterns in engorged ticks recovered from deer, cattle and goats vs. prevalence in questing ticks (62, 63). Therefore, it has been suggested that an increase in grazing domestic ruminants may lower the risk of Lyme disease acquisition in a certain area (62). However, this does not apply to all ruminants, as several *B. burgdorferi* s.l. species are resistant toward serum of sheep and their wild relatives, the mouflon (59), and sheep may sustain natural *B. burgdorferi* s.l. cycles in the absence of other tick hosts (64).

Despite their apparent ability to eliminate *B. burgdorferi* s.l. spirochaetes, active *B. burgdorferi* sensu stricto (s.s.), and *B. afzelii* infections with associated symptoms (skin erythema, fever, acute lameness due to arthritis) have been described in cattle in rare cases (65, 66). Other studies draw a connection between serological evidence of *B. burgdorferi* s.l. infection and clinical signs such as lameness and swollen joints (67), but causality in these cases is extremely questionable. Experimental infections of cattle with *B. burgdorferi* s.s., *B. garinii*, and *B. afzelii* produced no clinical signs (68). Similarly, clinical manifestations of LB have been suspected in sheep (69), but experimental infections failed to produce any symptoms (70). Regarding goats, neither clinical cases nor infection experiments have been published to the authors' knowledge. Overall, clinical relevance of *B. burgdorferi* s.l. for ruminants is questionable. Nevertheless, they seroconvert upon contact with the pathogen (68) and may therefore be regarded as sentinels for pathogen presence.

In the present survey, 12 studies reporting seroprevalence rates in cattle were retrieved (six from Germany, one each from France, Poland, Slovakia, Sweden, and Switzerland and one reporting data from Poland as well as Slovakia; **Supplementary Table 2**). Reported seroprevalences ranged from 1.1% in northern Sweden (71) to 66.0% in Germany (72). Five studies reported data on sheep (two from Sweden, one each from France, Norway and Slovakia), with seroprevalences ranging from 0.0% in healthy sheep in central Sweden to 84.6% in lambs with arthritis on the island of Gotland, Sweden (71). The highest seroprevalence in asymptomatic sheep was determined in France (56.5%) (73). The only study containing data on goats reported a 17.2% seroprevalence rate in this species in Slovakia (74). Direct pathogen detection, e.g., by PCR, was not reported for ruminants in the considered studies.

Horses

In horses, a broad spectrum of clinical manifestations, including arthritis, lameness, anterior uveitis, encephalitis, and abortion, has been attributed to *B. burgdorferi* s.l. infection; however, in many cases a causal relationship has not been conclusively proven (75). Experimental inoculations of ponies led to systemic infection, persisting for at least 9 months, but did not induce any clinical signs nor histopathological alterations, except for skin lesions (76, 77). More recently, however, several case reports of equine neuroborreliosis with *B. burgdorferi* s.l. detection in the central nervous system have been published (78–81). In one of these studies, the species was identified as *B. burgdorferi* s.s. and high spirochaetal loads were demonstrated in tissues with inflammation (79). However, all of these cases occurred in North America, thus, it remains unclear if European *B. burgdorferi* s.s. isolates and other LB agents are capable of causing clinical manifestations in horses. Evidence from *in vitro* studies suggests that all tested *B. burgdorferi* s.l. species are susceptible to inactivation by equine complement,

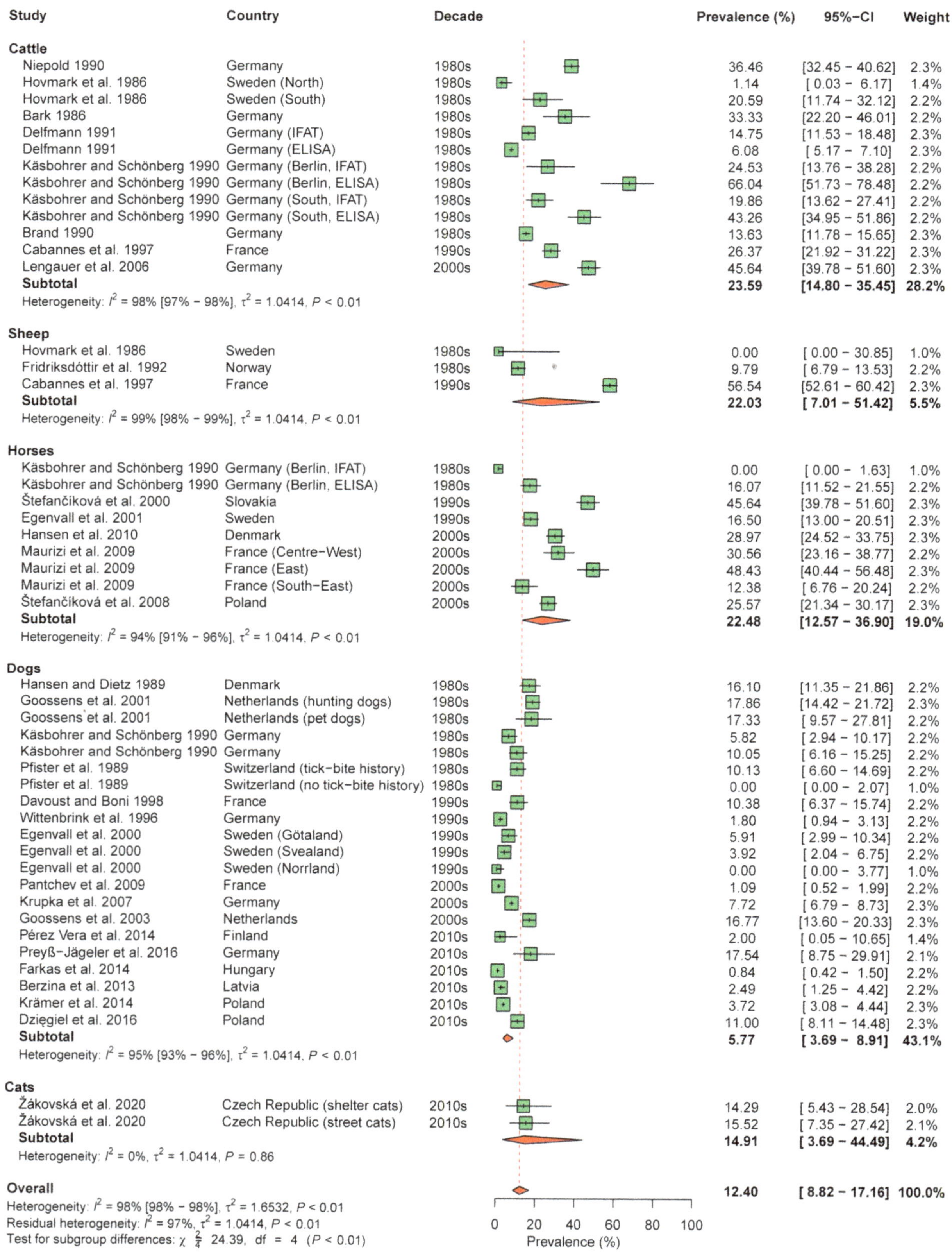

FIGURE 5 | Forest plot displaying the results of random-effects meta-analysis of *B. burgdorferi* s.l. seroprevalence in domestic animals, with subgroup analysis according to animal species. Individual study results are shown as green squares, corresponding in size to the weight of the study on the overall prevalence estimate. Error bars indicate 95% confidence intervals (CI). Pooled prevalences are shown as red diamonds and the red dotted vertical line indicates the estimated overall prevalence.

except for *B. burgdorferi* s.s. which displays an intermediate sensitivity (59).

In contrast to the paucity of conclusive clinical equine borreliosis cases in Europe, six studies evaluating seroprevalence rates in this species were retrieved (one each from Poland, Denmark, France, Germany, and Sweden and one reporting data from both Poland and Slovakia). Reported seroprevalence rates ranged from 12.4% in south-eastern to 48.4% in eastern France (82). Studies employing direct detection methods, e.g., PCR, were not retrieved.

Dogs and Cats

According to a consensus statement by the American College of Veterinary Internal Medicine (ACVIM), most *B. burgdorferi* s.l. seropositive dogs and cats display no clinical signs, neither after natural nor experimental infections (58). A small subset of dogs, however, may develop arthritis due to *B. burgdorferi* s.s. infection, as demonstrated by experimental infections (83–85). Furthermore, nephritis is putatively associated with *B. burgdorferi* s.s. infections, however, well-documented case reports are rare and no experimental studies exist in this regard (58). To the authors' knowledge, evidence for clinical manifestations due to other species of the *B. burgdorferi* s.l. complex in dogs is lacking to date, although *B. afzelii* has been isolated from a dog with clinical signs attributable to LB in Europe (86). Furthermore, DNA of *B. valaisiana* and *B. garinii* has been amplified from symptomatic dogs [(87, 88); see below]. In experimental studies, dogs have been shown to transmit borreliae to ticks, indicating a potential reservoir function (89). However, in the light of abundant wild reservoir hosts, such as rodents and birds, the impact of pet dogs on the natural epidemiological cycle is probably neglectable (90).

Cats have been infected experimentally and show seroconversion, but no clinical signs of infection (91, 92). Some case reports have attributed clinical signs in cats, such as cardiac arrhythmia and lameness, to *B. burgdorferi* s.l. infection based on seropositivity, PCR detection of the pathogen and/or resolution upon antibiotic treatment (93, 94); however, as in many other cases a causative relationship remains speculative.

Nevertheless, seroprevalence in domestic dogs and cats may provide an estimate of human LB risk. A strong association was found between canine seroprevalence and mean LB incidence on county level in the United States of America (95).

In the present survey, 38 studies reporting *B. burgdorferi* s.l. (sero-)prevalences in dogs were compiled (seven each from Germany and Poland, four from Sweden, three each from the Netherlands, Slovakia, and Switzerland, two each from the Czech Republic and France and one each from Austria, Denmark, Finland, Hungary, Latvia, Lithuania, and Norway). Seroprevalences ranging from 0.0% in northern Norway (96) to 57.5% in Bernese Mountain dogs in Switzerland (97) were reported. This dog breed seems to have a predisposition for *B. burgdorferi* s.l. infection, as demonstrated by several studies (97–99), although the reasons for this predisposition are unknown (58). As reported above, a significant effect of the utilized diagnostic test on the seroprevalence in dogs was found (section Tick-Borne Encephalitis Virus, **Supplementary Figure 1**), with lower rates determined by the most recently developed test, a C6-based rapid ELISA, than by conventional ELISA or IFAT (57).

Some studies also reported PCR detection rates in dogs, ranging from 0.0% in asymptomatic dogs (100) to 60.0% in animals with clinical signs attributable to borreliosis (87). DNA of *B. burgdorferi* s.s., *B. afzelii*, *B. valaisiana*, and *B. garinii* was amplified in these cases (87, 88).

Three studies reported data on cats (one each from the Czech Republic and the United Kingdom, one based on cats from different European countries). Two of these assessed seroprevalence, which ranged from 2.2% in symptomatic cats from different European countries, determined by a C6-based rapid ELISA (101), to 19.2% of cats presented at veterinary clinics in the Czech Republic, determined by conventional ELISA (102). The third study determined a 1.6% *B. burgdorferi* s.l. infection rate in systemically ill cats in the United Kingdom by PCR (103).

Borrelia miyamotoi

Borrelia miyamotoi was first isolated from *Ixodes persulcatus* in Japan in 1995 (19), but pathogenicity for humans was not recognized until 2011 (20). Since then, this pathogen has been known to cause a febrile illness (104) and, more recently, it has been associated with meningoencephalitis in immunocompromised patients (105, 106). Similar to *B. burgdorferi* s.l., rodents and birds seem to be reservoir hosts for this spirochaete (104). Little is known about the role of domestic animals regarding *B. miyamotoi* ecology. In contrast to *B. burgdorferi* s.l., prevalence of *B. miyamotoi* in ticks is not negatively affected by the presence of cattle (62, 107). *Borrelia miyamotoi* DNA has been detected in two healthy cats in the USA (108). However, infection of other domestic animals has not been documented so far to the authors' knowledge and no (sero-)prevalence studies have been conducted.

Anaplasma phagocytophilum

Anaplasma phagocytophilum is regarded as an important zoonotic pathogen, causing disease in humans, domestic ruminants, horses, dogs, and rarely in cats, while wild mammals act as reservoir hosts (109). This obligate intracellular rickettsial pathogen replicates in neutrophilic granulocytes and leads to thrombocytopenia, leukopenia, anemia, and immunosuppression associated with variable clinical signs (110). The epidemiology of *A. phagocytophilum* is complex due to the circulation of various strains and ecotypes, and shows considerable differences between Europe and North America (109). Human, equine, and canine granulocytic anaplasmosis have been described in Asia, Europe, and North America, while domestic ruminants only seem to be affected in Europe (109). Based on *groEL* genetic sequences, eight haplotype clusters of *A. phagocytophilum* were recently identified, and most isolates from humans and domestic animals belong to cluster 1, while other clusters, e.g., containing samples from roe deer, do not seem to be zoonotic (111).

Overall, 65 studies reporting (sero-)prevalence rates of *A. phagocytophilum* in domestic animals in the study region were retrieved (**Supplementary Table 3**). The meta-analysis based on seroprevalence rates of asymptomatic animals, including data on 35 animal cohorts (2x cattle, 3x sheep, 9x horses, 18x dogs, 3x cats) from 28 publications, yielded an estimated overall seroprevalence of 16.2% (95% CI: 11.7–22.0%), with a significant level of heterogeneity ($I^2 = 98.6\%$; 95% CI: 98.4–98.8%; $P < 0.001$). Although rather high seroprevalence rates were detected in sheep as compared to the other animal species, subgroup analyses indicated no significant difference (test for subgroup differences: $\chi^2 = 6.4$, df = 4, $P = 0.171$; **Figure 6**). Likewise, significant differences according to geographical region ($\chi^2 = 0.38$, df = 2, $P = 0.828$), the decades of sampling ($\chi^2 = 0.78$, df = 2, $P = 0.676$; **Figure 6**) or the type of diagnostic test were not detected ($\chi^2 = 4.98$, df = 2, $P = 0.083$).

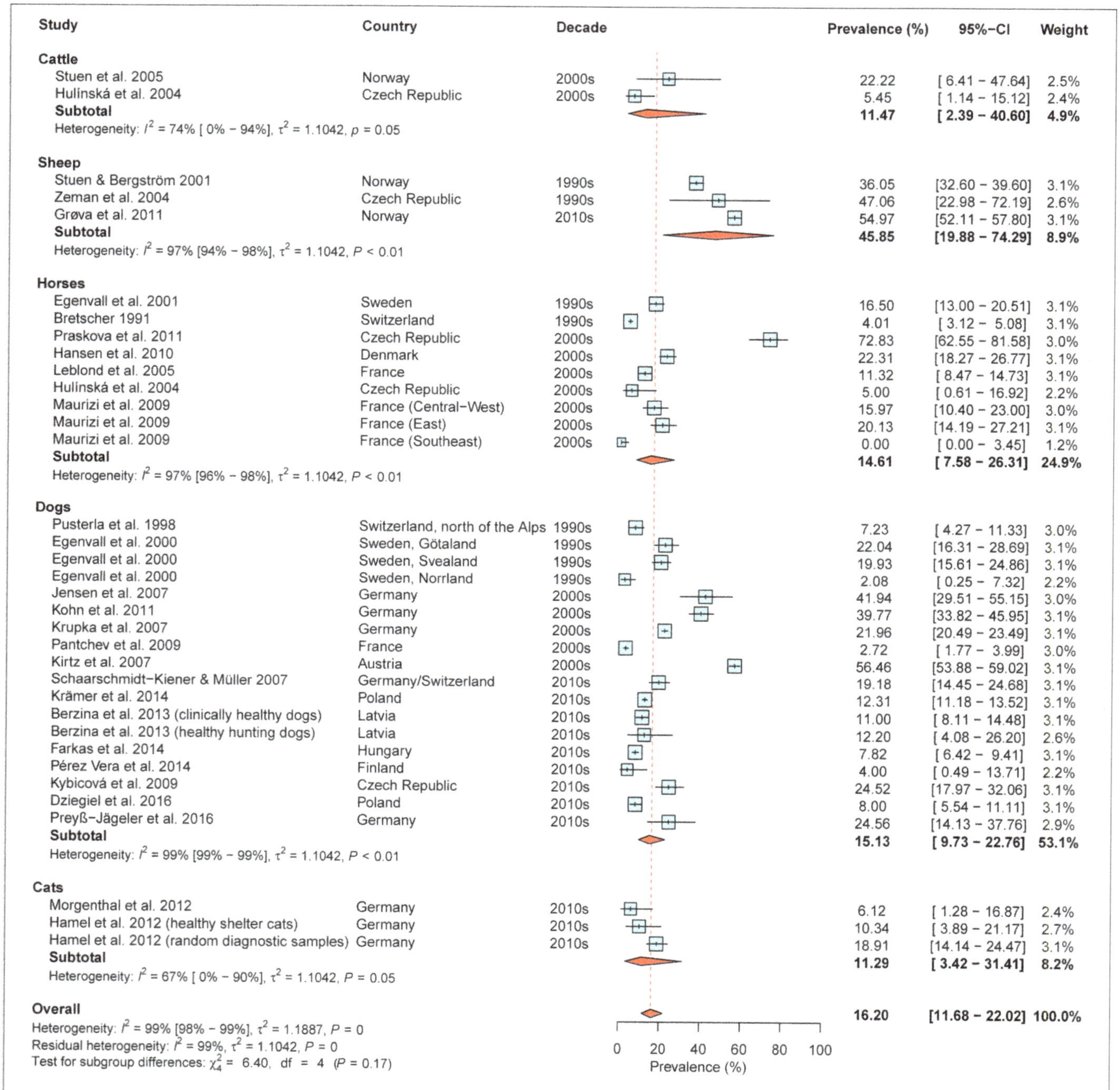

FIGURE 6 | Forest plot displaying the results of random-effects meta-analysis of *A. phagocytophilum* seroprevalence in domestic animals, with subgroup analysis according to animal species. Individual study results are shown as blue squares, corresponding in size to the weight of the study on the overall prevalence estimate Error bars indicate 95% confidence intervals (CI). Pooled prevalences are shown as red diamonds and the red dotted vertical line indicates the estimated overall prevalence.

Ruminants

In domestic ruminants, the disease caused by *A. phagocytophilum* is known as tick-borne fever and presents with fever, anorexia, abortion and a drop in milk production (109). In sheep but not in cattle, immunosuppression is also common, frequently resulting in secondary infections (112), which may be fatal in some cases (113). After recovery, sheep develop persistent infections with recurrent phases of high bacteraemia for at least 1 year, suggesting they may also act as a pathogen reservoir (114, 115). Furthermore, field data suggest that cattle can also become persistently infected or are frequently re-infected, indicating a possible reservoir function, which needs to be explored further (116). Recent genetic analyses have shown that *A. phagocytophilum* isolates from sheep and cattle in Europe cluster with isolates from humans, dogs, and horses (117).

In total, six studies reported (sero-)prevalence rates for cattle (two studies from Sweden and one study each from Belgium, the Czech Republic, Norway, and Switzerland), seven for sheep (two each from the Czech Republic and Norway, one each from Denmark, Germany and Sweden), and two for goats (Switzerland and United Kingdom, **Supplementary Table 3**).

In cattle, seroprevalence rates varied from 5.5% in the Czech Republic (118) to 100% in a clinically-affected herd in Norway (119). The highest published seroprevalence rate in asymptomatic cattle was 63.0% in a Swiss study (120). Three studies reported prevalence rates based on PCR, which ranged from 5.5% in the Czech Republic (118) to 85.7% in symptomatic animals in Sweden (121).

In sheep, prevalence of *A. phagocytophilum* antibodies ranged from 36.0% in Norway (122) to 100% in a flock in the Czech Republic (123). PCR-determined prevalence rates in sheep varied from 2.9% in the Czech Republic/Slovakia (124) to 41.9% in sheep flocks with high lamb morbidity and mortality in Sweden (43). Regarding goats, a PCR-determined prevalence of 5.6% was reported from Switzerland (125). In addition, four of five feral goats caught in Northern Ireland, UK, were PCR-positive (126).

However, (sero-)prevalence rates in ruminants may be difficult to compare between studies, since marked seasonal variation has been found. For example, in a Swiss study, seroprevalence of two cattle herds varied between 16% before and 63% at the end of the grazing season (120). As most ruminants are housed during winter, determined (sero-)prevalence rates greatly depend upon the season of sampling.

In addition, serologic cross-reactivity with other *Anaplasma* spp., e.g., *Anaplasma marginale* in cattle (127) and probably also *Anaplasma ovis* in sheep (128), needs to be considered. In Europe, *A. marginale* occurs mainly in the Mediterranean region, but also in Switzerland, Austria, and Hungary (129). *Anaplasma ovis* has been detected in France (130) as well as Slovakia (124) and Hungary (129).

Horses

In horses, *A. phagocytophilum* may cause an acute febrile disease with depression, anorexia, ataxia, icterus, and lower limb oedema, which is usually self-limiting (131). Similar to sheep, horses may develop persistent subclinical infections with recurrent bacteraemia after spontaneous recovery from acute disease (132). Notably, equine *A. phagocytophilum* strains seem to be similar or identical to those causing disease in humans and dogs (133).

Most equine granulocytic anaplasmosis (EGA) cases have been reported from European countries (131). In the present investigation, 11 studies reporting (sero-)prevalence rates of *A. phagocytophilum* in horses were identified, two each from the Czech Republic, France, and Sweden and one each from Denmark, France, the Netherlands, Switzerland, and Sweden. Another two studies reported data from Poland, Slovakia and the Ukraine and from Germany, Poland and the Ukraine, respectively. Reported seroprevalence rates ranged from 4.0% in Switzerland (134) to 72.8% in the Czech Republic (135). Remarkably, the latter study was based on healthy horses. Prevalences determined by PCR ranged from 0.0% in the Ukraine (136) to 62.9% in Sweden, whereby the latter study was based on horses presenting symptoms attributable to EGA.

Dogs and Cats

Canine granulocytic anaplasmosis (CGA) is regarded as one of the most important vector-borne diseases in Europe. While many cases are probably subclinical, acute febrile illness may also occur (137). Frequent clinical signs are lethargy, anorexia, and pale mucous membranes, sometimes accompanied by enlarged lymph nodes, bleeding (petechias, epistaxis), and immune-mediated arthritis (137). Similar symptoms may be seen in cats infected with *A. phagocytophilum*, although experimental studies indicate that symptoms are usually mild (138). Experimental infections have been shown to persist for at least $5^1/_2$ months in dogs (139) and 3 months in cats (91). The *A. phagocytophilum* strains causing disease in dogs seem to be zoonotic (117).

In total, 37 studies on *A. phagocytophilum* (sero-)prevalence in dogs were retrieved from the literature, including 10 from Germany, six from Poland, five from Sweden, two each from Austria, the Czech Republic, Hungary Slovakia, and Switzerland, and one study each from Finland, France, Latvia, Lithuania, and the United Kingdom. One study included dogs from Germany and Switzerland. Reported seroprevalence rates, determined either by IFAT or (rapid) ELISA, ranged from 2.1% in northern Norway (96) to 56.5% in Austria (140) (**Supplementary Table 3**). However, the latter study included dogs with symptoms possibly related to CGA. Since infection may not lead to clinical disease, and CGA is characterized by rather unspecific symptoms, several studies did not find a significant difference in seroprevalence between apparently healthy animals and those presenting some form of illness [e.g., (100, 141)]. Nevertheless, cohorts of symptomatic dogs were excluded from the meta-analysis on seroprevalence. Serologic tests available for assessing *A. phagocytophilum* exposure may cross-react with *Anaplasma platys* antibodies, therefore, seroprevalence may be overestimated. However, as *A. platys* transmission in Europe is restricted to Mediterranean countries (137), this pathogen only plays a role as an imported bacterium in the countries considered in this review, with the exception of southern France. Nevertheless, with increased travel activity and import of dogs by animal welfare organizations, this should be kept in mind when interpreting seroprevalence rates.

Prevalence rates determined by PCR ranged from 0.0% in Switzerland and Poland (142, 143) to 66.7% in dogs with symptoms attributable to CGA in Sweden (121). The highest prevalence in apparently healthy dogs was 12.2% in a group of Latvian hunting dogs (144).

Regarding cats, six studies were found (four from Germany, one from the United Kingdom and one from Ireland). These studies reported IFAT-determined seroprevalence rates from 6.1% in healthy cats (145) to 18.9% in random diagnostic samples (146). PCR detection rates varied from 0.0% in healthy cats (145) to 4.3% in necropsy samples from shelter cats (147).

Neoehrlichia mikurensis

Neoehrlichia mikurensis, a member of the family Anaplasmataceae, was first discovered in the early 2000s, recognized as a human pathogen in 2010 and recently cultivated in tick cell lines as well as human endothelial cells (148). It occurs in *I. ricinus* populations throughout Europe and human cases, mainly involving immunosuppressed patients, have been reported from several countries (149). Regarding domestic animals, knowledge on the relevance of *N. mikurensis* as a pathogenic agent and respective prevalence data are scarce.

In the present literature survey, five studies investigating *N. mikurensis* occurrence in domestic animals (four in dogs and one in cats) by PCR, but no seroprevalence studies, were obtained (**Table 1**). Infections in dogs seem to be rare, as only 0.3% of 1,023 dogs in Germany (151) and 0.1% of 889 dogs in Switzerland were infected (142). The positive dog in Switzerland was splenectomised (142). Another positive dog died of haemolytic anemia in the Czech Republic (150) and in a case report from Germany, canine *N. mikurensis* infection was associated with neutropenia and thrombocytopenia (23). However, the clinical relevance of *N. mikurensis* in dogs is still unclear (23, 142). A single study also tested spleen samples from 141 cats in Germany, but *N. mikurensis* was not detected (147). Other domestic animal species have not been investigated so far to the authors' knowledge.

Rickettsia spp.

Several tick-transmitted human-pathogenic *Rickettsia* spp. occur in Europe. While the causative agent of Mediterranean spotted fever, *Rickettsia conorii*, has been known since the beginning of the twentieth century, several further *Rickettsia* spp. and their associated syndromes were described in the 1990s and 2000s (153). In central and northern Europe, *R. helvetica*, transmitted by *I. ricinus*, is probably the most frequent species. It causes a mild febrile illness in humans and is only sometimes associated with skin rash (154). In addition, *I. ricinus* may transmit *Rickettsia monacensis*, which leads to a clinical picture similar to Mediterranean spotted fever (153). *Rickettsia slovaca* and *R. raoultii*, causative agents of scalp eschar and neck lymphadenopathy (SENLAT), are transmitted by *Dermacentor* species (153).

With the exception of dogs, domestic animals do not seem to be susceptible to disease caused by human-pathogenic *Rickettsia* species. In dogs, infection with *Rickettsia rickettsii*, which causes Rocky Mountain spotted fever in North America, leads to clinical signs similar to those in humans (155). In addition, *R. conorii* has been associated with canine febrile illness (156). Dogs are also capable of transmitting *R. conorii* to ticks and may thus exert a reservoir function (157). However, canine disease due to the *Rickettsia* spp. relevant in central and northern Europe or a respective reservoir function have not been reported to the authors' knowledge.

Overall, domestic animals can mainly be regarded as sentinels for human exposure to *Rickettsia* spp. in central and northern Europe. However, only nine studies were identified (three from Germany, two from Switzerland, one each from the Czech Republic, Ireland, Poland, and Sweden), reporting data on horses, dogs, and cats (**Table 2**). Regarding domestic ruminants, no studies on *Rickettsia* (sero-)prevalence in the considered geographical region were obtained. The only study on horses reported a 36.5% *R. helvetica* seroprevalence in Sweden (158).

In dogs, a high level of exposure to spotted-fever group rickettsiae was reported, with seroprevalence rates ranging from 17.0 to 93.9% (158, 160). When *R. helvetica*-specific antigens were used, seroprevalences of 17.0% (158) and 66.0% (160) were determined. Despite this high level of exposure, *Rickettsia* DNA (mainly *R. raoultii*) was found in only 0.8% of tested dogs in Germany (151), whereas two PCR-based studies from Switzerland (142, 162) and one study from Poland (161) reported

TABLE 1 | (Sero-)prevalence studies on *Neoehrlichia mikurensis* in domestic animals in temperate and cold regions of Europe.

Country	Region	Year(s) of sampling	Method(s)	Positive/total	Prevalence	Comment(s)	References
DOGS							
Czech Republic	NA	2009–2012	PCR	1/19	5.3%	Dogs with fatal immunhaemolytic anemia	(150)
Germany	Brandenburg	2013–2014	HRM PCR	3/1,023	0.3%		(151)
Hungary	Somogy	NA	PCR	0/90	0.0%	*Candidatus* Neoehrlichia lotoris-like detected in 6 dogs	(152)
Switzerland	Zurich	2005–2006	Real-time PCR	1/889	0.1%	The positive dog was splenectomised	(142)
CATS							
Germany	Berlin	2006–2008	HRM PCR	0/141	0.0%	Spleen samples from shelter cats	(147)

HRM PCR, high-resolution melt PCR.

TABLE 2 | (Sero-)prevalence studies on tick-transmitted *Rickettsia* spp. in domestic animals in temperate and cold regions of Europe.

Country	Region	Year(s) of sampling	Method(s)	Positive/total	Prevalence	Comment(s)	References
HORSES							
Sweden	NA	2010–2011	IFAT	23/63	36.5%	*R. helvetica* used as antigen	(158)
DOGS							
Czech Republic	NA	2009–2012	PCR	0/19	0.0%	Dogs with fatal immunhaemolytic anemia	(150)
Germany	Nationwide	2012–2014	ELISA[a]	469/602	77.9%	Dogs that never left Germany	(159)
	Nationwide	2012–2014	Micro-IFAT	568/605	93.9%	Same samples as in (159); clearly differentiable samples: 66.0% *R. helvetica*, 2.8% *R. raoultii*, 1.6% *R. slovaca*	(160)
	Brandenburg	2013–2014	PCR	8/1,021	0.8%	Identified species: 7x *R. raoultii*, 1x *R. felis*	(151)
Poland	North-Western Poland	NA	PCR	0/100 (group 1), 0/92 (group 2), 0/50 (group 3)	0.0% (group 1), 0.0% (group 2), 0.0% (group 3)	Group 1: healthy shelter dogs, group 2: suspected borreliosis, group 3: diagnosed babesiosis	(161)
Sweden	NA	2010–2011	IFAT	17/100	17.0%	*R. helvetica* used as antigen	(158)
Switzerland	Zurich	2005–2006	Real-time PCR[b]	0/889	0.0%		(142)
	Zurich	NA	Real-time PCR[b]	0/884	0.0%		(162)
CATS							
Ireland	Dublin	2008	PCR	0/121	0.0%		(163)
Sweden	NA	2010–2011	IFAT	19/90	22.1%	*R. helvetica* used as antigen	(158)

[a]*Commercially available, detects all spotted-fever group rickettsiae.*
[b]*Specific for R. helvetica.*
ELISA, enzyme-linked immunosorbent assay; IFAT, immunofluorescence antibody test.

0.0% prevalence. Similarly, *R. helvetica* antibodies were detected in 22.1% of tested cats in Sweden (158), but no *Rickettsia* DNA was amplified from 121 tested cats in Ireland (163). Therefore, it seems unlikely that dogs and cats contribute to the epidemiology of tick-transmitted rickettsioses as reservoir hosts in northern and central Europe.

Zoonotic *Babesia* spp.

Piroplasms of the genus *Babesia* are tick-transmitted protozoan parasites, which usually display a high degree of host specificity. Nevertheless, a few species are zoonotic, predominantly affecting immunocompromised patients (24). In Europe, most human infections are caused by the cattle parasite *B. divergens* (154). On the American continent, human babesiosis due to *Babesia microti*, which is rodent-associated, is more common. *Babesia microti* also occurs in Europe. However, clinically symptomatic human *B. microti* infections reported in Europe were mostly acquired in the Americas, so it is unclear whether European *B. microti* strains are human-pathogenic (154). Furthermore, *Babesia venatorum*, a parasite of deer, has been recognized as a human pathogen in immunocompromised patients in Europe (154).

Regarding domestic animals, only cattle are affected by and act as reservoirs for a *Babesia* spp. with zoonotic relevance, namely *B. divergens*, whereas the species parasitizing horses, sheep, goats, and dogs are not zoonotic. No cat-specific *Babesia* species are distributed in Europe. *Babesia microti* DNA has been detected in cats in southern Europe (e.g., in Italy) but the relevance of this finding remains unclear (164).

In cattle, *B. divergens* infection may lead to severe haemolytic anemia, which can be fatal (165, 166). Symptoms consist of fever, pale or jaundiced mucous membranes, anorexia, weakness, elevated heart and respiratory rates and hemoglobinuria, hence the colloquial name of the disease, "redwater" (165). Recovering animals acquire immunity, which is maintained by repeated pathogen exposure (165). Calves under the age of ~9 months display higher resistance toward clinical disease and are subsequently immunologically protected (167, 168), thus, clinical disease in endemic situations usually only occurs in immunologically naïve animals, which were either recently introduced to the area or had no access to pasture during the first year of life (165).

In the present survey, 18 studies reporting *Babesia* (sero-)prevalence data in cattle were retrieved (four each from France, Germany, and the United Kingdom, two from Belgium, and one each from Hungary, Norway, Sweden, and Switzerland; **Table 3**). Reported seroprevalence rates, determined mostly by IFAT, ranged from 0.0% in asymptomatic animals in Northern Germany (177) to 100% in animals presenting with acute babesiosis in France (172). The highest seroprevalence in randomly chosen individuals, but from a region where babesiosis was known to occur, was 90.6% at the end of the grazing season (167). The latter study also showed that seroprevalence varied throughout the year, similar to the pattern described above for *A. phagocytophilum* (120), making different studies difficult to compare. Keeping this draw-back in mind, an overall seroprevalence of 7.4% (95% CI: 2.6–19.2%) was estimated based on 11 healthy or randomly chosen

TABLE 3 | (Sero-)prevalence studies on zoonotic *Babesia* spp. in domestic animals in temperate and cold regions of Europe.

Country	Region	Year(s) of sampling	Method(s)	Positive/total	Prevalence	Comment(s)	Referencea
Cattle (*B. divergens*)							
Belgium	Central Belgium	1988	IFAT	136/1,721	7.9%		(169)*
	Southern Belgium	2010	IFAT	7/65 (spring), 13/65 (summer), 8/65 (autumn)	10.7% (spring), 20.0% (summer), 12.3% (autumn)	Farms with a known history of babesiosis or anaplasmosis	(170)
France	Nationwide	1988	Blood smears / inoculation in gerbils	374/424	88.2%	Animals treated for clinical babesiosis	(171)
	Sarthe	1991	ELISA	115/200	57.5%	Farms with clinical babesiosis during the last 5 years	(171)
	Ille-et-Vilaine	2001–2002	IFAT, *in vitro* culture	19/19 (IFAT, group 1), 31/77 (IFAT, group 2), 19/19 (culture, group 1), 31/77 (culture, group 2)	100% (IFAT, group 1), 40.3% (IFAT, group 2), 100% (culture, group 1), 40.3% (culture, group 2)	Group 1: acute babesiosis, group 2: asymptomatic	(172)*
	Mid-eastern France	2001–2002	IFAT, PCR	18/254 (IFAT), 12/254 (PCR)	7.1% (IFAT), 4.7% (PCR)		(173)*
	Western France	2007	IFAT	102/711	14.3%		(174)*
Germany	Bavaria	1982	IFAT, ELISA	211/1,616	13.1%		(175)*
	Northern Germany	1984–1985	IFAT	108/251	43.0%	Farms with history of babesiosis, includes vaccinated animals	(176)
	Northern Germany	1988–1990	IFAT	0/212 (group 1), 0/354 (group 2), 8/200 (group 3)	0.0% (group 1), 0.0% (group 2), 4.0% (group 3)	Group 1: *Borrelia*-positive animals, group 2: farms with suspected babesiosis, group 3: farms with history of babesiosis	(177)*
	Bavaria	2002	IFAT	1/287	0.4%		(178)*
Hungary	Northeastern Hungary	2005	IFAT	2/654	0.3%		(179)*
Norway	Southern Norway	2004–2005	IFAT	84/306	27.4%		(180)*
Sweden	Southern Sweden	NA	Real-time PCR	38/71	53.5%	Includes 39 cattle with symptoms of babesiosis	(181)
Switzerland	Jura Canton	1981	IFAT	98/289 (April), 190/327 (July), 309/341 (December)	33.9% (April), 58.1% (July), 90.6% (December)		(167)
United Kingdom	Scotland	1976	IFAT	290/368	78.8%	Two farms which experienced babesiosis outbreak	(182)
	Scotland	NA	IFAT	2,522/22,044	11.4%		(183)*
	Northern Ireland	1978	IFAT	5,731/18,000	31.8%		(184)*
	Scotland	2014	PCR	0/107	0.0%	Farms with a known history of babesiosis or anaplasmosis	(185)
SHEEP							
United Kingdom	Scotland	2014	PCR	11/93	11.8%	Identified as *B. venatorum*	(185)

**Included in meta-analysis of seroprevalence.*
ELISA, enzyme-linked immunosorbent assay, IFAT, immunfluorescence antibody test.

cattle cohorts (**Supplementary Figure 2**). A significant level of heterogeneity was detected ($I^2 = 99.6\%$; 95% CI: 99.6–99.7%; $P < 0.001$). No significant temporal change in seroprevalence was detected from the 1970s to the 2000s (test for subgroup differences, $\chi^2 = 0.96$, df = 2, $P = 0.619$), although a decline in bovine babesiosis prevalence and/or clinical incidence has been postulated for several European countries (179, 180, 186). This may be due to the fact that several studies reporting this decline were based on clinical incidence (179, 186) and were thus not included in the calculation. Furthermore, no difference according to geographical region was found ($\chi^2 = 5.8$, df = 3, $P = 0.121$).

A few studies also reported detection of *B. divergens* by PCR, with infection rates ranging from 0.0% in Scotland (185) to 53.5% among clinically symptomatic cattle in Sweden (181). In randomly selected cattle in France, an infection rate of 4.7% was determined by PCR (173).

In addition to cattle, sheep might act as reservoirs for zoonotic *Babesia* spp., as *B. venatorum* infections have recently been detected in 11.8% of 93 studied sheep in the United Kingdom, whereas the 107 tested cattle were negative (185).

DISCUSSION

The present survey aimed at presenting an overview of the most important zoonotic TBDs in domestic animals in temperate and cold regions of Europe, where *I. ricinus* is the predominant tick vector. While a rather large number of studies on *B. burgdorferi* s.l., *A. phagocytophilum* and TBEV were retrieved, studies on *Rickettsia* spp. in domestic animals were few, probably because *Rickettsia* spp. have not (yet) been associated with clinical disease in these species. Therefore, the prevalence and clinical relevance of *Rickettsia* spp. in domestic animals represent a knowledge gap. Similarly, only few studies exist on the relatively recently discovered pathogen *N. mikurensis* in domestic animals, although first reports indicate that this pathogen may be of clinical relevance for dogs (150). Studies on relevant zoonotic *Babesia* spp. were only found with regard to *B. divergens* in cattle, while only one study investigated *B. venatorum*, which is usually deer-associated, in cattle and sheep. As *Babesia* spp. are characterized by a high level of host-specificity (187), it was not surprising that no prevalence studies were conducted on rodent-associated *B. microti* in domestic animals in the considered regions.

In general, a high level of heterogeneity was detected in the datasets. To limit this heterogeneity in meta-analysis of seroprevalence, only animal cohorts asymptomatic for the considered pathogen or random diagnostic samples were included, and further restrictions were applied regarding the diagnostic test used for TBEV in all domestic animals and *B. burgdorferi* s.l. in dogs. Nevertheless, heterogeneity remained high, even after conducting subgroup analyses according to species, diagnostic test (if applicable), geographic region and decade. A significant effect was only found regarding species differences in *B. burgdorferi* s.l. infections, with higher rates in domestic ruminants and horses than in dogs. On the one hand, this might be due to the close relationship between dogs and their owners, resulting in better protection from TBDs due to treatment with (repellent) acaricides, and shorter duration of tick attachment, as ticks are probably noticed sooner on dogs than on horses or cattle. On the other hand, the choice of diagnostic test may have contributed to the significantly lower *B. burgdorferi* s.l. seroprevalence in dogs. Although no significant effect of diagnostic test was found in the overall dataset, analyzing the data subset on dogs alone revealed a significant effect, with lower rates determined by the most recently developed test, a rapid ELISA with a high sensitivity and specificity for antibodies against the *Borrelia* C6 antigen (57). This test was almost exclusively used in dogs, except for two studies on horses. This indicates that cross-reactivity with other pathogens, e.g., *Leptospira* spp. (74), may have been an issue, especially in older and in non-canine studies.

Regarding *A. phagocytophilum*, conspicuously high seroprevalence rates in sheep were reported. However, as the meta-analysis included only three studies on sheep, no significant species differences were found when conducting subgroup analysis. However, this should be investigated further, as granulocytic anaplasmosis is a severe, possibly fatal disease in sheep (113). In addition, sheep might constitute a reservoir for human-pathogenic *A. phagocytophilum* strains (114, 115, 117). Thus, more studies on *A. phagocytophilum* (sero-)prevalence in sheep seem warranted.

In addition to species differences and different diagnostic tests used, the chosen cut-off level to determine seropositivity, the source of the antigen in serological tests or the timing of sampling—as seroprevalences may increase during seasons of tick exposure (120, 171)—may have further increased heterogeneity of study results. These aspects, hampering the comparability of studies, may have contributed to the fact that no temporal changes in TBD seroprevalence in domestic animals were found. Possibly, a larger number of studies may have been necessary to detect a temporal trend under these conditions. Furthermore, there were large temporal gaps in the available seroprevalence studies. For example, studies on TBEV considered suitable for meta-analysis were mainly conducted as of the year 2000, with only one comparable study from the 1960s and none from the decades in between. Regarding *Babesia* spp., there was a gap in available screening studies on asymptomatic animals concerning the 1990s as well as the 2010s. Regarding *B. burgdorferi* s.l., most studies were conducted in the 1980s, following the initial description of the pathogen (188).

In consequence, the trend of increasing TBD incidence in humans was not reflected by the available data from domestic animals. Apart from the mentioned drawbacks that may have masked such a trend, it is also possible that seroprevalences in domestic animals are rather stable and that the increased TBD incidence in humans is due to factors which are not relevant for animals. For example, increased exposure due to more outdoor activities or increased awareness of patients and physicians for TBDs may lead to an increased disease incidence or more diagnoses of TBD infections in humans (2).

With regard to the geographical spread of zoonotic TBDs, e.g., concerning TBE, (sero-)prevalence in animals is usually not studied in a certain area until there is an indication of pathogen presence due to human cases. Therefore, it is difficult to ascertain when the pathogen emerged in animal populations in this area. As an example, no studies on TBEV in domestic animals in the United Kingdom were retrieved, where TBEV has only recently been detected (17).

CONCLUSIONS

This survey revealed a high heterogeneity in (sero-)prevalences of zoonotic TBDs in domestic animals in temperate and cold regions of Europe. In addition, temporal gaps in available studies were detected, e.g., for TBEV and *B. divergens*. The high level of heterogeneity as well as the temporal gaps make it difficult to assess long-term temporal trends for comparison with data on humans. Furthermore, only few studies were retrieved regarding *Rickettsia* spp. and the recently described pathogen *N. mikurensis*, and none regarding *B. miyamotoi*. Therefore, more studies investigating these neglected pathogens are warranted. Additionally, further surveillance studies employing highly sensitive and specific test methods and including hitherto non-investigated regions are needed to determine if and how a changing world impacts the frequency of neglected zoonotic tick-borne pathogens in domestic animals.

AUTHOR CONTRIBUTIONS

CS designed the study. AS, AG, and A-KT conducted the literature search. AS conducted statistical analyses and drafted the manuscript. All authors participated in data interpretation, reviewed the manuscript draft, read, and approved the final manuscript.

REFERENCES

1. WHO/FAO. *Joint FAO/WHO Expert Committee on Zoonoses [Meeting Held in Geneva from 6 to 12 December 1966]: Third Report.*World Health Organization, Geneva (1967).
2. Vayssier-Taussat M, Cosson JF, Degeilh B, Eloit M, Fontanet A, Moutailler S, et al. How a multidisciplinary 'One health' approach can combat the tick-borne pathogen threat in Europe. *Future Microbiol.* (2015) 10:809–18. doi: 10.2217/fmb.15.15
3. Rubel F, Brugger K, Pfeffer M, Chitimia-Dobler L, Didyk YM, Leverenz S, et al. Geographical distribution of *Dermacentor marginatus* and *Dermacentor reticulatus* in Europe. *Ticks Tick Borne Dis.* (2016) 7:224–33. doi: 10.1016/j.ttbdis.2015.10.015
4. Lički M, Fumačová Havlíková S, Slávikova M, Slovák M, Drexler JF, Klempa B. *Dermacentor reticulatus* is a vector of tick-borne encephalitis virus. *Ticks Tick Borne Dis.* (2020) 11:101414. doi: 10.1016/j.ttbdis.2020.101414
5. Hvidsten D, Frafjord K, Gray JS, Henningsson AJ, Jenkins A, Kristiansen BE, et al. The distribution limit of the common tick, *Ixodes ricinus*, and some associated pathogens in north-western Europe. *Ticks Tick Borne Dis.* (2020) 11:101388. doi: 10.1016/j.ttbdis.2020.101388
6. Jore S, Vanwambeke SO, Viljugrein H, Isaksen K, Kristoffersen AB, Woldehiwet Z, et al. Climate and environmental change drives *Ixodes ricinus* geographical expansion at the northern range margin. *Parasit Vectors.* (2014) 7:11. doi: 10.1186/1756-3305-7-11
7. Materna J, Daniel M, Metelka L, Harčarik J. The vertical distribution, density and the development of the tick *Ixodes ricinus* in mountain areas influenced by climate changes (The Krkonoše Mts., Czech Republic). *Int J Med Microbiol.* (2008) 298:25–37. doi: 10.1016/j.ijmm.2008.05.004
8. Mierzejewska EJ, Estrada-Peña A, Alsarraf M, Kowalec M, Bajer A. Mapping of *Dermacentor reticulatus* expansion in Poland in 2012–2014. *Ticks Tick Borne Dis.* (2016) 7:94–106. doi: 10.1016/j.ttbdis.2015.09.003
9. Dautel H, Dippel C, Oehme R, Hartelt K, Schettler E. Evidence for an increased geographical distribution of *Dermacentor reticulatus* in Germany and detection of *Rickettsia* sp. *RpA4. Int J Med Microbiol.* (2006) 296:149–56. doi: 10.1016/j.ijmm.2006.01.013
10. Paulauskas A, Radzijevskaja J, Mardosaite-Busaitiene D, Aleksandravičiene A, Galdikas M, Krikštolaitis R. New localities of *Dermacentor reticulatus* ticks in the baltic countries. *Ticks Tick Borne Dis.* (2015) 6:630–5. doi: 10.1016/j.ttbdis.2015.05.007
11. Drehmann M, Springer A, Lindau A, Fachet K, Mai S, Thoma D, et al. The spatial distribution of *Dermacentor* ticks (Ixodidae) in Germany - evidence of a continuing spread of *Dermacentor reticulatus. Front Vet Sci.* (2020) 7:578220. doi: 10.3389/fvets.2020.578220
12. Sykes RA, Makiello P. An estimate of lyme borreliosis incidence in Western Europe. *J Public Health.* (2017) 39:74–81. doi: 10.1093/pubmed/fdw017
13. Hofhuis A, van der Giessen JW, Borgsteede F, Wielinga PR, Notermans DW, van Pelt W. Lyme borreliosis in the Netherlands: strong increase in GP consultations and hospital admissions in past 10 years. *Eurosurveillance.* (2006) 11:2978. doi: 10.2807/esw.11.25.02978-en
14. Tulloch JSP, Christley RM, Radford AD, Warner JC, Beadsworth MBJ, Beeching NJ, et al. A descriptive epidemiological study of the incidence of newly diagnosed lyme disease cases in a UK primary care cohort, 1998-2016. *BMC Infect Dis.* (2020) 20:285. doi: 10.1186/s12879-020-05018-2
15. Süss J. Tick-borne encephalitis in Europe and beyond – the epidemiological situation as of 2007. *Eurosurveillance.* (2008) 13:18916. doi: 10.2807/ese.13.26.18916-en
16. Dekker M, Laverman GD, de Vries A, Reimerink J, Geeraedts F. Emergence of tick-borne encephalitis (TBE) in the Netherlands. *Ticks Tick Borne Dis.* (2019) 10:176–9. doi: 10.1016/j.ttbdis.2018.10.008
17. Holding M, Dowall SD, Medlock JM, Carter DP, Pullan ST, Lewis J, et al. Tick-borne encephalitis virus, United Kingdom. *Emerg Infect Dis.* (2020) 26:90–6. doi: 10.3201/eid2601.191085
18. Kernif T, Leulmi H, Raoult D, Parola P. Emerging tick-borne bacterial pathogens. In: Scheld WM, Hughes JM, Whitley RJ, editors. *Emerging Infections.* Washington, DC: American Society for Microbiology (2016). p. 295–310.
19. Fukunaga M, Takahashi Y, Tsuruta Y, Matsushita O, Ralph D, Mcclelland M, et al. Genetic and phenotypic analysis of *Borrelia miyamotoi* sp. nov., isolated from the ixodid tick *Ixodes persulcatus*, the vector for Lyme Disease in Japan. *Int J Syst Evol Microbiol.* (1995) 45:804–10. doi: 10.1099/00207713-45-4-804
20. Platonov AE, Karan LS, Kolyasnikova NM, Makhneva NA, Toporkova MG, Maleev VV, et al. Humans infected with relapsing fever spirochete *Borrelia miyamotoi*, Russia. *Emerg Infect Dis.* (2011) 17:1816–23. doi: 10.3201/eid1710.101474
21. Kawahara M, Rikihisa Y, Isogai E, Takahashi M, Misumi H, Suto C, et al. Ultrastructure and phylogenetic analysis of '*Candidatus* Neoehrlichia mikurensis' in the family Anaplasmataceae, isolated from wild rats and found in *Ixodes ovatus* ticks. *Int J Syst Evol Microbiol.* (2004) 54:1837–43. doi: 10.1099/ijs.0.63260-0
22. Welinder-Olsson C, Kjellin E, Vaht K, Jacobsson S, Wennerås C. First case of human "*Candidatus* Neoehrlichia mikurensis" infection in a febrile patient with chronic lymphocytic leukemia. *J Clin Microbiol.* (2010) 48:1956–9. doi: 10.1128/JCM.02423-09
23. Diniz PPVP, Schulz BS, Hartmann K, Breitschwerdt EB. "*Candidatus* Neoehrlichia mikurensis" infection in a dog from Germany. *J Clin Microbiol.* (2011) 49:2059–62. doi: 10.1128/JCM.02327-10
24. Gray J, Zintl A, Hildebrandt A, Hunfeld K-P, Weiss L. Zoonotic babesiosis: overview of the disease and novel aspects of pathogen identity. *Ticks Tick Borne Dis.* (2010) 1:3–10. doi: 10.1016/j.ttbdis.2009.11.003
25. Dobler G, Gniel D, Petermann R, Pfeffer M. Epidemiology and distribution of tick-borne encephalitis. *Wien Med Wochenschr.* (2012) 162:230–8. doi: 10.1007/s10354-012-0100-5
26. Schwarzer G. meta: an R package for meta-analysis. *R News.* (2007) 7:40–5.
27. R Core Team. *R: A Language and Environment for Statistical Computing.* 3.5.0 ed. Vienna: R Foundation for Statistical Computing (2018).
28. Maulik PK, Mascarenhas MN, Mathers CD, Dua T, Saxena S. Prevalence of intellectual disability: a meta-analysis of population-based studies. *Res Dev Disabil.* (2011) 32:419–36. doi: 10.1016/j.ridd.2010.12.018
29. Dobler G, Hufert F, Pfeffer M, Essbauer S. Tick-borne encephalitis: from microfocus to human disease. In: Mehlhorn H, editor. *Progress in Parasitology.* Berlin: Springer. (2011) p. 323–31. doi: 10.1007/978-3-642-21396-0_17

30. Imhoff M, Hagedorn P, Schulze Y, Hellenbrand W, Pfeffer M, Niedrig M. Review: sentinels of tick-borne encephalitis risk. *Ticks Tick Borne Dis.* (2015) 6:592–600. doi: 10.1016/j.ttbdis.2015.05.001
31. Roelandt S, Suin V, Gucht S, Stede Y, Roels S. Comparative tick-borne encephalitis (virus) surveillance in Belgium 2009-2015: experiences with diagnostic tests, sentinel species and surveillance designs. *J Zoonotic Dis Public Health.* (2017) 1:4.
32. Paulsen KM, Granquist EG, Okstad W, Vikse R, Stiasny K, Andreassen ÅK, et al. Experimental infection of lambs with tick-borne encephalitis virus and co-infection with *Anaplasma phagocytophilum*. *PLoS ONE.* (2019) 14:e0226836. doi: 10.1371/journal.pone.0226836
33. Balogh Z, Egyed L, Ferenczi E, Bán E, Szomor KN, Takács M, et al. Experimental infection of goats with tick-borne encephalitis virus and the possibilities to prevent virus transmission by raw goat milk. *Intervirology.* (2012) 55:194–200. doi: 10.1159/000324023
34. Balogh Z, Ferenczi E, Szeles K, Stefanoff P, Gut W, Szomor KN, et al. Tick-borne encephalitis outbreak in hungary due to consumption of raw goat milk. *J Virol Methods.* (2010) 163:481–5. doi: 10.1016/j.jviromet.2009.10.003
35. Brockmann S, Oehme R, Buckenmaier T, Beer M, Jeffery-Smith A, Spannenkrebs M, et al. A cluster of two human cases of tick-borne encephalitis (TBE) transmitted by unpasteurised goat milk and cheese in Germany, May 2016. *Eurosurveillance.* (2018) 23:17-00336. doi: 10.2807/1560-7917.ES.2018.23.15.17-00336
36. Böhm B, Schade B, Bauer B, Hoffmann B, Hoffmann D, Ziegler U, et al. Tick-borne encephalitis in a naturally infected sheep. *BMC Vet Res.* (2017) 13:267. doi: 10.1186/s12917-017-1192-3
37. Zindel W, Wyler R. Zeckenenzephalitis bei einer Ziege im untern Prättigau. *Schweiz Arch Tierheilkd.* (1983) 125:383–6.
38. Klaus C, Ziegler U, Kalthoff D, Hoffmann B, Beer M. Tick-borne encephalitis virus (TBEV) – findings on cross reactivity and longevity of TBEV antibodies in animal sera. *BMC Vet Res.* (2014) 10:78. doi: 10.1186/1746-6148-10-78
39. van der Poel WHM, van der Heide R, Bakker D, Looff MD, Jong JD, van Manen N, et al. Attempt to detect evidence for tick-borne encephalitis virus in ticks and mammalian wildlife in the Netherlands. *Vector Borne Zoonotic Dis.* (2005) 5:58–64. doi: 10.1089/vbz.2005.5.58
40. Šikutová S, Hornok S, Hubálek Z, DoleŽálková I, Juricová Z, Rudolf I. Serological survey of domestic animals for tick-borne encephalitis and Bhanja viruses in northeastern Hungary. *Vet Microbiol.* (2009) 135:267–71. doi: 10.1016/j.vetmic.2008.09.082
41. Paulsen KM, Stuen S, das Neves CG, Suhel F, Gurung D, Soleng A, et al. Tick-borne encephalitis virus in cows and unpasteurized cow milk from Norway. *Zoonoses Public Health.* (2019) 66:216–22. doi: 10.1111/zph.12554
42. Klaus C, Beer M, Saier R, Schau U, Moog U, Hoffmann B, et al. Goats and sheep as sentinels for tick-borne encephalitis (TBE) virus – epidemiological studies in areas endemic and non-endemic for TBE virus in Germany. *Ticks Tick Borne Dis.* (2012) 3:27–37. doi: 10.1016/j.ttbdis.2011.09.011
43. Grandi G, Aspán A, Pihl J, Gustafsson K, Engström F, Jinnerot T, et al. Detection of tick-borne pathogens in lambs undergoing prophylactic treatment against ticks on two Swedish farms. *Front Vet Sci.* (2018) 5:6. doi: 10.3389/fvets.2018.00072
44. Gao GF, Jiang WR, Hussain MH, Venugopal K, Gritsun TS, Reid HW, et al. Sequencing and antigenic studies of a Norwegian virus isolated from encephalomyelitic sheep confirm the existence of louping ill virus outside Great Britain and Ireland. *J Gen Virol.* (1993) 74:109–14. doi: 10.1099/0022-1317-74-1-109
45. Frimmel S, Löbermann M, Feldhusen F, Seelmann M, Stiasny K, Süss J, et al. Detection of tick-borne encephalitis virus antibodies in sera of sheep and goats in Mecklenburg-Western Pomerania (north-eastern Germany). *Ticks Tick Borne Dis.* (2019) 10:901–4. doi: 10.1016/j.ttbdis.2019.04.012
46. Casati Pagani S, Frigerio Malossa S, Klaus C, Hoffmann D, Beretta O, Bomio-Pacciorini N, et al. First detection of TBE virus in ticks and sero-reactivity in goats in a non-endemic region in the southern part of Switzerland (Canton of Ticino). *Ticks Tick Borne Dis.* (2019) 10:868–74. doi: 10.1016/j.ttbdis.2019.04.006
47. Salat J, Ruzek D. Tick-borne encephalitis in domestic animals. *Acta Virol.* (2020) 64:226–32. doi: 10.4149/av_2020_212
48. Waldvogel A, Matile H, Wegmann C, Wyler R, Kunz C. Tick-borne encephalitis in the horse. *Schweiz Arch Tierheilkd.* (1981) 123:227–33.
49. Klaus C, Hörügel U, Hoffmann B, Beer M. Tick-borne encephalitis virus (TBEV) infection in horses: clinical and laboratory findings and epidemiological investigations. *Vet Microbiol.* (2013) 163:368–72. doi: 10.1016/j.vetmic.2012.12.041
50. Pfeffer M, Dobler G. Tick-borne encephalitis virus in dogs - is this an issue? *Parasit Vectors.* (2011) 4:59. doi: 10.1186/1756-3305-4-59
51. Reiner B, Grasmück S, Steffen F, Djuric N, Schindler T, Müller W, et al. Prevalence of TBE antibodies in serum and CSF of dogs with inflammatory and non-inflammatory CNS disease. *Int J Med Microbiol.* (2002) 291(Suppl). 33:234. doi: 10.1016/S1438-4221(02)80069-8
52. Hekrlová A, Kubíček O, Lány P, Rosenbergová K, Schánilec P. Tick-borne encephalitis in dogs: application of "nested real-time RT-PCR" for intravital virus detection. *Berl Munch Tierarztl Wochenschr.* (2015) 128:397–401. doi: 10.23767/0005-9366-128-397
53. Margos G, Fedorova N, Becker NS, Kleinjan JE, Marosevic D, Krebs S, et al. *Borrelia maritima* sp. nov., a novel species of the *Borrelia burgdorferi* sensu lato complex, occupying a basal position to North American species. *Int J Syst Evol Microbiol.* (2020) 70:849–56. doi: 10.1099/ijsem.0.003833
54. Strnad M, Hönig V, Ružek D, Grubhoffer L, Rego ROM. Europe-wide meta-analysis of *Borrelia burgdorferi* sensu lato prevalence in questing *Ixodes ricinus* ticks. *Appl Environ Microbiol.* (2017) 83:e00609-17. doi: 10.1128/AEM.00609-17
55. Strle F, Stanek G, Strle K. Lyme borreliosis: the European perspective. In: Halperin JJ, editor. *Lyme Disease: An Evidence-based Approach.* 2 ed. Wallingford; Oxfordshire; Boston, MA: CAB International (2018). p. 105–23.
56. Tufts DM, Hart TM, Chen GF, Kolokotronis S-O, Diuk-Wasser MA, Lin Y-P. Outer surface protein polymorphisms linked to host-spirochete association in Lyme borreliae. *Mol Microbiol.* (2019) 111:868–82. doi: 10.1111/mmi.14209
57. Pantchev N, Pluta S, Huisinga E, Nather S, Scheufelen M, Vrhovec MG, et al. Tick-borne diseases (borreliosis, anaplasmosis, babesiosis) in German and Austrian dogs: status quo and review of distribution, transmission, clinical findings, diagnostics and prophylaxis. *Parasitol Res.* (2015) 114:19–54. doi: 10.1007/s00436-015-4513-0
58. Littman MP, Gerber B, Goldstein RE, Labato MA, Lappin MR, Moore GE. ACVIM consensus update on Lyme borreliosis in dogs and cats. *J Vet Intern Med.* (2018) 32:887–903. doi: 10.1111/jvim.15085
59. Lin Y-P, Diuk-Wasser MA, Stevenson B, Kraiczy P. Complement evasion contributes to Lyme borreliae–host associations. *Trends Parasitol.* (2020) 36:634–45. doi: 10.1016/j.pt.2020.04.011
60. Kurtenbach K, Sewell H-S, Ogden NH, Randolph SE, Nuttall PA. Serum complement sensitivity as a key factor in Lyme disease ecology. *Infect Immun.* (1998) 66:1248–51. doi: 10.1128/IAI.66.3.1248-1251.1998
61. Bhide MR, Travnicek M, Levkutova M, Curlik J, Revajova V, Levkut M. Sensitivity of *Borrelia* genospecies to serum complement from different animals and human: a host—pathogen relationship. *FEMS Immunol Med Microbiol.* (2005) 43:165–72. doi: 10.1016/j.femsim.2004.07.012
62. Richter D, Matuschka F-R. Elimination of Lyme disease spirochetes from ticks feeding on domestic ruminants. *Appl Environ Microbiol.* (2010) 76:7650–2. doi: 10.1128/AEM.01649-10
63. Lacombe E, Rand PW, Smith RP Jr. Disparity of *Borrelia burgdorferi* infection rates of adult *Ixodes dammini* on deer and vegetation. *J Infect Dis.* (1993) 167:1236–8. doi: 10.1093/infdis/167.5.1236
64. Ogden NH, Nuttall PA, Randolph SE. Natural Lyme disease cycles maintained via sheep by co-feeding ticks. *Parasitology.* (1997) 115:591–9. doi: 10.1017/S0031182097001868
65. Burgess EC, Gendron-Fitzpatrick A, Wright WO. Arthritis and systemic disease caused by *Borrelia burgdorferi* infection in a cow. *J Am Vet Med Assoc.* (1987) 191:1468–70.
66. Lischer CJ, Leutenegger CM, Braun U, Lutz H. Diagnosis of Lyme disease in two cows by the detection of *Borrelia burgdorferi* DNA. *Vet Rec.* (2000) 146:497. doi: 10.1136/vr.146.17.497

67. Štefančíková A, Štěpánová G, Derdáková M, Peťko B, Kyseľová J, Cigánek J, et al. Serological evidence for *Borrelia burgdorferi* infection associated with clinical signs in dairy cattle in Slovakia. *Vet Res Commun.* (2002) 26:601–11. doi: 10.1023/A:1020912618950
68. Tuomi J, Rantamäki LK, Tanskanen R. Experimental infection of cattle with several *Borrelia burgdorferi* sensu lato strains; immunological heterogeneity of strains as revealed in serological tests. *Vet Microbiol.* (1998) 60:27–43. doi: 10.1016/S0378-1135(97)00200-9
69. Fridriksdóttir V, Overnes G, Stuen S. Suspected Lyme borreliosis in sheep. *Vet Rec.* (1992) 130:323–4. doi: 10.1136/vr.130.15.323
70. Stuen S, Fridriksdóttir V. Experimental inoculation of sheep with *Borrelia burgdorferi. Vet Rec.* (1991) 129:315. doi: 10.1136/vr.129.14.315
71. Hovmark A, Åsbrink E, Schwan O, Hederstedt B, Christensson D. Antibodies to *Borrelia* spirochetes in sera from Swedish cattle and sheep. *Acta Vet Scand.* (1986) 27:479–85.
72. Käsbohrer A, Schönberg A. Serologic studies of the occurrence of *Borrelia burgdorferi* in domestic animals in Berlin (West). *Berl Munch Tierarztl Wochenschr.* (1990) 103:374–8.
73. Cabannes A, Hernandez JC, Lucchese F, Appriou M, Tribouley-Duret J. Epidemiology of Lyme disease in cattle and sheep, in Gironde (France). *Med Mal Infect.* (1997) 27:878–83. doi: 10.1016/S0399-077X(97)80242-9
74. Štefančíková A, Derdáková M, Škardová I, Szestáková E, Cisláková L, Kováčová D, et al. Some epidemiological and epizootiological aspects of Lyme borreliosis in Slovakia with the emphasis on the problems of serological diagnostics. *Biologia.* (2008) 63:1135–42. doi: 10.2478/s11756-008-0177-x
75. Divers TJ. Equine Lyme disease. *J Equine Vet Sci.* (2013) 33:488–92. doi: 10.1016/j.jevs.2013.03.187
76. Chang Y-F, Novosol V, McDonough SP, Chang C-F, Jacobson RH, Divers T, et al. Experimental infection of ponies with *Borrelia burgdorferi* by exposure to ixodid ticks. *Vet Pathol.* (2000) 37:68–76. doi: 10.1354/vp.37-1-68
77. Chang Y-F, Ku Y-W, Chang C-F, Chang C-D, McDonough SP, Divers T, et al. Antibiotic treatment of experimentally *Borrelia burgdorferi*-infected ponies. *Vet Microbiol.* (2005) 107:285–94. doi: 10.1016/j.vetmic.2005.02.006
78. James FM, Engiles JB, Beech J. Meningitis, cranial neuritis, and radiculoneuritis associated with *Borrelia burgdorferi* infection in a horse. *J Am Vet Med Assoc.* (2010) 237:1180–5. doi: 10.2460/javma.237.10.1180
79. Imai DM, Barr BC, Daft B, Bertone JJ, Feng S, Hodzic E, et al. Lyme neuroborreliosis in 2 horses. *Vet Pathol.* (2011) 48:1151–7. doi: 10.1177/0300985811398246
80. Wagner B, Glaser A, Bartol J, Mahar O, Johnson A, Divers T. A new sensitive Lyme multiplex assay to confirm neuroborreliosis in horses: a case report. In: *Proceedings of the 57th Annual Convention of the American Association of Equine Practitioners.* San Antonio, TX: American Association of Equine Practitioners (AAEP) (2011). p. 70–5.
81. Pecoraro HL, Felippe MJB, Miller AD, Divers TJ, Simpson KW, Guyer KM, et al. Neuroborreliosis in a horse with common variable immunodeficiency. *J Vet Diagn Investig.* (2019) 31:241–5. doi: 10.1177/1040638718824146
82. Maurizi L, Marié J-L, Aoun O, Courtin C, Gorsane S, Chal D, et al. Seroprevalence survey of equine Lyme borreliosis in France and in Sub-Saharan Africa. *Vector Borne Zoonotic Dis.* (2009) 10:535–7. doi: 10.1089/vbz.2009.0083
83. Appel MJG, Allan S, Jacobson RH, Lauderdale TL, Chang YF, Shin SJ, et al. Experimental Lyme disease in dogs produces arthritis and persistent infection. *J Infect Dis.* (1993) 167:651–4. doi: 10.1093/infdis/167.3.651
84. Chang Y-F, Novosel V, Chang C-F, Summers BA, Ma D-P, Chiang Y-W, et al. Experimental induction of chronic borreliosis in adult dogs exposed to *Borrelia burgdorferi*–infected ticks and treated with dexamethasone. *Am J Vet Res.* (2001) 62:1104–12. doi: 10.2460/ajvr.2001.62.1104
85. Summers BA, Straubinger AF, Jacobson RH, Chang YF, Appel MJG, Straubinger RK. Histopathological studies of experimental Lyme disease in the dog. *J Compar Pathol.* (2005) 133:1–13. doi: 10.1016/j.jcpa.2004.11.006
86. Speck S, Reiner B, Wittenbrink M. Isolation of *Borrelia afzelii* from dog. *Vet Rec.* (2001) 149:19–20. doi: 10.1136/vr.149.1.19
87. Hovius KE, Stark LA, Bleumink-Pluym NM, van de Pol I, Verbeek-de Kruif N, Rijpkema SG, et al. Presence and distribution of *Borrelia burgdorferi* sensu lato species in internal organs and skin of naturally infected symptomatic and asymptomatic dogs, as detected by polymerase chain reaction. *Vet Q.* (1999) 21:54–8. doi: 10.1080/01652176.1999.9694992
88. Skotarczak B, Wodecka B. Identification of *Borrelia burgdorferi* genospecies inducing Lyme disease in dogs from western Poland. *Acta Vet Hung.* (2005) 53:13–21. doi: 10.1556/avet.53.2005.1.2
89. Mather TN, Fish D, Coughlin RT. Competence of dogs as reservoirs for Lyme disease spirochetes (*Borrelia burgdorferi*). *J Am Vet Med Assoc.* (1994) 205:186–8.
90. Hovius KE. The protection of European dogs against infection with Lyme disease spirochaetes. In: Braks MAH, van Wieren SE, Takken W, Sprong H, editors. *Ecology and Prevention of Lyme borreliosis Ecology and Control of Vector-borne Diseases Vol 4.* Wageningen, NL: Wageningen Academic Publishers (2016). p. 409–26.
91. Lappin MR, Chandrashekar R, Stillman B, Liu J, Mather TN. Evidence of *Anaplasma phagocytophilum* and *Borrelia burgdorferi* infection in cats after exposure to wild-caught adult *Ixodes scapularis*. *J Vet Diagn Investig.* (2015) 27:522–5. doi: 10.1177/1040638715593598
92. Burgess EC. Experimentally induced infection of cats with *Borrelia burgdorferi*. *Am J Vet Res.* (1992) 53:1507–11.
93. Tørnqvist-Johnsen C, Dickson S-A, Rolph K, Palermo V, Hodgkiss-Geere H, Gilmore P, et al. First report of Lyme borreliosis leading to cardiac bradydysrhythmia in two cats. *JFMS Open Reports.* (2020) 6:1–6. doi: 10.1177/2055116919898292
94. Hoyt K, Chandrashekar R, Beall M, Leutenegger C, Lappin MR. Evidence for clinical anaplasmosis and borreliosis in cats in Maine. *Top Companion Anim Med.* (2018) 33:40–4. doi: 10.1053/j.tcam.2018.05.002
95. Liu Y, Nordone SK, Yabsley MJ, Lund RB, McMahan CS, Gettings JR. Quantifying the relationship between human Lyme disease and *Borrelia burgdorferi* exposure in domestic dogs. *Geospat Health.* (2019) 14:750. doi: 10.4081/gh.2019.750
96. Egenvall A, Bonnett BN, Gunnarsson A, Hedhammar A, Shoukri M, Bornstein S, et al. Sero-prevalence of granulocytic *Ehrlichia* spp. and *Borrelia burgdorferi* sensu lato in Swedish dogs 1991-94. *Scand J Infect Dis.* (2000) 32:19–25. doi: 10.1080/00365540050164164
97. Gerber B, Eichenberger S, Wittenbrink MM, Reusch CE. Increased prevalence of *Borrelia burgdorferi* infections in Bernese mountain dogs: a possible breed predisposition. *BMC Vet Res.* (2007) 3:15. doi: 10.1186/1746-6148-3-15
98. Preyß-Jägeler C, Müller E, Straubinger RK, Hartmann K. Prävalenz von Antikörpern gegen *Borrelia burgdorferi*, *Anaplasma phagocytophilum* und bestimmte *Leptospira-interrogans*-Serovare bei Berner Sennenhunden. *Tierarztl Prax Ausg K Kleintiere Heimtiere.* (2016) 44:77–85. doi: 10.15654/TPK-140962
99. Barth C, Straubinger RK, Sauter-Louis C, Hartmann K. Prevalence of antibodies against *Borrelia burgdorferi* sensu lato and *Anaplasma phagocytophilum* and their clinical relevance in dogs in Munich, Germany. *Berl Munch Tierarztl Wochenschr.* (2012) 125:337–44. doi: 10.2376/0005-9366-125-337
100. Kybicová K, Schánilec P, Hulínská D, Uherková L, Kurzová Z, Spejchalová S. Detection of *Anaplasma phagocytophilum* and *Borrelia burgdorferi* sensu lato in dogs in the Czech Republic. *Vector Borne Zoonotic Dis.* (2009) 9:655–61. doi: 10.1089/vbz.2008.0127
101. Pantchev N, Vrhovec MG, Pluta S, Straubinger RK. Seropositivity of *Borrelia burgdorferi* in a cohort of symptomatic cats from Europe based on a C6-peptide assay with discussion of implications in disease aetiology. *Berl Munch Tierarztl Wochenschr.* (2016) 129:333–9. doi: 10.2376/0005-9366-15088
102. Žákovská A, Schánilec P, Treml F, Dušková M, Agudelo RCF. Seroprevalence of antibodies against *Borrelia burgdorferi* s. l and *Leptospira interrogans* s. l. in cats in district of Brno and its environs, the Czech Republic. *Ann Agric Environ Med.* (2020) 27:356–60. doi: 10.26444/aaem/122804
103. Shaw SE, Binns SH, Birtles RJ, Day MJ, Smithson RC, Kenny MJ. Molecular evidence of tick-transmitted infections in dogs and cats in the United Kingdom. *Vet Rec.* (2005) 157:645. doi: 10.1136/vr.157.21.645
104. Cutler S, Vayssier-Taussat M, Estrada-Peña A, Potkonjak A, Mihalca AD, Zeller H. A new *Borrelia* on the block: *Borrelia miyamotoi* - a human health risk? *Eurosurveillance.* (2019) 24:1800170. doi: 10.2807/1560-7917.ES.2019.24.18.1800170

105. Gugliotta JL, Goethert HK, Berardi VP, Telford SR 3rd. Meningoencephalitis from *Borrelia miyamotoi* in an immunocompromised patient. *N Engl J Med.* (2013) 368:240-5. doi: 10.1056/NEJMoa1209039
106. Boden K, Lobenstein S, Hermann B, Margos G, Fingerle V. *Borrelia miyamotoi*-associated neuroborreliosis in immunocompromised person. *Emerg Infect Dis.* (2016) 22:1617–20. doi: 10.3201/eid2209.152034
107. Richter D, Matuschka F-R. Modulatory effect of cattle on risk for Lyme disease. *Emerg Infect Dis.* (2006) 12:1919–23. doi: 10.3201/eid1212.051552
108. Shannon AB, Rucinsky R, Gaff HD, Brinkerhoff RJ. *Borrelia miyamotoi*, other vector-borne agents in cat blood and ticks in Eastern Maryland. *EcoHealth.* (2017) 14:816–20. doi: 10.1007/s10393-017-1268-3
109. Dugat T, Lagree AC, Maillard R, Boulouis HJ, Haddad N. Opening the black box of *Anaplasma phagocytophilum* diversity: current situation and future perspectives. *Front Cell Infect Microbiol.* (2015) 5:61. doi: 10.3389/fcimb.2015.00061
110. Dumler JS, Choi K-S, Garcia-Garcia JC, Barat NS, Scorpio DG, Garyu JW, et al. Human granulocytic anaplasmosis and *Anaplasma phagocytophilum.* *Emerg Infect Dis.* (2005) 11:1828–34. doi: 10.3201/eid1112.050898
111. Jaarsma RI, Sprong H, Takumi K, Kazimirova M, Silaghi C, Mysterud A, et al. *Anaplasma phagocytophilum* evolves in geographical and biotic niches of vertebrates and ticks. *Parasit Vectors.* (2019) 12:328. doi: 10.1186/s13071-019-3583-8
112. Brown WC. Adaptive immunity to *Anaplasma* pathogens and immune dysregulation: implications for bacterial persistence. *Comp Immunol Microbiol Infect Dis.* (2012) 35:241–52. doi: 10.1016/j.cimid.2011.12.002
113. Stuen S, Nevland S, Moum T. Fatal cases of tick-borne fever (TBF) in sheep caused by several 16S rRNA gene variants of *Anaplasma phagocytophilum.* *Ann N Y Acad Sci.* (2003) 990:433–4. doi: 10.1111/j.1749-6632.2003.tb07407.x
114. Stuen S, Braten M, Bergström K, Bardsen K. Cyclic variation in lambs infected with *Anaplasma phagocytophilum.* *Vet Rec.* (2008) 163:338–9. doi: 10.1136/vr.163.11.338
115. Thomas RJ, Birtles RJ, Radford AD, Woldehiwet Z. Recurrent bacteraemia in sheep infected persistently with *Anaplasma phagocytophilum.* *J Compar Pathol.* (2012) 147:360–7. doi: 10.1016/j.jcpa.2012.02.005
116. Lagrée A-C, Rouxel C, Kevin M, Dugat T, Girault G, Durand B, et al. Co-circulation of different *A. phagocytophilum* variants within cattle herds and possible reservoir role for cattle. *Parasit Vectors.* (2018) 11:163. doi: 10.1186/s13071-018-2661-7
117. Scharf W, Schauer S, Freyburger F, Petrovec M, Schaarschmidt-Kiener D, Liebisch G, et al. Distinct host species correlate with *Anaplasma phagocytophilum* ankA gene clusters. *J Clin Microbiol.* (2011) 49:790–6. doi: 10.1128/JCM.02051-10
118. Hulínská D, Langrová K, Pejčoch M, Pavlásek I. Detection of *Anaplasma phagocytophilum* in animals by real-time polymerase chain reaction. *APMIS.* (2004) 112:239–47. doi: 10.1111/j.1600-0463.2004.apm11204-0503.x
119. Stuen S, Oppegaard AS, Bergström K, Moum T. *Anaplasma phagocytophilum* infection in north Norway. The first laboratory confirmed case. *Acta Vet Scand.* (2005) 46:167. doi: 10.1186/1751-0147-46-167
120. Pusterla N, Pusterla JB, Braun U, Lutz H. Serological, hematologic and PCR studies of cattle in an area of Switzerland in which tick-borne fever (caused by *Ehrlichia phagocytophila*) is endemic. *Clin Diagn Lab Immunol.* (1998) 5:325–7. doi: 10.1128/CDLI.5.3.325-327.1998
121. Engvall EO, Pettersson B, Persson M, Artursson K, Johansson KE. A 16S rRNA-based PCR assay for detection and identification of granulocytic *Ehrlichia* species in dogs, horses, and cattle. *J Clin Microbiol.* (1996) 34:2170–4. doi: 10.1128/JCM.34.9.2170-2174.1996
122. Stuen S, Bergström K. Serological investigation of granulocytic *Ehrlichia* infection in sheep in Norway. *Acta Vet Scand.* (2001) 42:331–8. doi: 10.1186/1751-0147-42-331
123. Zeman P, Januska J, Orolinova M, Stuen S, Struhar V, Jebavy L. High seroprevalence of granulocytic ehrlichiosis distinguishes sheep that were the source of an alimentary epidemic of tick-borne encephalitis. *Wien Klin Wochenschr.* (2004) 116:614–6. doi: 10.1007/s00508-004-0191-0
124. Derdáková M, Štefančíková A, Špitalská E, Taragelová V, Koštálová T, Hrklová G, et al. Emergence and genetic variability of *Anaplasma* species in small ruminants and ticks from central Europe. *Vet Microbiol.* (2011) 153:293–8. doi: 10.1016/j.vetmic.2011.05.044
125. Silaghi C, Scheuerle MC, Friche Passos LM, Thiel C, Pfister K. PCR detection of *Anaplasma phagocytophilum* in goat flocks in an area endemic for tick-borne fever in Switzerland. *Parasite.* (2011) 18:57–62. doi: 10.1051/parasite/2011181057
126. Harrison A, Brown KJ, Ian Montgomery W. *Anaplasma phagocytophilum* in feral goats in Northern Ireland. *Vet Rec.* (2012) 170:602–3. doi: 10.1136/vr.e3938
127. Dreher UM, de la Fuente J, Hofmann-Lehmann R, Meli ML, Pusterla N, Kocan KM, et al. Serologic cross-reactivity between *Anaplasma marginale* and *Anaplasma phagocytophilum.* *Clin Diagn Lab Immunol.* (2005) 12:1177–83. doi: 10.1128/CDLI.12.10.1177-1183.2005
128. de la Fuente J, Lew A, Lutz H, Meli ML, Hofmann-Lehmann R, Shkap V, et al. Genetic diversity of *Anaplasma* species major surface proteins and implications for anaplasmosis serodiagnosis and vaccine development. *Anim Health Res Rev.* (2005) 6:75–89. doi: 10.1079/AHR2005104
129. Hornok S, Micsutka A, Fernández de Mera IG, Meli ML, Gönczi E, Tánczos B, et al. Fatal bovine anaplasmosis in a herd with new genotypes of *Anaplasma marginale, Anaplasma ovis* and concurrent haemoplasmosis. *Res Vet Sci.* (2012) 92:30–5. doi: 10.1016/j.rvsc.2010.10.011
130. Dahmani M, Davoust B, Rousseau F, Raoult D, Fenollar F, Mediannikov O. Natural Anaplasmataceae infection in *Rhipicephalus bursa* ticks collected from sheep in the French Basque country. *Ticks Tick Borne Dis.* (2017) 8:18–24. doi: 10.1016/j.ttbdis.2016.09.009
131. Saleem S, Ijaz M, Farooqi SH, Ghaffar A, Ali A, Iqbal K, et al. Equine granulocytic anaplasmosis 28 years later. *Microbial Pathog.* (2018) 119:1–8. doi: 10.1016/j.micpath.2018.04.001
132. Franzén P, Aspan A, Egenvall A, Gunnarsson A, Karlstam E, Pringle J. Molecular evidence for persistence of *Anaplasma phagocytophilum* in the absence of clinical abnormalities in horses after recovery from acute experimental infection. *J Vet Intern Med.* (2009) 23:636–42. doi: 10.1111/j.1939-1676.2009.0317.x
133. Zeman P, Jahn P. An entropy-optimized multilocus approach for characterizing the strains of *Anaplasma phagocytophilum* infecting horses in the Czech Republic. *J Med Microbiol.* (2009) 58:423–9. doi: 10.1099/jmm.0.007831-0
134. Bretscher R. Serologische Untersuchungen zur Häufigkeit und Verbreitung der equinen Ehrlichiose in der Schweiz. *Schweiz Arch Tierheilkd.* (1991) 133:185.
135. Praskova I, Bezdekova B, Zeman P, Jahn P. Seroprevalence of *Anaplasma phagocytophilum* in horses in the Czech Republic. *Ticks Tick Borne Dis.* (2011) 2:111–5. doi: 10.1016/j.ttbdis.2011.01.002
136. Slivinska K, Víchová B, Werszko J, Szewczyk T, Wróblewski Z, Petko B, et al. Molecular surveillance of *Theileria equi* and *Anaplasma phagocytophilum* infections in horses from Ukraine, Poland and Slovakia. *Vet Parasitol.* (2016) 215:35–7. doi: 10.1016/j.vetpar.2015.10.025
137. Sainz Á, Roura X, Miró G, Estrada-Peña A, Kohn B, Harrus S, et al. Guideline for veterinary practitioners on canine ehrlichiosis and anaplasmosis in Europe. *Parasit Vectors.* (2015) 8:75. doi: 10.1186/s13071-015-0649-0
138. Pennisi MG, Hofmann-Lehmann R, Radford AD, Tasker S, Belák S, Addie DD, et al. *Anaplasma, Ehrlichia* and *Rickettsia* species infections in cats: European guidelines from the ABCD on prevention and management. *J Feline Med Surg.* (2017) 19:542–8. doi: 10.1177/1098612X17706462
139. Egenvall A, Lilliehöök I, Bjöersdorff A, Engvall EO, Karlstam E, Artursson K, et al. Detection of granulocytic *Ehrlichia* species DNA by PCR in persistently infected dogs. *Vet Rec.* (2000) 146:186–90. doi: 10.1136/vr.146.7.186
140. Kirtz G, Czettel B, Thum D, Leidinger E. *Anaplasma phagocytophilum* in einer österreischichen Hundepopulation: eine Prävalenz-Studie (2001–2006). *Kleintierpraxis.* (2007) 7:562–8.
141. Egenvall A, Franzén P, Gunnarsson A, Engvall EO, Vågsholm I, Wikström U-B, et al. Cross-sectional study of the seroprevalence to *Borrelia burgdorferi* sensu lato and granulocytic *Ehrlichia* spp. and demographic, clinical and tick-exposure factors in Swedish horses. *Prev Vet Med.* (2001) 49:191–208. doi: 10.1016/S0167-5877(01)00187-8
142. Hofmann-Lehmann R, Wagmann N, Meli ML, Riond B, Novacco M, Joekel D, et al. Detection of *Candidatus* Neoehrlichia mikurensis and other Anaplasmataceae and Rickettsiaceae in Canidae in Switzerland

and Mediterranean countries. *Schweiz Arch Tierheilkd.* (2016) 158:691–700. doi: 10.17236/sat00087

143. Bajer A, Mierzejewska EJ, Rodo A, Bednarska M, Kowalec M, Welc-Faleciak R. The risk of vector-borne infections in sled dogs associated with existing and new endemic areas in Poland: part 1: a population study on sled dogs during the racing season. *Vet Parasitol.* (2014) 202:276–86. doi: 10.1016/j.vetpar.2013.12.033
144. Berzina I, Capligina V, Bormane A, Pavulina A, Baumanis V, Ranka R, et al. Association between *Anaplasma phagocytophilum* seroprevalence in dogs and distribution of *Ixodes ricinus* and *Ixodes persulcatus* ticks in Latvia. *Ticks Tick Borne Dis.* (2013) 4:83–8. doi: 10.1016/j.ttbdis.2012.08.003
145. Morgenthal D, Hamel D, Arndt G, Silaghi C, Pfister K, Kempf VAJ, et al. Prävalenz von hämotrophen *Mycoplasma* spp., *Bartonella* spp. und *Anaplasma phagocytophilum* bei Katzen im Raum Berlin/Brandenburg. *Berl Munch Tierarztl Wochenschr.* (2012) 125:418–27. doi: 10.2376/0005-9366-125-11
146. Hamel D, Bondarenko A, Silaghi C, Nolte I, Pfister K. Seroprevalence and bacteremia [corrected] of *Anaplasma phagocytophilum* in cats from Bavaria and Lower Saxony (Germany). *Berl Munch Tierarztl Wochenschr.* (2012) 125:163–7. doi: 10.2371/0005-9311-125-113
147. Krücken J, Schreiber C, Maaz D, Kohn M, Demeler J, Beck S, et al. A novel high-resolution melt PCR assay discriminates *Anaplasma phagocytophilum* and *Candidatus* Neoehrlichia mikurensis. *J Clin Microbiol.* (2013) 51:1958–61. doi: 10.1128/JCM.00284-13
148. Wass L, Grankvist A, Bell-Sakyi L, Bergström M, Ulfhammer E, Lingblom C, et al. Cultivation of the causative agent of human neoehrlichiosis from clinical isolates identifies vascular endothelium as a target of infection. *Emerg Microbes Infect.* (2019) 8:413–25. doi: 10.1080/22221751.2019.1584017
149. Portillo A, Santibáñez P, Palomar AM, Santibáñez S, Oteo JA. *Candidatus* Neoehrlichia mikurensis in Europe. *New Microbes New Infect.* (2018) 22:30–6. doi: 10.1016/j.nmni.2017.12.011
150. Beck A, Huber D, Antolić M, Anzulović Ž, Reil I, Polkinghorne A, et al. Retrospective study of canine infectious haemolytic anaemia cases reveals the importance of molecular investigation in accurate postmortal diagnostic protocols. *Comp Immunol Microbiol Infect Dis.* (2019) 65:81–7. doi: 10.1016/j.cimid.2019.05.006
151. Liesner JM, Krücken J, Schaper R, Pachnicke S, Kohn B, Müller E, et al. Vector-borne pathogens in dogs and red foxes from the federal state of Brandenburg, Germany. *Vet Parasitol.* (2016) 224:44–51. doi: 10.1016/j.vetpar.2016.05.012
152. Hornok S, Horváth G, Takács N, Farkas R, Szoke K, Kontschán J. Molecular evidence of a badger-associated *Ehrlichia* sp., a *Candidatus* Neoehrlichia lotoris-like genotype and *Anaplasma marginale* in dogs. *Ticks Tick Borne Dis.* (2018) 9:1302–9. doi: 10.1016/j.ttbdis.2018.05.012
153. Oteo JA, Portillo A. Tick-borne rickettsioses in Europe. *Ticks Tick Borne Dis.* (2012) 3:271–8. doi: 10.1016/j.ttbdis.2012.10.035
154. Azagi T, Hoornstra D, Kremer K, Hovius JWR, Sprong H. Evaluation of disease causality of rare *Ixodes ricinus*-borne infections in Europe. *Pathogens.* (2020) 9:150. doi: 10.3390/pathogens9020150
155. Keenan KP, Buhles WC, Huxsoll DL, Williams RG, Hildebrandt PK. Studies on the pathogenesis of *Rickettsia rickettsii* in the dog: clinical and clinicopathologic changes of experimental infection. *Am J Vet Res.* (1977) 38:851–6.
156. Solano-Gallego L, Kidd L, Trotta M, Di Marco M, Caldin M, Furlanello T, et al. Febrile illness associated with *Rickettsia conorii* infection in dogs from Sicily. *Emerg Infect Dis.* (2006) 12:1985–8. doi: 10.3201/eid1212.060326
157. Levin ML, Killmaster LF, Zemtsova GE. Domestic dogs (*Canis familiaris*) as reservoir hosts for *Rickettsia conorii. Vector Borne Zoonotic Dis.* (2011) 12:28–33. doi: 10.1089/vbz.2011.0684
158. Elfving K, Malmsten J, Dalin A-M, Nilsson K. Serologic and molecular prevalence of *Rickettsia helvetica* and *Anaplasma phagocytophilum* in wild cervids and domestic mammals in the central parts of Sweden. *Vector Borne Zoonotic Dis.* (2015) 15:529–34. doi: 10.1089/vbz.2015.1768
159. Wächter M, Pfeffer M, Schulz N, Balling A, Chirek A, Bach JP, et al. Seroprevalence of spotted fever group *Rickettsiae* in dogs in Germany. *Vector Borne Zoonotic Dis.* (2015) 15:191–4. doi: 10.1089/vbz.2014.1715
160. Wächter M, Wölfel S, Pfeffer M, Dobler G, Kohn B, Moritz A, et al. Serological differentiation of antibodies against *Rickettsia helvetica, R raoultii, R. slovaca, R. monacensis* and *R. felis* in dogs from Germany by a micro-immunofluorescent antibody test. *Parasit Vectors.* (2015) 8:126. doi: 10.1186/s13071-015-0745-1
161. Rymaszewska A, Małgorzata A. Molecular evidence of vector-borne pathogens coinfecting dogs from Poland. *Acta Vet Hung.* (2011) 59:215. doi: 10.1556/avet.2011.008
162. Boretti FS, Perreten A, Meli ML, Cattori V, Willi B, Wengi N, et al. Molecular investigations of *Rickettsia helvetica* infection in dogs, foxes, humans, and *Ixodes* ticks. *Appl Environ Microbiol.* (2009) 75:3230–7. doi: 10.1128/AEM.00220-09
163. Juvet F, Lappin MR, Brennan S, Mooney CT. Prevalence of selected infectious agents in cats in Ireland. *J Feline Med Surg.* (2010) 12:476–82. doi: 10.1016/j.jfms.2010.02.003
164. Spada E, Proverbio D, Galluzzo P, Perego R, Bagnagatti De Giorgi G, Roggero N, et al. Frequency of piroplasms *Babesia microti* and *Cytauxzoon felis* in stray cats from northern Italy. *Biomed Res Int.* (2014) 2014:943754. doi: 10.1155/2014/943754
165. Zintl A, Mulcahy G, Skerrett HE, Taylor SM, Gray JS. *Babesia divergens,* a bovine blood parasite of veterinary and zoonotic importance. *Clin Microbiol Rev.* (2003) 16:622–36. doi: 10.1128/CMR.16.4.622-636.2003
166. Springer A, Höltershinken M, Lienhart F, Ermel S, Rehage J, Hülskötter K, et al. Emergence and epidemiology of bovine babesiosis due to *Babesia divergens* on a northern German beef production farm. *Front Vet Sci.* (2020) 7:649. doi: 10.3389/fvets.2020.00649
167. Gern L, Kindler A, Brossard M. Annual evolution of cattle immunity against *Babesia divergens* in northern Switzerland. *Prev Vet Med.* (1988) 6:9–16. doi: 10.1016/0167-5877(88)90021-9
168. Zintl A, Gray JS, Skerrett HE, Mulcahy G. Possible mechanisms underlying age-related resistance to bovine babesiosis. *Parasite Immunol.* (2005) 27:115–20. doi: 10.1111/j.1365-3024.2005.00748.x
169. Losson B, Lefevre F. La babesiose bovine en Belgique. Une enquête sérologique en zone d'endémie. *Ann Med Vet.* (1989) 133:421–6.
170. Lempereur L, Lebrun M, Cuvelier P, Sépult G, Caron Y, Saegerman C, et al. Longitudinal field study on bovine *Babesia* spp. and *Anaplasma phagocytophilum* infections during a grazing season in Belgium. *Parasitol Res.* (2012) 110:1525–30. doi: 10.1007/s00436-011-2657-0
171. L'Hostis M, Chauvin A, Valentin A, Precigout E, Gorenflot A. Survey of *Babesia divergens* antibody kinetics in cattle in western France. *Vet Res.* (1997) 28:481–8.
172. Malandrin L, L'Hostis M, Chauvin A. Isolation of *Babesia divergens* from carrier cattle blood using in vitro culture. *Vet Res.* (2004) 35:131–9. doi: 10.1051/vetres:2003047
173. Devos J, Geysen D. Epidemiological study of the prevalence of *Babesia divergens* in a veterinary practice in the mid-east of France. *Vet Parasitol.* (2004) 125:237–49. doi: 10.1016/j.vetpar.2004.08.004
174. Agoulon A, Malandrin L, Lepigeon F, Vénisse M, Bonnet S, Becker CAM, et al. A vegetation index qualifying pasture edges is related to *Ixodes ricinus* density and to *Babesia divergens* seroprevalence in dairy cattle herds. *Vet Parasitol.* (2012) 185:101–9. doi: 10.1016/j.vetpar.2011.10.022
175. Ullmann B. *Untersuchungen zum Vorkommen und zur serologischen Differenzierung von Babesien bei Rindern im westlichen Allgäu* (Dissertation). Ludwig-Maximilians-Universität München, Munich, Germany (1983).
176. Ganse-Dumrath D, Hannover TH. *Epidemiology of Babesia divergens infection in cattle in northern Germany* (Dissertation). Univerisity of Veterinary Medicine Hannover, Hanover, Germany (1986).
177. Niepold J. *Untersuchung von Rinderseren auf das simultane Vorkommen von Infektionen mit Borrelien (Borrelia burgdorferi) und Babesien (Babesia divergens).* (Dissertation). University of Veterinary Medicine Hannover, Hanover, Germany (1990).
178. Lengauer H, Just FT, Edelhofer R, Pfister K. Tick infestation and the prevalence of *Borrelia burgdorferi* and *Babesia divergens* in cattle in Bavaria. *Berl Munch Tierarztl Wochenschr.* (2006) 119:335–41.
179. Hornok S, Edelhofer R, Szotáczky I, Hajtós I. *Babesia divergens* becoming extinct in cattle of northeast Hungary: new data on the past and present

situation. *Acta Vet Hung.* (2006) 54:493–501. doi: 10.1556/AVet.54.2006.4.7

180. Hasle G, Bjune GA, Christensson D, Røed KH, Whist AC, Leinaas HP. Detection of *Babesia divergens* in southern Norway by using an immunofluorescence antibody test in cow sera. *Acta Vet Scand.* (2010) 52:55. doi: 10.1186/1751-0147-52-55
181. Andersson MO, Víchová B, Tolf C, Krzyzanowska S, Waldenström J, Karlsson ME. Co-infection with *Babesia divergens* and *Anaplasma phagocytophilum* in cattle (*Bos taurus*), Sweden. *Ticks Tick Borne Dis.* (2017) 8:933–5. doi: 10.1016/j.ttbdis.2017.08.005
182. Adam KMG, Blewett DA, Collins TJ, Edgar JT. Outbreaks of babesiasis on two farms in Scotland. *Br Vet J.* (1978) 134:428–33. doi: 10.1016/S0007-1935(17)33384-5
183. Adam KM, Blewett DA. A serological survey for *Babesia* in cattle in Scotland II. The occurrence of antibody in the population and the distribution of infected herds. *Ann Trop Med Parasitol.* (1978) 72:417–28. doi: 10.1080/00034983.1978.11719342
184. Taylor SM, Kenny J, Strain A. The distribution of *Babesia divergens* infection within the cattle population of Northern Ireland. *Br Vet J.* (1982) 138:384–92. doi: 10.1016/S0007-1935(17)30983-1
185. Gray A, Capewell P, Loney C, Katzer F, Shiels BR, Weir W. Sheep as host species for zoonotic *Babesia venatorum*, United Kingdom. *Emerg Infect Dis.* (2019) 25:2257–60. doi: 10.3201/eid2512.190459
186. Zintl A, McGrath G, O'Grady L, Fanning J, Downing K, Roche D, et al. Changing incidence of bovine babesiosis in Ireland. *Ir Vet J.* (2014) 67:7. doi: 10.1186/2046-0481-67-19
187. Chauvin A, Moreau E, Bonnet S, Plantard O, Malandrin L. *Babesia* and its hosts: adaptation to long-lasting interactions as a way to achieve efficient transmission. *Vet Res.* (2009) 40:37. doi: 10.1051/vetres/2009020
188. Johnson RC, Schmid GP, Hyde FW, Steigerwalt AG, Brenner DJ. *Borrelia burgdorferi* sp. nov.: etiologic agent of Lyme disease. *Int J Syst Evol Microbiol.* (1984) 34:496–7. doi: 10.1099/00207713-34-4-496

24

Asian Admixture in European *Echinococcus multilocularis* Populations: New Data from Poland Comparing EmsB Microsatellite Analyses and Mitochondrial Sequencing

Gérald Umhang [1], Jenny Knapp [2,3], Marion Wassermann [4], Vanessa Bastid [1], Carine Peytavin de Garam [1], Franck Boué [1], Tomasz Cencek [5], Thomas Romig [4] and Jacek Karamon [5]*

[1] Wildlife Surveillance and Eco-Epidemiology Unit, National Reference Laboratory for Echinococcus spp., Rabies and Wildlife Laboratory, ANSES, Malzéville, France, [2] UMR CNRS 6249 Laboratoire Chrono-Environnement, Université Franche-Comté, Besançon, France, [3] Department of Parasitology-Mycology, National Reference Centre for Echinococcoses, University Hospital of Besançon, Besançon, France, [4] Parasitology Unit, University of Hohenheim, Stuttgart, Germany, [5] Department of Parasitology, National Veterinary Research Institute, Pulawy, Poland

***Correspondence:**
Gérald Umhang
gerald.umhang@anses.fr

The cestode *Echinococcus multilocularis* is the causative agent of a severe zoonotic disease: alveolar echinococcosis (AE). The parasite is distributed over a vast area in northern Eurasia and North America, but the impact of AE on human health is highly uneven between different regions. One hypothetical reason for this difference in virulence may be the genetic structure of *E. multilocularis* which—based on mitochondrial sequences and EmsB microsatellite profiles—forms four distinct clades. These clades correspond approximately to their continents of origin: Asia, Europe, and North America, with a fourth clade apparently restricted to Mongolia and neighboring regions, even though this clade has not yet been described by EmsB genotyping. However, there are various records of genetic variants from the "wrong" region, e.g., "European" haplotypes in Western Canada, which may be the result of introduction or natural migration of host animals. One such example, prompting this study, is the recent record of an "Asian" mitochondrial haplotype in worms from foxes in Poland. At the time, this could not be confirmed by EmsB microsatellite analysis, a method that has proven to possess greater discriminatory power with the *E. multilocularis* nuclear genome than sequencing of mitochondrial markers. Therefore, worms collected from foxes in Poland were examined both by EmsB analysis and sequencing of the full mitochondrial *cox1* gene in order to allocate the samples to the European or Asian cluster. Based on EmsB analyses of 349 worms from 97 Polish red foxes, 92% of the worms clearly showed "European-type" EmsB profiles, but 27 worms (8%) from seven foxes showed profiles that clustered with samples of Asian origin. According to *cox1* sequences, a total of 18 worms from 8 foxes belonged to the Asian cluster of haplotypes. The two methods did not fully agree: only 13 worms from three foxes belonged to Asian clusters by both EmsB and *cox1*, whereas 18 worms from nine foxes belonged to different clusters, according to each marker. Cross-fertilization between worms of Asian origin and those from the European Polish population may explain these conflicting results. The presence of clearly Asian elements in the Polish *E. multilocularis* population could be the result of introduction of *E. multilocularis* with host animals (e.g., domestic dogs), or the migration of foxes. In the absence of genetic data from eastern European countries, especially those bordering Poland, it cannot be concluded whether this Asian admixture is typical for a larger area toward central/eastern Europe, or the Polish parasite population is the western extreme of a gradient where both European and Asian elements mingle. Further studies are needed on this subject, preferably using both mitochondrial sequencing and EmsB microsatellite analysis.

Keywords: *Echinococcus multilocularis*, Poland, EmsB microsatellite, mitochondrial sequencing, Asian origin, cross-fertilization

INTRODUCTION

The cestode *Echinococcus multilocularis* is the causative agent of a severe parasitic disease: alveolar echinococcosis (AE). This zoonotic disease is widely distributed throughout the northern hemisphere. China is considered the main focus of human AE cases, with an estimated 91% of all new cases per year worldwide; in contrast, the European proportion of the global load was estimated at <1%, representing 168 new AE cases annually (1). After the initial infection event, human disease is characterized by a long asymptomatic period (5–15 years), during which parasitic lesions develop in the liver, potentially extending or metastasizing to other organs. The mortality rate is >90% in untreated or inadequately treated cases within 10–15 years after diagnosis (2). Humans become infected through oral ingestion of *E. multilocularis* eggs dispersed into the environment. In the typical parasitic lifecycle, small mammals (often arvicoline rodents) ingest these eggs, leading to the development of hepatic lesions producing protoscoleces. The prey-predator relationship between these rodents and carnivores, in central and eastern Europe mainly red foxes, results in the colonization of the small intestines of carnivores by these protoscoleces, where they evolve to adult worms releasing eggs into the environment via the feces.

The impact of AE on human health is highly uneven between different regions. One hypothetical reason for this difference in virulence may be the genetic structure of *E. multilocularis*. A study based on sequencing of three complete mitochondrial genes *cox1*, *cob* and *nad2* (3,558 bp) of *E. multilocularis* samples resulted in the identification of four different geographical clades: Europe, Asia and North America, with a fourth clade apparently restricted to Mongolia and neighboring regions (3). The correlation between mitochondrial haplotype groups and geographical areas was recently demonstrated by different studies to be more complex, despite a still limited and inadequate geographical and numerical sampling coverage (4), with various records of genetic variants from the "wrong" region. European mitochondrial haplotypes were identified in Canada (5–8), but also in a captive primate from Russia (Moscow zoo), even though the latter probably did not correspond to autochthonous infection (9). Mongolian and North American mitochondrial haplotypes have been identified in Southern and Northern Siberia, respectively (9). Asian mitochondrial haplotypes were reported from the European part of Russia (9) and northwestern America (Alaska, Saint Lawrence island) (3).

Investigations of the genetic diversity of *E. multilocularis* were simultaneously to mitochondrial sequencing carried out using the EmsB microsatellite marker. This molecular tool has a very high discriminative power due to the quantitative exploitation of the amplification of about 40 copies located on chromosome 5 (10–12). EmsB studies confirmed the same geographical clades as those obtained by mitochondrial sequencing for Europe and Asia, although samples from various circumpolar locations above the Arctic Circle clustered with North American isolates, possibly due to long-distance mobility of Arctic foxes (11, 13, 14). EmsB profiles of the Mongolian clade have currently not been described, most probably due to the absence of EmsB genotyping of samples from this area. As for mitochondrial haplotypes, there are also some samples where the EmsB profiles do not correspond to their geographical origin. One *E. multilocularis* rodent sample from Canada and another from a human patient from Alaska shared the same EmsB profile with a Japanese isolate in the Asian clade (11). The exclusive presence in Svalbard of a single EmsB profile from the Arctic clade is coherent, despite it being geographically a part of Europe (14). Further European studies on the presence of *E. multilocularis* based on EmsB have revealed only profiles clustering together, therefore designated "European" profiles. The expansion of the parasite in Europe was investigated in the historical Alpine focus, with peripheral areas revealing mainland-island transmission ruled by founder events due to migration of red foxes (13). The presence of the parasite across France, but also in Denmark and Sweden, has confirmed this transmission scheme due to the identification of EmsB profiles previously reported from the historical focus in south-central Europe (15, 16). Microsatellite investigations of 301 worms from 87 foxes (one to five worms per fox) originating from all endemic provinces of Poland have resulted in the identification of 29 EmsB profiles and highlighted the influence of neighboring countries in the spatial expansion of the parasite (17). In the same period of the cited study, mitochondrial sequencing (*cox1*, *cob*, *nad2*) was carried out on 83 worms isolated from red foxes (one worm per fox) (18), almost all had previously been characterized by EmsB. Seven of these worms, all from the northeastern part of Poland, belonged to a haplotype with very close genetic proximity to haplotypes typical for Asia. However, five of these seven worms were considered to belong to EmsB profiles (Pol01, Pol03, Pol17, and Pol19) typical for Europe, while for technical reasons, no profile was obtained for the other two worms (17).

In many studies using EmsB as a tool to investigate genetic diversity in *E. multilocularis*, attention was focused on the national or regional context, especially in the construction of dendrograms which only include samples from that study. However, due to the nature of the marker and the unweighted pair group method with arithmetic mean (UPGMA) used, the clustering structure of the dendrogram may be influenced by the number and the individual variation of the samples used (19). To obtain information for a larger geographical context, it is therefore necessary to combine larger and spatially distant EmsB data sets.

The identification of mitochondrial haplotypes of the Asian cluster in Poland and the availability of EmsB data from the same worms attributed to the European cluster has prompted this study, focusing on Poland, where the described inconsistencies between mitochondrial sequencing and EmsB results had been observed. Additional sequencing of a mitochondrial target (full *cox1*) was carried out in order to evaluate the current epidemiological situation in Poland regarding a potential Asian admixture in European *E. multilocularis* populations.

MATERIALS AND METHODS

Sample Collection

The 301 worms from 87 Polish foxes previously analyzed for EmsB microsatellite genetic diversity in the studies carried out by Umhang et al. (17) were added to 46 worms from ten foxes genotyped by Knapp et al. (13) to construct a dendrogram that also includes samples of Asian and Arctic origin [i.e., China, Japan, Canada, Alaska, and Svalbard from (11, 14)]. The foxes were each identified by a number and each worm by the number of the fox followed by the number of the individual worm (from one to five), as practiced previously (13, 17). Worms with an Asian mitochondrial haplotype identified previously (18) without available EmsB profiles were re-examined by EmsB genotyping. In addition, EmsB microsatellite data from all other *E. multilocularis* samples previously genotyped [EWET Project, (20)] in Europe (13, 15, 16, 21) and available from the EmsB database (20) were used to visualize potential Asian origins by performing a hierarchical clustering analysis represented in a dendrogram.

EmsB Microsatellite Analyses and Clustering Dendrogram

EmsB PCR amplification was performed as previously reported (17). Capillary electrophoresis of PCR products was performed on a 3500 genetic analyzer (Life Technologies, Foster City, CA, USA). The size and height of each peak of the electrophoretic profile constituting the EmsB profiles were determined with the use of GeneMapper 4.1. The characterization of EmsB profiles composed of several peaks or alleles from 209 to 241 bp was carried out as previously described (11, 20). The hierarchical clustering analysis was done using the Euclidean distance and the average link clustering method (UPGMA) (22). The uncertainty of clusters was evaluated by multiscale bootstrap resampling (B = 1,000) and given by approximately unbiased *p*-values (AU), according to Shimodaira (23, 24). Clustering analyses were performed using R statistical software (25) and the pvclust library (26). In each dendrogram, EmsB microsatellite data from previously genotyped samples from the Arctic and Asian groups (11, 13) were added. The genetic threshold of 0.08 was used to determine the genotyping status of each sample (11), while two *E. granulosus sensu stricto* (G1) samples were used as the outgroup.

Mitochondrial Sequencing and Haplotype Analysis

The worm samples with an Asian EmsB profile identified were submitted to full *cox1* sequencing when the haplotype was not previously obtained by Karamon et al. (18). Sequencing of the full mitochondrial *cox1* gene (1,608 bp) was performed from amplicons obtained by PCR, as previously reported (27, 28). Nucleotide sequences of the *cox1* gene obtained were used in addition to those previously reported (3, 9, 18) to construct a TCS haplotype network (29) generated with PopART (http://popart.otago.ac.nz). The previously reported *cox1* haplotypes from Russia (9) and from Europe (Austria, France, Belgium, Slovakia, Germany), Asia (Kazakhstan, China), North America, and Mongolia (China: Inner Mongolia) (3) with their original identification were integrated into this network. Polish *cox1* haplotypes were designated bythe letter referring to the specific *cox1* haplotype [e.g., POL_Efor *cox1* E haplotype from Poland as in (18)].

RESULTS

The retrospective analyses of 935 EmsB genotyped samples from all European countries except Poland (France, Sweden, Denmark, Estonia, Germany, Switzerland, Czech Republic, Austria, and Slovakia) did not reveal the presence of any Asian EmsB profiles and confirmed the exclusive presence of European profiles (data not shown). A dendrogram was constructed including the 349 worms from 97 Polish red foxes previously genotyped using EmsB (13, 17) and also including the two worms with the Asian cox_E haplotype for *cox1* reported by Karamon et al. (18) (worms 13.1 and 76.1 not available in Umhang et al. (17) (**Figure 1**). The analysis confirmed that 92% of the Polish worms belonged to the European group, but 27 worms isolated from seven foxes clustered in the three EmsB profiles APol1 to APol3 from the Asian group. These three profiles cluster together and are more distant from the other samples of Asian origin from China and Japan. Profile APol1 is exclusively composed of six worms from two foxes from North Poland (13) (**Table 1**). Profile APol2 is represented by only one worm (76.1) and is close to profile APol3,

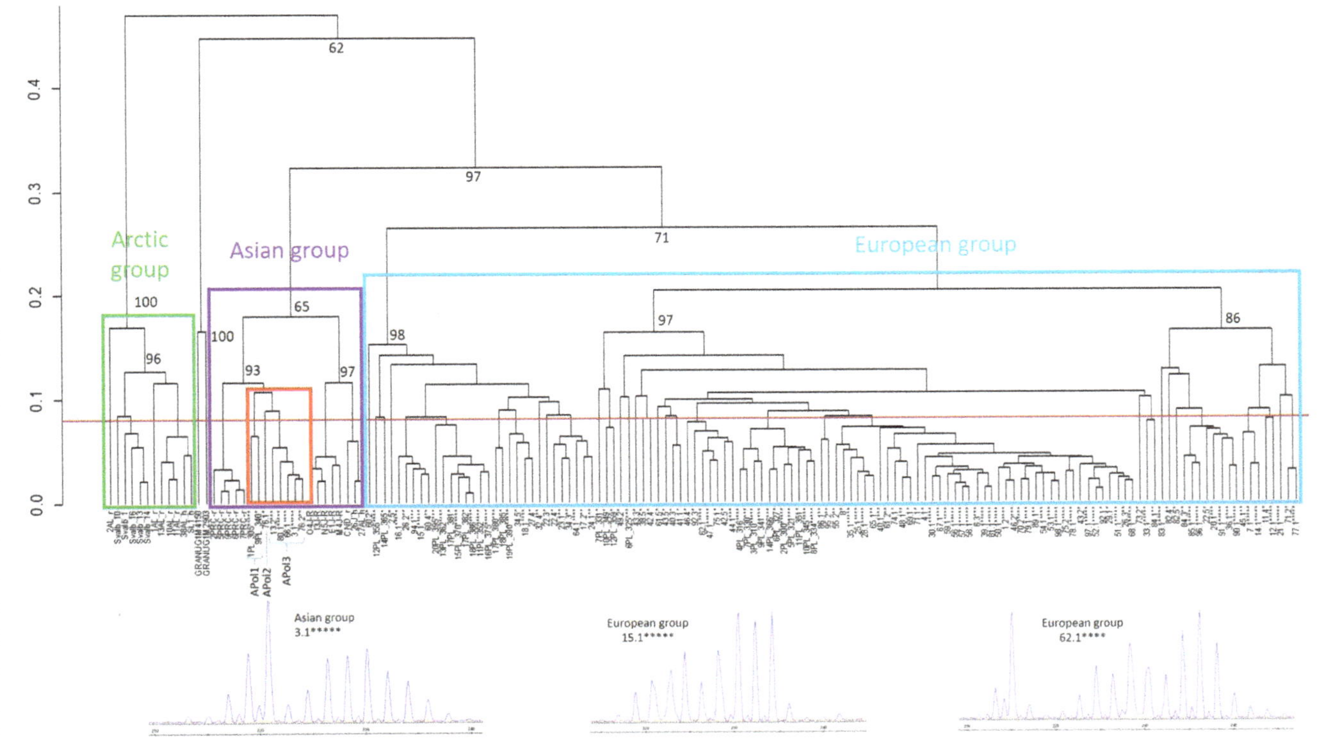

FIGURE 1 | Dendrogram constructed from EmsB data for Polish worm samples from Knapp et al. (13) and Umhang et al. (17). Worms from the same fox with the same profile were pooled to simplify the dendrogram, with the number of asterisks representing the number of worms concerned. Polish samples are indicated by the number of the fox and the representative worm, spaced by PL concerning samples from Knapp et al. (13). The outgroup control is made up of two samples of *Echinococcus granulosus sensu stricto* (G1). Samples from the EWET database were used for Asian (J: Japan, PRC: China, CND: Canada, AL: Alaska) and Arctic groups (AL: Alaska, Svalbard). The Polish samples with Asian profiles APol1 to APol3 are framed in red. The approximately unbiased *p*-values (black numbers on nodes, in percent) were calculated with multiscale bootstrap resampling (B = 1,000). A representative EmsB electrophoregram is provided for one Asian and two European profiles.

which is composed of 20 worms from 6 foxes genotyped in the national Polish study (17), with the exception of worm 13.1 which grouped with other worms from fox #13.

In addition to the ten nucleotide sequences of the full *cox1* gene already available (18), 19 others (including four partial sequences) were obtained from worms with an Asian EmsB profile (**Table 1**). The three *cox1* haplotypes A, B, and E previously reported by Karamon et al. (18) were identified in the 27 worms from the seven foxes, with the same haplotype for worms from the same fox. Haplotypes A and B of the European group differ in only one mutation and were identified in worms from foxes #1PL, #9PL, #13, and #80 (**Figure 2**). Haplotype E corresponds to a previously reported haplotype from Sichuan (China) and Altai (Russia) in the Asian group, and was identified in worms from foxes #3, #66, and #76. Karamon et al. (18) reported this haplotype previously from one worm each from five different foxes (40.1, 44.1, 77.1, 78.1, and 45.1), all of them showing European EmsB profiles, but also from one worm each from four different foxes (3.1, 13.1, 66.1, 76.1) showing Asian EmsB profiles (APol2 and Apol3), like the other worms from these foxes.

In total, worms from 12 foxes harbor an Asian mitochondrial haplotype and/or an Asian EmsB profile (**Table 1**, **Supplementary Table 1**). Thirteen worms isolated from three foxes (#3, #66, #76) belonged to Asian clusters by both EmsB and *cox1*. An Asian EmsB profile but a European mitochondrial haplotype was found in 13 worms from four foxes (#1PL, #9PL, #13, and #80), whereas an Asian mitochondrial haplotype and a European EmsB profile was obtained from the remaining five foxes. The geographic location of the foxes harboring worms from the Asian cluster (*cox1* haplotype and/or EmsB) concerned the provinces of Lubuskie (LB), Warmińsko-Mazurskie (WM), Kujawsko-Pomorskie (KP), Podlaskie (PD), and Mazowieckie (MZ).

DISCUSSION

Genetic variants of *E. multilocularis* from the "wrong" regions had previously been described from North America and Asia,

TABLE 1 | Results of full *cox1* sequencing and EmsB microsatellite analyses for Polish worm samples of Asian origin identified by at least one of the two molecular methods.

ID sample (fox_worm)	Province of Poland	Original study concerned	EmsB genotyping			Full *cox1* sequencing			Consensus origin
			Original profile	Study profile	Origin	Haplotype	GENBANK ID	Origin	EmsB/*cox1*
1PL_305	WM	Knapp et al. (13)	G01	APol1	Asian	POL_B (partial)	NA	European	Asian/European
1PL_306			G01	APol1	Asian	POL_B	MW255891	European	Asian/European
1PL_307			G01	APol1	Asian	NA	NA	NA	Asian/European
1PL_308			G01	APol1	Asian	POL_B	MW255892	European	Asian/European
1PL_309			G01	APol1	Asian	POL_B	MW255893	European	Asian/European
9PL340	WM	Knapp et al. (13)	G01	APol1	Asian	POL_A	MW255894	European	Asian/European
3.1	WM	Umhang et al. (17) and Karamon et al. (18)	P01	Apol3	Asian	POL_E	KY205685	Asian	Asian
3.2		Umhang et al. (17)	P01	Apol3	Asian	POL_E	MW255896	Asian	Asian
3.3			P01	Apol3	Asian	POL_E	MW255897	Asian	Asian
3.4			P01	Apol3	Asian	POL_E (partial)	NA	Asian	Asian
3.5			P01	Apol3	Asian	POL_E	MW255898	Asian	Asian
13.1	LB	Karamon et al. (18) and this study	NA	APol3	Asian	POL_A	KY205677	European	Asian/European
13.2		Umhang et al. (17)	P01	APol3	Asian	POL_A	MW255900	European	Asian/European
13.4			P01	APol3	Asian	POL_A	MW255901	European	Asian/European
66.1	PD	Umhang et al. (17) and Karamon et al. (18)	P01	APol3	Asian	POL_E	KY205685	Asian	Asian
66.2		Umhang et al. (17)	P01	APol3	Asian	POL_E (partial)	NA	Asian	Asian
66.3			P01	APol3	Asian	POL_E	MW255903	Asian	Asian
66.4			P01	APol3	Asian	POL_E	MW255904	Asian	Asian
66.5			P01	APol3	Asian	POL_E	MW255905	Asian	Asian
76.1	KP	Karamon et al. (18) and this study	NA	APol2	Asian	POL_E	KY205685	Asian	Asian
76.2		Umhang et al. (17)	P01	APol3	Asian	POL_E	MW255907	Asian	Asian
76.4			P01	APol3	Asian	POL_E (partial)	NA	Asian	Asian
80.1	MZ	Umhang et al. (17) and Karamon et al. (18)	P01	APol3	Asian	POL_A	KY205677	European	Asian/European
80.2		Umhang et al. (17)	P01	APol3	Asian	POL_A	MW255909	European	Asian/European
80.3			P01	APol3	Asian	POL_A	MW255910	European	Asian/European
80.4			P01	APol3	Asian	POL_A	MW255911	European	Asian/European
80.5			P01	APol3	Asian	NA	NA	NA	NA
40.1	WM	Umhang et al. (17) and Karamon et al. (18)	P19	EPol26	European	POL_E	KY205685	Asian	European/Asian
44.1	WM	Umhang et al. (17) and Karamon et al. (18)	P17	EPol22	European	POL_E	KY205685	Asian	European/Asian
77.1	MZ	Umhang et al. (17) and Karamon et al. (18)	P03	EPol34	European	POL_E	KY205685	Asian	European/Asian
78.1	MZ	Umhang et al. (17) and Karamon et al. (18)	P19	EPol26	European	POL_E	KY205685	Asian	European/Asian
45.1	WM	Umhang et al. (17) and Karamon et al. (18)	P24	EPol31	European	POL_E	KY205685	Asian	European/Asian

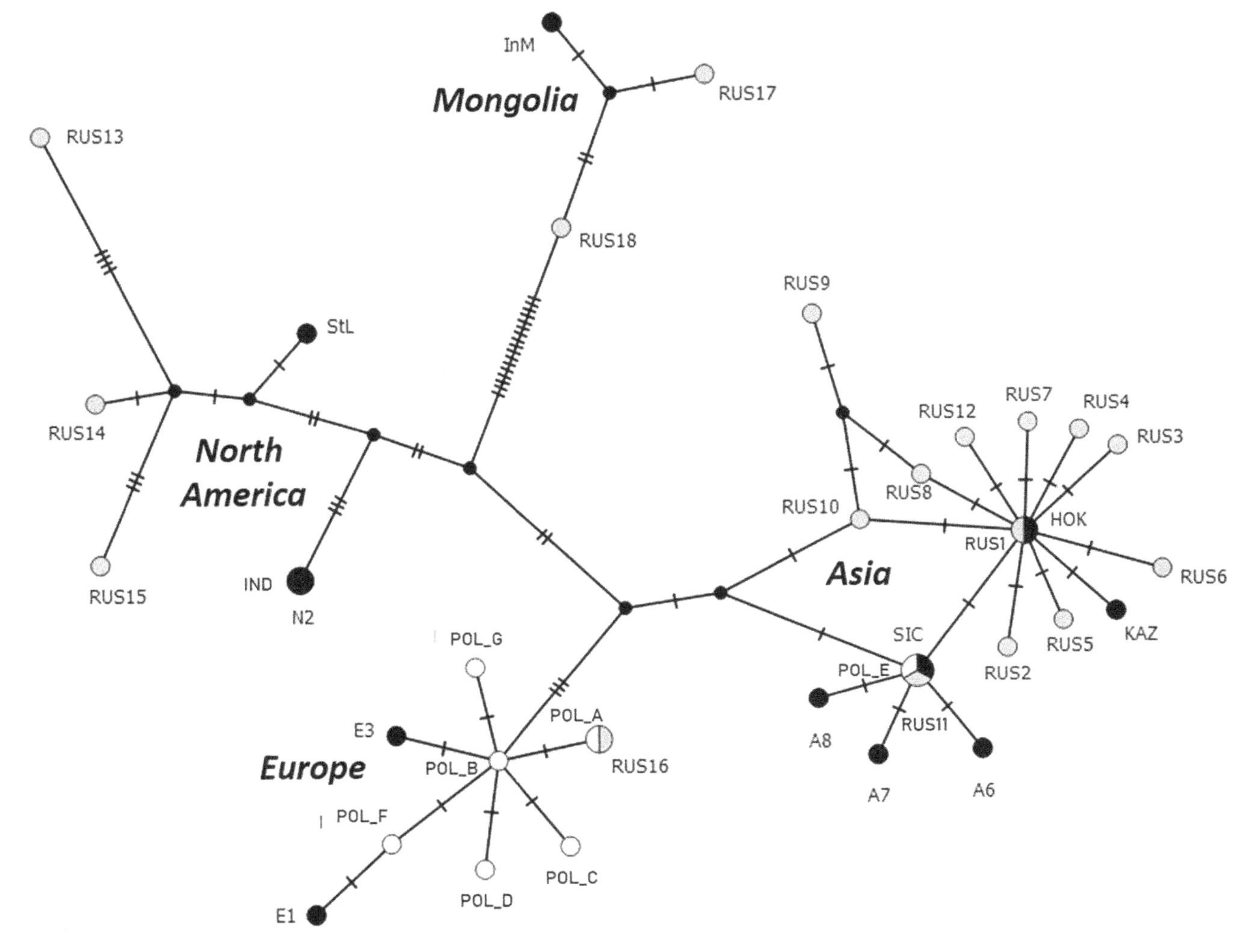

FIGURE 2 | Parsimonious network of *cox1* haplotypes of *E. multilocularis* samples from Poland (white) completed by others previously reported by Konyaev et al. (9) (gray) and Nakao et al. (3) (black), with their original identification of haplotypes. E, Europe; POL, Poland; RUS, Russia; InM, Chinese Inner Mongolia; StL, Alaska (St-Lawrence Island); SIC, China (Sichuan); HOK, Japan (Hokkaido); KAZ, Kazakhstan.

but this had never before concerned samples from non-Arctic Europe until the identification of a mitochondrial haplotype of Asian origin in Polish worms (18). Previous genetic analyses performed by mitochondrial sequencing had consistently identified European haplotypes in European samples (3, 21). In the same way, all the EmsB profiles previously reported from Europe were attributed to the European cluster (13, 15, 16, 20, 21). Here for the first time, both methods (representing the nuclear and the mitochondrial genomes) were used consistently with a larger set of samples. The results reveal the widespread and rather frequent presence in Poland of variants that belong to mitochondrial and/or EmsB clusters typical for Asia, and not known from anywhere else in Europe. Erroneously, profiles of certain samples had previously been allocated to the European cluster of EmsB profiles (13, 17), which could be shown to be an artifact due to the absence of samples from the Asian group in the dendrograms in that study. Attribution to one of the different clades (Europe, Asia, Arctic) using EmsB analyses requires systematic visual analysis of the electrophoretic profile and a hierarchical clustering analysis resulting in a dendrogram that includes samples from each of the different clades: Europe, Asia, and Arctic (including North America). Mitochondrial sequencing, unexpectedly, did not in all cases correspond to the EmsB status regarding the European or Asian clades. Only 13 worms from three foxes belonged to Asian clusters by both EmsB and *cox1*, whereas 18 worms from nine foxes belonged to different clusters according to each marker. However, the large majority (92%) of worms from Poland belonged to European clusters by both methods.

The two methods target mitochondrial or nuclear genomes corresponding to coding and non-coding regions, respectively. In contrast to the mitochondrial genome, the nuclear genome is subjected to recombination and is inherited by both male and female. Recent studies have confirmed that both cross-fertilization and self-fertilization occur within species of *Echinococcus*, including *E. multilocularis* (11, 30–32). Cross-fertilization between worms from two different strains may occur in the intestines, leading to production of eggs with the mitochondrial genome of female origin, but with a nuclear genome integrating genetic material of male origin ("male introgression"). Worms with discrepancies between mitochondrial sequencing and EmsB microsatellite analyses are assumed to result from cross-fertilization between worms of typically "European" and typically "Asian" genomes.

The presence of clusters of genetic variants (both mitochondrial and nuclear) that correspond to continental origins indicates prolonged evolution in these geographical areas, without significant genetic exchange. Our study from Poland is the first large-scale investigation where a zone of apparent overlap or co-existence of such variants was identified. Our data do not allow for an unequivocal explanation of this observation, i.e., whether the presence of different variants was caused by recent introduction (e.g., via traveling domestic dogs, or via migration of wild foxes), or whether this situation represents an ancient polymorphism that has been present in the area for a longer period. The presence of only three EmsB profiles and one mitochondrial haplotype of the Asian cluster argues for (a) sporadic introduction event(s), although our observation of a "mosaic" distribution of mitochondrial and nuclear variants appears to indicate prolonged presence of these variants in Poland with sufficient time for recombination. However, it cannot be ruled out that the Polish worms are the westernmost representatives of Asian variants, and there may be a gradient of progressively decreasing "Asian" components in the genome of *E. multilocularis* populations from East to West. To decide on this, additional genetic analyses in Western Asia and Eastern Europe will be needed. To date, only few data are available from this region: European haplotypes and EmsB profiles were obtained from worms isolated in raccoon dogs from Estonia (21), but no genetic data are available for neighboring countries such as Latvia, Belarus and Ukraine. Concerning Russia, the only *E. multilocularis* sample reported that belongs to the European cluster (according to full *cox1* sequencing) was from a captive primate (*Galago senegalensis*) from the Moscow zoo, where there was a strong suspicion of an infection source from Baltic countries through imported mulch spread as ground cover in the enclosure (9). All the other *E. multilocularis* samples from the European or Asian parts of the Russian Federation belonged to Asian, North American or Mongolian genetic clusters.

It will be interesting to study the geographical limits of this Asian admixture in European *E. multilocularis* populations outside of Poland. As shown in this study, the simultaneous use of both mitochondrial sequencing and EmsB analysis is relevant in order to increase sensitivity and to detect introgression events. As we mentioned, future studies will be particularly relevant in the eastern part of Europe, but sample sizes using the described approach are not large, even in well-known endemic areas of central Europe. Given the fact that Asian genetic components in Poland were found not to be limited to the Northeast of the country but extend as far as Lubuskie (LB) province on the border with Germany, it would not be surprising to detect this kind of admixture even further to the West.

It has been speculated that the presence of certain genetic variants of *E. multilocularis* may have an impact on public health via differences in infectivity or pathogenicity to humans (33). This hypothesis has for instance served as a hypothetical explanation for the low number of human AE cases in North America, despite widespread presence of the parasite in animal hosts. However, no conclusions have been reached on this, and our detection of widespread recombinations between nuclear and mitochondrial markers calls for an examination of human samples using both approaches, as pathogenicity factors will most likely be situated in the nuclear genome rather than the mitochondria, which are at present far more frequently used for genetic characterization of isolates and allocation to clusters. This is highly relevant for the area under study, as, like elsewhere in Europe, an increasing prevalence in red foxes was observed followed by an increase of AE human cases associated with high morbidity and mortality, resulting in a public health situation that is of concern (34 35).

AUTHOR CONTRIBUTIONS

GU, JKa, JKn, and TR: conceptualization. GU, JKa, and JKn: methodology. VB, CP, MW, GU, and JKa: investigation. JKa, TC, JKn, TR, MW, and GU: ressources. GU: writing original draft preparation and project administration. JKn, JKa, TR, MW, and FB: writing-review and editing. All authors contributed to the article and approved the submitted version.

REFERENCES

1. Torgerson PR, Keller K, Magnotta M, Ragland N. The global burden of alveolar echinococcosis. *PLoS Negl Trop Dis.* (2010) 4:e722. doi: 10.1371/journal.pntd.0000722
2. Torgerson PR, Schweiger A, Deplazes P, Pohar M, Reichen J, Ammann RW, et al. Alveolar echinococcosis: from a deadly disease to a well-controlled infection. Relative survival and economic analysis in Switzerland over the last 35 years. *J Hepatol.* (2008) 49:72–7. doi: 10.1016/j.jhep.2008.03.023
3. Nakao M, Xiao N, Okamoto M, Yanagida T, Sako Y, Ito A. Geographic pattern of genetic variation in the fox tapeworm *Echinococcus multilocularis*. *Parasitol Int.* (2009) 58:384–9. doi: 10.1016/j.parint.2009.07.010
4. Deplazes P, Rinaldi L, Alvarez Rojas CA, Torgerson PR, Harandi MF, Romig T, et al. Global distribution of alveolar and cystic echinococcosis. *Adv Parasitol.* (2017) 95:315–493. doi: 10.1016/bs.apar.2016.11.001
5. Gesy K, Hill JE, Schwantje H, Liccioli S, Jenkins EJ. Establishment of a European-type strain of *Echinococcus multilocularis* in Canadian wildlife. *Parasitology.* (2013) 140:1133–7. doi: 10.1017/S0031182013000607
6. Christiansen EF, Himsworth CG, Hill JE, Haulena M. Infection of a Goeldi's monkey (*Callimico goeldii*) with a european strain of *Echinococcus multilocularis* in a canadian institution. *J Zoo Wildl Med.* (2015) 46:378–81. doi: 10.1638/2014-0123R1.1
7. Massolo A, Klein C, Kowalewska-Grochowska K, Belga S, MacDonald C, Vaughan S, et al. European *Echinococcus multilocularis* identified in patients in Canada. *N Engl J Med.* (2019) 381:384–5. doi: 10.1056/NEJMc1814975

8. Schurer JM, Tsybina P, Gesy KM, Kolapo TU, Skinner S, Hill JE, et al. Molecular evidence for local acquisition of human alveolar echinococcosis in Saskatchewan, Canada. *J Infect Dis.* (2020) jiaa473. doi: 10.1093/infdis/jiaa473
9. Konyaev SV, Yanagida T, Nakao M, Ingovatova GM, Shoykhet YN, Bondarev AY, et al. Genetic diversity of Echinococcus spp. in Russia. *Parasitology.* (2013) 140:1637–47. doi: 10.1017/S0031182013001340
10. Bart JM, Knapp J, Gottstein B, El-Garch F, Giraudoux P, Glowatzki ML, et al. EmsB, a tandem repeated multi-loci microsatellite, new tool to investigate the genetic diversity of *Echinococcus multilocularis. Infect Genet Evol.* (2006) 6:390–400. doi: 10.1016/j.meegid.2006.01.006
11. Knapp J, Bart JM, Glowatzki ML, Ito A, Gerard S, Maillard S, et al. Assessment of use of microsatellite polymorphism analysis for improving spatial distribution tracking of *Echinococcus multilocularis. J Clin Microbiol.* (2007) 45:2943–50. doi: 10.1128/JCM.02107-06
12. Valot B, Knapp J, Umhang G, Grenouillet F, Millon L. Genomic characterization of EmsB microsatellite loci in *Echinococcus multilocularis. Infect Genet Evol.* (2015) 32:338–41. doi: 10.1016/j.meegid.2015.03.040
13. Knapp J, Bart JM, Giraudoux P, Glowatzki ML, Breyer I, Raoul F, et al. Genetic diversity of the cestode *Echinococcus multilocularis* in red foxes at a continental scale in Europe. *PLoS Negl Trop Dis.* (2009) 3:e452. doi: 10.1371/journal.pntd.0000452
14. Knapp J, Staebler S, Bar JM, Stien A, Yoccoz NG, Drögemüller C, et al. *Echinococcus multilocularis* in Svalbard, Norway: microsatellite genotyping to investigate the origin of a highly focal contamination. *Infect Genet Evol.* (2012) 12:1270–4. doi: 10.1016/j.meegid.2012.03.008
15. Umhang G, Knapp J, Hormaz V, Raoul F, Boué F. Using the genetics of *Echinococcus multilocularis* to trace the history of expansion from an endemic area. *Infect Genet Evol.* (2014) 22:142–9. doi: 10.1016/j.meegid.2014.01.018
16. Knapp J, Umhang G, Wahlström H, Al-Sabi MNS, Ågren EO, Enemark HL. Genetic diversity of *Echinococcus multilocularis* in red foxes from two Scandinavian countries: Denmark and Sweden. *Food Waterborne Parasitol.* (2019) 14:e00045. doi: 10.1016/j.fawpar.2019.e00045
17. Umhang G, Karamon J, Hormaz V, Knapp J, Cencek T, Boué F. A step forward in the understanding of the presence and expansion of Echinococcus multilocularis in Eastern Europe using microsatellite EmsB genotyping in Poland. *Infect Genet Evol.* (2017) 54:176–82. doi: 10.1016/j.meegid.2017.07.004
18. Karamon J, Stojecki K, Samorek-Pierog M, Bilska-Zajac E, Rozycki M, Chmurzynska E, et al. Genetic diversity of *Echinococcus multilocularis* in red foxes in Poland: the first report of a haplotype of probable Asian origin. *Folia Parasitol.* (2017) 64:2017.007. doi: 10.14411/fp.2017.007
19. Knapp J, Gottstein B, Bretagne S, Bart JM, Umhang G, Richou C, et al. Genotyping *Echinococcus multilocularis* in human alveolar echinococcosis patients: an EmsB microsatellite analysis. *Pathogens.* (2020) 9:4. doi: 10.3390/pathogens9040282
20. Knapp J, Damy S, Brillaud J, Tissot JD, Navion J, Mélior R, et al. EWET: data collection and interface for the genetic analysis of *Echinococcus multilocularis* based on EmsB microsatellite. *PLoS ONE.* (2017) 12:e0183849. doi: 10.1371/journal.pone.0183849
21. Laurimaa L, Süld K, Moks E, Valdmann H, Umhang G, Knapp J, et al. First report of the zoonotic tapeworm *Echinococcus multilocularis* in raccoon dogs in Estonia, and comparisons with other countries in Europe. *Vet Parasitol.* (2015) 212:200–5. doi: 10.1016/j.vetpar.2015.06.004
22. Legendre P, Legendre L. *Numerical Ecology*. Amsterdam: Elsevier (1998).
23. Shimodaira H. An approximately unbiased test of phylogenetic tree selection. *Syst Biol.* (2002) 51:492–508.
24. Shimodaira H. Approximately unbiased tests of regions using multistep-multiscale bootstrap resampling. *Ann Stat.* (2004) 32:2616–41.
25. R Development Core Team. *R: A language and environment for statistical computing*. Vienna: The R Foundation for Statistical Computing (2005).
26. Suzuki R, Shimodaira H. Pvclust: an R package for assessing the uncertainty in hierarchical clustering. *Bioinformatics* (2006) 22:1540–2.
27. Hüttner M, Nakao M, Wassermann T, Siefert L, Boomker JD, Dinkel A, et al. Genetic characterization and phylogenetic position of *Echinococcus felidis* (Cestoda: Taeniidae) from the African lion. *Int J Parasitol.* (2008) 38:861–8. doi: 10.1016/j.ijpara.2007.10.013
28. Addy F, Wassermann M, Banda F, Mbaya H, Aschenborn J, Aschenborn O, et al. Genetic polymorphism and population structure of *Echinococcus ortleppi. Parasitology.* (2017) 144:450–8. doi: 10.1017/S0031182016001840
29. Clement M, Posada D, Crandall, KA. TCS: a computer program to estimate gene genealogies. *Mol Ecol.* (2000) 9:1657–9. doi: 10.1046/j.1365-294x.2000.01020.x
30. Nakao M, Sako Y, Ito A. Isolation of polymorphic microsatellite loci from the tapeworm *Echinococcus multilocularis. Infect Genet Evol.* (2003) 3:159–63. doi: 10.1016/S1567-1348(03)00070-4
31. Knapp J, Guislain MH, Bart JM, Raoul F, Gottstein B, Giraudoux P, et al. Genetic diversity of *Echinococcus multilocularis* on a local scale. *Infect Genet Evol.* (2008) 8:367–73. doi: 10.1016/j.meegid.2008.02.010
32. Lymbery AJ. Phylogenetic pattern, evolutionary processes and species delimitation in the genus Echinococcus. *Adv Parasitol.* (2017) 95:111–45. doi: 10.1016/bs.apar.2016.07.002
33. Romig T, Deplazes P, Jenkins D, Giraudoux P, Massolo A, Craig PS, et al. Ecology and life cycle patterns of Echinococcus species. *Adv Parasitol.* (2017) 95:213–314. doi: 10.1016/bs.apar.2016.11.002
34. Marcinkute A, Šarkunas M, Moks E, Saarma U, Jokelainen P, Bagrade G, et al. Echinococcus infections in the Baltic region. *Vet Parasitol.* (2015) 213:121–31. doi: 10.1016/j.vetpar.2015.07.032
35. Bagrade G, Deksne G, Ozolina Z, Howlett SJ, Interisano M, Casulli A, et al. *Echinococcus multilocularis* in foxes and raccoon dogs: an increasing concern for Baltic countries. *Parasit Vectors.* (2016) 9:615. doi: 10.1186/s13071-016-1891-9

Toxocara canis Differentially Affects Hepatic MicroRNA Expression in Beagle Dogs at Different Stages of Infection

Yang Zou[1], *Wen-Bin Zheng*[2], *Jun-Jun He*[2], *Hany M. Elsheikha*[3], *Xing-Quan Zhu*[2,4*] and *Yi-Xin Lu*[1*]

[1] *Heilongjiang Key Laboratory for Zoonosis, College of Veterinary Medicine, Northeast Agricultural University, Harbin, China,* [2] *State Key Laboratory of Veterinary Etiological Biology, Key Laboratory of Veterinary Parasitology of Gansu Province, Lanzhou Veterinary Research Institute, Chinese Academy of Agricultural Sciences, Lanzhou, China,* [3] *Faculty of Medicine and Health Sciences, School of Veterinary Medicine and Science, University of Nottingham, Loughborough, United Kingdom,* [4] *College of Veterinary Medicine, Shanxi Agricultural University, Taigu, China*

Correspondence:
Yi-Xin Lu
luyixin@neau.edu.cn
Xing-Quan Zhu
xingquanzhu1@hotmail.com

Toxocara canis is a neglected zoonotic parasite, which threatens the health of dogs and humans worldwide. The molecular mechanisms that underlie the progression of *T. canis* infection remain mostly unknown. MicroRNAs (miRNAs) are small non-coding RNAs that have been identified in *T. canis*; however, the regulation and role of miRNAs in the host during infection remain incompletely understood. In this study, we determined hepatic miRNA expression at different stages of *T. canis* infection in beagle dogs. Individual dogs were infected by 300 embryonated *T. canis* eggs, and their livers were collected at 12 hpi (hours post-infection), 24 hpi, and 36 dpi (days post-infection). The expression profiles of liver miRNAs were determined using RNA-sequencing. Compared to the control groups, 9, 16, and 34 differentially expressed miRNAs (DEmiRNAs) were detected in the livers of infected dogs at the three infection stages, respectively. Among those DEmiRNAs, the novel-294 and cfa-miR-885 were predicted to regulate inflammation-related genes at the initial stage of infection (12 hpi). The cfa-miR-1839 was predicted to regulate the target gene TRIM71, which may influence the development of *T. canis* larvae at 24 hpi. Moreover, cfa-miR-370 and cfa-miR-133c were associated with immune response at the final stage of infection (36 dpi). Some immunity-related Gene Ontology terms were enriched particularly at 24 hpi. Likewise, Kyoto Encyclopedia of Genes and Genomes pathway analysis showed that many significantly enriched pathways were involved in inflammation and immune responses. The expression level of nine DEmiRNAs was validated using quantitative real-time PCR (qRT-PCR). These results show that miRNAs play critical roles in the pathogenesis of *T. canis* during the hepatic phase of parasite development. Our data provide fundamental information for further investigation of the roles of miRNAs in the innate/adaptive immune response of dogs infected by *T. canis*.

Keywords: *Toxocara canis*, miRNAs, beagle dogs, liver, RNA-seq

INTRODUCTION

Toxocariasis, mainly caused by *Toxocara canis* infection in dogs (1), is a neglected zoonosis worldwide. Dogs, as the definitive hosts of *T. canis*, can excrete eggs with feces, leading to environment contamination (2, 3). Humans can be infected by *T. canis* via ingestion of food contaminated with embryonated eggs or larvae (2, 4). The larvae hatch inside the intestinal tract of the host and then migrate to the other parts of the body, leading to serious health problems, such as visceral larva migrans, ocular larva migrans, and neurotoxocariasis (5, 6). Owing to non-specific symptoms in human infection and the diagnostic challenges (7), the public health impact caused by *T. canis* infection may be ignored. More efforts are needed to achieve better understanding of the pathogenesis of toxocariasis (1).

In recent years, multiple approaches, such as genomics, transcriptomics, and proteomics, have been applied to characterize the biological and molecular features of *T. canis* (8–11). However, there is a dearth of information regarding the interaction between *T. canis* and its host. MicroRNAs (miRNAs) are endogenous, small, non-coding RNAs that have received significant attention from the scientific community due to their involvement in many and diverse biological processes, such as apoptosis, proliferation, metabolism, and immune response (12). miRNAs together with transcription factors have been considered key regulators that modulate the expression levels of almost all genes that mediate various pathophysiological processes (13, 14). Also, parasites can alter the expression level of host miRNAs in order to regulate gene expression of the target tissues (15–17). miRNAs can repress mRNA expression through binding to the 3′ untranslated regions of target genes or by enhancing mRNA degradation (18). A previous study showed that *T. canis* miRNAs, Tc-let-7-5p, Tc-miR-34, and Tc-miR-100, play roles in host–parasite interactions (8). However, the regulation of miRNAs and their roles in the pathogenesis of *T. canis* during the hepatic phase of infection remains mostly unknown.

Therefore, the present study aimed to investigate the alteration of miRNA expression profiles in the livers of beagle dogs infected by *T. canis* at different stages of infection using small RNA transcriptome sequencing and bioinformatics analysis. The study findings revealed that some differentially expressed miRNAs (DEmiRNAs) play roles in the regulation of inflammatory and immune responses of puppies against *T. canis* infection.

MATERIALS AND METHODS

Experimental Infection of Dogs

The adult *T. canis* worms were collected from naturally infected dogs in Rongchang District, Chongqing Municipality, China, and female adult *T. canis* were identified based on gross morphology. The eggs of *T. canis* were obtained from the uteri of female *T. canis* worms. The unembryonated eggs were incubated with 0.5% formalin solution at 28°C (85–95% humidity) for 28 days, and then the eggs were harvested and filtered through a 200-mesh screen. The finally embryonated eggs were stored in 1% formalin solution at 4°C. Eighteen beagle puppies (6–7 weeks old) were provided by the National Canine Laboratory Animal Resource Center and housed following Good Laboratory Practice (GLP) in an animal facility, according to the GB standard (GB 14922.2-2011) of China. All puppies had tested negative for *T. canis* infection by indirect ELISA, using larval ES antigen, before the start of the experiment. Feces of individual puppies were collected daily and examined using a standard sugar floatation method. Puppies were equally allocated into three experimental and three control groups (three puppies per group). The puppy groups were housed separately and were provided with similar conditions including access to the same water source and food supply. Each puppy was orally infected with 300 embryonated eggs in 1 ml normal saline solution, while the control puppies were inoculated with the same amount of saline but without any eggs.

Detection of *T. canis* Infection

Blood samples of each puppy were collected from the jugular vein into sterile tubes containing EDTA-K2 and tubes without anticoagulant. The *T. canis* IgG antibody was detected using indirect ELISA as previously described (19). Light microscopy was also used to observe whether *T. canis* larvae are present in the livers of puppies. The genomic DNA of infectious eggs (used to infect puppies), larvae (isolated from the liver of infected puppies), and adult *T. canis* (recovered from the small intestine of infected puppies) were isolated using a DNA extraction kit (TianGen™, Beijing, China) according to the manufacturer's instruction. The isolated DNA samples were analyzed using PCR with primer sequences specific to the internal transcribed spacer (ITS) region (partial sequence of ITS-1 and ITS-2) (20). The positive PCR products were sequenced by Sangon Biotech (Shanghai, China), and the obtained sequences were searched against similar sequences available in the GenBank database using Nucleotide BLAST (https://blast.ncbi.nlm.nih.gov/Blast.cgi).

Sample Collection, RNA Extraction, and Quantification

Infected puppies ($n = 9$) and naive (control) puppies ($n = 9$) were killed by potassium chloride (KCl) under a general anesthetic [50 mg/kg tiletamine-zolazepam (Zoletil®), Virbac, France]. The liver samples were collected from all puppies at 12 h post-infection (hpi), 24 hpi, and 36 days post-infection (dpi) according to methods described in our previous study (21). Three biological replicates were examined in each group at each time point post-infection. The collected liver samples were quickly stored in liquid nitrogen until used for RNA extraction. The larvae were recovered from the remaining fresh liver sample of each puppy using the modified Baermann funnel method as previously described (22). The total RNA was extracted from the liver samples of puppies using TRIZOL (Life Technologies, CA, USA). The genomic DNA was removed using DNase I (NEB, Ipswich, USA). RNA concentration was measured using the Qubit® RNA Assay Kit and Qubit® 2.0 Fluorometer (Life Technologies, CA, USA). The integrity of RNA was assessed by the RNA Nano 6000 Assay Kit and the Agilent Bioanalyzer 2100 system (Agilent Technologies, CA, USA). The purity of RNA was examined using

TABLE 1 | Primers used in microRNA (miRNA)–specific quantitative real-time PCR (qRT-PCR) analysis.

miRNAs	Primer	Sequence (5′ to 3′)
U6	Forward primer	CGCTTCGGCAGCACATATAC
Cfa-miR-381	Forward primer	CTGGGTCTGGTATACAAGGGCAAGCTCTC
Cfa-miR-10b	Forward primer	CTGGGTCTGGTATACAAGGGCAAGCTCTC
Cfa-miR-194	Forward primer	CTGGGTCTGGTGTAACAGCAACTCCATGT
Cfa-miR-125a	Forward primer	CTGGGTCTGGTCCCTGAGACCCTTTAAC
Cfa-miR-371	Forward primer	CTGGGTCTGGACTCAAAAAATGGCGGCA
Cfa-miR-16	Forward primer	CTGGGTCTGGTAGCAGCACGTAAATATTGG
Cfa-miR-10a	Forward primer	CTGGGTCTGGTACCCTGTAGATCCGAA
Cfa-miR-146a	Forward primer	CTGGGTCTGGTGAGAACTGAATTCCATGGG

the NanoPhotometer® spectrophotometer (IMPLEN, CA, USA). High-quality RNA samples with RNA integrity numbers (RINs) >8.0 were used to construct the sequencing library.

Small RNA Library Preparation and Sequencing

A total of 3 μg RNA of each sample was used for the construction of the small RNA library by using the NEBNext® Multiplex Small RNA Library Prep Set for Illumina® (NEB, USA). The constructed libraries were sequenced on an Illumina Hiseq 2500 platform. The reads that contain poly N, 5′ adapter contaminants, without 3′ adapter or the insert tag (including poly G, C, A, or T and low-quality reads) were filtered from raw data using custom perl and python scripts. The clean reads that ranged from 18 to 35 nt were mapped against the reference sequence by Bowtie (23). The mapped sRNAs were searched against miRBase20.0 data to identify known miRNAs. In addition, mirdeep2 (24) and miREvo (25) were used to identify potential novel miRNAs. The novel miRNA was predicted by the characteristics of the hairpin structure of the miRNA precursor. The expression levels of miRNA were estimated by TPM (transcript per million) (26). Differential expression analysis was performed using the DESeq R package (1.8.3). A P-value < 0.05 was used as the significance threshold value of differential expression.

Bioinformatics Analysis of DEmiRNA

The target genes of miRNAs were predicted by RNAhybrid, PITA tools, and miRanda (27). To predict the function of the target gene of DEmiRNAs, GOseq R package (28), and KOBAS software (29, 30) were used for Gene Ontology (GO) enrichment and Kyoto Encyclopedia of Genes and Genomes (KEGG) pathway analysis, respectively. A P-value < 0.05 was considered as significantly enriched.

Verification of miRNA Expression by Quantitative Real-Time PCR

Quantitative real-time PCR (qRT-PCR) was performed to confirm the upregulation and downregulation of nine miRNAs randomly selected for verification of the RNA-seq results. qRT-PCR was performed using an miRcute enhanced miRNA qRT-PCR Kit (TianGen, Beijing, China) on a LightCycler480 (Roche, Basle, Switzerland). The cDNA of miRNA was synthesized using an miRcute enhanced miRNA cDNA first chain synthesis Kit (TianGen, Beijing, China). Then, 1 μl cDNA was used for qRT-PCR as follows: initial denaturation at 95°C for 15 min, followed by 40 cycles of 94°C for 20 s and 60°C for 34 s. All primers are listed in **Table 1**. The U6 small nuclear RNA (snRNA) was used as an internal control gene. Melting curve analysis (95°C for 10 s, 65°C for 1 min, and progressive increase from 65°C to 95°C) was performed to ensure specific amplification in each reaction. Each reaction included a blank control to rule out the presence of contamination. The relative expression quantity was analyzed by the $^{2-\Delta\Delta}$Ct method (31, 32).

RESULTS

Detection of *T. canis* Infection in Beagle Dogs

A blood sample of each puppy was collected and tested for IgG antibody against *T. canis*. The IgG antibodies of *T. canis* were detected in infected puppies at 36 dpi. At 12 hpi, *T. canis* larvae were recovered from the livers of three infected puppies, and at 24 hpi, *T. canis* larvae were recovered from the livers of all infected puppies. At 36 dpi, *T. canis* larvae were detected in the liver of one infected puppy, and adult *T. canis* were recovered in the small intestine of all infected puppies. Furthermore, no *T. canis* larvae and anti–*T. canis* IgG antibodies were found in the control puppies. The sequences obtained from the embryonated eggs, larvae, and adult worms were found to match the sequence of *T. canis* (GenBank Accession No. JF837169.1).

Characteristics of the Sequenced Data

In each miRNA library, 142,605,411 raw reads and 7.131 Gb raw data were obtained from infected puppy groups, whereas 136,764,149 raw reads and 6.898 Gb raw data were obtained from the control groups. More than 99% of reads had sequencing quality >Q20 (**Table 2**). The clean reads with appropriate 18–35 nt lengths were selected for further analysis. Moreover, 52.72–65.17 and 0.17–0.24% unique reads were confirmed as known and novel miRNAs, respectively. In addition, 22.16–29.70% non-annotated reads were found in this study (**Supplementary Table 1**), suggesting that these non-annotated reads could be involved in the pathogenesis and progression of *T. canis* infection.

Differentially Expressed Hepatic miRNAs (DEmiRNAs) at Different Infection stages

A total of 59 DEmiRNAs were identified at three infection stages, including 9, 16, and 34 DEmiRNAs at 12 hpi, 24 hpi, and 36 dpi, respectively. Details of DEmiRNAs are shown in **Supplementary Table 2**. Among these DEmiRNAs, 23 DEmiRNAs were upregulated, whereas 36 DEmiRNAs were downregulated (**Figure 1**). However, no common miRNA was found at the three infection stages (**Figure 2**).

Target Gene Prediction and Functional Analysis

Candidate target genes of DEmiRNAs of beagle dog livers were predicted by RNAhybrid, miRanda, and PITA tools. The

TABLE 2 | Summary of the quality control parameters of the reads.

Groups	Samples	Raw reads	Clean reads	Bases	Error rate (%)	Q20 (%)	Q30 (%)	GC content (%)
12 hpi	A12hT1	17,052,302	16,734,756	0.853G	0.01	99.72	99.28	49.61
	A12hT2	15,050,522	14,632,243	0.753G	0.01	99.69	99.24	49.39
	A12hT3	15,753,780	15,606,433	0.788G	0.01	99.70	99.21	49.92
	A12hC1	18,499,157	18,320,368	0.925G	0.01	99.72	99.27	49.75
	A12hC2	15,502,426	15,346,075	0.775G	0.01	99.64	99.09	49.73
	A12hC3	13,471,115	13,320,106	0.674G	0.01	99.65	99.13	49.71
24 hpi	B24hT1	16,220,657	16,074,374	0.811G	0.01	99.57	98.92	49.48
	B24hT2	14,587,167	14,466,523	0.729G	0.01	99.69	99.20	49.60
	B24hT3	17,146,312	16,980,582	0.857G	0.01	99.62	99.04	49.76
	B24hC1	14,239,211	14,125,501	0.712G	0.01	99.64	99.10	49.01
	B24hC2	15,619,834	15,495,519	0.781G	0.01	99.58	98.97	49.15
	B24hC3	14,913,621	14,810,484	0.746G	0.01	99.70	99.23	49.20
36 dpi	D36dT1	18,000,592	17,826,356	0.900G	0.01	99.57	98.93	49.39
	D36dT2	15,372,801	15,223,534	0.769G	0.01	99.72	99.26	49.52
	D36dT3	13,421,278	13,326,515	0.671G	0.01	99.79	99.45	49.33
	D36dC1	13,738,157	13,648,316	0.687G	0.01	99.73	99.31	49.23
	D36dC2	15,012,200	14,900,388	0.751G	0.01	99.73	99.32	49.51
	D36dC3	16,947,963	16,797,392	0.847G	0.01	99.75	99.36	49.26

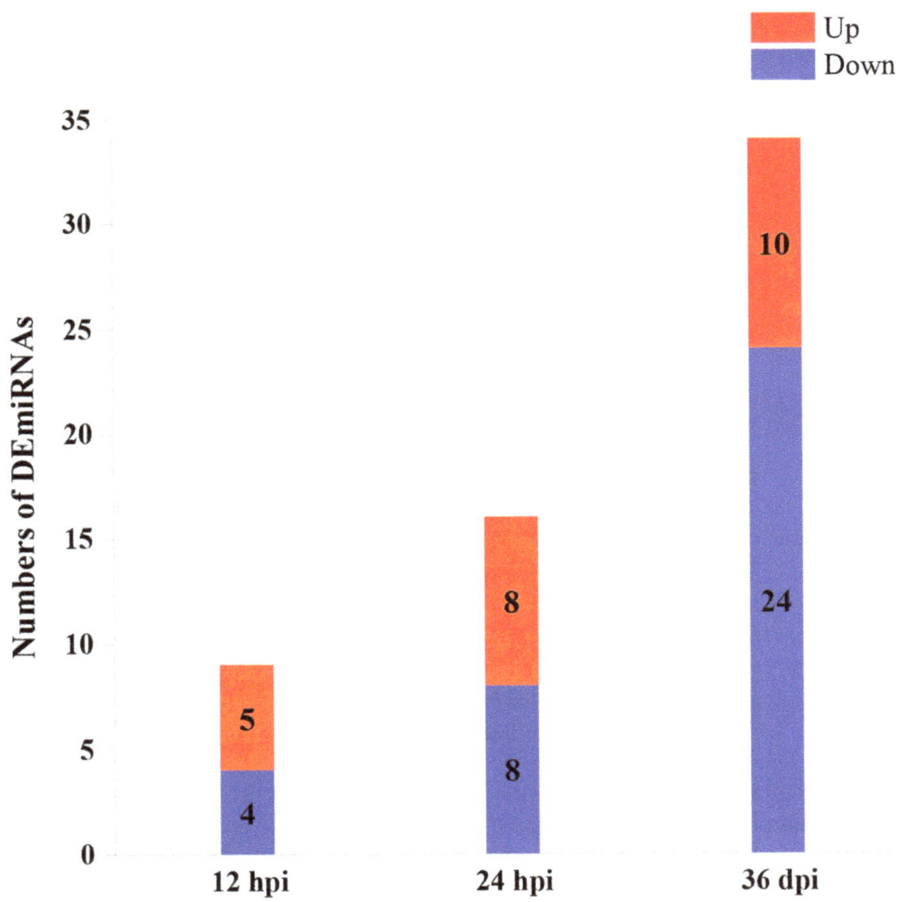

FIGURE 1 | The numbers of differentially expressed microRNAs (DEmiRNAs) at three infection stages [12 h post-infection (hpi), 24 hpi, and 36 days post-infection (dpi)]. The red and blue colors represent the upregulated and downregulated miRNAs, respectively.

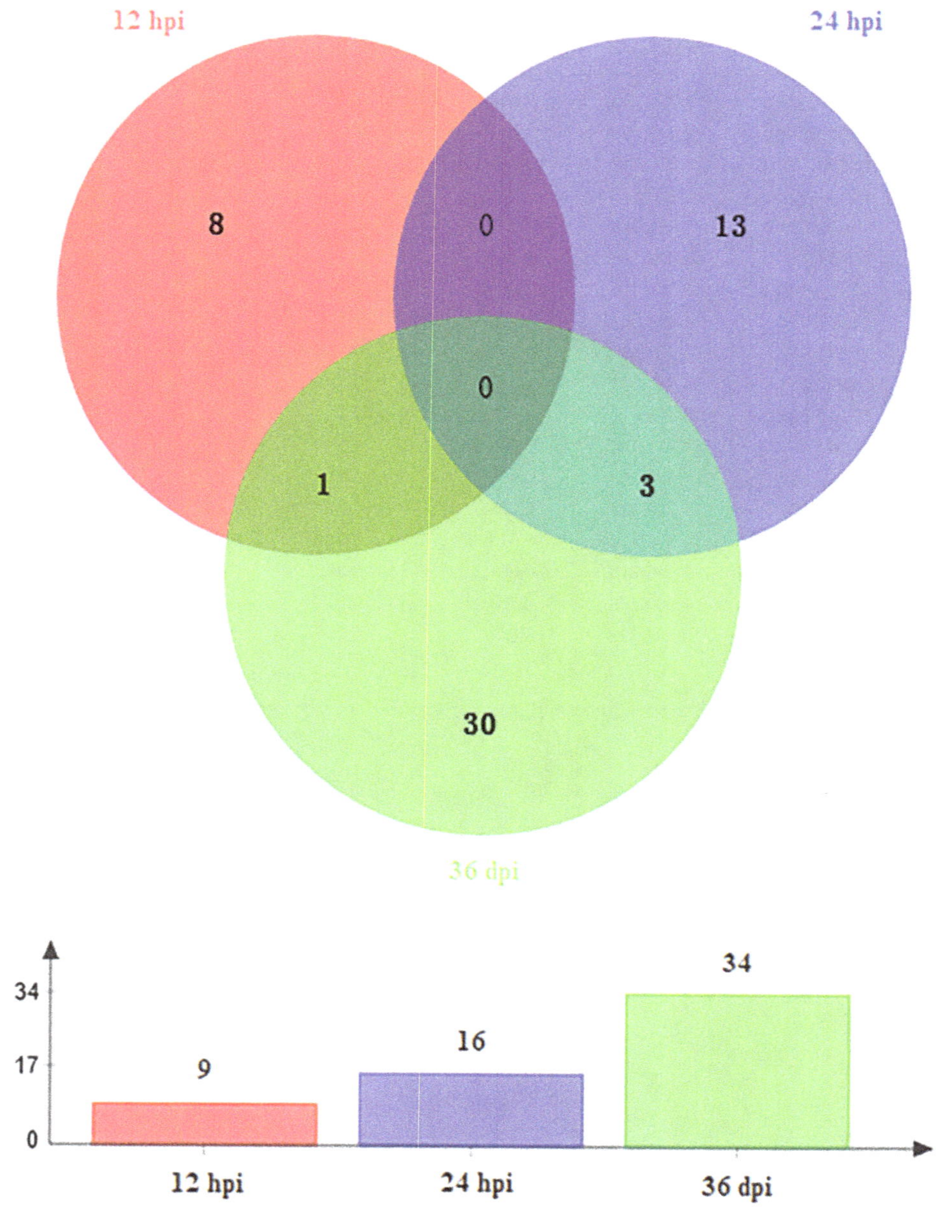

FIGURE 2 | Venn diagram showing the shared and unique DEmiRNAs at different time points after infection (12 hpi, 24 hpi, and 36 dpi).

prediction results showed that a total of 384, 518, and 1,225 hepatic genes were targeted by DEmiRNAs at 12 hpi, 24 hpi, and 36 dpi, respectively. The immunoglobulin superfamily (IgSF) is a molecular superfamily with an immunoglobulin-like domain, and most members of IgSF are found on the surface of lymphocytes and participate in various immune activities. In this study, the IgSF genes were predicted to be regulated by some miRNAs, such as novel-294, cfa-miR-25, cfa-miR-15b, cfa-miR-145, cfa-miR-150, cfa-miR-497, cfa-miR-1839 and cfa-miR-151, cfa-miR-133c, novel-337, cfa-miR-127, cfa-miR-205, and cfa-miR-194 (**Supplementary Table 3**). The GO enrichment analysis showed that 9 DEmiRNAs were significantly enriched in 797 GO terms at 12 hpi; 16 DEmiRNAs were significantly enriched in 768 GO terms at 24 hpi; and 34 DEmiRNAs were significantly enriched in 665 GO terms at 36 dpi ($P < 0.05$) (**Supplementary Table 4**). The top 30 most significant GO terms ($P < 0.05$) belonging to biological process and molecular function at each time point are shown in **Figure 3**. Among of these GO terms, the immune-related GO terms were found in infected livers (**Supplementary Table 5**). At 12 hpi, one DEmiRNA was related to three immune-related GO terms, including natural killer (NK) cell differentiation involved in immune response (GO:0002325), regulation of NK cell differentiation involved in immune response (GO:0032826),

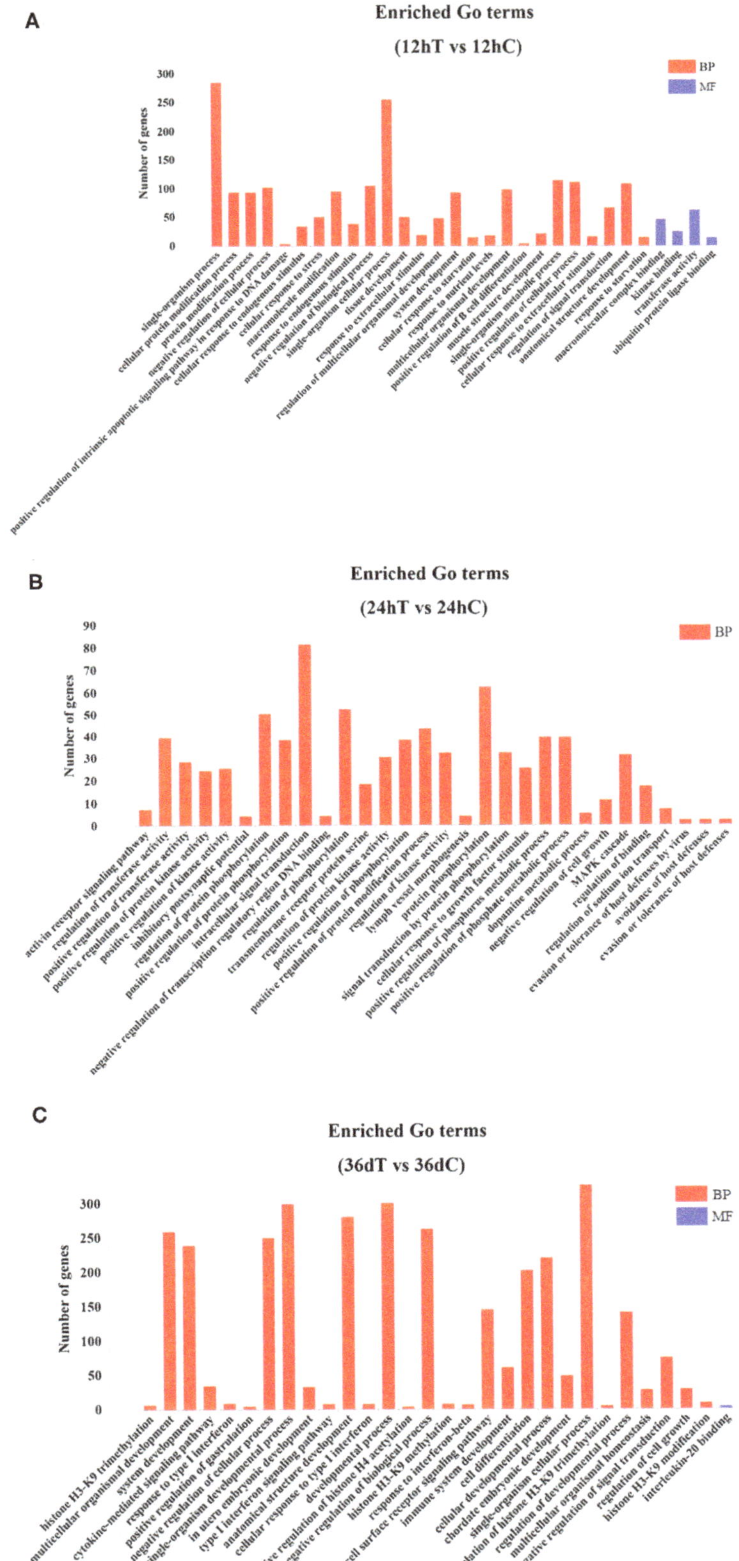

FIGURE 3 | The top 30 Gene Ontology (GO) terms of the DEmiRNAs. **(A)** The significantly enriched biological process (BP) and molecular function (MF) terms of the target genes of DEmiRNAs at 12 hpi. **(B)** The significantly enriched BP terms of target genes of DEmiRNAs at 24 hpi. **(C)** The significantly enriched BP and MF terms of target genes of DEmiRNAs at 36 dpi.

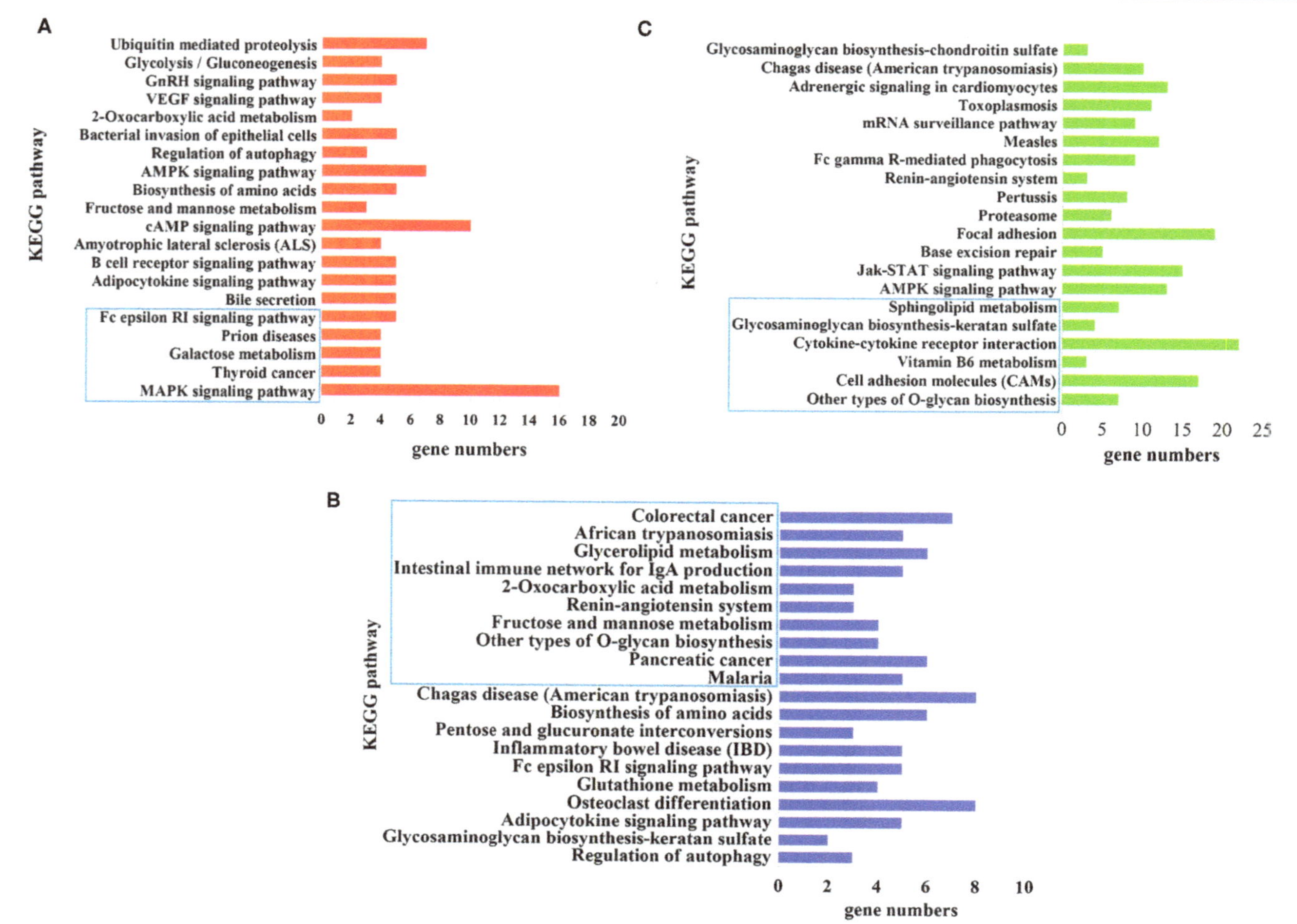

FIGURE 4 | The top 20 signaling pathways enriched by the target genes of differently expressed microRNAs (miRNAs) at **(A)** 12 hpi, **(B)** 24 hpi, and **(C)** 36 dpi. The X-axis labels denote the gene numbers, and the Y-axis labels represent the names of Kyoto Encyclopedia of Genes and Genomes (KEGG) pathways. The pathways enclosed within the blue rectangle represent the significantly enriched pathways.

and negative regulation of NK cell differentiation involved in immune response (GO:0032827). At 24 hpi, six DEmiRNAs were significantly related to 32 immune-related GO terms, including positive regulation of B-cell–mediated immunity (GO:0002714), positive regulation of immunoglobulin-mediated immune response (GO:0002891), positive regulation of leukocyte-mediated immunity (GO:0002705), positive regulation of lymphocyte-mediated immunity (GO:0002708), and regulation of innate immune response (GO:0045088). At 36 dpi, 12 DEmiRNAs were significantly related to four immune-related GO terms, including immune system development (GO:0002520), negative regulation of innate immune response (GO:0045824), positive regulation of immune system process (GO:0002684), and negative regulation of immune response (GO:0050777) (**Supplementary Table 5**).

KEGG Pathway Analysis

KEGG pathway analysis revealed that 5, 10, and 6 pathways were significantly enriched ($P < 0.05$) at 12 hpi, 24 hpi, and 36 dpi, respectively (**Supplementary Table 6**). The top 20 targeted pathways of DEmiRNAs are shown in **Figure 4**. At 12 hpi, some immune-related pathways were significantly enriched, including the mitogen-activated protein kinase (MAPK) signaling pathway (cfa04010) and Fc epsilon RI signaling pathway (cfa04664) (**Figure 4A**). The highly enriched pathways at 24 hpi (**Figure 4B**) included glycerolipid metabolism (cfa00561), the renin–angiotensin system pathway (cfa04614), and other types of O-glycan biosynthesis (cfa00514). Moreover, significantly inflammation-related pathways were found at 36 dpi, including cell adhesion molecules (CAMs) (cfa04514), vitamin B6 metabolism (cfa00750), cytokine–cytokine receptor interaction (cfa04060), and glycosaminoglycan biosynthesis–keratan sulfate (cfa00533) (**Figure 4C**).

qRT-PCR Validation of RNA-Sequencing Data

Nine miRNAs were randomly selected for qRT-PCR verification (**Figure 5**), including cfa-miR-381, cfa-miR-10b, cfa-miR-146,

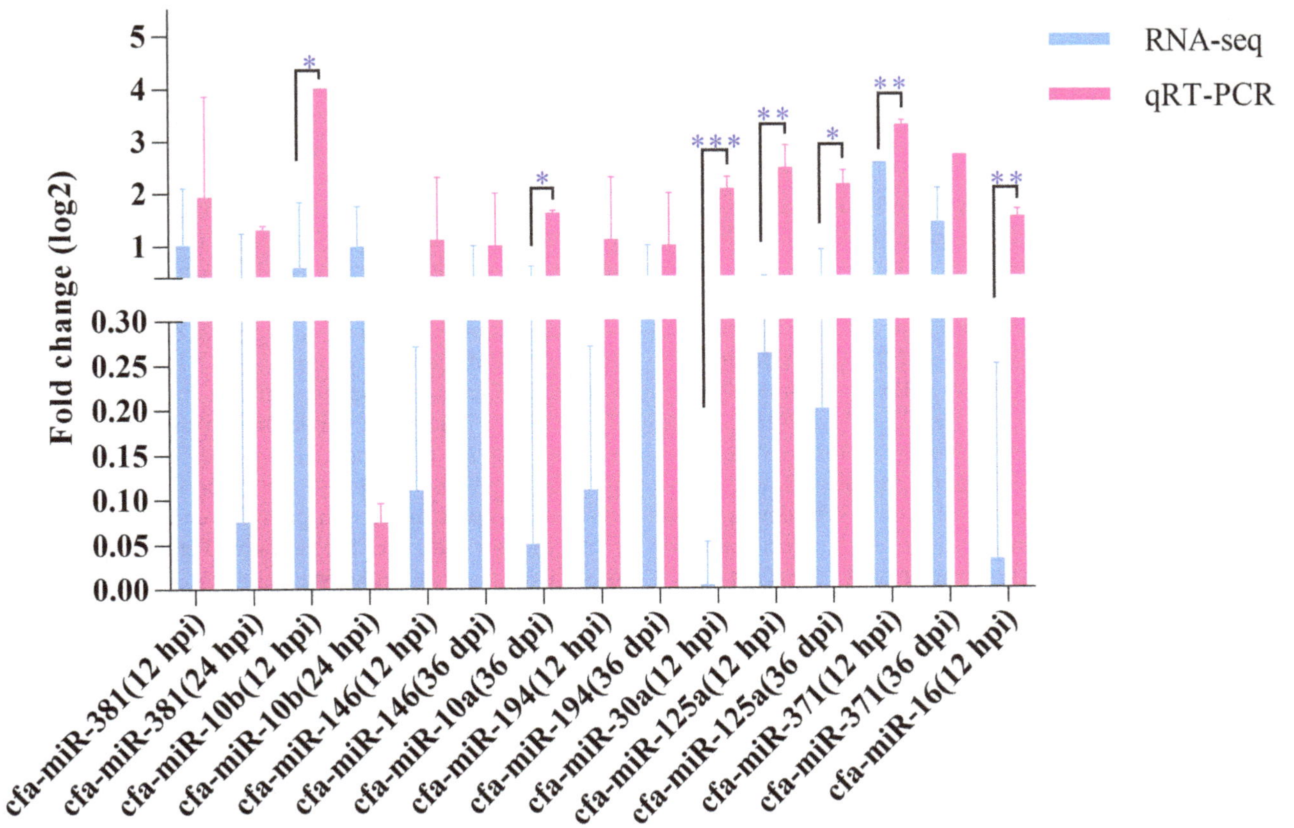

FIGURE 5 | Quantitative real-time PCR. The Y-axis shows the relative change of miRNA levels expressed as fold increase compared with the control U6 small nuclear RNA (snRNA). The X-axis shows the name of the nine miRNAs used in the cross-validation of expression analysis. *$P < 0.05$; **$P < 0.01$; ***$P < 0.001$.

cfa-miR-10a, cfa-miR-194, cfa-miR-30a, cfa-miR-125a, cfa-miR-371, and cfa-miR-16. Although the expression levels of the nine miRNAs obtained by qRT-PCR were slightly higher those obtained by RNA-sequencing, the expression trends obtained by both methods were consistent, which suggested an increased expression of the examined miRNAs.

DISCUSSION

In this study, hepatic miRNA expression patterns of beagle dogs during *T. canis* infection were investigated using RNA-sequencing analysis. A total of 59 DEmiRNAs were identified, including 9, 16, and 34 DEmiRNAs at 12 hpi, 24 hpi, and 36 dpi, respectively. Most of the downregulated DEmiRNAs were found in the infected group at 36 dpi (**Figure 1**). This finding suggested that miRNAs were negatively regulated to alter the expression of the target genes during the later stage of infection in infected puppies' livers. Moreover, among the dysregulated miRNAs, only one and three were common between 12 hpi and 36 dpi and between 24 hpi and 36 dpi, respectively (**Figure 2**). This finding indicates that the expression of hepatic miRNAs of beagle dogs evolves during the *T. canis* infection. Two important miRNAs, novel-294 and cfa-miR-885, were differentially expressed at the initial stage of infection (12 hpi) (**Supplementary Table 2**). Furthermore, the IgSF gene *FGFR1* was predicted to be regulated by miRNA novel-294 at 12 hpi (**Supplementary Table 3**). A previous study found that *FGFR1* expression improved beta-cell survival in cytokine-induced inflammation (33). Hence, we speculated that the upregulation of the novel-294 in puppies' livers promotes the immune response of puppies to *T. canis* infection *via* increasing the expression of *FGFR1*. miRNA cfa-miR-885 was predicted to regulate *IGSF3* gene of the IgSF (**Supplementary Table 3**). The IgSF and leukocyte integrins play an important role in the regulation of leukocyte recruitment to the inflammation sites (34). These findings suggest that cfa-miR-885 plays a protective role during *T. canis* infection.

At 24 hpi, 16 miRNAs were found differentially expressed in infected livers (e.g., cfa-miR-1839). The cfa-miR-1839 was downregulated at 24 hpi, and TRIM71, the predicted target gene of cfa-miR-1839 (**Supplementary Table 3**), regulates juvenile-to-adult transition events in nematodes and mammals (35). The majority of *T. canis* larvae reach the liver at 24 hpi (36); subsequently, the larvae migrate to lung, muscle, and brain tissue *via* the circulation (36). However, some larvae cannot continue to migrate and are trapped in the hepatic capillaries (36). Thus, we assumed that the downregulation of hepatic cfa-miR-1839 possibly regulates the juvenile-to-adult development of *T. canis* larvae in the puppies' livers. Whether cfa-miR-1839 regulates juvenile-to-adult transition of *T. canis* larvae remains to be further investigated.

cfa-miR-370 and cfa-miR-133c were significantly downregulated at 36 dpi (**Supplementary Table 2**). The target gene prediction showed that cfa-miR-370 targets the *CD3E* gene (**Supplementary Table 3**). *CD3E*, the T-cell antigen receptor epsilon subunit gene, is essential for TCR signaling and T-cell differentiation (37, 38). In our study, cfa-miR-370 was downregulated in the infected livers at 36 dpi, indicating that the downregulation of cfa-miR-370 may represent an immunoreaction to resist *T. canis* infection. In addition, two differently expressed miRNAs, cfa-miR-370 and cfa-miR-133c, were predicted to regulate the *ARRDC1* gene (**Supplementary Table 3**). Additionally, cfa-miR-133c was predicted to regulate the *IL18R1* gene. Previous research found that *IL-18R/MyD88* plays a crucial role in the development of a robust Th1 response during *Trypanosoma cruzi* infection (39). Therefore, the abnormal expression of cfa-miR-133c seems to be a potential candidate for further study of the role of cfa-miR-133c in promoting a protective Th1 immune response to *T. canis* infection.

GO enrichment analysis showed that 797, 769, and 665 GO terms were significantly enriched at 12 hpi, 24 hpi, and 36 dpi, respectively (**Supplementary Table 4**). Based on the analysis of the 797 significantly enriched GO terms at 12 hpi, nine DEmiRNAs were mainly involved in the signal-related biological process, including instance single-organism processes, single-organism cellular process, and single-organism metabolic process (**Figure 3A**). These processes are involved in acute liver injury (40). At 24 hpi, 16 DEmiRNAs were mainly associated with biological processes, such as protein phosphorylation, intracellular signal transduction, regulation of phosphorylation, and regulation of protein phosphorylation (**Figure 3B**). Some phosphorylated proteins were related to TNF-α signaling (41), which regulate immune response (42). At 36 dpi, 10 upregulated and 24 downregulated miRNAs were involved in response to stress, positive regulation of the immune system process, and regulation of nervous system development (**Figure 3C**). Moreover, a total of 39 immunization-related GO terms were significantly enriched at three time points (**Supplementary Table 5**). These results show that *T. canis* larvae can elicit a significant immune response after infecting the liver.

The top 20 enriched pathways are shown in **Figure 4**. The target genes of the DEmiRNAs were significantly enriched in the MAPK signaling pathway, galactose metabolism, and Fc epsilon RI signaling pathway at 12 hpi (**Figure 4A**). The MAPK signaling pathway participated in diverse cellular responses, such as inflammation, differentiation, proliferation, and apoptosis (43). Additionally, the MAPK signaling pathway is involved in the development, reproduction, and survival of *Schistosoma mansoni* (44). The Fc epsilon RI is the primary receptor in mast cells, which can influence the synthesis of proinflammatory cytokines and other molecules that are involved in inflammatory responses (45) (**Figure 4A**). These findings suggested that *T. canis* can cause inflammatory responses in puppy livers at the initial stage. At 24 hpi, the glycerolipid metabolism pathway, renin–angiotensin system pathway, and other types of O-glycan biosynthesis pathways were significantly enriched (**Figure 4B**). The glycerolipid metabolism pathway could perturb the host immune system and metabolism following anisakid infection (46). Further, the renin–angiotensin system pathway influences a range of processes from inflammation and immune responses to longevity (47). A previous study found that the O-glycoprotein biosynthesis pathway was associated with the immune response of dendritic cells (48). According to these findings, we assumed that *T. canis* larvae can trigger the immune responses in the infected host liver at 24 hpi. Some inflammation-related pathways were significantly enriched at 36 dpi, such as the cell adhesion molecules (CAMs) pathway, vitamin B6 metabolism pathway, cytokine–cytokine receptor interaction pathway, and glycosaminoglycan biosynthesis–keratan sulfate pathway (**Figure 4C**). The CAMs can direct mediate leukocyte migration, which is essential for generating effective inflammatory responses (49). Previous research found that vitamin B6 as a co-factor was involved in the inflammation response (50). It was reported that a high level of cytokine–cytokine motif chemokine ligand 1 could enhance and prolong the inflammatory response (51). The glycosaminoglycan pathway interacts with multiple ligands, which play an essential role in the inflammatory reaction (52). These results indicated that the puppies' livers may trigger inflammatory responses at the late stage of *T. canis* infection.

CONCLUSION

The present study, for the first time, revealed the hepatic miRNA expression patterns of beagle dogs at three *T. canis* infection stages. A total of 59 DEmiRNAs were identified in the infected livers. The functional enrichment analysis of predicted target genes showed that miRNA cfa-miR-1839 could be related to the juvenile-to-adult transition of *T. canis* larvae. KEGG pathway analysis found that some significantly enriched pathways were related to the inflammatory response at 12 hpi and 36 dpi. Several miRNAs, such as novel-294, cfa-miR-88, cfa-miR-370, and cfa-miR-133c, were associated with immune responses. These findings should enrich our understanding of the interactions between *T. canis* and its definitive host. Further studies to elucidate the detailed molecular mechanisms and the physiological functions of the DEmiRNAs in the pathogenesis of *T. canis* infection are warranted.

ETHICS STATEMENT

The animal study was reviewed and approved by the Animal Administration and Ethics Committee of Lanzhou Veterinary

Research Institute, Chinese Academy of Agricultural Sciences (Approval No. 2018-015). The dogs used in the study were handled in accordance with good animal practices required by the Animal Ethics Procedures and Guidelines of the People's Republic of China.

AUTHOR CONTRIBUTIONS

Y-XL and X-QZ conceived and designed the experiments. YZ and W-BZ performed the experiments. YZ analyzed the data and wrote the paper. J-JH and HME participated in improving the English of the manuscript. HME, X-QZ, and Y-XL critically revised the manuscript. All authors have read and approved the final version of the manuscript. All authors contributed to the preparation of the manuscript.

FUNDING

Project support was provided by the International Science and Technology Cooperation Project of Gansu Provincial Key Research and Development Program (Grant No. 17JR7WA031) and the Agricultural Science and Technology Innovation Program (ASTIP) (Grant No. CAAS-ASTIP-2016-LVRI-03).

ACKNOWLEDGMENTS

We thanked Novogene Bioinformatics Technology Co., Ltd. (Beijing, China) for technical support.

REFERENCES

1. Chen J, Zhou DH, Nisbet AJ, Xu MJ, Huang SY, Li MW, et al. Advances in molecular identification, taxonomy, genetic variation and diagnosis of *Toxocara* spp. *Infect Genet Evol.* (2012) 12:1344–8. doi: 10.1016/j.meegid.2012.04.019
2. Overgaauw PA, van Knapen F. Veterinary and public health aspects of *Toxocara* spp. *Vet Parasitol.* (2013) 193:398–403. doi: 10.1016/j.vetpar.2012.12.035
3. Holland CV. Knowledge gaps in the epidemiology of *Toxocara*: the enigma remains. *Parasitology.* (2017) 144:81–94. doi: 10.1017/S0031182015001407
4. Macpherson CN. The epidemiology and public health importance of toxocariasis: a zoonosis of global importance. *Int J Parasitol.* (2013) 43:999–1008. doi: 10.1016/j.ijpara.2013.07.004
5. Ma G, Holland CV, Wang T, Hofmann A, Fan CK, Maizels RM, et al. Human toxocariasis. *Lancet Infect Dis.* (2018) 18:14–24. doi: 10.1016/S1473-3099(17)30331-6
6. Fan CK, Liao CW, Cheng YC. Factors affecting disease manifestation of toxocarosis in humans: genetics and environment. *Vet Parasitol.* (2013) 193:342–52. doi: 10.1016/j.vetpar.2012.12.030
7. Rubinsky-Elefant G, Hirata CE, Yamamoto JH, Ferreira MU. Human toxocariasis: diagnosis, worldwide seroprevalences and clinical expression of the systemic and ocular forms. *Ann Trop Med Parasitol.* (2010) 104:3–23. doi: 10.1179/136485910X12607012373957
8. Ma G, Luo Y, Zhu H, Luo Y, Korhonen PK, Young ND, et al. MicroRNAs of *Toxocara canis* and their predicted functional roles. *Parasit Vectors.* (2016) 9:229. doi: 10.1186/s13071-016-1508-3
9. Sperotto RL, Kremer FS, Aires Berne ME, Costa de Avila LF, da Silva Pinto L, Monteiro KM, et al. Proteomic analysis of *Toxocara canis* excretory and secretory (TES) proteins. *Mol Biochem Parasitol.* (2017) 211:39–47. doi: 10.1016/j.molbiopara.2016.09.002
10. Zheng WB, Zou Y, Zhu XQ, Liu GH. *Toxocara* "omics" and the promises it holds for medicine and veterinary medicine. *Adv Parasitol.* (2020) 109:89–108. doi: 10.1016/bs.apar.2020.01.002
11. Zhu XQ, Korhonen PK, Cai H, Young ND, Nejsum P, von Samson-Himmelstjerna G, et al. Genetic blueprint of the zoonotic pathogen *Toxocara canis*. *Nat Commun.* (2015) 6:6145. doi: 10.1038/ncomms7145
12. Cai Y, Yu X, Hu S, Yu J. A brief review on the mechanisms of miRNA regulation. *Genom Proteom Bioinform.* (2009) 7:147–54. doi: 10.1016/S1672-0229(08)60044-3
13. Chen K, Rajewsky N. The evolution of gene regulation by transcription factors and microRNAs. *Nat Rev Genet.* (2007) 8:93–103. doi: 10.1038/nrg1990
14. Hobert O. Gene regulation by transcription factors and microRNAs. *Science.* (2008) 319:1785–6. doi: 10.1126/science.1151651
15. Deng M, Lancto CA, Abrahamsen MS. *Cryptosporidium parvum* regulation of human epithelial cell gene expression. *Int J Parasitol.* (2004) 34:73–82. doi: 10.1016/j.ijpara.2003.10.001
16. Sturm A, Amino R, van de Sand C, Regen T, Retzlaff S, Rennenberg A, et al. Manipulation of host hepatocytes by the malaria parasite for delivery into liver sinusoids. *Science.* (2006) 313:1287–90. doi: 10.1126/science.1129720
17. McDonald V, Korbel DS, Barakat FM, Choudhry N, Petry F. Innate immune responses against *Cryptosporidium parvum* infection. *Parasite Immunol.* (2013) 35:55–64. doi: 10.1111/pim.12020
18. Ambros V. The functions of animal microRNAs. *Nature.* (2004) 431:350–5. doi: 10.1038/nature02871
19. Regis SC, Mendonça LR, Silva Ndos S, Dattoli VC, Alcântara-Neves NM, Barrouin-Melo SM. Seroprevalence and risk factors for canine toxocariasis by detection of specific IgG as a marker of infection in dogs from Salvador, Brazil. *Acta Trop.* (2011) 120:46–51. doi: 10.1016/j.actatropica.2011.05.011
20. Mikaeili F, Mathis A, Deplazes P, Mirhendi H, Barazesh A, Ebrahimi S, et al. Differentiation of *Toxocara canis* and *Toxocara cati* based on PCR-RFLP analyses of rDNA-ITS and mitochondrial cox1 and nad1 regions. *Acta Parasitol.* (2017) 62:549–56. doi: 10.1515/ap-2017-0066
21. Zheng WB, Zou Y, Elsheikha HM, Liu GH, Hu MH, Wang SL, et al. Serum metabolomic alterations in Beagle dogs experimentally infected with *Toxocara canis*. *Parasit Vectors.* (2019) 12:447. doi: 10.1186/s13071-019-3703-5
22. Takamiya S, Mita T. Large-scale purification of active liquid-cultured *Caenorhabditis elegans* using a modified Baermann apparatus. *Parasitol Int.* (2016) 65:580–3. doi: 10.1016/j.parint.2016.03.013
23. Langmead B, Trapnell C, Pop M, Salzberg SL. Ultrafast and memory-efficient alignment of short DNA sequences to the human genome. *Genome Biol.* (2009) 10:R25. doi: 10.1186/gb-2009-10-3-r25
24. Friedländer MR, Mackowiak SD, Li N, Chen W, Rajewsky N. miRDeep2 accurately identifies known and hundreds of novel microRNA genes in seven animal clades. *Nucleic Acids Res.* (2012) 40:37–52. doi: 10.1093/nar/gkr688
25. Wen M, Shen Y, Shi S, Tang T. miREvo: an integrative microRNA evolutionary analysis platform for next-generation sequencing experiments. *BMC Bioinformatics.* (2012) 13:140. doi: 10.1186/1471-2105-13-140
26. Zhou L, Chen J, Li Z, Li X, Hu X, Huang Y, et al. Integrated profiling of microRNAs and mRNAs: microRNAs located on Xq27.3 associate with clear cell renal cell carcinoma. *PLoS ONE.* (2010) 5:e15224. doi: 10.1371/journal.pone.0015224
27. Enright AJ, John B, Gaul U, Tuschl T, Sander C, Marks DS. MicroRNA targets in Drosophila. *Genome Biol.* (2003) 5:R1. doi: 10.1186/gb-2003-5-1-r1
28. Chen CM, Lu YL, Sio CP, Wu GC, Tzou WS, Pai TW. Gene Ontology based housekeeping gene selection for RNA-seq normalization. *Methods.* (2014) 67:354–63. doi: 10.1016/j.ymeth.2014.01.019

29. Kanehisa M, Araki M, Goto S, Hattori M, Hirakawa M, Itoh M, et al. KEGG for linking genomes to life and the environment. *Nucleic Acids Res.* (2008) 36:D480–4. doi: 10.1093/nar/gkm882
30. Mao X, Cai T, Olyarchuk JG, Wei L. Automated genome annotation and pathway identification using the KEGG Orthology (KO) as a controlled vocabulary. *Bioinformatics.* (2005) 21:3787–93. doi: 10.1093/bioinformatics/bti430
31. Livak KJ, Schmittgen TD. Analysis of relative gene expression data using real-time quantitative PCR and the $2^{-\Delta\Delta C_T}$ method. *Methods.* (2001) 25:402–8. doi: 10.1006/meth.2001.1262
32. Adnan M, Morton G, Hadi S. Analysis of rpoS and bolA gene expression under various stress-induced environments in planktonic and biofilm phase using $2^{-\Delta\Delta C_T}$ method. *Mol Cell Biochem.* (2011) 357:275–82. doi: 10.1007/s11010-011-0898-y
33. Regeenes R, Silva PN, Chang HH, Arany EJ, Shukalyuk AI, Audet J, et al. Fibroblast growth factor receptor 5 (FGFR5) is a co-receptor for FGFR1 that is up-regulated in beta-cells by cytokine-induced inflammation. *J Biol Chem.* (2018) 293:17218–28. doi: 10.1074/jbc.RA118.003036
34. Wetzel A, Chavakis T, Preissner KT, Sticherling M, Haustein UF, Anderegg U, et al. Human Thy-1 (CD90) on activated endothelial cells is a counterreceptor for the leukocyte integrin Mac-1 (CD11b/CD18). *J Immunol.* (2004) 172:3850–9. doi: 10.4049/jimmunol.172.6.3850
35. Aeschimann F, Neagu A, Rausch M, Großhans H. let-7 coordinates the transition to adulthood through a single primary and four secondary targets. *Life Sci Alliance.* (2019) 2:e201900335. doi: 10.26508/lsa.201900335
36. Schnieder T, Laabs EM, Welz C. Larval development of *Toxocara canis* in dogs. *Vet Parasitol.* (2011) 175:193–206. doi: 10.1016/j.vetpar.2010.10.027
37. Le Deist F, Hivroz C, Partiseti M, Rieux-Laucat F, Debatin KM, Choquet D, et al. T cell activation deficiencies. *Clin Immunol Immunopathol.* (1995) 76:163–4. doi: 10.1016/S0090-1229(95)90072-1
38. Soudais C, De Villartay JP, Le Deist F, Fischer A, Lisowska-Grospierre B. Genetic analysis of the human CD3-epsilon gene in a T cell receptor/CD3 immunodeficiency. *Immunodeficiency.* (1993) 4:117–9. doi: 10.1038/ng0193-77
39. Oliveira AC, Gomes-Neto JF, Barbosa CD, Granato A, Reis BS, Santos BM, et al. Crucial role for T cell-intrinsic IL-18R-MyD88 signaling in cognate immune response to intracellular parasite infection. *Elife.* (2017) 6:e30883. doi: 10.7554/eLife.30883
40. Wang G, Jin S, Ling X, Li Y, Hu Y, Zhang Y, et al. Proteomic profiling of LPS-induced macrophage-derived exosomes indicates their involvement in acute liver injury. *Proteomics.* (2019) 19:e1800274. doi: 10.1002/pmic.201800274
41. Oliveira KC, Carvalho ML, Bonatto JM, Schechtman D, Verjovski-Almeida S. Human TNF-α induces differential protein phosphorylation in Schistosoma mansoni adult male worms. *Parasitol Res.* (2016) 115:817–28. doi: 10.1007/s00436-015-4812-5
42. Pereira-Fonseca DCM, Oliveira-Rovai FM, Rodas LAC, Beloti CAC, Torrecilha RBP, Ito PKRK, et al. Dog skin parasite load, TLR-2, IL-10 and TNF-α expression and infectiousness. *Parasite Immunol.* (2017) 39:e12493. doi: 10.1111/pim.12493
43. Kim L, Butcher BA, Denkers EY. *Toxoplasma gondii* interferes with lipopolysaccharide-induced mitogen-activated protein kinase activation by mechanisms distinct from endotoxin tolerance. *J Immunol.* (2004) 172:3003–10. doi: 10.4049/jimmunol.172.5.3003
44. Gava SG, Tavares NC, Falcone FH, Oliveira G, Mourão MM. Profiling Transcriptional regulation and functional roles of schistosoma mansoni c-Jun N-Terminal Kinase. *Front Genet.* (2019) 10:1036. doi: 10.3389/fgene.2019.01036
45. Kraft S, Bieber T. Fc epsilon ri-mediated activation of transcription factors in antigen-presenting cells. *Int Arch Allergy Immunol.* (2001) 125:9–15. doi: 10.1159/000053791
46. Liu K, Yin D, Shu Y, Dai P, Yang Y, Wu H. Transcriptome and metabolome analyses of *Coilia nasus* in response to Anisakidae parasite infection. *Fish Shellfish Immunol.* (2019) 87:235–42. doi: 10.1016/j.fsi.2018.12.077
47. Sparks MA, Crowley SD, Gurley SB, Mirotsou M, Coffman TM. Classical Renin-Angiotensin system in kidney physiology. *Compr Physiol.* (2014) 4:1201–28. doi: 10.1002/cphy.c130040
48. Tomek MB, Maresch D, Windwarder M, Friedrich V, Janesch B, Fuchs K, et al. A general protein O-glycosylation gene cluster encodes the species-specific Glycan of the oral pathogen *Tannerella forsythia*: O-Glycan biosynthesis and immunological implications. *Front Microbiol.* (2018) 9:2008. doi: 10.3389/fmicb.2018.02008
49. Golias C, Tsoutsi E, Matziridis A, Makridis P, Batistatou A, Charalabopoulos K. Review. Leukocyte and endothelial cell adhesion molecules in inflammation focusing on inflammatory heart disease. *In Vivo.* (2007) 21:757–69.
50. Ueland PM, McCann A, Midttun Ø, Ulvik A. Inflammation, vitamin B6 and related pathways. *Mol Aspects Med.* (2017) 53:10–27. doi: 10.1016/j.mam.2016.08.001
51. Zhou Y, Qiao H, Yin N, Chen L, Xie Y, Wu J, et al. Immune and cytokine/chemokine responses of PBMCs in rotavirus-infected rhesus infants and their significance in viral pathogenesis. *J Med Virol.* (2019) 91:1448–69. doi: 10.1002/jmv.25460
52. Morla S. Glycosaminoglycans and Glycosaminoglycan mimetics in cancer and inflammation. *Int J Mol Sci.* (2019) 20:1963. doi: 10.3390/ijms20081963

Permissions

All chapters in this book were first published by Frontiers; hereby published with permission under the Creative Commons Attribution License or equivalent. Every chapter published in this book has been scrutinized by our experts. Their significance has been extensively debated. The topics covered herein carry significant findings which will fuel the growth of the discipline. They may even be implemented as practical applications or may be referred to as a beginning point for another development.

The contributors of this book come from diverse backgrounds, making this book a truly international effort. This book will bring forth new frontiers with its revolutionizing research information and detailed analysis of the nascent developments around the world.

We would like to thank all the contributing authors for lending their expertise to make the book truly unique. They have played a crucial role in the development of this book. Without their invaluable contributions this book wouldn't have been possible. They have made vital efforts to compile up to date information on the varied aspects of this subject to make this book a valuable addition to the collection of many professionals and students.

This book was conceptualized with the vision of imparting up-to-date information and advanced data in this field. To ensure the same, a matchless editorial board was set up. Every individual on the board went through rigorous rounds of assessment to prove their worth. After which they invested a large part of their time researching and compiling the most relevant data for our readers.

The editorial board has been involved in producing this book since its inception. They have spent rigorous hours researching and exploring the diverse topics which have resulted in the successful publishing of this book. They have passed on their knowledge of decades through this book. To expedite this challenging task, the publisher supported the team at every step. A small team of assistant editors was also appointed to further simplify the editing procedure and attain best results for the readers.

Apart from the editorial board, the designing team has also invested a significant amount of their time in understanding the subject and creating the most relevant covers. They scrutinized every image to scout for the most suitable representation of the subject and create an appropriate cover for the book.

The publishing team has been an ardent support to the editorial, designing and production team. Their endless efforts to recruit the best for this project, has resulted in the accomplishment of this book. They are a veteran in the field of academics and their pool of knowledge is as vast as their experience in printing. Their expertise and guidance has proved useful at every step. Their uncompromising quality standards have made this book an exceptional effort. Their encouragement from time to time has been an inspiration for everyone.

The publisher and the editorial board hope that this book will prove to be a valuable piece of knowledge for researchers, students, practitioners and scholars across the globe.

List of Contributors

Elena Izquierdo-Rodriguez and Natalia Martin-Carrillo
Instituto Universitario de Enfermedades Tropicales y Salud Pública de Canarias, Universidad de La Laguna, San Cristóbal de La Laguna, Spain

Basilio Valladares and Pilar Foronda
Instituto Universitario de Enfermedades Tropicales y Salud Pública de Canarias, Universidad de La Laguna, San Cristóbal de La Laguna, Spain
Departament Obstetricia y Ginecología, Pediatría, Medicina Preventiva y Salud Pública, Toxicología, Medicina Legal y Forense y Parasitología, Universidad de La Laguna, San Cristóbal de La Laguna, Spain

Clara Marin, Laura Lorenzo-Rebenaque, Omar Laso and Santiago Vega
Facultad de Veterinaria, Instituto de Ciencias Biomédicas, Universidad Cardenal Herrera-CEU, CEU Universities, Alfara del Patriarca, Spain

José Villora-Gonzalez
Selvätica Veterinary Clinic, Valencia, Spain Salmonella

Lucy A. Parker
Departamento de Salud Pública y Ginecología, Universidad Miguel Hernández de Elche, Alicante, Spain
CIBER Epidemiología y Salud Pública, Madrid, Spain

Lucrecia Acosta and Fernando Jorge Bornay-Llinares
Área de Parasitología, Departamento de Agroquímica y Medio Ambiente, Universidad Miguel Hernández de Elche, Alicante, Spain

Mariana Noel Gutierrez
Veterinary Centre "Dame la Pata", Posadas, Argentina

Israel Cruz
National School of Public Health, Instituto de Salud Carlos III, Madrid, Spain

Javier Nieto
WHO Collaborating Centre for Leishmaniasis, Servicio de Parasitología, Centro Nacional de Microbiología, Instituto de Salud Carlos III, Madrid, Spain

Enrique Jorge Deschutter
Facultad de Ciencias Exactas, Químicas y Naturales, Universidad Nacional de Misiones, Posadas, Argentina

Lilas Mercuriali, Pere Simón and Eva Masdeu
Agència de Salut Pública de Barcelona (ASPB), Barcelona, Spain

Tomás Montalvo, David Palma, Joan-Pau Millet and Cristina Rius
Agència de Salut Pública de Barcelona (ASPB), Barcelona, Spain
Centro de Investigación Biomédica en Red en Epidemiología y Salud Pública (CIBER-ESP), Madrid, Spain

Jordi Figuerola
Centro de Investigación Biomédica en Red en Epidemiología y Salud Pública (CIBER-ESP), Madrid, Spain
Estación Biológica de Doñana (EBD-CSIC), Sevilla, Spain

Rubén Bueno-Marí
Department of Research and Development (R&D), Laboratorios Lokímica, Valencia, Spain
Parasitology Area, Department of Pharmacy and Pharmaceutical Technology and Parasitology, University of Valencia, Valencia, Spain

Magdalena E. Wysmołek, Ewa Długosz, Maciej Klockiewicz and Marcin Wiśniewski
Division of Parasitology, Department of Preclinical Sciences, Institute of Veterinary Medicine, Warsaw University of Life Sciences-SGGW, Warsaw, Poland

Artur Dobrzyński and Piotr Jurka
Department of Small Animal Diseases and Clinic, Institute of Veterinary Medicine, Warsaw University of Life Sciences-SGGW, Warsaw, Poland

Michał Czopowicz
Division of Veterinary Epidemiology and Economics, Institute of Veterinary Medicine, Warsaw University of Life Sciences-SGGW, Warsaw, Poland

Santiago Vega, Clara Marin and Rosana Domingo
Facultad de Veterinaria, Instituto de Ciencias Biomédicas, Universidad Cardenal Herrera-CEU, CEU Universities, Alfara del Patriarca, Spain

Fernando Fariñas
Instituto de Inmunología Clínica y Enfermedades Infecciosas. Grupo One Health, Malaga, Spain

Iván Rodríguez-Escolar and Rodrigo Morchón
Zoonotic Infections and One Health GIR, Laboratory of Parasitology, Faculty of Pharmacy, University of Salamanca, Salamanca, Spain

Patricia Pérez Pérez
Zoonotic Infections and One Health GIR, Laboratory of Parasitology, Faculty of Pharmacy, University of Salamanca, Salamanca, Spain
Instituto Universitario de Enfermedades Tropicales y Salud Pde Canarias (IUETSPC), Departamento de Obstetricia y Ginecolog, Pediatría, Medicina Preventiva y Salud Pública, Toxicología, Medicina Legal y Forense y Parasitología, Universidad de La Laguna, La Laguna, Tenerife, Spain

Jacob Lorenzo-Morales
Instituto Universitario de Enfermedades Tropicales y Salud Pde Canarias (IUETSPC), Departamento de Obstetricia y Ginecolog, Pediatría, Medicina Preventiva y Salud Pública, Toxicología, Medicina Legal y Forense y Parasitología, Universidad de La Laguna, La Laguna, Tenerife, Spain
CIBER de Enfermedades Infecciosas, Instituto de Salud Carlos III, Madrid, Spain

Elena Carretón and José Alberto Montoya-Alonso
Internal Medicine, Faculty of Veterinary Medicine, Research Institute of Biomedical and Health Sciences, University of Las Palmas de Gran Canaria, Las Palmas de Gran Canaria, Spain

José Ángel Sánchez Agudo
Grupo de Investigación en Biodiversidad, Diversidad humana y Biología de la Conservación, Universidad de Salamanca, Salamanca, Spain

Maciej Klockiewicz and Marcin Wiśniewski
Division of Parasitology and Parasitic Diseases, Department of Pre-Clinical Sciences, Institute of Veterinary Medicine, Warsaw University of Life Sciences, Warsaw, Poland

Małgorzata Sobczak-Filipiak
Department of Pathology and Veterinary Diagnostics, Institute of Veterinary Medicine, Warsaw University of Life Sciences, Warsaw, Poland

Lavinia Ciuca, Paola Pepe, Antonio Bosco, Giuseppe Cringoli, Maria Paola Maurelli and Laura Rinaldi
Department of Veterinary Medicine and Animal Production, University of Naples Federico II, Naples, Italy

Simone Mario Caccio and Anna Rosa Sannella
European Union Reference Laboratory for Parasites, Department of Infectious Diseases, Istituto Superiore di Sanità, Rome, Italy

Alice Vismarra, Laura Kramer and Marco Genchi
Department of Veterinary Science, University of Parma, Parma, Italy

Sara Savić, Marina Zekic Stosic and Doroteja Marcic
Scientific Veterinary Institute "Novi Sad", Novi Sad, Serbia

Isabel Hernández
Group of Animal and Human Dirofilariasis, Faculty of Pharmacy, Campus Miguel Unamuno, University of Salamanca, Salamanca, Spain

Aleksandar Potkonjak
Department of Veterinary Medicine, Faculty of Agriculture, University of Novi Sad, Novi Sad, Serbia

Suzana Otasevic
Faculty of Medicine, University of Nis, Nis, Serbia

Maja Ruzic
Clinic for Infectious Diseases, Faculty of Medicine, Clinical Center of Vojvodina, University of Novi Sad, Novi Sad, Serbia

Keneth Iceland Kasozi
Infection Medicine, Deanery of Biomedical Sciences, College of Medicine and Veterinary Medicine, The University of Edinburgh, Scotland, United Kingdom
School of Medicine, Kabale University, Kabale, Uganda

Tianren Shen and Susan Christina Welburn
Infection Medicine, Deanery of Biomedical Sciences, College of Medicine and Veterinary Medicine, The University of Edinburgh, Scotland, United Kingdom

Zhejiang
University-University of Edinburgh Institute, Zhejiang University School of Medicine, Zhejiang University, Haining, China

Gerald Zirintunda and Leonard Omadang
Department of Animal Production and Management, Faculty of Agriculture and Animal Sciences, Busitema University Arapai Campus, Soroti, Uganda

Helen N. Nakimbugwe
Department of Animal Production and Management, Faculty of Agriculture and Animal Sciences, Busitema University Arapai Campus, Soroti, Uganda
Department of Agriculture, Faculty of Vocational Studies, Kyambogo University, Kampala, Uganda

Fred Ssempijja and Juma John Ochieng
Faculty of Biomedical Sciences, Kampala International University Western Campus, Bushenyi, Uganda

Bridget Buyinza, Wycliff Matovu and David Paul Nalumenya
College of Veterinary Medicine Animal Resources and Biosecurity, Makerere University, Kampala, Uganda

Khalid J. Alzahrani
Department of Clinical Laboratories Sciences, College of Applied Medical Sciences, Taif University, Taif, Saudi Arabia

Kevin Matama
School of Pharmacy, Kampala International University Western Campus, Bushenyi, Uganda

Luay Alkazmi
Biology Department, Faculty of Applied Sciences, Umm Al-Qura University, Makkah, Saudi Arabia

David Onanyang
Department of Biology, Faculty of Science, Gulu University, Gulu, Uganda

Paul Bogere
Faculty of Agriculture and Environmental Science, Muni University, Arua, Uganda

Saher Islam
Department of Biotechnology, Lahore College for Women University, Lahore, Pakistan

Gaber El-Saber Batiha
Department of Pharmacology and Therapeutics, Faculty of Veterinary Medicine, Damanhour University, Damanhour, Egypt

Lawrence Obado Osuwat
School of Medicine and Health Sciences, Soroti University, Soroti, Uganda

Mahmoud Abdelhamid
Department of Parasitology, Faculty of Veterinary Medicine, Aswan University, Aswan, Egypt

Josué Martínez-de la Puente, Ramón Soriguer and Jordi Figuerola
Estación Biológica de Doñana (EBD-CSIC), Sevilla, Spain

Juan Carlos Senar
Evolutionary and Behavioural Ecology Research Unit, Museu de Ciències Naturals de Barcelona, Barcelona, Spain

Rubén Bueno-Mari
Laboratorios Lokímica, Departamento de Investigación y Desarrollo (I+D), Valencia, Spain

Hans-Peter Fuehrer, Feodora Natalie Kayikci and Bita Shahi Barogh
Department of Pathobiology, Institute of Parasitology, University of Veterinary Medicine, Vienna, Austria

Ana Margarida Alho and Luís Madeira de Carvalho
CIISA - Centro de Investigação Interdisciplinar em Sanidade Animal, Faculdade de Medicina Veterinária, Universidade de Lisbon, Lisbon, Portugal

Hugo Rosa, José Tomás and Hugo Rocha
Guarda Nacional Republicana, Lisbon, Portugal

Josef Harl
Department of Pathobiology, Institute of Pathology, University of Veterinary Medicine, Vienna, Austria

Daniel Salazar-Rodríguez and Yamilé Aleaga-Santiesteban
Department of Clinical Microbiology Diagnostic, Hospital Center of Institute of Tropical Medicine "Pedro Kourí," Havana, Cuba

Enrique Iglesias
Departamento de Vacunas, Centro de Ingeniería Genética y Biotecnología, Havana, Cuba

Arturo Plascencia-Hernández and Héctor R. Pérez-Gómez
Centro Universitario de Ciencias de la Salud de la Universidad de Guadalajara, Guadalajara, Mexico

Enrique J. Calderón
Instituto de Biomedicina de Sevilla, Hospital Universitario Virgen del Rocío/Consejo Superior de Investigaciones Científicas/Universidad de Sevilla, Centro de Investigación Biomédica en Red de Epidemiología y Salud Pública (CIBERESP), Seville, Spain

José A. Vázquez-Boland
Microbial Pathogenesis Group, Edinburgh Medical School (Biomedical Sciences - Infection Medicine), University of Edinburgh, Edinburgh, United Kingdom

Yaxsier de Armas
Department of Clinical Microbiology Diagnostic, Hospital Center of Institute of Tropical Medicine "Pedro Kourí," Havana, Cuba
Pathology Department, Hospital Center of Institute of Tropical Medicine "Pedro Kourí," Havana, Cuba

José-Manuel Ramos-Rincón
Clinical Medicine Department, University Miguel Hernández de Elche, Alicante, Spain
Internal Medicine Service, General University Hospital of Alicante-ISABIAL, Alicante, Spain

Sonia Ortiz-Martínez
Medical Practice El Ballestero, Health Service of Castilla La Mancha, Albacete, Spain

María-Esteyner Vásquez-Chasnamote
Natural Resources Research Center, Peruvian Amazon National University, Iquitos, Peru

Olga-Nohelia Gamboa-Paredes
Research Assistant, Amazon Rainforest Civil Association, Iquitos, Peru

Viviana-Vanessa Pinedo-Cancino
Molecular Biology and Immunology Laboratory of the Specialized Unit of LIPNAA-CIRNA, Peruvian Amazon National University, Iquitos, Peru

Cesar Ramal-Asayag
Infectious Diseases and Tropical Medicine Service, Loreto Regional Hospital, Iquitos, Peru
School of Medicine, National University of the Peruvian Amazon, Iquitos, Peru

Miguel Górgolas-Hernández-Mora
Infectious Disease Division, University Hospital Foundation Jiménez Díaz, Madrid, Spain
Medicine Department, Autonomous University of Madrid, Madrid, Spain

Martin Casapía-Morales
Infectious Diseases and Tropical Medicine Service, Loreto Regional Hospital, Iquitos, Peru
School of Medicine, National University of the Peruvian Amazon, Iquitos, Peru
Medical Department, Amazon Rainforest Civil Association, Iquitos, Peru

Lucrecia Acosta Soto
Área de Parasitología del Departamento de Agroquímica y Medioambiente, Universidad Miguel Hernández de Elche, Alicante, Spain

Lucy Anne Parker
Departamento de Salud Pública Historia de la Ciencia y Ginecología, Universidad Miguel Hernández de Elche, Alicante, Spain
Centro de Investigación Biomédica en Red de Epidemiología y Salud Pública (CIBERESP), Madrid, Spain

María José Irisarri-Gutiérrez
Área de Parasitología, Dpto. Farmacia y Tecnología Farmacéutica y Parasitología, Facultat de Farmàcia, Universitat de València, Valencia, Spain
Dpto. de Ciencias de la Salud, Facultad de Ciencias Biomédicas, Universidad Europea de Madrid, Madrid, Spain

Carla Muñoz-Antoli and José Guillermo Esteban
Área de Parasitología, Dpto. Farmacia y Tecnología Farmacéutica y Parasitología, Facultat de Farmàcia, Universitat de València, Valencia, Spain

Javier Arturo Bustos and Héctor Hugo García
Cysticercosis Unit, Instituto Nacional de Ciencias Neurológicas, Lima, Peru
Center for Global Health, Universidad Peruana Cayetano Heredia, Lima, Peru

Erika Perez
Cysticercosis Unit, Instituto Nacional de Ciencias Neurológicas, Lima, Peru

Yesenia Castillo
Center for Global Health, Universidad Peruana Cayetano Heredia, Lima, Peru

Santiago Mas-Coma, Ilra R. Funatsu, Patricio, Artigas M. Adela Valero and M. Dolores Bargues
Departamento de Parasitología, Facultad de Farmacia, Universidad de Valencia, Valencia, Spain

Paola Buchon
Unidad de Limnología, Instituto de Ecología, Universidad Mayor de San Andrés (UMSA), La Paz, Bolivia

Rene Angles
Cátedra de Parasitología, Facultad de Medicina, Universidad Mayor de San Andrés (UMSA), La Paz, Bolivia

Cristina Mas-Bargues
Departamento de Fisiología, Facultad de Medicina, Universidad de Valencia, Valencia, Spain

Tsegahun Manyazewal
Center for Innovative Drug Development and Therapeutic Trials for Africa (CDT-Africa), College of Health Sciences, Addis Ababa University, Addis Ababa, Ethiopia

Senait Belay
Center for Innovative Drug Development and Therapeutic Trials for Africa (CDT-Africa), College of Health Sciences, Addis Ababa University, Addis Ababa, Ethiopia
Faculty of Veterinary Medicine, Hawassa University, Hawassa, Ethiopia

Mirutse Giday
Center for Innovative Drug Development and Therapeutic Trials for Africa (CDT-Africa), College of Health Sciences, Addis Ababa University, Addis Ababa, Ethiopia
Aklilu Lemma Institute of Pathobiology, Addis Ababa University, Addis Ababa, Ethiopia

Julia Rivero, Cristina Cutillas and Rocío Callejón
Department of Microbiology and Parasitology, Faculty of Pharmacy, University of Seville, Seville, Spain

Alfonso J. Rodriguez-Morales
Grupo de Investigación Biomedicina, Faculty of Medicine, Fundacion Universitaria Autonoma de las Americas, Pereira, Colombia
Emerging Infectious Diseases and Tropical Medicine Research Group, Instituto para la Investigación en Ciencias Biomédicas - Sci-Help, Pereira, Colombia
Coordinación Nacional de Investigación, Universidad Privada Franz Tamayo (UNIFRANZ), Cochabamba, Bolivia
Master Program on Clinical Epidemiology and Biostatistics, Universidad Científica del Sur, Lima, Peru

Jaime A. Cardona-Ospina
Grupo de Investigación Biomedicina, Faculty of Medicine, Fundacion Universitaria Autonoma de las Americas, Pereira, Colombia
Emerging Infectious Diseases and Tropical Medicine Research Group, Instituto para la Investigación en Ciencias Biomédicas - Sci-Help, Pereira, Colombia

Lucia E. Alvarado-Arnez
Coordinación Nacional de Investigación, Universidad Privada Franz Tamayo (UNIFRANZ), Cochabamba, Bolivia

Jorge L. Maguiña
Master Program on Clinical Epidemiology and Biostatistics, Universidad Científica del Sur, Lima, Peru

Alberto E. Paniz-Mondolfi
Department of Pathology, Molecular and Cell-Based Medicine, Laboratory of Microbiology, Icahn School of Medicine at Mount Sinai, New York, NY, United States
Instituto de Investigaciones Biomédicas IDB/Incubadora Venezolana de la Ciencia, Barquisimeto, Venezuela

Álvaro A. Faccini-Martínez
Department of Pathology, University of Texas Medical Branch, Galveston, TX, United States

Andrés F. Henao-Martínez
Department of Medicine, Division of Infectious Diseases, School of Medicine, University of Colorado Denver, Aurora, CO, United States

Julian Ruiz-Saenz
Grupo de Investigación en Ciencias Animales - GRICA, Facultad de Medicina Veterinaria y Zootecnia, Universidad Cooperativa de Colombia, Bucaramanga, Colombia

Marlen Martinez-Gutierrez
Grupo de Investigación en Ciencias Animales - GRICA, Facultad de Medicina Veterinaria y Zootecnia, Universidad Cooperativa de Colombia, Bucaramanga, Colombia
Infettare, Facultad de Medicina, Universidad Cooperativa de Colombia, Medellín, Colombia

Jorge E. Gomez-Marin
Grupo de Estudio en Parasitologia Molecular (GEPAMOL) Group, Facultad de Ciencias de la Salud, Universidad del Quindío, Armenia, Colombia

Ruben Bueno-Marí
Departamento de Investigación y Desarrollo (I+D), Laboratorios Lokímica, Paterna, Spain
Área de Parasitología, Departamento de Farmacia y Tecnología Farmaceútica y Parasitología, Universidad de Valencia, Burjasot, Spain

Yenddy Carrero
Facultad de Ciencias de la Salud, Carrera de Medicina, Universidad Técnica de Ambato, Ambato, Ecuador

Wilmer E. Villamil-Gomez
Infectious Diseases and Infection Control Research Group, Hospital Universitario de Sincelejo, Sincelejo, Colombia
Programa Del Doctorado de Medicina Tropical, SUE Caribe, Universidad Del Atlántico, Barranquilla, Colombia

D. Katterine Bonilla-Aldana
Semillero de Investigación en Zoonosis (SIZOO), Grupo de Investigación BIOECOS, Fundacion Universitaria Autonoma de las Americas, Pereira, Colombia

Ubydul Haque
Department of Biostatistics and Epidemiology, University of North Texas Health Science Center, Fort Worth, TX, United States

Juan D. Ramirez
Centro de Investigaciones en Microbiología y Biotecnología-UR (CIMBIUR), Facultad de Ciencias Naturales, Universidad del Rosario, Bogotá, Colombia

Juan-Carlos Navarro
Research Group of Emerging Diseases, Ecoepidemiology and Biodiversity, Health Sciences Faculty, Universidad Internacional SEK, Quito, Ecuador

Susana Lloveras
Sección Zoopatología Médica, Hospital de Infecciosas FJ Muñiz, Buenos Aires, Argentina

Kovy Arteaga-Livias
Master Program on Clinical Epidemiology and Biostatistics, Universidad Científica del Sur, Lima, Peru
Faculty of Medicine, Universidad Nacional Hermilio Valdizán, Huánuco, Peru

Cristina Casalone
Istituto Zooprofilattico del Piemonte, Torino, Italy

Angel A. Escobedo
Department of Epidemiology, Institute of Gastroenterology, Havana, Cuba

Marylin Hidalgo
Infectious Diseases Group, Facultad de Ciencias, Pontificia Universidad Javeriana, Bogotá, Colombia

Antonio C. Bandeira
Faculdade de Medicina, UniFTC, Salvador, Brazil

Salim Mattar
Instituto de Investigaciones Biologicas del Tropico, Universidad de Cordoba, Monteria, Colombia

Jose A. Suárez
Investigador SNI Senacyt Panamá, Instituto Conmemorativo Gorgas de Estudios de la Salud (ICGES), Panama, Panama University of North Texas Health Science Center, Fort Worth, TX, United States

Qian Chen, Kunlun Wang, Yongchun Zhou, Dongfang Li, Yuancai Chen and Yongshuai Peng
College of Animal Science and Veterinary Medicine, Henan Agricultural University, Zhengzhou, China

Ke Shi, Yaqun Yan, Fuchang Yu, Longxian Zhang and Changshen Ning
College of Animal Science and Veterinary Medicine, Henan Agricultural University, Zhengzhou, China
International Joint Research Laboratory for Zoonotic Diseases of Henan, Zhengzhou, China

Junqiang Li
College of Animal Science and Veterinary Medicine, Henan Agricultural University, Zhengzhou, China
Scientific Research Experiment Center & Laboratory Animal Center, Henan University of Chinese Medicine, Zhengzhou, China

Krzysztof Skowron, Katarzyna Grudlewska-Buda, Natalia Wiktorczyk-Kapischke, Zuzanna Bernaciak and Eugenia Gospodarek-Komkowska
Department of Microbiology, Ludwik Rydygier Collegium Medicum in Bydgoszcz, Nicolaus Copernicus University in Toruń, Bydgoszcz, Poland

Justyna Bauza-Kaszewska
Department of Microbiology and Food Technology, Jan and Jędrzej Śniadecki University of Technology in Bydgoszcz, Bydgoszcz, Poland

Maciej Zacharski
Department of Biochemistry and Molecular Biology, Wrocław University of Environmental and Life Sciences, Wrocław, Poland

Andrea Springer, Antje Glass, Anna-Katharina Topp and Christina Strube
Institute for Parasitology, Centre for Infection Medicine, University of Veterinary Medicine Hannover, Hanover, Germany

Gérald Umhang, Vanessa Bastid, Carine Peytavin de Garam and Franck Boué
Wildlife Surveillance and Eco-Epidemiology Unit, National Reference Laboratory for Echinococcus spp, Rabies and Wildlife Laboratory, ANSES, Malzéville, France

Jenny Knapp
UMR CNRS 6249 Laboratoire Chrono-Environnement, Université Franche-Comté, Besançon, France
Department of Parasitology-Mycology, National Reference Centre for Echinococcoses, University Hospital of Besançon, Besançon, France

Marion Wassermann and Thomas Romig
Parasitology Unit, University of Hohenheim, Stuttgart, Germany

Tomasz Cencek and Jacek Karamon
Department of Parasitology, National Veterinary Research Institute, Pulawy, Poland

Yang Zou and Yi-Xin Lu
Heilongjiang Key Laboratory for Zoonosis, College of Veterinary Medicine, Northeast Agricultural University, Harbin, China

Wen-Bin Zheng and Jun-Jun He
State Key Laboratory of Veterinary Etiological Biology, Key Laboratory of Veterinary Parasitology of Gansu Province, Lanzhou Veterinary Research Institute, Chinese Academy of Agricultural Sciences, Lanzhou, China

Hany M. Elsheikha
Faculty of Medicine and Health Sciences, School of Veterinary Medicine and Science, University of Nottingham, Loughborough, United Kingdom

Xing-Quan Zhu
State Key Laboratory of Veterinary Etiological Biology, Key Laboratory of Veterinary Parasitology of Gansu Province, Lanzhou Veterinary Research Institute, Chinese Academy of Agricultural Sciences, Lanzhou, China
College of Veterinary Medicine, Shanxi Agricultural University, Taigu, China

Index

www.ingramcontent.com/pod-product-compliance
Lightning Source LLC
Chambersburg PA
CBHW081215180926
51613CB00003B/245
* 9 7 8 1 6 4 1 1 6 8 4 3 4 *